Covid-19 and Pregnancy

Covid-19 and Pregnancy

Editor: Camelia Bamford

FOSTER ACADEMICS
www.fosteracademics.com

www.fosteracademics.com

FOSTER ACADEMICS

Cataloging-in-Publication Data

Covid-19 and pregnancy / edited by Camelia Bamford.
p. cm.
Includes bibliographical references and index.
ISBN 978-1-64646-597-2
1. Pregnancy. 2. COVID-19 (Disease). 3. Pregnancy—Complications. I. Bamford, Camelia.
RG556 .C68 2023
618.2--dc23

Foster Academics,
118-35 Queens Blvd., Suite 400,
Forest Hills, NY 11375, USA

ISBN 978-1-64646-597-2 (Hardback)

Contents

Preface

Over the recent decade, advancements and applications have progressed exponentially. This has led to the increased interest in this field and projects are being conducted to enhance knowledge. The main objective of this book is to present some of the critical challenges and provide insights into possible solutions. This book will answer the varied questions that arise in the field and also provide an increased scope for furthering studies.

Coronavirus disease 2019 (Covid-19) refers to a type of contagious disease caused by the severe acute respiratory syndrome coronavirus 2. The signs and symptoms of Covid 19 might vary but commonly include coughing, breathing difficulties, fever, loss of taste, headaches, loss of smell and exhaustion. The physical changes that occur in women's bodies due to pregnancy may make them prone to respiratory viruses like Covid-19. The risk of getting infected with Covid-19 in case of expectant mothers is generally minimal. However, exposure to this virus during pregnancy has been linked to a higher risk of premature delivery. Women who have Covid-19 during pregnancy may be more prone to other pregnancy issues, like delivering a stillborn infant. Pregnant women who are overweight, older or already have certain medical disorders like diabetes or hypertension are more likely to suffer from negative effects of Covid-19. This book unravels the recent studies on the relationship between Covid-19 and pregnancy. Its extensive content will provide the readers with a thorough understanding of the topic.

I hope that this book, with its visionary approach, will be a valuable addition and will promote interest among readers. Each of the authors has provided their extraordinary competence in their specific fields by providing different perspectives as they come from diverse nations and regions. I thank them for their contributions.

Editor

1

Pregnancy During the Global COVID-19 Pandemic: Canadian Experiences of Care

Sarah Rudrum *

Department of Sociology, Acadia University, Wolfville, Canada

Correspondence:
Sarah Rudrum
sarah.rudrum@acadiau.ca

Drawing on journal entries written by a cohort of pregnant Canadians, this article explores how responses to the COVID-19 pandemic shaped access to and experiences of maternity care. Variance in practices among jurisdictions and among provider groups meant that participants had diverse experiences. Nevertheless, I identify clear shared concerns, including fear over giving birth with no familial support, the need for better communications, and challenges entailed when needing to switch providers or travel for care during a state of emergency. Despite a universal health care system, there are gaps and inequities in access to appropriate maternity care in Canada; the pandemic exposed existing access challenges.

Keywords: Canada, maternity care, pandemic (COVID-19), midwifery, gender, health

INTRODUCTION: CANADIAN EXPERIENCES OF PREGNANCY CARE DURING THE PANDEMIC

When states of emergency were declared in Canada as a result of COVID-19, many non-essential health services were suspended. Maternity and delivery care of course continued, with changes made to protect patients and to streamline health care toward the pandemic. General practitioners, obstetricians, midwives, and interdisciplinary teams are among the publicly funded primary care options available in Canada. At the best of times, however, access to primary care—as well as to specialist and allied care—varies significantly based on jurisdiction and other factors. In particular, access to midwifery care can be poor outside of urban centers in larger provinces, while in rural areas, access to specialist and sometimes even primary health care can require travel.

To learn about the experiences of pregnant people during the early stages of the pandemic, I recruited individuals who were pregnant in April 2020 to participate in journaling about their care; thus I learned about which practices were helpful or concerning at this time. While jurisdiction and provider type remained important, clear communications and continuity of care were essential: women remarked on the difficulties caused by their absence or were grateful for their presence, identifying *communication* and *continuity* as central to feeling cared for. Good communications practices were idiosyncratic, in that they were not concentrated solely in particular jurisdictions or provider types, though midwives were more frequently cited as providing clear communications. As the pandemic continues, or in the event of another health system crisis, communications and care continuity are areas to prioritize.

TABLE 1 | Participant Demographics.

Demographic category	Count	Percent (%)
Ethnicity/race		
European/white	24	92
White and first nations	1	4
Métis and hispanic	1	4
Indigenous (national population: 4.9%)		
Yes	2	8
No	24	92
Gender		
Woman	24	96
X	1	4
Sexuality		
Straight	21	84
Bisexual/pansexual	4	16
Marital Status		
Married/common-law	23	92
Single	2	8
Income (household, annual)		
Less than $25K+	2	8
$25–49K	2	8
$50–74K	2	8
$75–99K	5	20
$100K+	14	56
Urban/rural		
Urban	17	68
Rural	8	32
Expected care provider		
Family Doctor	6	24
Midwife	8	32
Obstetrician	11	44
Other children		
Yes	13	52
No	10	40
No response	2	8
Total (n)	25	

METHODOLOGY: JOURNALING CARE

For 10 weeks between April and July 2020, I undertook a mixed-methods, primarily qualitative study in which pregnant Canadians completed journal entries in response to prompts, with at least four entries required for inclusion. At the end of the ten-week period, participants were offered the option to complete any additional weekly entries, responding to a generic prompt, as well as one entry post-delivery, reflecting on their delivery and initial post-partum experiences. Participants completed a demographic survey after consenting to participate and before receiving the first journal prompt. As well as capturing the demography of participants, the survey helped me to reach pregnant individuals across Canada and to recruit a higher number of participants, as I anticipated that over a 10-week period there would be some attrition. In the survey, participants were asked for demographic information such as age, province of residence, weeks pregnant, and other children. Recruitment was via Facebook, with posts to pregnancy and maternity care groups in all provinces and territories. The survey did not include questions about maternity care, which was instead explored over ten-weeks of journal prompts. In the prompts, I asked about experiences of care including changes to care, sources of information, and changing plans. I began with a draft set of prompts, which I revised in response to emerging conditions, including changes to public health protocols and restrictions. I read journal entries each week as they were submitted. At the close of the study, I read all data, first reading all entries by each participant to understand full narratives over time, and then by prompt, in order to begin to identify shared experiences. I identified and grouped themes and for the purposes of this article, have focused extensively on those relating to health care and to a lesser extent social support.

Of the 56 people who completed the survey, 24 went on to complete at least four responses. Among them, six lived in Nova Scotia; four in Ontario; three each in British Columbia and Manitoba; two each in New Brunswick and Prince Edward Island; and one each in Alberta, Newfoundland, Saskatchewan, and Yukon. Their demographic information is included in **Table 1**, below. Most participants self-identified as white; one was white and First Nations and one was Hispanic and Métis. The percentage of Indigenous people in the study, 8%, was almost double the national percentage: 4.9% of people in Canada are Indigenous (Government of Canada, Statistics Canada, 2017), while Latinx people make up 1.3% of the Canadian population (Government of Canada, Statistics Canada, 2016). Participants ranged in age from 21 to 40 with an average age of 32. One participant indicated their gender as X; all others self-identified as women. There was some diversity of sexuality, with 20 straight participants, three bisexual, and one queer pansexual. Two participants were single, while the rest were married or in common-law relationships. Via postal code classification, I determined whether participants lived in a rural or urban setting. Most participants had one or more children. Ten participants were expecting their first child, among them women who identified that they had previously miscarried. While I worked toward diversity in recruitment, I did not seek for this small study to be representative of the Canadian population. The lack of racialized Canadians—with the exception of the Métis-Hispanic and White-First Nations participants is a limitation of the study, in particular for understanding racialized dimensions of healthcare. However, the diversity among participants in terms of provinces and territories, rural and urban, and intended care providers is a strength of the study. One participant was a second-time surrogate. Pseudonyms, selected by participants and revised if they repeated each other or were actual names, are used throughout. I received ethical approval for the study from Acadia University.

BACKGROUND: ACCESS TO UNIVERSAL CARE

Across the Canadian provinces and territories, public health responses to COVID-19 have varied, partly due to different courses of disease outbreak but also in relation to their political and economic characteristics. Similarly, while universal health care is national, specific policies and practices surrounding maternity care and particularly midwifery vary significantly among jurisdictions, with differences magnified during the pandemic response. Unregulated and extralegal throughout much of the 20th century, midwifery is now regulated and funded in most of Canada—a process that occurred province-by-province between the mid-1990s and today, and whose reach remains uneven. Midwifery demand tends to outstrip its availability, particularly in rural areas or jurisdictions where regulation is recent and scale-up slow. In most settings, midwives are the only provider type to offer home birth—a difference that gained significance during the pandemic.

As states of emergency were announced in the spring of 2020, some provinces banned home births while others supported the uptick in demand for them. The government of Nova Scotia suspended home births on March 30, despite increased demand and without consulting the midwives' professional association. While no rationale was reported, it occurred during a time when Nova Scotians were being instructed to stay at home and avoid having guests in the home. The suspension was met by protest and was lifted after a month (Grant, 2020; MacLean, 2020; Sibonney, 2020). Quebec also announced but quickly reversed a homebirth ban, opting instead for specific safety measures for home births (Sibonney, 2020). In Ontario, there was no ban, but some seeking midwifery care were turned away due to lack of capacity (Viau, 2020). The College of Midwives of British Columbia recruited retired and non-practicing midwives to meet demand (Midwives Association of British Columbia, 2020). In most Canadian provinces, there are not enough midwives in ordinary times (Viau 2020); demand for options during the pandemic further exposed the existing shortfall.

Increased interest in home birth, as elsewhere, was a response to two major factors: fear of exposure to the virus in hospitals and concern over restrictions on support people at delivery. All provinces and territories introduced limits to non-medical support people, typically allowing only one. Families were also watching the international context, in which some hospitals, including in New York, demanded that women give birth alone (Caron and Van Syckle, 2020), leading New York's Governor to issue an executive order on rights during labor (Cuomo and Andrew, 2020; Van Syckle and Caron, 2020) and the World Health Organization to affirm laboring women's right to a "companion of choice (World Health Organization, 2020b). Newfoundland allowed one support person but required that they leave after the delivery with no in-and-out privileges (Bradbury, 2020; Gillis, 2020). BC's Center for disease Control stated that one person would be permitted, while BC Women's Hospital in Vancouver allowed a doula plus one additional support person, stating that doulas are members of the health team (Pole 2020); Yukon hospitals took a similar approach (Yukon Hospitals, 2020). Inconsistency over the role of doulas demonstrates the lack of clarity experienced by pregnant people navigating the emerging policy context during COVID-19. Canada's three Northern territories had low numbers of COVID-19 cases, likely due to their remote locations and restrictions on gathering and travel (CBC News, 2020; Dawson, 2020; D'entremont et al., 2020), yet nevertheless followed similar guidelines of permitting one support person (Northwest Territories Health and Social Services Authority, 2020; Pearce, 2020; Savikataaq, 2020).

The potential need to travel for emergency or specialist care is an additional concern throughout the Canadian North and in some other rural regions—a prospect made more stressful and costly during the pandemic. Restrictions challenged movements to better support Indigenous births, as protocols often include extended family; however Indigenous advocates worked to create tailored advice (Piapot, 2020). For example, a BC report on cultural safety (First Nations Health Authority and Prinatal Services BC, 2020) acknowledged that the virus was likely to have a disproportionate impact in Indigenous communities, and that health care settings and the wearing of PPE had the potential to retraumatize patients due to the impact of both past disease outbreak and of a painful history with medical personnel and practices in residential schools and other settings. It included specific resources for connecting patients to culturally appropriate resources, such as online smudging or ceremony during social distancing and to a funded Indigenous doula program, as well as more general advice, such as working to build connection despite the need for PPE.

Maternity and neonatal care in Canada remained largely safe from COVID-19 during the study period. A hospital in Alberta had confirmed cases among maternity staff in April 2020 (Rieger, 2020), and a neonatal unit in Vancouver had an outbreak in July 2020 (Daflos, 2020). Such outbreaks, thankfully, remained the exception rather than the norm. For all pregnant individuals, however, the care and support normally available during pregnancy and labor changed, whether through changes to provider type, shifting care online, limiting partners, and/or requiring additional costs or steps.

FINDINGS AND DISCUSSION: PERINATAL CHALLENGES

I have organized my data to follow the course of a pregnancy, from prenatal experiences through labor and delivery and into the post-partum period. I discuss primary health care, allied health care, and social supports in each phase. While there are through-lines of concern—including the desire for continuity of care, good communications, and some access to social support—I found that participants characterized each stage according to distinct challenges, discussed below.

Prenatal Challenges

All provider types in Canada offer comprehensive prenatal care, which monitors health status and facilitates diagnostics. For low-risk pregnancies, the Society of Obstetricians and Gynecologists of Canada recommends care on a schedule with increasing frequency as the due date draws near, with visits every 4 weeks during the first thirty weeks, then moving to every 2 weeks until 37 weeks, at which point a weekly appointment is recommended (Ontario, 2020). Prenatal care experiences varied dramatically among participants, depending on province, timing, and their care needs. Prominent concerns regarding primary care included: the need to switch providers and/or provider-types (due to preference or through necessity as their doctors prioritized emergency work during COVID and reduced their caseloads to protect patients), in-person appointments moving to virtual ones, gaps in care, and traveling for care. As well as for primary care, participants discussed changes in access to allied health care services, which also became harder to access during the pandemic. People's journal entries recounted experiences with prenatal care that ranged from "frustrating" to "exceptional."

Continuity of care is a tenet of quality maternity care, as it helps meet medical and psychosocial needs (Perdok et al., 2018; World Health Organization, 2018). However, it is not unusual to switch providers during pregnancy. Midwifery clinics often run waitlists; an opening might precipitate a mid-pregnancy move. A switch to an obstetrician might be necessitated by a newly identified risk factor. Those with no care provider at the outset of pregnancy might move from a temporary to a regular provider. The pandemic increased the potential for changes to care, particularly as in order to avoid exposing patients, some doctors working in multiple settings, including emergency rooms, transferred their pregnant patients to other providers, and at the same time, some patients sought midwifery care to be able to avoid hospital and/or clinical settings (MacLean, 2020; Sibonney, 2020).

Catrina, expecting her first baby in Nova Scotia, was among those who experienced a provider change. She was moved to a new doctor, as hers was working in emergency care and did not want to risk exposing patients. She had since begun to contact midwives in her area because she was worried that she would "be made to do something I hadn't planned on without proper explanation or without having my options laid out for me." She found it difficult to contact her care team, which was frustrating. Polly, expecting her second child on Prince Edward Island, also had a change in care, to a nurse-practitioner (NP), as her doctor was similarly "prioritizing in-patients at the hospital." Primary care NPs tend to work in a collaborative care model with other providers; their training and recruitment has been emphasized to ease doctor shortages and improve access to care (Peckham et al., 2018). Polly was happy with the arrangement, saying, "I've had two appointments to date with my NP and I believe I received more thorough care at these two appointments than I ever have. Because most patients were being triaged or seen virtually, but prenatal care was continuing in person, she ... was able to spend over an hour with me at each appointment. I was pleasantly surprised." However, not all care was available within Catrina's home province, and, when she later had to later travel to Nova Scotia, she found it stressful, as, unlike during pre-COVID times, she had to complete the round trip in 1 day, in order to be exempt from a 14-days quarantine requirement.

While some patients were required to change providers due to COVID-19, others were hoping for a change. Gwen, a White and First Nations woman expecting her first child in Nova Scotia, did not have a family doctor as is the case with many Canadians. She wrote: "Luckily, I was seeing this OBGYN already for follow up from a surgery ... and she agreed to take me on ... Otherwise, I think I may have had to wait several weeks into my pregnancy before being seen." While Gwen felt lucky to have any primary care, it was not ideal, as the pandemic affected access. Communicating with her health care team was stressful and frustrating, as for Catrina, and Gwen experienced gaps in healthcare provision. She wrote:

> I have had follow-up appointments canceled. Since COVID-19 started, there have been weeks at a time where my OB's office is closed; they do not have a voicemail at their clinic, so there is no way to get in touch with them. This was very stressful when I was becoming increasingly ill with vomiting and was unable to get help. I am hoping that a midwifery group will take me on at 20 weeks, but as there are no midwives in my area, I would have to travel over an hour to a different "health zone" and I am unsure of the likelihood that they will take me on.

Only three sites offer midwifery care in Nova Scotia, all oversubscribed, so the experience of seeking care far away and being waitlisted is, unfortunately, common. Later, Gwen did get a midwife. She updated her journal, writing:

> My midwife presented all options and risks and benefits for every choice I had to make. Everything was explained to me in detail. My midwife was very easily accessible to me via phone or email. I wish I had made the switch from OB to midwife much earlier as the experience was much better. Particularly, communication and allowing me to make informed choices was much better. The care I am receiving from my midwife empowers me, vs. the care from my OB, which was anxiety-provoking due to poor communication and lack of information.

Again, communication stood out as important aspect of quality prenatal care.

Wendy, a bisexual doula who lived in Manitoba and was carrying her first child, also had a midwife—a source of reassurance. She wrote: "I'm not concerned (for myself) about how COVID is impacting hospital policies, because I have been extremely fortunate and got placed with a midwife. I've always wanted a home birth anyway—huge dream—so this is about as perfect as perfect gets." This framing of midwifery access as something to hope for and feel lucky about, expressed by Catrina, Gwen, and Wendy, is a discourse I have observed in previous research (Rudrum and Frank, 2021). Despite the Canada Health Act stating that Canadians must have "reasonable access" to insured services, the positioning of midwifery as a special privilege, unlike other kinds of primary care, reflects the lack of sufficient numbers of midwives in Canada. The responses I gathered suggest that there should be a sufficient number of practicing midwives to serve as primary care providers for all who want their services.

Lila, who identified their gender as X, was a second-time surrogate living in southern Ontario, with a modest household income between $25,000 and $49,000. They would have liked to include midwives in their care, but did not. They explained:

> Last pregnancy, I used midwives, but my care was transferred in the last week before I gave birth by C-section (at 36 weeks) due to pre-eclampsia and high blood pressure. Due to those complications, the

> fertility doctor [...] recommended that I use my OB for [this] entire pregnancy [...] I am bound by legal contract to follow the fertility doctor's medical advice, so I am using my OB for this pregnancy. I like my OB, but I prefer the care midwives provide.

While Lila could have opted to include midwives in a support role, since they wanted their husband and the intended fathers present during delivery, they chose not to, making a similar calculation about doula care: "the fewer people involved, the better." As with several others, Lila identified a gap in their care, in their case partly because they were waiting for a COVID-19 test result.

For Maria, expecting her first child in Ontario, a gap in her care meant that a healthy ultrasound came as a great relief, demonstrating that during breaks in care, people were not only waiting but also worrying: "I was also very happy after our 20 weeks ultrasound, since there had been almost 10 weeks since my last appointment. I felt so much relief and joy." The maximum recommended time between two appointments is 4 weeks, so this was indeed a long break in care. Cjay, a Latina and Métis woman in Manitoba, also found extended periods between appointments stressful, writing: "All these changes have me a little stressed out because there's more precautions to take when leaving the house but also because there's less check-ups and appointments." She found that social supports had also changed, writing: "There is a prenatal nutrition program at the health center where they give you a $40 voucher to spend on healthy foods at the food mart. They used to hand out $10 vouchers every week but they've changed it to one for the month so you don't have to go in as much." Cjay was in her early 20s and one of two participants listing a low household income (under $25,000); this support was likely important to her family.

Among participants whose appointments were moved to a virtual format, some appreciated the time saved by not having to travel or wait, while others experienced virtual care as akin to a gap in care. Harper, who lived in BC and was planning a homebirth, the same as with her older child, appreciated the extra time that virtual care afforded, but stated, "I miss community, connecting with other pregnant women, feeling connected to practitioners." Larah, expecting her third child in Saskatchewan, wrote:

> This pregnancy has been difficult for me and I could of really used the extra care appointment at around 16 weeks, but our midwives office moved to the WHO's prenatal schedule and cut out that appointment. I had an appointment around 12 weeks but I felt I didn't need an in-person visit (the pandemic was new and scary) so I opted for a phone appointment instead. I have not seen my midwife since my initial visit at around 9 weeks pregnant, my next appointment is after my 20 weeks ultrasound in 2–3 weeks. It's been a long stretch.

Again, the space between appointments exceeded the recommended minimum of an appointment every four weeks during this stage of pregnancy. In particular, Larah was concerned about the potential need for specialist care, and worried that if she needed a fetal echocardiogram (which uses reflected ultrasonic waves to examine the structures and functioning of the heart), as she had during her previous pregnancy, she might have to travel to the nearest major city. This did become necessary, and she described the visit:

> The hospital was on lockdown and it was almost eerie how slow everything was. My appointment was 4 h later than it should of been and there was nowhere to go and grab a snack while I waited [...]. I had to sit in a room by myself for the entire time. I had the nurse check on me twice in 4 h, but it was pretty depressing and lonely to have to go through the appointment by myself for that length of time.

The need to travel for care is always disproportionately experienced among people in rural communities, with the pandemic exacerbating its stresses and discomforts. While Larah appreciated being checked on by the nurse during her wait, the length of the wait made those efforts at communication feel insufficient.

Ann, expecting her second child in Nova Scotia, received empathetic and supportive prenatal care from her health team. She wrote:

> Despite restrictions and new protocols as a result of COVID, I have felt nothing but supported by the health care system during this pregnancy. On three separate occasions I had concerns with the baby (lack of movement and unexplained pain) .... I called the [care provider] and they encouraged me to not hesitate to come in. I was greeted by a fully masked nurse each time who was nothing but empathetic and helpful ... These visits brought such a peace of mind and I was never made to feel as if they were too busy, or that I was overreacting. They always ended each visit urging me to come back if I ever had any concerns again. My OB was also very supportive.

Ann's overwhelmingly positive experience of prenatal care, however, stood out as an exception.

As well as changes to primary care, changes in access to allied health care services created worry. Previous infertility or pregnancy loss added to the reliance on care from alternative and allied health professions for some. For example, Margaret, who lived in Yukon and was expecting a first child, wrote of her naturopath that "She was instrumental in identifying hormonal and thyroid problems that were keeping us from getting pregnant, so to have this consistent, positive support essentially cut off at the beginning of a pregnancy was extremely stressful." Kelly, a single woman in her early 40s living in New Brunswick, was expecting a first child after having experienced a previous miscarriage, and her disappointment about missing acupressure was shared in this context.

Alexandra, expecting her second child in BC, also relied on allied health treatments, and was frustrated to have them canceled, noting the cost of paying insurance for unavailable care:

> For almost 3 months now, most pregnancy-related appointments I had scheduled have been cancelled—not even rescheduled or postponed, simply canceled indefinitely. It is incredibly frustrating not being able to go to the chiropractor or acupuncturist to relieve pregnancy pains, let alone prenatal registered massages. Especially when you are paying into insurance for such benefits.

Alexandra is referring to employee benefits, which cover some health services not funded under the Canada Health Act and are typically paid via a combination of employer and employee contributions. Services that are not designated as primary care are typically costly to access in Canada, with fees billed privately or to insurance. The pandemic made such treatments less accessible, even to those with insurance.

Challenges in Labor

Participants wrote about their plans for delivery, and later, about the delivery itself. Birth location (home vs. hospital) was important to some, though not all, participants. A worry over who would be permitted to be present was prevalent. While all jurisdictions allowed at least one support person, being forced to birth without family support remained a fear.

Harper shared that: "I did a home birth with my first, and I am (more) motivated to do the same with this child, just to stay away from the hospital .... The hospital nearest to me was diverting their maternity cases to another hospital. I'm not sure what the current situation is, but expect to get that information from my midwife closer to my due date."

Harper's motivation to stay away from the hospital echoed trends reported in the media, but was not shared by all participants. For example, Kristen, a mother of one living in Manitoba, was flexible:

> My birth plan is not terribly specific; I plan to go to the hospital and have a baby. It doesn't matter to me what happens in between, I just want the baby to be healthy and me to be healthy (in that order). For women who have very specific birth plans, I think they may be feeling more anxious and frustrated with the unknown ... At this point I have accepted that these are exceptional times, and I will do whatever is required to ensure the safety of my family (in terms of public health recommendations).

During her surrogate pregnancy, Lila was particularly worried about who could be present, as her partner and the intended parents all seemed essential. They wrote of hearing about:

> ... a hospital in Quebec [that] told all pregnant people they had to sign a form agreeing to undergo a c-section or they could not deliver at that hospital. This goes against human rights and is NOT acceptable. I am already worried about who I will be able to have in the delivery room, as I want my husband and BOTH parents to be there, if they want to be.

Lila also worried over whether the intended parents would have to quarantine after arriving from Europe. Cjay too worried about family support at delivery:

> Lately I've found myself worrying about when it comes time to give birth. The first time I had my boyfriend G. and my mom with me, so I hope they can both be there again, or if I'm only allowed one person this time that's alright too. I just don't want to be in there alone. I always think something's gonna go wrong because I've read so many awful stories.

Ann similarly wrote that her biggest worry was that her husband would be absent. Margaret shared this worry:

> I am terrified that there is a chance that if things get very bad that my partner will not be allowed at the birth of our child. There is no reason to think this is likely to be the case, especially since there is a lot of pressure to keep one support person with labouring mothers, but it's always in the corner of my mind, especially when I know so many people are not taking any precautions.

That *no* partner would be permitted seemed unlikely, given that policies throughout Canada allowed at least one person. Nevertheless, this was a prevalent fear, demonstrating how a short-lived poor practice in another jurisdiction, such as New York in the early peak of the pandemic (Caron and Van Syckle 2020), could contribute to fears elsewhere.

Brin was expecting her third child in Alberta. She felt that much of the information around pregnancy and COVID-19 was unclear, and wrote:

> My OB has told me that 3 weeks prior to my due date, myself and my immediate family need to self-isolate completely to ensure that no one has COVID and we are able to have a healthy and safe delivery with my husband. This is helpful because it's a clear guideline. It's not necessarily easy, but it's clear, which I appreciate.

Later on, when asked to reflect on what had been difficult or helpful about care during this time, she noted that the requirement felt onerous. She wrote:

> I'm nervous about doing a full self-isolation at 36 weeks and having both of our young children at home while I try to finish out my last 3 weeks of work. I feel like this will really make the last portion of the pregnancy extra stressful and I'm just not sure if I'll be able to work as long as I'd like to, but I understand the risks associated.

Self-isolation 3 weeks before the due date was *not* indicated by public health sources in Alberta or elsewhere, to my knowledge, nor was it mentioned by other participants. It is possible that the information conveyed was a personal preference of the obstetrician or practice, and not based on a public health directive. While participants repeatedly referred to their gratitude for providers who shared information and answered questions, a potential weakness of relying on providers to convey public health advice is that the advice offered might be inconsistent, and, as in this case, might be more onerous to patients than what was recommended by public health directives. Ann had a household income over $100,000, perhaps mitigating the consequences of extended self-isolation, but nevertheless the request felt hard to manage. For many patients, this advice to self-isolate for 3 weeks might be impossible due to work demands, the health care needs of family members, family and household structure or other reasons.

Kristen noticed differences between her previous delivery and birthing during the pandemic; she found these differences to be frustrating at worst, while at best she found that, with fewer people on site, the hospital environment was somewhat calmer than usual:

> When we arrived at the hospital, I was in active labor. In addition to all of the standard questions they ask you in triage, I also had to answer COVID screening questions while having contractions. This was very frustrating as I felt it held up the process and delayed my admission. All health care workers wore masks at all times ... Thankfully, I was not required to wear a mask while labouring as I had answered "no" to all of the screening questions. I was the only patient in the shared recovery room, but I am unsure if it just worked out that way or if patients were being deliberately placed in separate rooms.
>
> I was allowed to have two support people, but I chose to just have my husband. I am unsure if there were visitors allowed at the hospital, however my husband's family and I were in agreement that no one should come to the hospital to see the baby. Therefore, my husband and I were the only ones at the hospital during our stay. This was a marked difference from when my son was born 3 years ago, when we had many visitors and stayed 3 days in the hospital. This time I only stayed overnight. Again, not sure if that was a coincidence or COVID precautions. The hospital itself was very quiet. There was no background din of a busy hallway. There were no people in the hallways. It was a bit strange but also very relaxing. It seemed like there were not any visitors for anyone else, either.

Restrictions on visitors created a calm, if somewhat surreal, birth environment. Lilith, a first-time expectant mother in Ontario, found that other than the lack of nitrous oxide, which she had wanted but been previously advised was not being used due to COVID, delivery care went smoothly. She wrote: "We felt welcomed with our delivery team and did not feel like the care was any different from how it would be normally. Usually our hospital offers a follow-up check in the hospital but unfortunately this is now being offered just by phone, so this likely will not be as thorough, and requires us to then have a hearing test done at a later date that would normally be completed at that follow up." Most of the changes would come post-partum.

Challenges in Postpartum Plans

Postpartum care—care for the mother-infant dyad in the 6 weeks after delivery—is an essential part of maternity care throughout Canada, while it varies by jurisdiction and by provider type. Those whose primary care is with a physician may see their doctor once in this period, at the doctor's office (HealthLinkBC, 2020); in contrast, "quality, continuous care" is built into the midwifery model and, for example, Ontario midwives reported seeing their patients over six times on average in the post-partum period, typically in home visits (Association of Ontario midwives, 2019). When planning for delivery, experienced parents were less worried as a group than first-time parents, yet more worried about loss of medical and social support postpartum. They were able to look back on their previous experiences and the value of the care they received. Feelings about fewer visitors were mixed: here too, some experienced parents remembered that visits can be exhausting as well as supportive. Feelings about support networks also depended on the presence or absence of built-in support, particularly among single mothers. Alongside COVID-19 restrictions, which were easing across Canada at the end of June when the question was asked, concern over a potential "second wave" was prominent. While participants mostly had a manageable post-partum plan, words like "anxiety" and "stress" came up frequently. One way of coping with less access to clinical care was to purchase equipment usually provided in a health care setting such as scales for weighing the baby—a move that depended on a degree of financial security.

For most, postpartum plans included fewer people, though this didn't necessarily mean feeling less supported. In Nova Scotia, Lynne, who was expecting a second child, welcomed the fact the hospital might not be admitting many visitors. She was anticipating a second wave, and wrote:

> I am much more comfortable to have limited visitors at the hospital due to that. Recovery from childbirth is challenging, and being in the hospital with the baby uninterrupted is such a short time, that I don't necessarily want to have numerous visitors in the hospital this time. I found with my first birth, it prolonged the recovery as there were so many visitors coming to see the baby, which caused unneeded physical stress on me while I am trying to heal from surgery and learn to breastfeed my child.

Wendy also mentioned the potential for a second wave and also recognized the advantage of limits to visitors, writing "our available support network is more than adequate, and ... if anything, finding polite ways to secure time alone with the baby as parents will be the tricky part." She lived with her parents and near her in-laws, and hoped to have a frank conversation about managing contact in the event of a second wave. With local in-laws and parents in an adjacent province, Margaret wrote: "I worry that [the pandemic] means my parents might not be able to visit for a long time after the baby comes, but my partner's family will pressure us to spend time with them even if I feel unsafe (I will put my foot down if I need to)." She echoed Wendy in planning ahead for difficult conversations in order to manage contact.

Gwen pointed out the link between uncertain postpartum support and anxiety, particularly for first-time parents, writing:

> I am nervous I will not know how to be a good parent. I've never been good with kids and haven't ever enjoyed babysitting. Despite that, I've always wanted a child or children of my own. I think that it is normal for a person who is having their first baby to feel nervous. I do think I might feel less nervous if it wasn't so uncertain what supports will be available to me (thinking support groups, my family, my partners' family) in the first few weeks of my baby's life.

Gwen's isolation added to the worries of a first-time pregnancy.

Among the participants were two single mothers, both expecting their first child. Kelly's plans hadn't greatly changed: her mother was certain to be there for the labor and the following week. However, Sinclair, a queer pansexual woman with an income under $25,000, lived in Toronto, a COVID hotspot in the Canadian context (Shah, 2020) and her plan to rely on friends for support was made difficult by the pandemic. She too worried about a second wave:

> I don't even have family that can open their bubble to me so I'm not sure if anyone besides my midwives will even be able to be there. Originally my community was going to come and help me out as a single mother, but that's a huge risk during this time. I do not feel currently adequately supported and if this continues to when I give birth I definitely won't feel adequately supported.

Lila had found the post-partum period challenging after their previous surrogacy, and was planning to spend time with their husband and their journal, with a therapist available as needed. In ordinary times, the health care system relies on family, and the precarity of this reliance became apparent during COVID.

Participants anticipated that visits with health care providers might be limited, and as this cohort began to have their babies, this turned out to be the case. Alexandra, who was supported by midwives, spoke for many when she wrote:

> I have been mostly concerned with having a lack of postpartum care following being discharged from the hospital. I remember with my first birthing experience, I had the most wonderful and attentive care both in and out of the hospital as there weren't any crazy protective measures being taken at the time. I received visits from public health nurses regularly to ensure I was well on my way to recovery. However this time, I have been warned there will not be the same sort of care, perhaps only a telephone call once in awhile to check in. So that is certainly a bit concerning! I remember my fears the first time around breastfeeding and the amount of blood I was losing, etc., which was so relieving to be physically examined and reassured that all was well with both baby and I. The support a mother receives postpartum I believe is quite crucial to her emotional, mental and physical well-being and road to recovery.

Others also mentioned potential lack of breastfeeding support as central among post-partum concerns.

Kristen described changes to her post-partum care compared to her previous pregnancy, starting with a public health nurse visit the day after taking her daughter home, which included protocols like mask wearing and sanitizing. She had to monitor her baby's weight, because, as with her first, she was slow to gain. Kristen described that the places she would have gone to had been closed or allocated to COVID testing. Instead, she describes: "I had to take her to a walk-in clinic to be weighed, which made me nervous as I did not want to bring her around anyone who was sick. I ended up ordering a baby scale online so I would not have to bring her to any clinics or the hospital to be weighed." Similar to purchasing sonograms, buying a scale was a way to keep care safe at home; the ability to do so relied on having expendable income.

Like other parturient women, these participants were working to balance their needs for privacy, recovery, and connection to the baby with their needs for support and a social network, and doing so in the context of various degrees of isolation due to the pandemic.

Throughout their prenatal, delivery, and post-partum care, participants demonstrated patience and acceptance of changes to care during COVID-19 in their journals about their experiences. Nevertheless, some changes were frustrating and unsettling. Most notably, it was difficult for participants to experience changes to care, gaps in care and poor communication during the pre-natal period and decreased supports in the postpartum period. Prior clinical and social factors shaped how care during COVID was experienced: where shortcomings in care were evident, their impacts were most strongly felt by those with prior pregnancy losses or difficult pregnancies, singles without access to their usual social network during COVID, and to an extent first time parents-to-be.

CONCLUSION: COVID STRESS AND THE IMPORTANCE OF COMMUNICATION, CONTINUITY OF CARE, AND COMMUNITY SUPPORT

While this is an exceptional time to be pregnant, needs during pregnancy have not changed: childbearing participants confirmed that they are still seeking clear, reassuring information, autonomy over where and with whom they seek care and give birth, and social and familial support. This study, which drew on journal entries over a ten-week period, shows that whether or not those needs were met within the pandemic response varied considerably, depending on province, outbreak conditions, provider type, and other factors. Many pressing concerns, including difficulty accessing their provider type of choice, the need to travel for care, and waiting for care, resulted from and highlighted pre-existing shortcomings in the health care system. Some problems, such as the need to change providers or travel for care, were multiplied or heightened by pandemic conditions.

The principles of autonomy, choice, and continuity of care are recognized as contributing to a high standard of maternity care in Canada (Sandall, 1995; McCourt and Stevens, 2006; Vedam et al., 2019), and each of these areas suffered to an extent during the pandemic. Participants approached necessary changes to their health care with flexibility and patience, while continuing to highly value clear communications, continuity of care, and community supports. Some participants mitigated changes to care by purchasing their own quasi-medical equipment such as sonograms or scales. It was when participants experienced long gaps in care, were unable to contact their care team, or were unclear about necessary public health protocols that the stress of pandemic pregnancy was exacerbated. The value placed on communication and the continuous, quality care built into the midwifery model of care, and midwives' singularity of focus on childbearing, meant that pregnant people seen by midwives experienced fewer major disruptions to care, adding to the case for investment in midwifery care. As pandemic states of emergency continue, or in the event of another health system disruption, it is clear that to support birthing women, communications and continuity of care must be prioritized, and any limits to choice and autonomy of care and location be made cautiously, if at all.

ETHICS STATEMENT

The studies involving human participants were reviewed and approved by Acadia University Research Ethics Board 2020. The participants provided their written informed consent to participate in this study.

AUTHOR CONTRIBUTIONS

The author confirms being the sole contributor of this work and has approved it for publication.

REFERENCES

Association of Ontario Midwives. (2019). *Postpartum visit schedules: guidelines for timing postpartum visits.* Toronto, Canada: Association of Ontario Midwives.

Bradbury, T. (2020). Hospital visitation rules are unfair: expectant mother. Available at: https://www.thetelegram.com/news/local/hospital-visitation-rules-are-unfair-expectant-mother-433198/ (Accessed May 14, 2020).

Caron, C., and Van Syckle, K. (2020). Some pregnant women in New York city will have to deliver babies alone. Available at: https://www.nytimes.com/2020/03/24/parenting/coronavirus-labor-birth.html (Accessed July 27, 2020).

CBC News (2020). Yukon has 2 confirmed cases of COVID-19, the 1st in the territory. Available at: https://www.cbc.ca/news/canada/north/yukon-covid-19-1.5506363 (Accessed July 26, 2020).

Cuomo, G., and Andrew, M. (2020). No. 202.12: continuing temporary suspension and modification of laws relating to the disaster emergency. Available at: https://www.governor.ny.gov/news/no-20212-continuing-temporary-suspension-and-modification-laws-relating-disaster-emergency (Accessed July 29, 2020).

Daflos, P. (2020). Baby tests positive for COVID-19 in vancouver newborn ICU outbreak. Available at: https://bc.ctvnews.ca/baby-tests-positive-for-covid-19-in-vancouver-newborn-icu-outbreak-1.5028867#_gus&_gucid=&_gup=Facebook&_gsc=SdEmQVD (Accessed July 17, 2020).

Dawson, T. (2020). Nunavut confirms first case of COVID-19: "It was only a matter of time". Available at: https://nationalpost.com/news/canada/cp-newsalert-nunavut-confirms-first-case-of-covid-19-in-pond-inlet?utm_source=Twitter&utm_medium=organic_fb_tw&utm_campaign=broadsheet_promo (Accessed July 26, 2020).

D'Entremont, D., Walter, S., and Hwang, P. (2020). N. W. T. shuts its borders as 1st case of COVID-19 confirmed in territory. Available at: https://www.cbc.ca/news/canada/north/nwt-first-case-covid19-1.5505701 (Accessed July 26, 2020).

First Nations Health Authority and Perinatal Services BC (2020). *Perinatal health, cultural safety in COVID-19.* Vancouver, Canada: First Nations Health Authority and Perinatal Services BC.

Gillis, H. (2020). Expectant mother says COVID-19 restrictions unduly harsh to pregnant women and partners. Available at: https://www.cbc.ca/news/canada/newfoundland-labrador/expectant-mother-support-person-birth-covid19-1.5573894 (Accessed May 26, 2020).

Government of Canada, Statistics Canada (2017a). *Aboriginal identity (9), age (20), registered or treaty Indian status (3) and Sex (3) for the population in private households of Canada, provinces and territories Census Metropolitan areas and Census Agglomerations, 2016 Census—25% sample data.* Ottawa, Canada: Government of Canada, Statistics Canada.

Government of Canada, Statistics Canada (2017b). *Immigration and ethnocultural diversity highlight tables.* Ottawa, Canada: Government of Canada, Statistics Canada.

Grant, T. (2020). Nova Scotia suspends home births during COVID-19 pandemic. Available at: https://www.cbc.ca/news/canada/nova-scotia/nova-scotia-home-births-suspended-covid-19-1.5514941 (Accessed April 3, 2020).

HealthLinkBC.(2020). *Post-Pactum: the first 6 weeks after childbirth.* Victoria, Canada: HealthLinkBC.

Maclean, A. (2020). Coronavirus: N.S. couple calls for home birth suspension to be reversed. Available at: https://globalnews.ca/news/6805759/coronavirus-nova-scotia-home-birth/?fbclid=IwAR2oJyyVvVbIxhC0KXqmv9MbQS90__4VDe4bE0pthC14suBvzhJCGRDL90Y (Accessed April 17, 2020).

McCourt, C., and Stevens, T. (2006). Continuity of carer–what does it mean and does it matter to midwives and birthing women? *Can. J. Midwifery Res. Pract.* 4 (3), 10–20.

Midwives Association of British Columbia (2020). Pregnant in a pandemic: expectant mothers change birth plans due to COVID-19. Vancouver, Canada: Midwives Association of British Columbia.

Northwest Territories Health and Social Services Authority (2020). Visitor restrictions and processes during COVID-19. Available at: https://www.nthssa.ca/en/services/coronavirus-disease-covid-19-updates/visitor-restrictions-and-processes-during-covid-19 (Accessed June 29, 2020).

Ontario (2020). Routine prenatal care. Available at: https://www.ontarioprenataleducation.ca/routine-prenatal-care/.

Pearce, N. (2020). What to expect when you're expecting amid COVID-19. Available at: https://nnsl.com/yellowknifer/what-to-expect-when-youre-expecting-amid-covid-19/ (Accessed June 30, 2020).

Peckham, A., Ho, J., and Marchildon, G. P. (2018). *Policy innovations in primary care across Canada.* Toronto, Canada: North American observatory on health systems and policies.

Perdok, H., Verhoeven, C., and van Dillen, J. (2018). Continuity of care is an important and distinct aspect of childbirth experience: findings of a survey evaluating experienced continuity of care, experienced quality of care and women's perception of labor. *BMC Pregnancy Childbirth.* 18, 13. doi:10.1186/s12884-017-1615-y

Piapot, N. (2020). Birthing a nation' during a pandemic: indigenous doulas try to maintain practices and protocols from Afar. Available at: https://www.cbc.ca/news/canada/saskatchewan/saskatchewan-indigenous-doulas-covid-19-response-1.5588786 (Accessed June 10, 2020).

Pole, A. (2020). "We'll have to face time our parents": COVID-19 changes delivery plans for women about to give birth. Available at: https://www.cbc.ca/news/health/coronavirus-covid-19-pandemic-pregnancy-1.5505198 (Accessed April 3, 2020).

Rieger, S. (2020). Foothills maternity staff test positive for COVID-19. Available at: https://www.cbc.ca/news/canada/calgary/covid19-foothills-maternity-1.5533955 (Accessed April 17, 2020).

Rudrum, S., and Frank, L. (2021). " Reproducing the rural citizen: barriers to rural birthing and maternity care," in *The right to Be Rural.* Editors K. R. Foster, and J. Jarman, (Edmonton, Canada: University of Alberta Press).

Sandall, J. (1995). Choice, continuity and control: changing midwifery, towards a sociological perspective. *Midwifery* 11 (4), 201–209. doi:10.1016/0266-6138(95)90005-5

Savikataaq, J. (2020). Covid-19 Update. Available at: https://www.premier.gov.nu.ca/en/news-releases/covid-19-gn-update-may-1-2020.

Shah, M. (2020). With 62% of Canada's coronavirus deaths, quebec remains hardest hit province. Available at: https://globalnews.ca/news/6979155/canada-coronavirus-cases-deaths-may-23/ (Accessed July 26, 2020).

Sibonney, C. (2020). Nova scotia has cancelled all home births – could it happen in other provinces? Available at: https://www.todaysparent.com/pregnancy/giving-birth/cancelled-home-births-coronavirus/?fbclid=IwAR1ck2siS8A2hdcBC6JqtU-E47ZEnUd4oY8aqbheJoyj5x5bfahzlMkfMCQ (Accessed April 3, 2020).

Van Syckle, K., and Caron, C. (2020). "Women will not be forced to be alone when they are giving birth". Available at: https://www.nytimes.com/2020/03/28/parenting/nyc-coronavirus-hospitals-visitors-labor.html (Accessed July 29, 2020).

Viau, J. (2020). Midwives inundated with home birth requests amid COVID-19 pandemic. Available at: https://www.cbc.ca/news/canada/windsor/midwives-ontario-influx-patients-1.5536904 (Accessed May 27, 2020).

Vedam, S., Stoll, K., McRae, D. N., Korchinski, M., Velasquez, R., Wang, J., et al. (2019). Patient-led decision making: measuring autonomy and respect in canadian maternity care. *Patient Educ. Counsel.* 102 (3), 586–594. doi:10.1016/j.pec.2018.10.023

World Health Organization (2020a). Clinical management of COVID-19: interim guidance Available at https://www.who.int/publications/i/item/clinical-management-of-covid-19 (Accessed July 25, 2020).

World Health Organization (2020b). Pregnancy, childbirth, breastfeeding and COVID-19. Available at: https://www.who.int/reproductivehealth/publications/emergencies/COVID-19-pregnancy-ipc-breastfeeding-infographics/en/ (Accessed July 28, 2020).

World Health Organization (2018). WHO recommendation on continuity of care for a positive childbirth experience. Available at: https://extranet.who.int/rhl/guidelines/who-recommendations-intrapartum-care-positive-childbirth-experience (Accessed July 24, 2020).

Yukon Hospitals (2020). COVID-19 updates. Available at: https://yukonhospitals.ca/covid-19-updates (Accessed July 28, 2020).

2

"They Would have Stopped Births, if they Only Could have": Short -and Long-Term Impacts of the COVID-19 Pandemic

Brenda Benaglia[1]* *and Daniela Canzini*[2]

[1]*University of Bologna, Bologna, Italy,* [2]*Voci di Nascita Birth Community, Bologna, Italy*

***Correspondence:**
Brenda Benaglia
brenda.benaglia@unibo.it

This article addresses the short-term impacts of the COVID-19 pandemic in Italy and hints at its potential long-term effects. Though many might want it to, birth does not stop during a pandemic. In emergency times, birth practices need to be adjusted to safeguard the health of birthing mothers, babies, birth providers, and the general population. In Bologna, Italy, one of the emergency measures employed by local hospitals in response to COVID-19 was to suspend women's right to be accompanied by a person of their choice for the whole duration of labor and childbirth. In this work, we look at how this measure was disputed by the local activist birth community. Through the analysis of a social campaign empowered by Voci di Nascita—an association of parents, birth providers, and activists—we examine how social actors negotiated the balance between public health and reproductive rights in a time of crisis. We argue that this process unveils several structural issues that characterize maternity care at the local and national levels, including the (re)medicalization of birth, the discourse on risk and safety, the internal fragmentation of Italian midwifery, and the fragility of reproductive rights. The Covidian experience forced the reshaping of the birth carepath during the peak of the emergency. We suggest that it also offered an opportunity to rethink how birth is conceived, experienced, and accompanied in times of unprecedented global uncertainty—and beyond.

Keywords: birth, maternity care, COVID-19, covidian, reproductive rights, midwifery, public health, Italy

INTO THE FIELD: COVID-19 IN ITALY

The first case of an Italian contracting COVID-19 was documented on February 21, 2020. "Patient 1" is a 38-year-old man from a small town near Milan whose wife was pregnant. In the turmoil of the breaking news, this detail was often repeated. Our thoughts—as a medical anthropologist and an activist mother engaged in the field of birth—ran to this mother-to-be, who was abruptly separated from her husband when he was confined to intensive care. We felt frightened and powerless, thinking about the health risk to her and their baby. Very little was then known about SARS-CoV-2, let alone about its effects during pregnancy. At that time, we could not imagine that separation, isolation, and loneliness would become trademarks of how we give birth—and die—during a pandemic.

This was also when the national hunt for the "culprit" (Moretti, 2020) began. Attempts were made to trace the chain of contagion, in the hope of exorcising the growing fear that it was too late to stop it.

Before February 21, the only two confirmed cases of the novel coronavirus in Italy dated back to January 30 and were related to two Chinese tourists on holiday in Rome. Until then, the media portrayed the virus as something lethal but exotic, still distant enough to leave all of us living in privileged old Europe substantially safe. A lethal mix of ethnocentric shortsightedness, structural issues in some parts of the Italian National Health Service, and the imponderability of nature created the perfect environment for the virus to proliferate in the country.

"Patient 1" and his pregnant wife were the tip of an iceberg that would soon reveal its magnitude. At the end of February, a frightening scenario was emerging: thousands of people were exposed to the risk of being infected, including hundreds of women who were soon to become mothers. Hospitals—where 99.9% of births occur in Italy (Ministero della Salute, 2019)—were quickly identified as dangerous contagion hotbeds. Health services, including the entire birth carepath, required urgent reorganization. Protocols had to be rewritten and interpersonal relationships reshaped in light of the sudden need for social distancing. Drastic measures were to be implemented, as births could not be stopped.

ETHNOGRAPHY IN THE TIME OF COVID-19: ENGAGEMENT *VS.* SOCIAL DISTANCING

This study looks at maternity care in Bologna, Italy, during the Italian COVID-19 lockdown. To describe this lockdown, an early op-ed in the *New York Times* was provocatively titled: "Even Mass Is Canceled" (Parks, 2020). From March 9 to May 18, 2020, all citizens not involved in primary activities (such as health care, food production and distribution, vital logistics, law enforcement and security) had to follow one simple rule: stay at home.

From our own domestic quarantines, we observed the turmoil that was swirling around maternity care in Bologna through texts, calls, photos, and accounts coming from "outside." These were the voices of soon-to-be parents and birth providers—hospital midwives in particular—confronting this new Covidian world and enduring its immediate effects. On April 17—a full month into the total lockdown—the association Voci di Nascita sent a formal letter to the local political and healthcare authorities in representation of parents, birth professionals, and birth activists[1]. The goal was to denounce the temporary suspension of women's right to be accompanied by a person of choice during labor and childbirth in the city hospitals. Dozens of parents followed suit, enclosing a copy of the letter in their inquiries to the public relations departments of the hospitals where they were planning to give birth. The authorities responded, opening up a dialogue with the association and its members. Shortly after that, along with the gradual decrease in the emergency and the progressive systematization of the scientific evidence, the most restrictive measures were modified.

This article, like our engagements in the field of birth, is driven by our shared desire to contribute to fostering positive cultural change and social impact (Low and Merry, 2010). Such an aspiration proves more urgent than ever in times of social distancing and temporary restriction of reproductive rights: timely and informed critique is vital to the constant maintenance process that public health deserves in a democratic setting. This was also the primary driving factor for the social campaign empowered by Voci di Nascita and the reason why we decided to analyze that campaign and its repercussions on the community and on maternity care.

Anthropological work normally requires prolonged participation in the research field and direct engagement in relationships with interlocutors and research collaborators. Given social distancing measures, this was not possible for us. Therefore, we designed a short-term ethnographic research plan, which included two online questionnaires, in-depth conversations between we two authors, informal exchanges with local birth providers, participation in relevant webinars, and a review of the latest literature on the topic. Our study combines the analysis of data derived from such sources and unfolds on the basis of previous engagements in the field—both Daniela's as an activist mother and Brenda's as an anthropologist (Benaglia 2013, Benaglia, 2016, Benaglia, 2018, Benaglia, 2020).

ONLINE QUESTIONNAIRES: GOALS AND PRELIMINARY RESULTS

For the purposes of this research, we designed and disseminated two different online questionnaires: one addressed to parents, the other to midwives. We narrowed our core sample to individuals directly related to the social campaign empowered by Voci di Nascita (people who had joined it, asked for information, expressed support, and/or shared spontaneous testimonies). All of our primary respondents had written at least once to the campaign's official email address during the lockdown period (March-May). Additionally, parents had to have given birth during that time or immediately afterward. A secondary sample is composed of parents and midwives from outside of Bologna who had not been directly involved in the local campaign. Because of their efforts in reacting spontaneously to the survey, we decided to include their input in the broader context of our analysis.

Both questionnaires were open from July 4 to August 4, 2020 on the web-based platform Qualtrics. The invitation to participate in the questionnaire for parents was sent by email from the dedicated address of the association Voci di Nascita to 62 parents. Afterwards, we published a post on the Facebook page of Voci di Nascita, thus introducing the work to a broader audience. Information on the campaign and the link to the survey then circulated among secondary recipients outside Bologna.

[1]The full letter, in Italian, can be found on the association's Facebook page (https://www.facebook.com/vocidinascita, accessed August 20, 2020). Abstracts of the letter cited in this article, as well as quotes from questionnaires, have been translated into English by the authors.

We emailed the invitation to participate in the second questionnaire to 12 midwives, all of them active in the city of Bologna. The message included a request to forward the email to colleagues potentially interested in participating in the study. Another email was sent to the local College of Midwives and, a few days later, a post with the link to our survey appeared on their Facebook page. The announcement was reposted on Voci di Nascita's Facebook page.

The goal of the questionnaire dedicated to parents was to collect stories of those who gave birth during the lockdown in Bologna and how the emergency restrictions reshaped their experiences before, during, and after the birth. We focused our queries on the presence/absence of the partner or support person during labor and childbirth, as this was the issue we were most interested in exploring. Most inquiries were directed to birthing mothers; however, a final question was dedicated to the partners (among our respondents these were all fathers, except for one, who was a second mother). We asked no personal details apart from the parents' age, and whether it was the first birth. We set up the survey using the strictest anonymity settings, and no additional sensitive data was recorded.

The mothers' questionnaire received 49 complete or partially complete responses (more than 60% filled in). These 49 accounts constitute the sample taken for analysis. Of these responses, 29 concern the Bologna area, and 20 are from other parts of Italy. The average age of the respondents (mothers) was 35 for the Bologna area and 34.6 for the whole national area. The average age of the partners was 36.3 and 36.7, respectively. The percentage of primiparas in the Bologna area was 22% and 30% for the whole national area. 27 of the Bolognese births took place in a hospital, 1 in a maternity home, and 1 at home. In the rest of the national territory, 15 births occurred in a hospital or clinic, three at home, and in 2 cases the place of birth was not declared. In Bologna, 2% of the respondents gave birth in a different place from the one planned and/or desired; this percentage rises to 6% in the rest of the country. Before the emergency, the desired labor companion(s) in Bologna was: the partner for 23 women, the partner and the parturient's mother for 3, and the partner together with the midwife for 3. On the national scale, these numbers are 37, 6 and 6, respectively. In Bologna, 21% of women stated that they were left alone during labor and childbirth (similar to the national percentage, 22%).

The goal of the questionnaire dedicated to midwives was to gather their personal views on how obstetric practice and care changed in response to the pandemic and collect accounts of their direct experiences accompanying women and births in times of COVID-19. Particular focus in the midwives' questionnaire was also on the temporary prohibition/limitation of partners in the birthing room; additionally, it addressed midwives's needs during the crisis. Again no sensitive personal data was requested, aside from age and city. However, to better understand and contextualize the responses of our interlocutors, we asked midwives to describe their professional environment and experience, and to name the three words that they most associate with midwifery. Finally, we invited midwives to share their thoughts about the future of birth and maternity care.

The questionnaire for midwives received 18 full responses, constituting the sample taken for analysis. Of these, eight concern the Bologna area and the other 10 the rest of Italy. The average age of the respondents in the Bologna area is 31.6 years; the total national average age is 36.6. In Bologna, four responding midwives work at a hospital, 1 in a family clinic, and 3 as freelance professionals. These numbers at the national level are 9, 2, and 7, respectively. The three words most frequently associated with midwifery by respondents were "listening," "empathy," and "compassion."

THE *VOCI DI NASCITA* BIRTH COMMUNITY AND ITS SOCIAL CAMPAIGN

Voci di Nascita means "voices of birth" and was founded on International Women's Day of 2017. The birth of the association is related to the personal experience of becoming a mother and a doula of the founder and president, co-author Daniela Canzini. For her, the direct encounter with motherhood suddenly revealed a personal lack of "birth culture," which, she felt, demanded an active stance at the individual and social levels. From its beginning, the association's fundamental aim was to create and promote "culture" around birth and parenthood through various forms of social activism and services to birthing families. Midwives were progressively identified as the strategic actors of their local birth communities. Together with women, Italian midwives are directly engaged in the biosocial process of birth and largely operate within the biomedical environment. In the association's view, midwives' voices—largely unheard—called for a dialogue with parents, institutions, and within midwifery as well.

During the initial phase of the lockdown, dialogue appeared urgent yet almost impossible to achieve. This was the frantic time in which major emergency adjustments to the birth carepath were adopted, along with the broader reorganization of hospital spaces and services. Information on the new procedures for parents and staff appeared swiftly, increasing everyone's anxiety and stress. Homemade signs popped up on the doors of maternity wards with vague communications such as "Due to the COVID-19 emergency, it is no longer possible to allow the accompaniment of women during the whole duration of labor." In late March, a worried mother-to-be saw such an announcement during a prenatal visit at the hospital and sent a picture of it to Voci di Nascita to share her disorientation. Although other city hospitals had not employed the same restrictive measure (yet), the general feeling was that things could only worsen, and there was talk of the possibility of separating mother from child after the birth. Luckily, that did not happen. Eventually, on April 7, all three city hospitals adjusted to the strictest rule: the birth partner was not allowed during labor and was only to be admitted at the expulsion stage of birth. This left no choice to parents who, until then, could weigh their hospital options and decide to give birth where the partner or person of choice was still allowed to be with the mother and support her during labor as well.

The association decided it was necessary to demand that parents' and birth professionals' voices be taken into consideration, despite—and, in virtue of—the current emergency. A few midwives had already shared their concerns and expressed their feelings of being impotent, voiceless, and stuck in a violent defensive mechanism with no clear direction. On April 17, Daniela Canzini signed and sent out a letter to the authorities in charge of local health and hospital services, social politics (in the fields of welfare, infant rights, and birth), and to the president of the Emilia-Romagna Region.

The letter was successful in opening a dialogue and receiving formal feedback. Daniela was invited to be duly informed on the situation with the local health authorities. The most restrictive measures were corrected: starting from April 27, partners could be present from the beginning of active labor up until after the birth.

Of course, the campaign's immediate impact should also be read in light of the progressive decrease in the COVID-19 emergency and the consolidation of the scientific evidence. However, the social campaign did mark a turning point and created an important precedent. Moreover, the letter hinted at several structural issues that characterize the local culture of maternity care and birth, which the experience of COVID-19 unveiled. In the following sections, we will discuss these, combining the responses given by parents and midwives to our questionnaires with selected abstracts from the letter itself.

SEPARATION AND PROHIBITIONS: HOSPITALS AND COVID-19

Since the beginning of the pandemic, one of the risks associated with the reorganization of the birth carepath on the basis of the principle of social and physical distancing was the obstetric tendency to "revert back" to "deeply held belief systems" (Davis-Floyd, et al., 2020). This risk included the reinforcement of technocratic practices through the employment of restrictive measures. Davis-Floyd (2001, 2018) has identified "separation" as the underyling principle of the technocratic model of medicine (Davis-Floyd and St. John, 2001). Since modernization, rationalism, mechanicity, and determinism—all resting on the basic *principle of separation*—have significantly shaped Western scientific thought, and that of biomedicine in particular. One of the side effects of its development has been a progressive medicalization process, which affects multiple aspects of society through forms of biopolitical control of bodily experiences (Foucault, 1963; Canguilhem, 1966; Illich, 1976). Pregnancy and childbirth are no exception (Martin, 1987; Lock, 2004).

The "principle of separation" unfolds in the technocratic paradigm of birth, which is predominantly male-centered, sees the body as a machine, the birthing process as inherently mechanical and prone to dysfunction, the hospital as a factory, the baby as a product, and the environmental and relational aspects of childbirth as irrelevant (Davis-Floyd, 1987, Davis Floyd, 2001, Davis Floyd, 2003). Despite considerable progress toward less restrictive, more humanistic approaches and the revaluation of midwifery care, this model still shapes birth "management" in hospitals, and over-medicalization generally characterizes birth practices in the country, although with significant regional differences (Scavini and Molinari, 2015)[2].

In pre-Covidian and Covidian times, hospital spaces, protocols, and hierachies do rest on the principle of separation, which is complementary to what we are calling the *principle of prohibition*. The biomedical choice to remove the birth partner from the birth scene shows that both principles were amplified in practice during the peak of the crisis.

Giuseppe Battagliarin, renowned obstetrician and president of the regional Birth Commission, recently suggested a connection between COVID-19, the hospital environment, and the "principle of prohibition." During a public webinar[3], he stated that "This virus has authorized more than any other the right to prohibit." Battagliarin noted that COVID-19 turned ordinary things, such as walking around or shaking hands, into something forbidden—inconceivable in ordinary times. In his view, the power and authority of hospitals and doctors is structurally related to the power to set limitations and to prohibit. According to Battagliarin, the decision not to allow partners to participate in the whole birthing process partly stemmed from an "instinct" to prohibit, structured into the biomedical approach: a tangible instance of the aformentioned risk of regressing to former times when women were never allowed birth companions, their human rights were ignored, and birth practices were more controlling and less sensitive to women's protagonism and psychosocial needs.

In his speech, Battagliarin also mentioned and praised a "letter from women"—probably referring to the campaign of Voci di Nascita—and synthesized the overall situation that health institutions were facing in the peak of the crisis. The ever-present inner risk inherent to the bodily experience of pregnancy and birth was confronted with the outer, diffused, and violent risk of contagion. Risk was everywhere: social and physical distancing became key, turning separation into the driving principle of all emergency measures, including those regarding birth companionship—despite long-established evidence on the importance of not leaving birthing mothers unsupported. The letter of Voci di Nascita repeatedly draws attention to the importance of continuity of supportive care throughout the birth process. It stresses that the continuous presence of a trusted person of choice is an undeniable right of all women, including during pandemics, and that removing

[2]It must be aknowledged that, so far, at least deliveries among women affected by COVID-19 do not show an increase in medicalization procedures, such as unnecessary c-sections (Maraschini et al., 2020). While this is certainly an achievement, it must be highlighted that the vast majority of birthing women are not SARS-CoV-2 positive and are being exposed to an environment that, directly or indirectly, tends towards over-medicalization.

[3]The online conference Becoming Parents Together in the Era of COVID-19 was organized within the framework of the activities of the PARENT project. The full recording is available at https://www.facebook.com/watch/?v=893690627805177 (accessed August 11, 2020). PARENT, an acronym for Promotion, Awareness-raising and Engagement of Men in Nurture Transformations, is a European project that aims at enhancing gender equality and reducing violence against women by promoting fathers' nurturing care, starting from pregnancy itself (OECD, 2016; Luppi and Rosina, 2019).

this right is detrimental to the health of mother and baby, and to the bonding process:

> There is no such thing as a moment which is more important than the other. Childbirth is a very delicate process that should be protected in the continuity of intimacy. [This process] is built over time, and requires minimum environmental changes, especially in the expulsive phase. The solution [to the current emergency] cannot be at the expense of the experience of those who are born, those who give birth, and those who are there to support the most delicate and powerful beginning of one's social and relational life (Voci di Nascita, April 17, 2020).

The restrictive measures failed to consider the authoritative evidence available on birth companionship (Bohren et al., 2017) and its effects in biological and social terms—both in the short and long run. Moreover, during birth and the early stages of parenthood, the very concepts of separation and physical distancing represent "conceptual and biological nonsense" (Coscia et al., 2020), as childbirth, breastfeeding, and nurturing care necessitate close physical contact. Such early physical relations are the very first social relations as well, and both aspects have repercussions on babies' neuro-cognitive development (WHO, 2018). Yet, in the frantic peak of the emergency, a semantic—albeit essential—*quid pro quo* occurred: the terms "visitor," "relative," "support person," and "parent" were suddenly mixed, with the result that partners were cut off just where their relationship with their newborns normally begins (Coscia et al., 2020). Emergency procedures assumed that "the other parent" could be separated from the birthing mother and their newborn. These new restrictions and prohibitions implied that childbirth could be regarded as a single, specific moment that could be separated from the broader process of becoming parents, thus technocratically devaluing its relational, social, and political entanglements.

EVIDENCE, RISK, AND SAFETY DURING THE EMERGENCY

During the early times of the emergency, it was difficult to navigate the scientific evidence on the new virus, which was "being produced, published, and disseminated at a rate never seen before" (Renfrew et al., 2020). For this reason, the Italian Istituto Superiore di Sanità[4] issued systematic reviews weekly from the end of February. The final report, published on May 31, acknowledges that, initially, local health services had to react on the basis of their organizational availability and that until March, the scientific evidence was still poor and not always consistent (Giusti et al., 2020).

The Voci di Nascita letter acknowledged the medical staff's efforts in responding to the unprecedented needs that appeared during the pandemic and expressed trust in the good conscience of decision-makers confronted with extraordinary responsibilities. The letter also raised questions as to how the evidence was interpreted and used to drive the implementation of emergency measures. For instance, the letter quotes the WHO infographics[5] and abstracts from the guidelines for birth professionals issued by the Emilia-Romagna Regional Health Service, which suggested that one person could accompany the mother during labor and birth[6]. Why then limit the duration of the presence of the birth partner to the expulsion phase? On the basis of what evidence had similar hospitals in the same city proposed different rules?

Such inquiries recall the accounts of some midwife respondents to the questionnaire, who could not understand the rationale for restricting access to "husbands who had been with women up until 1 min before entering the hospital." Many interpreted this security measure in terms of a poorly informed, reactionary rule devaluing parents' rights and babies' wellbeing—and also complicating midwives' job during labor and birth. For instance, one midwife wrote:

> Restricting access to the delivery room to fathers or an accompanying person has been detrimental to the mother's rights, the newborn baby, the father. It has undoubtedly harmed the delicate process of birth at various levels. Increasing anxiety and fear in pregnant mothers, altering the dynamics and timing of labor and childbirth, exposing the mother to an excessive emotional and psychological burden postpartum, creating a fertile ground for emotional and psychological repercussions for the mother (Midwife #17).

Another commented that:

> The exclusion of partners was an absurdity experienced with anguish by women who sometimes turned towards alternatives in the wake of fear instead of awareness—a measure with absolutely no scientific basis: an action against human rights, a violence against parents and babies (Midwife #7).

[4]The Istituto Superiore di Sanità (ISS) is the main center for technical-scientific research on public health in Italy. It serves the Italian National Health Service and the Ministry of Health. In this article, we use the website of the ISS and its publications as our primary reference for epidemiological data. Complete information on the impacts of COVID-19 in terms of cases, deaths, and recoveries in the national territory is produced and constantly updated by the ISS through an integrated surveillance system (https://www.epicentro.iss.it/en/coronavirus/sars-cov-2-dashboard, accessed August 10, 2020).

[5]The WHO infographic states that "All women have the right to a safe and positive childbirth experience, whether or not they have a confirmed COVID-19 infection. Respect and dignity; a companion of choice, clear communication by maternity staff; pain relief strategies; mobility in labor where possible and birth position of choice" (https://www.who.int/reproductivehealth/publications/emergencies/Pregnancy-3-1200x1200.png?ua=1, accessed August 20, 2020).

[6]The document was published on March 22, 2020 and is available online (https://www.saperidoc.it/flex/cm/pages/ServeAttachment.php/L/IT/D/1%252F3%252F2%252FD.1aa8e5fc6fd8fcdde5c6/P/BLOB%3AID%3D1402/E/pdf, accessed August 20, 2020).

This midwife raises several crucial issues, including that birthing parents could end up changing their birthplace because of fear. A mother confirmed that she and her partner eventually changed hospitals because "she could not even think" of giving birth without her husband. Some parents in our study wrote that, during COVID-19, they felt out-of-hospital birth could be safer. However, no one planning a hospital birth actually shifted to homebirth. On the other hand, the women who gave birth at home (1 in Bologna and 3 nation-wide)—having previously decided to do so—said that their greatest fear was an emergency transfer to the hospital because they knew they might end up laboring alone.

22% of the birthing mothers in our survey declared that they were, in fact, left alone in the hospital during labor and birth. For example, one woman said that, although she had been assured that her partner could be there, he was only called into the room just after the birth. Partners usually remained outside the hospital premises, waiting to be called by the birthing mother herself or—more likely, given the circumstances—by the midwife on duty. A father said that this situation made him feel "powerless" and the typical scene is decribed by another man, who wrote:

> I spent the whole night outside the hospital on the phone with my wife to make her feel my presence and give her courage, even though I was afraid. I left my wife at 9 p.m., and I saw her again at 3 a.m., after labor. I was able to experience the emotion of childbirth during the pushing phase. Despite the restrictions, I was lucky to be there and see my daughter being born (Partner #20).

Fear and luck are recurring expressions in both mothers' and fathers' accounts, and a midwife noted that:

> Most women have an attitude of acceptance of the restrictions. Some of us received official complaints from inpatients when they realized that we broke the rules when necessary. We endured continuous disputes with our superiors, and we feared being reported by other colleagues. Nowadays, it is more us than women who have been asking for more openness and urging them to stand up for themselves. Fear has been the master, lately (Midwife #11).

This statement echoes the general feeling that most mothers expressed about their birthing experience: in the chaotic times of COVID-19, many women entered the hospital already "tired," "stressed," "fearful," and "disillusioned." Referring to the initial phase of the emergency, when protocols were not clear and could change from one day to the next, one mother said:

> During the last few weeks of pregnancy, we feared that my partner could not be present at the birth. This made me really upset. Luckily, things changed shortly before the birth, and he was able to be there. Otherwise, I would have considered it as violence (Mother #25).

In their accounts, almost all mothers expressed disappointment with regards to the prohibition. Some of them specifically pointed at the impossibility of reaching the necessary intimacy with partners during childbirth because they could only be there for the very final moments. And yet—while expressing frustration, sadness, and loneliness—most birthing mothers accepted the restrictive measure for the sake of "safety" and because they saw no feasible alternative. Some also pointed to the fact that they were "lucky" this was not their first birth, suggesting a diffused perception that the quality of assistance and care is ultimately a matter of luck (Campisi, 2015), rather than a well-established right worth fighting for.

MIDWIVES AT WAR

The "war" metaphor has been employed in mainstream media to describe the scenario generated by COVID-19, especially inside hospital wards. We chose to adopt this metaphor herein because it mirrors the words used by many midwives in our study when describing their experiences during the pandemic. Midwife respondents agreed that empathetic care is essential for birthing women. They were vocal in denouncing the risks connected to leaving mothers alone and depriving them of personalized midwifery care, which requires presence, empathy, and close contact. They also believe that such care is an essential safety factor, especially in critical times. Most midwives seemed to suggest that COVID-19 restrictions endangered a double right to quality midwifery care: for women to receive it, and for midwives to provide it, safely.

During the lockdown in Italy, the first "battle" for midwives began with instructions to abide by emergency measures "without being asked what they thought about them"—as the letter by Voci di Nascita points out. One midwife in particular felt that, by adhering to the new rules, she was (re)producing violence against women—suggesting the urgent need to further analyze the forms of obstetric violence (Quattrocchi, 2019) that birth practitioners simultaneously perform and suffer (Liese et al., 2021). Moreover, midwives in leadership and coordination roles highlighted their "frustration" at having to control their midwifery colleagues by forcing them into practices with which they disagreed. Hospital prohibitions hit midwives hard and, partially due to their lack of power and authority in the biomedical hierarchy (Davis-Floyd and Sargent, 1997), their response was weak.

Midwives' second battle, shared with all other medical staff, was the initial lack or inappropriateness of personal protective equipment (PPE). This was particularly hard for freelance out-of-hospital midwives who had no direct access to PPE. Although facemasks were deemed necessary, midwives reported that these played a detrimental role in their relationships with women by disguising facial expressions; furthermore, recalling the experience of a birthing mother, a midwife commented that "birthing with a facemask was asphyxiating."

The third and most structural battle midwives have had to endure over the past few months is their intra-professional conflicts. Respondents testifed to the fact that not all midwives disagreed with the most restrictive measures and that, because of their own fear and exhaustion, some actually thought that it was better to exclude partners from the birthing room. Generational issues should also be factored in, as younger hospital midwives tend to be more enthusiastic about their jobs. Older, more experienced midwives who had already fought for decades for mothers' rights were often tired and disillusioned by the fact that women themselves sometimes only care about not feeling pain or having a "souvenir" photo of their birth. Unfortunately, none of these midwives filled out our survey and therefore we cannot further elaborate on their perspectives. However, a young midwife wrote:

> The fact that there are no partners is seen by the majority as safer. For me, this emergency showed who loves their job, and who does it only for money. I am not saying that we should go out and die for midwifery, but neither that we have to carry out illogical and absurd procedures. For me it does not have to be like that: every mother is different, and we have to remember that we are not there to cure them but to accompany them. I think some of my colleagues are in burnout (Midwife #1).

Anxiety and burnout are very likely to increase during emergency situations. Adequate psychological support for hospital staff is structurally lacking in regular times, let alone during the pandemic. Yet women's needs for emotional support and reassurance grow during times of crisis, and midwives should be adequately prepared to respond (O'Connell et al., 2020), even though "healthcare staff did not sign up to be heroes fighting on the frontline" (Renfrew et al., 2020).

The key to understanding this broader "cold war" is structural in nature and goes well beyond midwives' experiences of COVID-19. It interrogates the very status of the midwifery profession in Italy, which has been defined a "semi-profession" due to a lack of collective identity and professional autonomy, and for its internal fragmentation (Spina, 2012). This "pre-existing condition" simply emerged more evidently during the pandemic. One midwife concluded her account by saying: "I have strong concerns about the future of my profession."

More broadly, when questioned about the future of birth and maternity care in post-Covidian times, midwives raised a number of issues. Some were afraid that fear might normalize the strictest rules and that the medicalization of birth might increase at the expense of midwifery care. Others worried about the quality of virtual antenatal and postnatal care and feared that women will end up being even more isolated. Some hope for the development of social policies to support out-of-hospital birth for normal physiologic pregnancies. One midwife summarized the feeling of most respondents: "An unfortunate scenario has opened up: the little importance given to being born as a form of relationship."

FINAL REMARKS: A "MESSAGE" TO CONSIDER

As elsewhere, as also demonstrated in other articles in this Special Issue, the experience of COVID-19 exposed pre-existing structural issues in Italian maternity care, especially within the hospital environment. Under the initial epidemiological pressure, emergency measures reshaped the birth carepath in ways that highlighted the delicate balance between safeguarding public health and guaranteeing reproductive rights (Yuill, 2020). In this sense, COVID-19 might be recalled as "a watershed moment for birth rights" (Drandić and Van Leeuwen, 2020).

Well past the first and hopefully last Covidian summer, a generalized feeling of uncertainty still characterizes the entire Italian scenario. There has not been a "second wave" of emergency and, therefore, no further lockdowns. The contagion at the national level seems relatively under control, particularly compared with other European countries (France and Spain, for instance). However, it is hard to make predictions for the upcoming weeks and months, and a serious threat remains. For this reason, at the Bolognese level, the "semi-restrictive" rules implemented in local hospitals after the campaign of Voci di Nascita still apply: women can be accompanied by a person of choice from the beginning of active labor only. According to informal testimonies we continue to receive, hospital staff seem to be more flexible than during emergency times, and their approaches—whether more or less medicalized—tend to resemble those in place before the pandemic. The situation could be rapidly shifting, and it is too early to confirm any stable changes in midwifery practice in the hospitals of Bologna, let alone at the broader national level.

In our study, we could not analyze what happened outside of the hospital during the emergency, in private homes, family clinics, and birthing centers. Parents and midwives who participated in our survey raised several themes that also deserve further attention, such as the need to design supportive out-of-hospital birth policies at the local and national levels (Quattrocchi, 2018); the role of partners during prenatal and postnatal care; the revaluation or deterioration of interpersonal relationships during quarantine; the virtualization of community services; the relationship between birth and death in times of crisis; and the risk of retroceding on progress in honoring women's rights by reinforcing unbalanced domestic and affective workloads in family life; and other related issues (Coxon et al., 2020).

Our work suggests that the pandemic has been a touchstone, or pivotal moment, for local in-hospital birthcare. It shows how easy it is to go back to over-medicalized birth practices that had been considered outdated and not evidence-based; how fragile is the awareness of parents of their reproductive rights; how paralyzing is the internal fragmentation of the midwifery profession. On the other hand, the social campaign empowered by Voci di Nascita represented a strong example of activist strategy during emergency times. It pronounced the needs for clear communication of the new rules and protocols, appropriateness of evidence-based emergency measures, recognition of professional roles and responsibilities among birth providers, and the guarantee of parents' rights. Respectfully, yet firmly, the letter demanded that the voices of all actors involved in the birth process be taken into consideration during times of crisis. It also created an opportunity to reclaim engaged parenthood.

The immediate achievement of the social campaign probably rests on the fact that it came from outside the hospital environment and that it was openly political. However, medium- and long-term effects of COVID-19 on maternity care practices and policies cannot be clearly foreseen and will be largely determined by the active and direct involvement of birth providers, health authorities, and parents in the aftermath of the emergency. In the words of one of the midwives in our study, it is a matter of whether the "message sent out by COVID-19 is understood, or not." COVID-19 dramatically exposed structural issues that characterize the multilayered experience of giving birth and accompaning the births of babies and parents. Oddly enough, the virus forced an eye to the socio-cultural implications of the process of birth as rooted in—yet not limited to—the biological experience.

Postscript (December 2020). At the time of submission for review of this article (October 2020), a second wave of COVID-19 had not yet hit Italy and we anticipated that no clear predictions could be made and that uncertainty and fear were still dominant. Indeed, a second wave did hit Europe and Italy did not escape it. The semi-restrictive rules described in our work are still in place, and no further significant progress has been made in the longed-for engagement towards an alliance of the actors involved for the safeguarding of appropriate and well-rounded practices in maternity care.

ETHICS STATEMENT

Ethical review and approval was not required for the study on human participants in accordance with the local legislation and institutional requirements. Written informed consent for participation was not required for this study in accordance with the national legislation and the institutional requirements.

AUTHOR CONTRIBUTIONS

BB and DC designed the survey, analyzed data and interpreted findings. BB wrote the original draft and revisions; DC contributed to editing the manuscript. Both authors read and approved the final work. Please see here for full authorship criteria.

ACKNOWLEDGMENTS

The authors wish to thank all mothers, fathers, and midwives, who took the time to share their personal experiences through our questionnaires. Warm appreciation also goes to other professionals, such as physicians, epidemiologists, doulas, and birth activists who have informally shared precious insights on the complicated relationship between the COVID-19 pandemic and maternity care.

REFERENCES

Benaglia, B. (2016). "Doula e maternità tra spazio pubblico e privato. Considerazioni dal campo su attivismo, ricerca e cambiamento,," in *Going Public. Percorsi di antropologia pubblica in Italia. I. Severi.* Editor Italia (Bologna, Italy: CIS—Dipartimento di Filosofia e Comunicazione; Università di Bologna), 65–88.

Benaglia, B. (2013). La cicogna sono io. Una etnografia dell'accompagnamento alla vita nell'Ecuador contemporaneo. *Intrecci. Quaderni di antropologia culturale.* 1, 41–54.

Benaglia, B. (2020). La cura invisibile: potenzialità e limiti della pratica della doula. *Antropologia e teatro.* 12, 59–83. doi:10.6092/issn.2039-2281/10885

Benaglia, B. (2018). "'Mothering the mother': doulas and the affective space," in *Everyday world-making: toward an understanding of affect and mothering.* Editors J. Lane and E. Joensuu (Bradford, England: Demeter Press), 238–259.

Bohren, M., Hofmeyr, G., Sakala, C., Fukuzawa, R., and Cuthbert, A. (2017). Continuous support for women during childbirth. *Cochrane Database Syst. Rev.* 7, CD003766. doi:10.1002/14651858.CD003766.pub6

Campisi, R. (2015). *Partorirai con dolore.* Milano, Italy: Rizzoli.

Canguilhem, G. (1966). *Le normal et le pathologique.* Paris, France: Presses Universitaires de France.

Coscia, A., Cavicchioli, P., and Strola, P. (2020). "Così lontano, così vicino": nascere ai tempi del coronavirus Medico e Bambino pagine elettroniche XXIII, 95–98. Available at:https://www.medicoebambino.com/?id=CM2005_10.html.

Coxon, K., Turienzo, C. F., Kweekel, L., Goodarzi, B., Brigante, L., Simon, A., et al. (2020). The impact of the coronavirus (COVID-19) pandemic on maternity care in Europe. *Midwifery* 88, 102779–102785. doi:10.1016/j.midw.2020.102779

Davis-Floyd, R. (2003). *Birth as an American rite of passage.* Berkeley, CA: University of California Press.

Davis-Floyd, R. E. (1987). The technological model of birth. *J. Am. Folklore.* 100, 479–495. doi:10.2307/540907

Davis-Floyd, R., Gutschow, K., and Schwartz, D. A. (2020). Pregnancy, birth and the COVID-19 pandemic in the United States. *Med. Anthropol.* 39, 413. doi:10.1080/01459740.2020.1761804

Davis-Floyd, R., and Sargent, C. F. (1997). *Childbirth and authoritative knowledge: cross-cultural perspectives.* Berkeley; London: University of California Press.

Davis-Floyd, R., and St. John, G. (2001). *From doctor to healer: the transformative journey.* New Jersey, NJ: Rutgers University Press.

Davis-Floyd, R. (2018). The technocratic, humanistic, and holistic paradigms of birth and health care. in *Ways of knowing about birth: mothers, midwives, medicine, and birth activism by Robbie davis-floyd.* Long Grove, IL: Waveland Press, 3–44.

Davis-Floyd, R. (2001). The technocratic, humanistic, and holistic paradigms of childbirth. *Int. J. Gynaecol. Obstet.* 75 Suppl 1, S5. doi:10.1016/S0020-7292(01)00510-0

Ministero della Salute (2019). Certificato di assistenza al parto (CeDAP). Analisi dell'evento nascita–anno 2016. Available at: http://www.salute.gov.it/portale/documentazione/p6_2_2_1.jsp?lingua=italiano&id=2881.

Drandić, D., and Van Leeuwen, F. (2020). COVID-19: a watershed moment for women's rights in childbirth. *Medical Anthropology Quarterly Rapid Response Blog Series.* 1. Available at: http://medanthroquarterly.org/?p=536.

Foucault, M. (1963). *Naissance de la clinique.* Paris, France: Presses Universitaires de France.

Giusti, A., Zambri, F., Marchetti, F., Sampaolo, L., Taruscio, D., Salerno, P., et al. (2020). *Indicazioni ad interim per gravidanza, parto, allattamento e cura dei piccolissimi di 0-2 anni in risposta all'emergenza COVID-19. Versione 31 maggio 2020.* (Roma: Istituto Superiore di Sanitá. (Rapporto ISS COVID-19 n. 45/2020).

Illich, I. (1976). *Limits to medicine. Medical nemesis: the expropriation of health.* London, England: Boyars.

Liese, K., Davis-Floyd, R., Stewart, K., and Cheyney, M. (2021). "Obstetric Iatrogenesis in the United States: The Spectrum of Disrespect, Violence, and Abuse." *Anthropology & Medicine*, Special Issue on "Medicine's Shadowside," eds. Emma Varley and Saiba Varma (in press).

Lock, M. (2004). Medicalization and the naturalization of social control. *Encyclopedia of Medical Anthropology.*, 116–125. doi:10.1007/0-387-29905-x_13

Low, S. M., and Merry, S. E. (2010). Engaged anthropology: diversity and dilemmas. *Curr. Anthropol.* 51, S203–S226. doi:10.1086/653837

Luppi, F., and Rosina, A. (2019). "From a single breadwinner model to two breadwinners to double earner/carer – do we need a new model?" in *New visions for gender equality 2019.* Editors N. Crowley and S. Sansonetti Brussels, Belgium: European Commission, 20–24.

Maraschini, A., Corsi, E., Salvatore, M. A., and Donati, S. (2020). *Coronavirus and birth in Italy: results of a national population-based cohort study.* London, England: British Medical Associationdoi:10.1006.11.2012865210.1101/2020.06.11.20128652

Martin, E. (1987). *The woman in the body: a cultural analysis of reproduction.* Boston, MA: Beacon Press.

Moretti, C. (2020). *Il senso della colpa ai tempi del Covid-19.* Milano, Italy: Nottetempo.

OECD (2016). Policy brief. Parent leave: where are the fathers? Available at: https://www.oecd.org/policy-briefs/parental-leave-where-are-the-fathers.pdf.

O'Connell, M., Crowther, S., Ravaldi, C., and Homer, C. (2020). Midwives in a pandemic: a call for solidarity and compassion. *Women Birth.* 33, 205–206. doi:10.1016/j.wombi.2020.03.008

Parks, T. (2020). This is life under lockdown in Italy. *The New York Times.* Available at: https://www.nytimes.com/2020/03/09/opinion/italy-coronavirus.html.

Quattrocchi, P. (2018). *Oltre i luoghi comuni: partorire e nascere a domicilio e in casa maternità.* Firenze, Italy: Editpress.

Quattrocchi, P. (2019). Violenza ostetrica. Le potenzialità politico-formative di un concetto innovativo. *EtnoAntropologia* 7, 125–148. ISSN: 2284-0176.

Renfrew, M. J., Cheyne, H., Craig, J., Duff, E., Dykes, F., Hunter, B., et al. (2020). Sustaining quality midwifery care in a pandemic and beyond. *Midwifery* 88, 102759–102767. doi:10.1016/j.midw.2020.102759

Scavini, M., and Molinari, C. (2015). in *"Italy" in* Maternity services and policy in an international context: risk, citizenship and welfare regimes. Editors P. Kennedy and N. Kodate (New York, NY: Routledge), 179–204.

Spina, E. (2012). An evaluation of the professional status of Italian midwives. *Evid. Base Midwifery.* 10, 88–93.

WHO (2018). *Nurturing care for early child development.* Geneva, Switzerland: World Health Organization.

Yuill, C. (2020). Reproductive rights in the time of COVID-19. Somatosphere. *Somatosphere*, 1–7. Available at: http://somatosphere.net/2020/reproductive-rights-in-the-time-of-covid-19.html/.

3

Born in Captivity: The Experiences of Puerto Rican Birth Workers and their Clients in Quarantine

Emaline Reyes *†

Department of Anthropology, Temple University, Philadelphia, PA, United States

***Correspondence:**
Emaline Reyes
emalinereyes@gmail.com

In this article, I seek to understand how the COVID-19 pandemic has impacted childbirth in Puerto Rico, an island that was already in recovery following the occurrence of two devastating hurricanes in the fall of 2017 and a major earthquake in the winter of 2020. Thus, I argue that it is important to discuss not only how individual disasters impact birth, but also how their compounding effects do so. In order to address these research questions, I conducted remote interviews with Puerto Rican birth workers and researchers. During times of crisis, this pandemic included, home and midwife-attended births have become increasingly more popular. However, Puerto Rican midwives and doulas currently have less institutional support than ever. In a time of quarantine when home births are rising, we need to consider whether society is designed to facilitate these models of care. In Puerto Rico, pre-pandemic, there was a less than 1% home birth rate and there still is a lack of legal recognition and protections for homebirth midwives. As this article demonstrates, an acknowledgment of the near-invisible labors of these birth workers is needed, in addition to supplies, support, and protections for them—and not just in times of "crisis."

Keywords: COVID-19, Home birth, midwifery model, reproductive justice, obstetric violence

INTRODUCTION: DISASTERS AND DELIVERIES

From Ebola to Zika, a primary concern in recent epidemics has been how infectious disease impacts pregnant women and infants. The COVID-19 crisis is no different, with headlines across the nation reporting on women who have decided to labor in their homes (Freytas-Tamura, 2020) or on doulas who were barred from entering hospitals (Meyerson, 2020)—in addition to the more biologically-focused questions of how COVID impacts the pregnant body and infant development. Puerto Rico, a US territory with a legacy of colonial control and exploitation, is in a particularly vulnerable position when it comes to COVID and maternal wellbeing, as its citizens have historically struggled with reproductive justice and access to adequate healthcare (Briggs, 2002; Lopez, 2008; Córdova, 2017). Most recently, before COVID, Puerto Rico was in the process of recovering from the 2017 Hurricanes Irma and Maria and the 2020 earthquakes. These left the population in a precarious position in regard to their economy and infrastructure and have certainly complicated their COVID responses (from what I have observed). What we see in Puerto Rico are incomplete recovery and the compounding effects of multiple and ongoing disasters. I have found that the impacts of COVID on childbirth in Puerto Rico are similar to the impacts seen in those prior disasters, and that the responses to these events have been strikingly similar as well. Furthermore, I argue that these patterns seen in disaster response and experience in Puerto Rico reflect the patterns observed in other disasters in other countries (Wick and Hassan, 2012; Ivry et al., 2019; Saulnier et al., 2020; Davis,

2021), now including COVID. In what follows, I will discuss how these disasters, and in particular COVID, have been lived, experienced, and managed—paying special attention to how COVID-19 has impacted childbirth in Puerto Rico, as well as maternal care systems and the labors of local birth workers who are often on the frontlines of disaster care.

BACKGROUND

When Hurricanes Irma and Maria hit Puerto Rico in 2017, many laboring women were unable to get in touch with their primary providers or to get to the hospital (Stein, 2017). During this time, midwives were on the frontlines, leading disaster response and relief both in maternity and community care (Dieppa, 2018), as midwives in other countries have also frequently done[1]. Midwives and home births in Puerto Rico were being covered by the mainstream media in ways previously unseen, creating more awareness of the work that homebirth midwives do and the diverse birth options available (to some) (Liautaud et al., 2017). Independent midwives were assisting in more home deliveries than ever before. There are only about two dozen practicing independent midwives in Puerto Rico, all of whom are certified professional midwives (CPMs), who are not allowed to practice in hospitals, and the pre-COVID homebirth rate in Puerto Rico was <1%; it remains to be seen how much that rate has risen during the pandemic[2]. Less than 2.5 years after Hurricanes Irma and Maria, when extreme earthquakes rocked the southern region of the island, these independent midwives were once again first responders. Though they are adamant that no births occurred in the "tent cities" (due to safety concerns), they did provide prenatal and postnatal care for the women of the community—many of whom were still having difficulty recovering from the earthquakes[3], both emotionally and physically. During COVID, we once again observe an increased reliance on midwives and a shift of births from the hospital to the home, due in large part to fears of infection, similar to the fear of leaving the home witnessed at the height of the Zika epidemic (Rodriguez, 2017). But we also must acknowledge the complications in this shift, for both midwives and their clients, as I will later discuss.

METHODS

In order to understand how COVID impacted birth in Puerto Rico, and how this differed from or was similar to previous disasters, I conducted remote interviews with 11 Puerto Rican women working in the fields of reproductive health and justice, including: 5 midwives, a doula, a clinical psychologist working in a Neonatal Intensive Care Unit (NICU), a social worker focused on combating gender violence, a child birth photo journalist, a midwifery student, and a fellow researcher. As midwives, doulas, and their allies are often found on the frontlines of disasters, working directly with laboring people, they are most knowledgeable about how these adverse events impact birth. I conducted these interviews via Zoom and on the phone, primarily in English (a second language for the birth workers) with some Spanish spoken intermittently. Individual interviews were conducted multiple times to track how the pandemic and responses to it changed over the April to August 2020 timespan. During this time, I closely monitored the media on birth experiences in quarantine and continued to review the literature on maternal services in times of disaster.

This project was granted exemption status from the Temple University Institutional Review Board because it consists entirely of interviews that are more in the tradition of journalism or oral history (and thus do are not subject to IRB oversight), and because there are adequate provisions in place to protect the privacy of any respondents who wish to remain anonymous. Verbal consent was obtained.

FINDINGS: BIRTH LOCATION, POWER DYNAMICS, SOCIAL REALITIES, AND PAST, PRESENT AND FUTURE ISSUES AROUND COVID-19, MIDWIVES, AND BIRTH

Interview results were mixed, with some stories of difficulty and despair and some messages of hope and resilience. I will describe and analyze these findings in terms of four emergent themes: birth location; vulnerability and isolation; advantages and disadvantages of telehealth; and midwives' reaction to obstetrician's increased domain protection. The information presented below comes directly from the accounts of my interlocutors (unless otherwise cited).

Locating Birth

Regarding birth location, my midwife interlocutors informed me that home births have become more popular and by extension, their services have been in high demand. However, they note that these services are still not accessible to everyone. This is especially true for those of a lower socioeconomic status—whether they want to or not, often they have no choice but to deliver at no cost in the public hospitals, where COVID cases are worst. The exceptions are those who are able to access free or reduced-cost midwifery and doula services, which some of my interlocutors offer. This issue of access is due to both the lack of insurance coverage of midwives and home birth and to the lack of stable housing and necessary resources such as clean water, clean surfaces, and supplies. Many people lost their homes during the hurricanes and the earthquakes; home birth is impossible for those who are home-*less*, and hospital and clinic births are the default. Even for those who have homes, blue tarp "roofs" are not

[1]See Davis-Floyd (2021) for descriptions of "low-tech, skilled touch" midwifery disaster care following the 2004 Aceh tsunami, the 2013 Hurricane Haiyan in the Philippines, and the Great Japanese Earthquake of 3/11/11.

[2]It is worth noting that in recent years the home birth rate has risen to closer to 2% in the United States as a whole.

[3]See Ivry et al. (2019) for a discussion of childbirth experiences *during* an earthquake (in Japan).

uncommon following Maria, and the additional economic constraints put in place by COVID have made it difficult to access necessary supplies and safe, secure, sanitary spaces.

For those who *are* able to give birth within the home, home births and midwifery services have been significantly altered by the virus, as my interlocutors have explained. Midwives must wear gowns, face masks and face shields, and of course gloves. If they are visiting homes for prenatal or postnatal check-ups in person, they must practice social distancing, wash their hands persistently, and keep hand sanitizer with them at all times. Some are simply using telehealth for these appointments (leading up to and following delivery). During labor and birth, all midwife care must obviously be administered in person, cautiously. Similar to the in-person appointments, social distancing guidelines are followed, and protective gear is worn. Midwives keep their distance as much as they can, relying heavily on the family to offer physical support to the laboring woman. They have to be close when the baby comes, so that they can catch and attend to it, but some say that they have heard stories of women being taught to catch their own babies while under the supervision of trained midwives. The company of healthy family members and doulas is encouraged, but smaller group sizes are preferred. This differs drastically from pre-COVID home births in which family, friends, and neighbors alike were all encouraged to attend, and midwives provided hands-on care throughout.

Additionally, for the protection of midwives, their clients, and the community, the screening process is much more intense—including inquiring about COVID symptoms and contact with infected individuals. Many midwives had to wait for their own test results before they could serve their clients. I was not told whether or not these midwives required that their clients get tested, but one midwife informed me that the midwives have great difficulties in accessing rapid COVID tests. Other articles in this Special Issue echo the accounts of my interlocutors.

While home birth may be challenging amid COVID, for those who give birth within the hospital, labor can be even more challenging. My interlocutors have reported that, unfortunately, during this time, cases of obstetric violence have increased. The isolation of birthing women has most likely contributed to this problem. Doulas are being banned in most hospitals on the island (with the exception of one hospital, identified by a doula I spoke with) along with other support persons. The lack of company, advocacy, and thus provider accountability has left many women vulnerable to the abusive practices of hospital personnel. Yet part of the poor treatment and care that women are receiving in hospitals is due to negligence rather than direct abuse. Hospitals are overburdened by COVID and were already dealing with a shortage of personnel as a result of the mass exodus that followed Hurricane Maria. One midwife told me about a client of hers who was transferred to the hospital, only to have her baby die there:

One of my clients called me in May and said she hadn't felt the baby move. I went to check up on her and could hear movement but could also tell that something was wrong. So I took my client to the hospital and called and told them about what was going on and how this woman needed a nurse to check her vitals and physically examine her...the thing is they (the hospitals) aren't hiring nurses and other personnel like they should be. So, I spoke with a nurse and said, "I'm sending my client and you need to do these things" and she (my client) showed up at the hospital and they didn't do anything.

Guess what? There was one nurse on that floor. In the end the baby died in the hospital, she had a stillbirth. They (the hospitals) need more people, things would have been different if there was a nurse who could have attended to my client. It probably would have been a C-section, but that baby would be alive today. There are less and less people in the hospitals. This has been such an issue and continues to be one. And the people who are there are giving worse care too. They are overextended because so many left—the mass exodus after Maria. You can feel that.

While this midwife wished to remain anonymous in regard to this specific account (for fear of retaliation from the clinical community--a conflict resulting from the power struggle between midwives and clinicians that will be discussed below), she was determined that I share it, noting how crucial it is for people to hear about these preventable tragedies. I was told that, shockingly, some maternal deaths may have been attributed to COVID with insufficient evidence. Midwives fear that the virus is being used to cover up malpractice and justify any maternal deaths for which the hospital does not want to be held liable. COVID has also given practitioners justifications for many unnecessary and excessive practices; when negligence is not the issue, increased intervention is. Most notably, the performance of more inductions and cesareans is being reported, with the justification that these move women more quickly through the system, thereby limiting potential viral exposure (Davis-Floyd, 2021; Davis-Floyd et al., 2020). Mothers and infants are often separated following cesarean birth, and even when delivered vaginally in hospitals, many mothers and infants are being separated post-birth due to fear of COVID transmission, though *in the absence of a positive test result or evidence that demonstrates mother-infant viral transfer.* Immediate skin-to-skin contact is thus often disallowed, making breastfeeding initiation difficult, both of which can seriously impact maternal-infant health and relationships, as well as postpartum recovery, and can force use of expensive formula often unavailable to the poor, or can result in cheap powdered formula being mixed with contaminated water—a potentially deadly situation for infants.

When I discussed this issue with a clinical psychologist, she was adamant that the harm of initial separation is not irreparable—you can still bond and breastfeed once you are finally reunited with your infant. She reminded me that this resilience perspective is crucial for survival, something she learned working in the NICU:

I do believe in immediate breastfeeding initiation and skin-to-skin contact and bonding, but I think that we need to be very careful to communicate to mothers that they can still connect and still breastfeed even after separation. They do not "miss" that one opportunity, they can make the best of the situation from there...I guess I have this perspective from working in the NICU, because (compared to these most recent COVID separations) we *always* have to separate the mothers and infants and yet we still try to encourage these practices (breastfeeding, skin-to-skin) in the long run. Even if a baby has been in the NICU for 7 months they can develop a close relationship with their parents and can still be successful in breastfeeding after they finally get to go home...this is difficult for people to comprehend if they haven't seen it. But we've seen it, and we know.

While birth location can certainly impact experiences and outcomes, it is important to remember that these beneficial practices can be utilized and encouraged at various stages and in many places.

Cultural and "Covidian" Concerns for Homebirth Midwives and Their Clients: Vulnerability and Isolation

Puerto Rican midwives have worked tirelessly to gain respect and recognition. In addition to navigating a pandemic, they must also dispel myths that midwives are "dirty," unsanitary, uneducated, and ill-equipped." They face stereotypes that date back centuries in Latin America and the Caribbean and are often associated with the race and ethnicity of the midwife, especially African ancestry and Indigeneity. Even as their work becomes more visible, local birth workers such as midwives and doulas are not recognized as healthcare professionals; therefore, they have not been given the same support (financial and political), supplies, and PPE as other healthcare workers. This has left them in a very vulnerable place, given that their services are in demand now more than ever. And it is also a dangerous time for them to be working and coming into contact with so many different people (their patients, their patients' families). Midwives worry about contracting COVID, both for themselves and for the safety of their own families. They talk about having to take everything off before entering the home, having to shower thoroughly and wash laundry multiple times, being cautious around their own children. Many worry that midwives will contract COVID at higher rates than any other essential workers. One midwife I spoke with, Tamara, wondered how many COVID cases we would see among midwives in the coming months:

Even if the Puerto Rican government doesn't want to acknowledge that we're health providers, we *are*. Midwives are acknowledged in other parts of the world, but they're not *seen* here. Because we aren't classified as healthcare providers, disaster funding goes to doctors but not to us. We are working for free and risking ourselves...We are having a lot of difficulty accessing COVID rapid tests. . .Because we don't have access, we are exposing ourselves going into the houses of these women who need our help. Other healthcare providers are given the tests and essential supplies but we have only gotten them through donations (we have had to buy supplies as well)...I think in September or October we could look back, gather our statistics, and say "our midwives got sick even when they used protection" because no one supported us. Right now, we're dealing with something that affects us all and it's pretty darn scary.

This constant stress and anxiety can take a serious toll on the mental health of community birth workers, as can the physical distance from their patients and the separation/disconnection that they feel due to protective measures such as masks and face guards. A number of midwives told me that one of the most difficult things about COVID has been not being able to embrace the baby after it is born. It saddens them that they cannot hold it, hug it, smell it, place a kiss on its forehead. There is sadness for both the mothers and the midwives in these home births.

COVID can be an incredibly lonely and isolating time, not only for midwives, but also for those who are about to or who have just given birth. One interlocutor told me that in Puerto Rico, pregnant women and new mothers are more than anyone else are self-isolating; they are worried for themselves, their babies, and their families. This isolation and constant worry can be detrimental to the mental health of both pregnant women and new mothers. What used to be a celebration is now a time of grave concern. They are lacking support in so many ways. They cannot have their older relatives (parents, grandparents) present for the birth; they must be careful of how many people they allow to attend the delivery or visit afterward, and they even have to be cautious around their own birth workers. One midwife, Gina, told me that one of her clients rejected postpartum care because she was so fearful of having anyone (other than herself and her immediate family) come into contact with her newborn baby:

Pregnant families are taking care of themselves the most. They are the ones quarantining in the house. I had a client who canceled her appointment with me 6 weeks away because she was worried about COVID. I had worked with her leading up to her birth, which ended up being a c-section, but even after a c-**section 1** do the postpartum care. She declined these last visits because she wanted to protect the baby. She wasn't letting anyone visit, even me as a midwife. But I respected her wishes and said "Okay. I hope you are both safe and healthy."

In this general environment of fear and uncertainty, mothers are anxious about bringing children into this world and about allowing them to interact with others. This stress surely impacts the birth experience itself. Many mothers in Puerto Rico and elsewhere are dealing with postpartum depression, which is not uncommon following a trauma or disaster, but has been compounded by the crushing loneliness and despair of COVID. And quality of care can be seriously compromised—especially in the hospitals; some women are coming out of their pandemic hospital births more traumatized than ever due to the obstetric violence—and/or the neglect--they experience there.

Telehealth: Advantages and Disadvantages

Over time, as the virus has been better understood and managed in some regions, families have begun to feel slightly less anxious. As government restrictions on the island have begun to relax, so too have citizens. Accordingly, some women may begin to feel less fearful, which could significantly reduce the stress that has been present in their deliveries. Most hospitals have started letting support persons into the delivery room (at the least a family member/partner), with the exception of one hospital (identified by my hospital doula contact) that continues to ban any support persons.

The telehealth journey has been particularly interesting, with arguments for both its advantages and disadvantages. For medical professionals, the implementation and use of telehealth could be seen as shifting power differentials. Patients are now in the position where they are the ones taking their own vitals, monitoring their own pregnancies, and guiding their own (virtual) appointments, leading up to and in preparation[4] for birth. This is a level of patient agency and autonomy previously unseen in Puerto Rican maternity care, and in most of Western medicine as well. In this way, telehealth could be considered empowering for patients. One midwife, Yariana told me:

With telehealth and remote appointments there is a lot of emphasis on self-care and being aware of your health-it is empowering for women. Parents use to be taught how to take their blood pressure and things like that, but now they are learning about fetal heart monitoring and measuring their own belly. Telehealth, telemedicine teaches them (parents) those things. Being very hands on with health can change a lot in you and make you very conscious.

This account was echoed by the researcher I spoke with, and these initial interactions had me under the impression that telehealth could be a positive experience within the clinical context; however, some midwives worry that telehealth may actually be abused by medical professionals. They are concerned that doctors are exploiting this new system in order to "not do their job and still get paid," and that now that doctors realize this is an option and something they could have been doing all along, they will continue to find reasons to do it more and more. This was the sentiment of one midwife I spoke with, Zulgeil:

I don't like to use telehealth; I think it is pretty dangerous actually. I worry that it's being abused by a lot of the doctors who are using it. Because they think, "oh, I don't even have to touch someone, and I can still make money from my home?" It's negligent really. I will do my initial interview through telehealth, but I will not recruit clients online, and then after that I will go in person and wear a mask and screen the clients and discuss ethics and protocols. But these doctors, they were doing 5-min appointments anyway, even before COVID! Now it's like nothing. I mean I know some midwives are doing it, especially birth centers, and it's a choice, but I'm just not comfortable with that. I'm following protocols in person, and anything I can do additionally online, I will. I just worry that now that telehealth is an option, it is just going to continue to be abused.

This is a legitimate concern that Zulgiel spoke to, and while telehealth is primarily used for prenatal and postnatal check-ups (with the exception of its use by doulas and other support persons in labor-a practice intended to circumvent restrictive hospital policies, or even to ensure proper social distancing in home births), limited attention in birth and lack of continuity of care can be real issues in the hospital, just as brief, condensed appointments are.

For midwives, telehealth has had little impact on the power differentials between practitioners and patients, as midwives already prided themselves on embracing a model of care that treated mothers as equals. Even before COVID, midwives were conscientious in supporting mothers to be active agents in their own pregnancies and births, constantly educating and involving them in decision-making. This client involvement is still there; however, some midwives argue that COVID, social distancing, and telehealth have impacted crucial patient-practitioner interactions in more negative ways. The midwifery model of care is based on humanistic and holistic care that relies heavily on physical, social, emotional, mental, and spiritual support (see Davis-Floyd 2018a for a full description of this model). Midwives argue that with telehealth and social distancing, this presence is missing, and, equally as important, so are their keen, trained eyes and informed touch. While the midwives I spoke with acknowledge the competence and intelligence of their patients, trusting them to take charge of their own care, they argue that this is their job, this is what they are "paid for"[5], this is the kind of care they are supposed to offer (and what separates them from medicalized practitioners). They are adamant that they simply need to be there, to be able to offer hands-on support. The lack of their physical presence and ability to connect as human beings is detrimental both to these midwives and to their clients and could potentially negatively shape birth experiences.

The Home/Hospital and Midwife/Obstetrician Divide: Obstetrician's Increased Domain Protection and Midwives' Responses

The pandemic has impacted the medical culture in Puerto Rico, emboldening doctors to "protect" their "domain," which appears to be threatened by the growing preference for midwives. While some few humanistic obstetricians (one midwife approximated that their number was somewhere close to 4 out of 84) are being supportive of community birth workers during this time, especially doulas (whom they see as allies)[6], overall, COVID has only served to further the divide between midwives and medical professionals. I have been told that this conflict existed before, but is exacerbated in times of crisis, including during COVID. From the very beginning of the pandemic, OBs have seen how preference for midwife-attended home births has increased and have responded by launching a campaign against home deliveries and the midwives performing them. In an extreme overreaction on an island with only 24 homebirth midwives and a pre-pandemic homebirth rate of 1%, medical professionals have taken to social media, recording videos through Facebook Live, and have gone on the news to argue that the absolute safest place to give birth is the hospital. They claim that this is especially true given the current pandemic, which they believe has made birth even *more* risky and

[4]This preparation could potentially impact psychological and physiological birth preparedness.

[5]Though, as previously discussed, during the pandemic some of my interlocutors are offering services for free or at reduced cost, and when responding to disasters such as the hurricanes and the earthquakes, they must volunteer and rely on donations.

[6]Doulas (unlike independent midwives) can attend hospital births in Puerto Rico, do not serve as competition for "catching the baby," and provide emotional and social support to patients that clinicians most often do not have the time for. In this way doulas may assist in their work without truly threatening it.

pathological (more of a disease, more worthy of being medicalized). The midwifery student whom I spoke with explained to me that:

Parents are being guilted if they choose home birth. Doctors tell them that this is dangerous, negligent, abusive. They say it is the start of bad parenting and a bad childhood...many of these arguments are not evidence-based, they are fear-based. This is not, and should not be, a moral issue. This pressure was already there, but COVID is just a way in which they (the doctors) are reinforcing their message, which they already felt justified in promoting. Some people are emboldened during the time of the virus though

Some midwives worry that the precautions taken during COVID are leading the way to midwifery becoming "too clinical."[7] What makes homebirth midwifery so special and unique, they argue, is that it is based on humanity and spirituality in a way that sets it apart from the clinical, technocratic model (Gaskin, 2002; Davis-Floyd, 2018a; Davis-Floyd and Davis, 2018). Midwives distinguish between those who choose home birth because they truly want "natural" births and those who are just afraid of hospital contagion; they are unsure whether the increased preference for home birth and doula-attended births[8] that they are currently seeing will persist, or whether this increase is a temporary result of the pandemic. Issues of accessibility also may determine whether or not higher rates of midwife-attended home births will continue over time, and many in Puerto Rico also want freestanding birth centers, yet so far none have emerged.

Most midwives want to be able to work alongside the local institutions, rather than against them, and they do want institutional recognition, but they also realize that such recognition may risk the values and standards they have set for themselves as community birth workers. Gaining the approval of the government will mean that they will essentially have to unionize, offer standardized care, all be on exactly the same page, and be governed by a set of laws/principles and protocols imposed by technocratic medicine[9].

Additionally, it would be difficult for midwives to work with an institution that does not want to work with them. The divide between medicine and midwifery existed pre-COVID but is more exaggerated now and characterized by vitriol and intolerance. The midwives call their increased persecution by the Puerto Rican obstetric community "a witch hunt," "a fear campaign," and "a crusade against midwives." The birth workers I spoke with agreed overall that more than anything, COVID has been making matters of reproductive health and justice more polarized. The virus is also making more evident the extreme structural inequalities between the wealthy and the poor that already existed but are more visible now, and more severe due to the fragile state of the economy during the pandemic.

As COVID has been making matters of inequality and injustice more visible—including the divide between midwives and the medical community and the economic disparities among clients--this visibility is integral to structural reform and change. For example, doula's rights were temporarily restricted at the beginning of the pandemic, making many feel that the island's maternity care system had "regressed," "lost progress," and "gone backwards" in a number of ways. They also worried that these changes would be difficult to reverse (and that the journey back would be just as long as the journey there had been). However, doulas, mothers, and allies alike rallied to have support persons recognized and protected, and they eventually were allowed to return back to the labor and delivery wards (as noted above)[10]. With disaster, there is inevitably destruction, but also a chance to rebuild. While there are still a number of barriers to overcome, midwives are glad that people are at least more aware of these options now and hope that families may embrace and fight for these alternatives in the future.

DISCUSSION: THE IMPACTS OF DISASTERS

In Puerto Rico, the impacts that COVID has had on birth have been very similar to the impacts of previous disasters—the hurricanes and earthquakes. During all of these events, midwives have been and continue to be primary disaster responders; home births have increased (either through choice or necessity—as is the case when people are physically unable to leave their homes); and pregnant people (and the general public) continue to become more aware of this alternative option. This growing awareness is due in large part to the Puerto Rican media coverage of midwifery care and home birth during disasters, which has continued to increase over these past three years (see **section 2**). Yet the sensationalization of infectious disease in the media has also instilled fear in soon-to-be, laboring, and new mothers that has prompted them to self-quarantine and made them hesitant to leave their homes. We are seeing this now with COVID, but we also saw this happen with Zika for a long time in Puerto Rico, especially around the time of Hurricane Maria when there were issues with flooding and standing water (National Institute of Health, 2017). These fears of infectious diseases (Zika, COVID) may not only prompt women to prefer home birth, they may actually lead to extreme isolation and restricted mobility outside of the home. The "turf war" between medical professionals and midwives, seen as well during the hurricanes and the earthquakes, persists and seems to intensify with each disaster as pregnant Puerto Rican women increasingly embrace the midwifery model of care.

[7]See Davis-Floyd and Johnson (2006) for a recounting of these same struggles in the mainland United States.

[8]While doulas have been restricted during COVID from accessing clinical spaces, the emotional/social support that they provide in labor is still invaluable. Fearing having to choose between a partner or doula as the "one sole support person" (in the hospital) was a driving force behind the increase in preference for home birth—a space where doulas continue to be welcome.

[9]See Hays and Prepas (2015) for a discussion of the institutionalization and standardization of midwives in disaster response.

[10]See Yakovi Gan-Or (2020) for a discussion of the legislation surrounding birth assistants in the states (and globally) during the pandemic.

So many of these impacts observed in Puerto Rico can also be witnessed in disaster responses worldwide. Globally, and historically, we see that midwives are often the first to respond in the immediate aftermath of disasters, as they are trained in "low-tech/skilled touch" (Davis-Floyd, 2021) methods and can make do with the most basic supplies. We have also seen destruction to hospitals and absence of medical professionals during these events, furthering the need for local birth workers' assistance (ibid.). Among these events is our current COVID pandemic, which has had similar impacts and responses worldwide. In Puerto Rico, the US, and a number of nations, there has been an increase in demand for midwives, home births have become more popular and preferable as fear of COVID makes women wary of hospitals, and frustration over restrictions on support persons prompt women to abandon the medical model altogether (Davis-Floyd, 2021; Davis-Floyd et al., 2020). However, this rapid surge also causes a shortage of community birth workers, as many of the areas in which home births and midwifery are in high demand do not support and encourage midwifery nor facilitate home births. While the new-found appreciation for midwifery is certainly encouraging, serious changes need to be implemented if midwifery care and home births are to be truly accessible to all, and widely available during times of disaster, when their "low-tech, skilled touch" care is needed most. In order to facilitate this midwife disaster response, Wick and Hassan (2012) suggest "Planning for emergency care by mapping the location of midwives, supplying them with basic equipment and medications, and legitimizing their profession with an appropriate scope of practice, licensing, back-up, and incentives . . . "

CONCLUSION: QUESTIONS AND CONSIDERATIONS

As I demonstrate in this article, COVID, among other disasters, has shifted a great deal of childbirth to the care of Puerto Rican community birth workers such as doulas and midwives. As the other articles in this special issue show, this is a pattern observed worldwide as well, and one that inspires hope for a future that embraces humanistic birth practices that incorporate necessary technologies (Davis-Floyd, 2018b; Davis-Floyd, 2021). However, this transition to home birth (in societies that do not facilitate it and are not designed for it) is not without its complications for both midwives and birthing women. In these uncertain times, there is still so much we are unsure of and so many questions that have yet to be answered. We will not know until we are truly on the other side of this pandemic, and have had the time to conduct more research, just how much it has impacted us and the women and children of our communities.

Moving forward, we will need to consider: How high did the home birth rate go during the pandemic? The induction and cesarean rates? What can be done about birth workers' increased risk of contracting COVID? What are the impacts? Will the transition to home birth and midwifery be sustainable (with regard to government support, policy changes, and increased accessibility)? Will midwifery be altered by the pandemic, made more official and therefore more clinical? Will problematic hospital practices persist? And of course, the people of Puerto Rico are constantly asking "What about the next catastrophe?" As I write, they have been coping with more earthquakes, weathering severe storms, and are preparing for a hurricane season that they know will be complicated by this ongoing pandemic. It is already being hypothesized that COVID will make hurricane response more difficult, due to a declining economy, compromised infrastructure, and fear of spreading disease (Canales, 2020).

And, unfortunately, the people of Puerto Rico are not alone in asking the question, "What next?" Worldwide in this Anthropocene Era, we are seeing disasters, including epidemics and pandemics, increase as a result of human-driven climate change (Wallace-Wells, 2020; Davis-Floyd, 2021). Whether we are prepared or not, these events will continue to arrive, sometimes overlapping with one another. This is why it is so crucial that we study how disasters impact human health, including reproductive health. In understanding what impacts past disasters have had, and how they have been successfully managed (or mis-managed), we can better prepare for the future and hopefully ensure the health and wellbeing of mothers, babies, and birth workers everywhere.

ETHICS STATEMENT

Ethical review and approval was not required for the study on human participants in accordance with the local legislation and institutional requirements. Written informed consent for participation was not required for this study in accordance with the national legislation and the institutional requirements. Written informed consent was not obtained from the individual(s) for the publication of any potentially identifiable images or data included in this article.

AUTHOR CONTRIBUTIONS

ER conducted remote interviews, reviewed the literature on the affects of COVID-19 on pregnancy and birth, and wrote the article manuscript.

REFERENCES

Briggs, L. (2002). *Reproducing empire: race, sex, science, and US imperialism in Puerto Rico*. Berkely, SC: Univ. of California Press, 337.

Córdova, I. M. (2017). *Pushing in silence: modernizing Puerto Rico and the medicalization of childbirth*. Texa, US: University of Texas Press, 249.

Canales, J. (2020). Puerto Rico leaders prepare for hurricane season amid coronavirus crisis. Available at: https://www.baynews9.com/fl/tampa/sports-news/2020/06/09/puerto-rico-preps-for-hurricane-season-coronavirus (Accessed June 30, 2020).

Davis, F. (2021). "Effective maternity disaster care: low tech, skilled touch," in *Sustainable birth in disruptive times*. Editors K. Gutschow, R. Davis-Floyd, and B. A. Daviss (New York, US: Springer Nature), 271.

Davis Floyd, R., and Johson, C. B. (2006). *Mainstreaming midwives: the politics of change*. New Brunswick NJ: Rutgers University Press, 572.

R. Davis-Floyd (Editor) (2021). *Birthing techno-sapiens: human-technology Co-evolution and the future of reproduction*. London, England: Routledge, in press.

Davis-Floyd, R., and Davis, E. (2018). "Intuition as authoritative knowledge in midwifery and home birth," in *Ways of Knowing about birth: mothers, midwives, medicine, and birth activism by robbie davis-floyd*. Editor R. Davis-Floyd (Long Grove IL: Waveland Press), 189–220.

Davis-Floyd, R., Gutschow, K., and Schwartz, D. A. (2020). Pregnancy, birth and the COVID-19 pandemic in the United States. *Med. Anthropol.* 39 (5), 413–427. doi:10.1080/01459740.2020.1761804

Davis-Floyd, R. (2018a). "The midwifery model of care: anthropological perspectives," in *Ways of Knowing about birth: mothers, midwives, medicine, and birth activism by robbie davis-floyd*. Editor R. Davis-Floyd (Long Grove IL: Waveland Press), 165–188.

Davis-Floyd, R. (2018b). "The technocratic, humanistic, and holistic paradigms of birth and health care," in *Ways of Knowing about birth: mothers, midwives, medicine, and birth activism by robbie davis-floyd*. Editor R. Davis-Floyd (Long Grove IL: Waveland Press), 3–44.

Dieppa, I. S. (2018). Midwives & doulas were critical healthcare providers after hurricane Maria - and are still filling A gap today. Available at: https://www.bustle.com/p/midwives-doulas-were-critical-healthcare-providers-after-hurricane-maria-are-still-filling-a-gap-today-11768875 (Accessed June 15, 2020).

Freytas-Tamura, K. D. (2020). Pregnant and scared of 'covid hospitals,' they're giving birth at home. Available at: https://www.nytimes.com/2020/04/21/nyregion/coronavirus-home-births.html (Accessed June 14, 2020)

Gaskin, I. M. (2002). *Spiritual midwifery*. 4th Edn. Summertown TN: The Book Publishing Company.

Hays, K. E., and Prepas, R. (2015). The professionalization of international disaster response: it is time for midwives to get ready. *J. Midwifery Womens Health* 60 (4), 348–359. doi:10.1111/jmwh.12339

Ivry, T., Takaki-Einy, R., and Murotsuki, J. (2019). What disasters can reveal about techno-medical birth: Japanese women's stories of childbirth during the 11 March, 2011 earthquake. *Health Risk Soc.* 21 (3-4), 164–184. doi:10.1080/13698575.2019.1643827

Liautaud, A., Giraldo, C., and Paoli, T. (2017). Delivering babies–and saving lives–in Puerto Rico after Maria. Available at: https://news.vice.com/en_us/article/j5dd74/delivering-babies-and-saving-lives-in-puerto-rico-after-maria (Accessed June 17, 2020).

López, I. O. (2008). *Matters of choice: Puerto Rican women's struggle for reproductive freedom*. New Brunswick NJ: Rutgers University Press.

Meyerson, C. (2020). Doulas are going virtual. Available at: https://nymag.com/intelligencer/2020/04/doulas-are-laboring-under-coronavirus-restrictions.html (Accessed June 30, 2020).

National Institute of Health (2017). Spotlight: Zika research after hurricane Maria. Available at: https://www.nichd.nih.gov/news/resources/spotlight/112017-zika (Accessed June 23, 2020).

Rodriguez, C (2017). Puerto Rico, the joy of pregnancy is tempered by fear of Zika. Available at: https://khn.org/news/in-puerto-rico-the-joy-of-pregnancy-is-tempered-by-fear-of-zika/ (Accessed June 30, 2020).

Saulnier, D. D., Hean, H., Thol, D., Ir, P., Hanson, C., Von Schreeb, J., and Alvesson, H. M. (2020). Staying afloat: community perspectives on health system resilience in the management of pregnancy and childbirth care during floods in Cambodia. *BMJ. Glob. Health.* 5 (4), e002272. doi:10.1136/bmjgh-2019-002272

Stein, M. (2017). Pregnant women in Puerto Rico are stranded without OB-GYNs - here's how you can help. Available at: https://www.romper.com/p/puerto-ricos-maternity-care-is-in-jeopardy-following-hurricane-maria-its-heartbreaking-5507323 (Accessed June 15, 2020).

Wallace-Wells, D. (2020). *The uninhabitable earth: life after warming*. New York, NY: Tim Duggan Books, 320.

Wick, L., and Hassan, S. (2012). No safe place for childbirth: women and midwives bearing witness, Gaza 2008-09. *Reprod. Health Matters* 20 (40), 7–15. doi:10.1016/S0968-8080(12)40648-6

Yakovi Gan-Or, N. (2020). Going solo: the law and ethics of childbirth during the COVID-19 pandemic. *J. L. Biosci.* 7 (1). doi:10.1093/jlb/lsaa079

4

On the Outside Looking In: A Global Doula Response to COVID-19

Julie Johnson Searcy[1]* *and Angela N. Castañeda*[2]

[1]Department of History and Anthropology, Butler University, Indianapolis, IN, United States, [2]Department of Sociology and Anthropology, DePauw University, Greencastle, IN, United States

***Correspondence:**
Julie Johnson Searcy
jsearcy@butler.edu

From around the world, doulas report the impact of new COVID-19 restrictions on their ability to provide continuous emotional, physical, and informational support to pregnant people and their families. In a qualitative survey conducted in March and April 2020, we heard from over 500 doulas in 24 countries. Doulas practicing across the world revealed rapid changes to hospital policies. Even accounting for different public health responses across countries, the doulas in our study pointed to one common theme - their absence at births and the subsequent need to support birthing people virtually. In a follow-up survey and in interviews we conducted in July, we reconnected with doulas from our initial study to track their access to institutional birthing spaces. As countries experienced the effects of "flattening the curve," we found that doulas were still not considered "essential" workers and the majority could not attend births. Our research shows that doulas have ambiguous feelings about the efficacy of virtual support, that they raise concerns about the long-term impact of COVID on their profession and that they are concerned about mistreatment and obstetric violence as birthing people enter hospitals alone.

Keywords: doulas, birth, COVID-19, reproduction, pandemic

INTRODUCTION AND METHODOLOGY: A CHANGING BIRTH LANDSCAPE

Months into the global COVID-19 pandemic, communities across the globe continue to adapt to new rules and regulations surrounding birth culture. In particular, data gathered in the United States highlights how quickly policy changes have shifted for pregnant people, families and providers (Davis-Floyd et al., 2020). This includes the global community of birth workers known as doulas, who herein report the impact of new COVID-19 restrictions on their ability to provide continuous emotional, physical, and informational support to pregnant people and their families (Castañeda and Johnson Searcy., 2020).

This research focuses on the experiences of doulas drawn from a qualitative survey conducted in March and april of 2020, which collected over 500 responses from doulas in 23 countries. The survey included a mix of fixed-choice and open-ended questions, including asking doulas about the spaces they practiced in, if they worked in urban, rural or suburban areas, and an open-ended question about which area of the world they practiced in. The other open-ended questions in the survey asked doulas to reflect on and describe different aspects of their work in relation to COVID-19. The survey also included the option of indicating interest in a follow-up interview. We posted this survey on 24 doula Facebook groups, including general groups (Love What You Doula, Doula Talk); geographic-specific groups (i.e., Doulas of CA, Doula Connect - FL) and demographic specific groups (Doulas and Midwives of Color, Doula Latina, Queer Doula Network). We also conducted internet searches for doula organizations and collectives in countries outside of the US and sent emails explaining and attaching the survey and asking for the survey to be distributed to interested doulas.

We received response from 515 doulas. 373 of these responses came from doulas in the United States from 42 of the 50 states. The remaining survey responses came from 22 different countries (South Africa, Canada, New Zealand, Australia, Germany, Italy, Finland, Hungary, Portugal, Ireland, Sweden, Denmark, Japan, United Kingdom, Taiwan, Israel, Peru, India, Dubai, Mexico, Argentina, Bolivia). The responses we received from each of these countries varied from 80 to a handful, making it difficult to create a statistically significant comparative analysis. In addition, not all respondents indicated their geographic location. To analyze these qualitative responses, we separately coded each survey response, line by line, looking for themes and concepts and prioritizing the language doulas used to describe their work during this pandemic. We then compared and triangulated the themes for analysis. We conducted a follow-up qualitative survey and interviews in July 2020 to see how doulas saw the pandemic continuing to affect their ability to "mother the mother." Response to this survey was much smaller and included 52 doulas from the US, Canada, South Africa, Argentina, Spain, Japan and New Zealand. Of these respondents, 43 of the respondents had taken our first survey. We repeated the same coding process with this survey and then compared themes to the first survey. What became apparent while coding were the similar experiences, fears and challenges doulas described both in the early days of the pandemic and a few months further in. The follow-up survey confirmed and elaborated on themes that were present in the first survey. While we recognize the variation in context for many of the responding doulas and the limitations of the survey to capture all of the differences among regions of the world, we were struck by the commonality of the themes doulas described of disruption and rupture to the very nature of their work.

Doulas practicing across the world reported rapid changes in hospital policies with the onset of COVID-19. Despite the variation in public health strategies reported from different countries, the doulas in our studies were most concerned about their absence at births. The overwhelming and near-universal restrictions on doula support in hospitals, and even in some birth centers and at home births, spanned six continents and held across the time span between our two surveys—and aligned with a sharp increase in virtual doula-ing. Comparing each country lies outside the scope of this article; instead we focus here on the common themes and patterns doulas describe about the continuing impact of COVID-19 restrictions on these birth workers. We found that doulas raised concerns around three themes: 1) the efficacy (or lack thereof) of virtual care; 2) the impacts of pandemic restrictions on doulas as a profession coalescing around the politics of "*The essential*"; and 3) the concerns about increasing obstetric violence without a birth partner to bear witness. Our research asks us to consider how doulas' experiences around the globe can help us understand the power of a pandemic to influence birth culture.

NEW HOSPITAL RESTRICTIONS AND POLICY CHALLENGES: THE POLITICS OF "THE ESSENTIAL"

COVID-19 ushered in new hospital restrictions across the globe leading to new configurations about who counted as "essential" at a birth. In the context of labor and birth, essential workers became defined by changing hospital protocols, health provider preferences, and new stay-at-home orders from local and national governments (Castañeda and Johnson Searcy 2020). Doulas initially reported a dizzying flurry of shifting policies that ultimately kept most doulas out of the hospital. The majority of respondents commented on changes to hospital protocols, as with this doula from Germany:

> "Hospital policies are constantly changing as far as birth support. All hospitals have a maximum of one accompanying person. In some places, the partner must be from the same household (so doulas not allowed). Some allow this partner to be present for (the) entire labor (while) some just for the pushing phase. Most hospitals allow very limited postpartum accompaniment. Most hospitals are releasing newborn/mom as early as possible."

Doulas pointed out how erratic the policies were and that they differed among hospitals. A doula in Portugal described it this way, "Hospital policies are totally different. I cannot enter, and in some cases, women cannot have their phones with them. They have to go alone, so we can't even talk with the father." If any labor support was allowed, laboring people were often forced to choose only one person. A doula in the Ireland described this choice:

> "I have lost some clients who were interested in hiring a doula as they don't want to have to choose between their partner or doula for labor and also finances have been affected so maybe now paying for a doula is not affordable any longer."

Doulas watched as hospital policies asked birthing people to choose only one support person. Many doulas told us it wasn't a fair choice for families to make because they understood the importance of the partner being there. A South African doula explained this dilemma:

> "My Doula business has been declared a Non-Essential role in the Birth Team. The Hospital refused my assistance in the Labor Ward so I had to go back home. The Mother had to choose between me and her husband as if we play the same role at the Birth..Oh, she eventually had to undergo an "emergency" Caesarean operation."

In this example, the doula clearly points out how hospital policies do not fully take into account the difference *and* mutual relationship between a doula and partner. This neglects how both a doula and partner work together with a laboring person. Doulas draw on a partner's intimate knowledge of the laboring person and thus the partner becomes an integral source of help to the doula to best assist the laboring person.

Doulas have always faced questions about the economic worth of what they do. This pandemic has heightened that issue as people consider whether virtual doula work is worth the cost. Doulas have long had to work to convince people that a supportive witness at birth can shift outcomes (Kayne et al., 2001; Hunter 2012; Bohren et al., 2019). Doulas have come up against barriers in their work in clinical spaces and scholars have written about the liminal space they occupy (Kayne et al., 2001; Everson and Cheney, 2015). Some doulas argue that their presence is necessary because a biomedical model of birth does not attend to (or often acknowledge) people's emotional and physical needs during labor. Because a biomedical model sees birth from a narrow framework, doulas have long had to fight for their place at the side of birthing people. And it is only very recently (in the last 5 years) that we find widespread institutional acknowledgment of the importance of a birth partner (WHO). COVID-19 policies that keep doulas away from people in labor and necessitate virtual doula support make doulas afraid that they will be re-framed as unimportant—as they originally were—and that this will impact women in profound ways. Doulas moved online as pandemic policies required, but worried about the fallout for those giving birth. {moved from *Economic Instability* per the reviewer's recommendation}

From Policy to Personal Obstacles

Doulas faced challenges beyond entering hospitals. The ability to travel and attend to clients in their homes depended on whether a doula either self-identified as "essential" or had access to supportive documentation or support from a health worker. In South Africa, a doula shared, "I am armed with a copy of my ID and Permit when I go on the road to visit my postnatal and Antenatal clients at their homes." Another doula reported, "Officially no private or government hospitals allow doulas in South Africa any longer. Some doctors have given permission, and mothers with no birth partner may do so but the new doula restrictions are strongly enforced." Another issue was whether there was even local transportation available, as shared in this case from Peru:

> "My work is difficult now especially due to transit being restricted. I was just a doula at a birth two days ago in the local public hospital, and I had to return from there walking to my house! I had to have permission to travel since there is a curfew from 6pm every day."

Doulas often managed to work around these challenges. They talked about which training organizations could certify them, with as little money and time as possible, in order to procure certification that would allow them in the hospitals. Some had influential clients helping them secure permission to travel. And despite being shut out from hospital births, doulas still found ways to continue their care, for example in the form of "care-box drop offs with herbs and ingredients for Ayurvedic recovery recipes" (South Africa).

Even as doulas pivoted to adjust to the ways in which the pandemic was changing the conditions of their work, they also expressed concern for their clients and for their own personal challenges that working as a doula now entailed. One doula in Canada told us, "I am navigating my relationship with my profession in a fundamentally different way. This is leading to both fulfillment and compassion fatigue. Birth work could use some shaking up, but the environment of fear is becoming rampant and toxic leaving (particularly students and new parents) in a lot of uncertainty."

Tracing doulas' responses to the pandemic through its first six months, we heard multiple patterns of concern. Alongside the emotional stress doulas carry as they work to provide intimate labor to their clients, they must simultaneously navigate near-impossible work-life constraints. From Germany, a doula summarized the situation: "It's a huge challenge. I have less clients, less income, and it's hard to have a quiet space at home while I myself have two young children who are also stuck at home." A doula in the US told us, "When I'm home I'm less available even if I'm physically present because I'm preoccupied. Previously I would leave to support. Now I support from the couch, which looks different to [my] children who can't understand the circumstances." And from Mexico a doula shared, "Doulas are agents of security and serenity for our clients but now, we are tasked with this in all new levels for our own families as well." Doulas also worried about moving their support for people in labor to a virtual platform; this was often their only option, given the global policies around attending births in most places.

VIRTUAL DOULAS

Doula practice is rooted in accepting change, remaining flexible and adapting to new scenarios (Hunter 2012; Castañeda and Johnson Searcy., 2020). Birth is different with every client; comfort techniques that work for one woman may not work for another. To be effective, a doula must learn to read what an individual in labor needs. For example, doulas often maneuver through relational dynamics - mothers-in-law who aren't welcomed by the birthing person or tension between partners or spouses. Because doulas most often follow women to their chosen birth location, doulas may attend births in multiple places: different hospitals, birth centers, and homes. Adaptation and flexibility are necessary for navigating each of these spaces. The degree to which doulas are required to adapt and change their practice drastically increased during COVID. Doulas reported that the pandemic necessitated a quick transition online. Doulas told us that they used a variety of platforms including Zoom, Facetime, Skype, Whatsapp, and Slack. One doula described how virtual work was transforming doula care. She said, "I shifted to fully virtual for hospital clients, a completely new experience for me. I am unable to physically be with my clients for prenatal visits, birth, or postpartum. Losing this aspect of my work is heartbreaking. Of course, any new consultations are taking place virtually as well" (USA). Doulas grieved the loss of physical presence and understood virtual support to require something very different from them. A Canadian doula told us, "All of it is online. It was not as simple as just taking what we used to do in putting it online. It is a completely different service now." Doulas had to rethink their practices of support and presence and refashion them for virtual formats. Doulas relayed how they made Whatsapp calls, sent voice messages and birth affirmations, and provided flash drives with hypnobirthing music. In our follow-up responses, it was clear that doulas were continuing to rely on virtual support to access their clients. One South African doula shares her approach:

> "I explain in depth what virtual support looks and feels like. I help set up the technology necessary and practice ahead of time that we can get good camera angles etc. and I "attend" the birth pretty much as if I were there in person. I watch and listen and offer suggestions to the partner. If no partner is allowed, I have the birthing person put on earphones to hear me supporting and encouraging etc."

Yet even virtual presence at a birth can be broken. One Canadian doula told us that she was present via a laptop that had been set up so she could see the room and talk with the laboring woman and her partner. When the woman reached the second stage and was ready to push, the doctor entered the room and shut the computer screen, rendering this doula useless in those important moments.

Because attending a birth virtually can be difficult, doulas also now practice with much more focus on prenatal care. The emphasis on new ways of working often involved greater participation from a pregnant person's partner. Doulas managed their absence during birth by emphasizing the importance of education and preparation. Some doulas reported success with this approach:

> "I've realized that preparing my clients ahead of time and suggesting techniques to use has proven much more useful than I could have known. A client recently delivered her baby in the driveway on the way to the hospital because she was so focused [from prenatal preparation], she didn't realize that she was in labor until her waters broke, and from that point, she gave birth within 40 min (South Africa)."

Doulas described examples of preparing partners as stand-in labor support when doulas are unable to attend a birth. A New Zealand doula recounts how her new practice involves, "Directing instruction specifically to the birth partner and encouraging the couple to actively practice techniques of massage, breathing, relaxation, and affirmations." And in Canada, a doula detailed the changes involved in becoming a virtual doula:

> "We used to have two prenatal sessions and then in person support. We now have five prenatal sessions because we need to train the couple in a lot more things when it comes to preparing for Birth and bringing home a baby. We are basically teaching the partner to be a Doula and then guide them periodically throughout the labor experience to help the partner recall the information and techniques."

Despite the stark differences in virtual vs. in-person doula care, some doulas were adamant about their ability to "hold space" for intimate care, as explained by a doula from South Africa: "Holding space does not need to be done in person. Being available to clients and encouraging and guiding them to be self-empowered is now my focus. Preparation prior to birth is of utmost importance." Some doulas worked to bring in personal practices to create and "hold space" virtually, focusing on their own breathing, ensuring a quiet, calm space on their end of a virtual connection, hoping that calmness would transfer to their client in the hospital.

Efficacy of Virtual Doula Support

While our surveys confirm that the majority of doulas made the switch to virtual labor support, the efficacy of this new approach remains unclear. As a doula in Italy wrote, "I'm trying with the online but it is not the same ... " A German doula noted the important emotional labor that her work entailed and said, "It's much more difficult to engage in heartfelt conversations. It feels like the virtual platform transforms the prenatal sessions into more of a lecture or informational class rather than a collective, emotional discussion." Other doulas felt that the virtual medium itself was not congruent with helping a person in labor. They were concerned about interjecting more technology into an already heavily technology-driven hospital. For example, one doula from South Africa shared, "No, I don't do virtual. I only trust the amazing womanly body that knows how to birth and teach women to listen to their bodies. Not a new technique but quite forgotten." And another South African doula explained, "I do not enjoy virtual support as I find it's too much neocortex stimuli for the birthing person, and I find technology around internet connection expensive and unreliable." Doulas in the US drew attention to equity issues, concerned that people who most needed the support would not have the kind of access required to make virtual doula work effective (Searcy and Castañeda 2020).

All of the challenges around virtual doula work resulted in some doulas reporting to us that they outright did not like it. One Canadian doula who attended a birth virtually felt she could not effectively participate or provide support. She told us, "I felt like I was just a fly on the wall." Another doula in Japan was much more explicit in her dislike for working virtually: "I actually hate virtual birth work. It is not the same. I now firmly believe doulas improve outcomes because they are there in person. It's been very frustrating for me and very lonely and scary for my clients." Doulas lament the restrictions on their ability to attend births and help new-formed families, with one doula from India affirming, "This is a field you can't [have] without touch." These doulas saw their presence as a critical component of the support they provide women; research on birth partners confirms the benefits of a physically present birth attendant and shows that the well-known "doula effect" of shortening length of labor, minimizing interventions, and increasing psychological satisfaction only holds if the doula is indeed physically present throughout the labor and birth (Sauls, 2002; Gruber et al., 2013; Steel et al., 2015).

Economic Instability

Doulas' pivot to virtual support required them to navigate uncharted territory and to deal with increasing financial stress. Doulas repeatedly pointed to the COVID-19 policies as the cause of the new economic instability they were experiencing. As many hospital policies precluded doulas from being present at births, they could no longer charge for the support they offered in person. One doula from Portugal described the drastic changes to her economic identity as "the fragility of my income." As lockdown orders went into effect and hospital policies changed, doulas dealt with canceled contracts or scrambled to rewrite contracts and refund payments for incomplete services. We heard repeatedly about increased stress, as for this United Kingdom doula: "Lots of stress and worries about how this will impact financially and whether I will be able to provide the services I have already been hired for." A South African a doula shared, "Clients are more anxious and need more emotional support, my income has diminished just about completely and I need to refigure how to charge clients in a climate like this." Doulas struggled to translate the value of their virtual services to current and potential clients, saying "My clients' income has reduced, and now they are reluctant to pay [for] even online support" (South Africa). A doula in Canada noted that "a significant aspect of my approach to support was physical, however, I'm exploring the other aspects of my support tool kit—information gathering, spiritual support and emotional guidance. Navigating payment has also significantly shifted and I find myself doing significantly more unpaid work." If doula services were categorized as a "luxury" before COVID-19, they most definitely would be after the start of this pandemic, as people all over the world saw their incomes negatively impacted: "Financially it will take a long time to recover from COVID-19 as people's income has been affected and we are a 'luxury' spend" (New Zealand). Here again we see the debate over whether doulas are essential workers or not, which we have called "the politics of the essential" at play: this New Zealand doula sees doulas as non-essential "luxuries."

IMPACTS ON THE DOULA PROFESSION AND THE POLITICS OF "ESSENTIAL" WORKERS

As governments across the globe worked to contain the COVID-19 pandemic, including implementing new stay-at-home orders for non-essential personnel, doulas have struggled to find a sense of belonging in the rapidly changing birth landscape. A consistent theme heard across doula responses was frustration with how these new restrictions limited their work, most often attributed to doulas finding themselves forced into a debate about their role as essential workers. One doula from New Zealand put this succinctly when she said, "We were totally disregarded as 'essential' which was heartbreaking." Another doula from South Africa reported:

> "We have been fighting very hard to show doulas' worth here, and in a second called us "non-essential" and closed all the doors to us again. This shows me that any change or gain we made was not based on merit or the research that showed all the benefits of a doula, and so it would never have been a lasting change."

Pandemic policies that restricted doulas' access to hospitals illuminated a much longer and larger struggle doulas have had globally as they try to assert the importance of the services they provide to birthing people. Doulas, like the South African one quoted above, felt the sting of being labeled "non-essential" during the pandemic, in part because that is how doulas have often been seen in biomedical spaces (Gilliland, 2002; Norman and Katz Rothman, 2007; Stevens et al., 2011; Neel et al., 2019). Doulas often occupy a liminal space, moving between multiple worlds, crossing boundaries (Everson and Cheney 2015; Horstman et al., 2017). Doulas' presence in hospitals often hinges on carefully cultivated relationships with local hospitals, as doulas seek to demonstrate the importance of their role during labor and birth. With no official recognition or role within the biomedical system, doulas have long worked to assert themselves as "essential" (Norman and Katz Rothman, 2007; Roth et al., 2016; World Health Organization, 2019). Being rendered "non-essential" during a pandemic heightens the tension on the tightrope doulas already walk. A doula in Canada captured this tension when she told us, "It has been incredibly stressful navigating constant changes in a system that doesn't recognize that we exist—no official public health body has named doulas as a profession/industry and therefore have not provided clear instructions to us." As this doula points out, the pandemic amplified doulas tenuous and often liminal status. Despite doulas efforts to professionalize, as evidenced by the many doula certifying and continuing education options now available to them, there is no outside institutional consensus or recognition of doulas professional role (National Academies of Science Engineering and medicine, 2020) making their status as essential always up for debate.

The void in clear direction created by the rapid change in hospital protocols left many doulas scrambling to make sense of their role at births and revealed deeper intrinsic debates among doulas about their role. South African doulas demonstrated the way this rapid change foregrounded the debate within the doula community about where doulas belong and what world they are a part of. One doula from South Africa wrote:

> "Some doulas are willing to support clients at their homes, before going to the hospital, during our lockdown. I wasn't, so that is why a client transferred to another doula who was willing to come to her home. There has been a huge debate about whether doulas are healthcare workers and whether they are essential. The "permission" we got to travel during the lockdown, in my opinion doesn't really give us permission, as we are

> deemed not essential and not medical persons. It's a sad state of affairs for doulas, but some are not willing to accept this as the current state."

This resulted in a split across doula communities, with some identifying as essential workers and wanting to be on the front lines, while others saw their scope outside of "essential worker" parameters and agreed to being sidelined during the pandemic. Another doula from South Africa found this divide to be one of the biggest challenges:

> "Convincing other doulas that they need to do the socially responsible thing and NOT attend births or client visits in person, that's what's most challenging. I run the local doula organization and this has been by far the biggest challenge. Despite legal definitions and new laws, Doulas continue to fight the system and attempt to find loopholes, committing fraud to do it."

This doula refers to reports of doulas in South African (and other places including the US) who used loopholes in hospital pandemic policy to get into hospitals as fraud. From her perspective, doulas who hastily put together paperwork that could appear as some kind of certification and thus grant them entry into a hospital, was fraud and beyond the scope of practice doulas should undertake. Another South African doula also saw the decision to not provide in-person doula care as the right thing to do:

> "I applaud hospitals for both realizing the value of Doulas but also being aware of their limitations during a pandemic. Contrary to popular belief, doulas are NOT medical professionals and as such, although a wonderful part of a birthing team, they are not essential healthcare workers. Doulas are not trained to prevent the spread of any virus and while it is infinitely sad to all of us (and our clients!) that we may not attend births anymore as we are not an essential service, it is the socially responsible thing to do!"

Thus, we can see that some doulas felt strongly that it was in their best interest and that of their clients to act according to public health rules and recommendations and so were in conflict with those who felt their role was essential at births. Some doulas felt that complying with public health policies that mandated doulas as "nonessential" was a "sad state of affairs" but the necessary reality. Other doulas felt that attending births was crucial to demonstrating the critical nature of a doula's role. In the doula community, the debate over who is "essential" demonstrates the political stakes; doulas who wanted to claim "essential" worker status hoped to do so as part of an ongoing effort to secure their role in reproductive care.

Many doulas also expressed concern about how current restrictions on doula presence would shape their profession moving forward. As one doula in Germany pointed out, "It is a difficult time that is testing my ability to do this work. The scariest part is that after the full 'crisis' is over, will hospitals continue to implement these restrictions and limitations on birthing support?" The uncertainty with the future was coupled with current frustration and grief due to changing hospital protocols, as a doula in South Africa lamented, "I feel we have worked so hard to be known and seen by medical staff, we've been always walking on a slippery slide and now we have been pushed down when women need our support more than ever." Doulas work to stay in the moment at birth, but the uncertainty of their future was repeatedly cited as occupying the forefront of their concerns. "It's going to be hard picking up the pieces when this is finally over. It's already been hard to build up trust and build relationships with doctors and hospitals in South Africa. Doulas are losing income and clients lose support." The global trend of classifying doulas as non-essential continues to keep doulas concerned about their professional standing in clinical settings.

CONCERNS ABOUT OBSTETRIC VIOLENCE

Doulas' concern about losing their place at the table of reproductive care was in part because of their fears that mistreatment and obstetric violence would escalate without their presence. We heard this theme come up again and again as doulas around the world reflected on the ongoing pandemic and restrictions. Doulas saw hospital protocols that required birthing people to be alone without anyone accompanying them as "a basic human right being taken away from parents" (South Africa). Another doula from South Africa said, "I am unable to support women in the government hospitals who are from township areas and have no support at all. They are alone and don't know what is happening to them." A doula in Ireland shared, "Hospitals have a one birth partner only restriction and some hospitals have banned all partners and mums have to go through labor alone," and from Hungary, "Doulas were excluded first, now fathers too. This means more obstetric violence and more vulnerable women." Other doulas in our study also expressed concern about increasing rates of obstetric violence occurring due to COVID-19 restrictions. A doula in Argentina affirmed, "Everything that happened before the pandemic in a pandemic worsens, grows bigger. Obstetric violence became more severe," as well as from Spain where "birth has involved emotional and physical obstetric violence." Doulas in the US were concerned about marginalized populations, describing how pandemic policies meant that "There is a lack of personal contact I would normally be allowed to provide. Basic human rights are being taken away and women are afraid. I work with young moms who are being talked into procedures they previously didn't want." Another US doula told us that the changes had a significant impact on her clients, whom, she felt, were at increased risk without doula support:

> "My clients are young, single, clinic patients who are typically women of color. Their care within the hospital

> is not given with dignity and respect. I have seen it with my own eyes. Without having a doula there for support, these girls are at the mercy of the doctors and nurses, as they don't feel empowered enough to speak up or question anything. It saddens me greatly, as this was why I got into doula-work."

Doulas saw themselves as witnesses to institutional mistreatment and violence and as providers of support to people who received such treatment. They also stressed that their presence at birth as witnesses is a deterrent to obstetric violence, disrespect, and abuse.

With the incorporation of virtual technology, doulas are now witnessing obstetric violence through a new lens. We heard this perspective from a doula in Japan, "My clients are treated much differently when I'm not in the room. I never fully understood this until virtual work." From Canada to South Africa, doulas reported examples of obstetric violence, including clients "overlooked due to shortages," as well as experiencing "lack of consent" and "fear mongering being used to get them to do a cesarean." In particular, South African doulas affirmed, "I feel as if women are now treated even harsher than before. More like a production line at hospitals now," and "Also, a lot of obstetricians are convincing moms of the ridiculous idea that C-sections are the safest option in this time." The results of these stressful experiences are visible during and after birth, as one doula reported, "I see stress taking over and partners worried during labor and postpartum" (South Africa). Without the power of witnessing and of supportive touch, whether in birth or postpartum with breastfeeding help, doulas worry about the damage being done to new families. This situation, described by one doula as "a recipe for postpartum depression" (South Africa) is leaving doulas to work virtually with new parents who are scared and concerned. A US doula confirmed:

> "My clients are terrified to not have a doula with them, and be stuck using virtual platforms. I have experienced obstetric violence, mistreatment, emotional abuse, lack of informed consent over virtual platforms. The presence of a doula alone causes an increase in true informed consent sessions, and therefore better outcomes. So with doulas being limited to virtual platforms, a few of my clients have experienced coercion and negative outcomes. One of them was pretty traumatized by the treatment she received, which means I am now watching her closely for postpartum depression. With the first postpartum visit usually being around 6 weeks, I now feel it is my duty to go above and beyond to make sure she is safe."

Preliminary research suggests that COVID's impact on postpartum depression is real (Davenport et al., 2020), and additional long-term studies will reveal the consequences of COVID policies that restrict support for birthing people.

DOULAS AND THE HOME BIRTH INCREASE

While many doulas described feeling "defeated" or "hopeless" with the pandemic situation, we also found areas of positive engagement, including more interest in home birth. Doulas reported a sharp increase in requests for home birth and information on midwifery models of care. As a South African doula explained:

> "This situation seems to have low risk birthing families to contact, discuss and look to midwife led facilities. Home births are being considered more also. This pleases me so much as it's directing birth back to where it belongs—with midwives and midwifery led units and at home."

This situation has also changed how some doulas serve clients by expanding their scope of practice. For example, "I no longer volunteer at the local government hospital maternity ward. I work with a midwife and we are snowed under with requests to support our midwife led birth unit, and we now do home births for women who can't travel across provincial borders" (South Africa). Another South African doula wrote:

> "At the midwifery unit we now do home births which we didn't do before. We have taken on another midwife and are looking for another doula. We are busier than ever before. I have not been to a government hospital for 4 weeks and no longer can support families at private hospitals. The main private hospitals have officially declared "No Doulas.""

According to Davis-Floyd et al., (2020), as COVID swept the country, numbers of US childbearers made a rapid switch to home birth to flee hospital contagion and also to avoid having to labor alone or to be forced to choose between partner and doula. One of our a US doula respondents stressed the latter reason as she shared her experience with the rise in home births:

> "The number of home births in our area went up astronomically in the past few months. Women who had never considered a home birth before, or had considered it but never made the leap, switched to home at the last minute. I was a part of 4 of these births in the past two months, and every one of them gave the same reason for switching—not that they were afraid of COVID exposure, but that they didn't want to be refused doula support in the hospital. Wow!! I think that speaks to the importance of doulas at births, and how badly women want them there."

Faced with mounting uncertainties both with the virus and changing hospital policies, pregnant people turned to doulas for help navigating the possibilities of home birth and midwifery models of care.

CONCLUSION: THE NEED TO INCREASE DOULA CARE

Research with doulas shows the power of the pandemic to intensify and homogenize biomedical, technocratic models of birth (Davis-Floyd 2003). As a South African doula described, "It reveals that psychological, practical, and emotional care during birth is still not considered a priority." We recognize the need for doulas to have training in infectious disease as well as proper personal protective equipment in order to serve their clients and safeguard other medical personnel. As one doula shared, "In uncertain times, doula care is even more important for mothers. If both parties desire, I believe there are safe ways to provide in person care for healthy families and doulas" (United Arab Emirates). Working within these parameters in person, doulas increase emotional and social support for laboring people as well as alleviate some of the stress of caring for them for hospital management. This sentiment was echoed by a South African doula:

> "While I understand that doulas are not medical professionals, and respect the need for distance and protection, we make essential differences to the birth experience for parents. Our responsible presence at births would make it so much easier, not only for the parents, but also the entire medical team during this time of fear and uncertainty."

Many doulas called on medical institutions to recognize and legitimize the support they bring to birth, and to code them as truly "essential."

As countries around the world continue to deal with varying rates of COVID-19 infections, from "flattening the curve" to second or third waves, many unanswered questions remain. This uncertainty is reflected in our most recent responses from international doulas. While some international respondents reported affirmatively that doulas were indeed readmitted as birth workers in hospitals, they were in the minority, as many others confirmed the continued exclusion of doulas. The answers to our questions were not bound by national borders, as we gathered differing responses from doulas within the same national territory and similar responses from around the globe. These responses only further reinforce our understanding that this virus knows no political borders—national, regional or local. Instead, what we can affirm from our international responses is that doulas around the world are continuing to support laboring people, sometimes in person and other times virtually, and that their commitment to a holistic form of care is rooted in their belief that the liminal moments of birth are both transformational and lasting. Doulas are expanding and increasing their intimate labor across platforms as they move online to continue to invite others to "breathe with me." A doula in Australia put it this way:

> "I really hope that rules and regulations recognize the important work doulas do in this time. I feel like they are the ones stepping up right now and trying to fill all the voids left in this strange time. Creating online mothers' groups, connecting new mums up with each other so they don't feel so alone, and being there consistently to talk to expecting mums. Please don't forget them and please acknowledge what the doula network is doing right now."

Now more than ever we need to recognize and support the essential work that doulas do, as well as invest in strategies that increase access to doula care for women worldwide in sustainable ways.

ETHICS STATEMENT

The studies involving human participants were reviewed and approved by the DePauw University IRB. The patients/participants provided their written informed consent to participate in this study.

AUTHOR CONTRIBUTIONS

Both authors conducted and coded the qualitative survey on which the article is based. AC put ethnographic data into document and wrote a rough draft. JJS then added to the rough draft. After a discussion, JJS then wrote and revised and edited the manuscript. AC read over it and made small changes.

REFERENCES

Bohren, M. A., Berger, B. O., Munthe-Kaas, H., and Tunçalp, Ö. (2019). Perceptions and experiences of labour companionship: a qualitative evidence synthesis. *Cochrane Database Syst. Rev.* 3, CD012449. doi:10.1002/14651858.CD01244910.1002/14651858.CD012449.pub2

Castañeda, A. N., and Johnson Searcy, J. (2020). Forthcoming "shifting landscapes of Belonging: Birth Doulas and COVID-19." *Practicing Anthropology.* 42:4, 5-10. doi:10.17730/0888-4552.42.4.5

Davenport, M. H., Sarah MeyerMeah, V. L., Strynadka, M. C., and Rshmi, K. (2020). Moms are not ok: COVID-19 and maternal mental health. *Frontiers in global women's health.* doi:10.3389/fgwh.2020.00001

Davis-Floyd, R. (2003). *Birth as an American rite of passage.* 2nd Edn. Berkeley, CA: University of California Press.

Davis-Floyd, R., Gutschow, K., and Schwartz, D. A. (2020). Pregnancy, birth and the COVID-19 pandemic in the United States. *Med. Anthropol.* 39 (5), 413–427. doi:10.1080/01459740.2020.1761804

Everson, C., and Cheney, M. (2015). "Between two worlds: doula care, liminality and the power of mandorla spaces." in *Douglas and intimate labor: boundaries,*

Bodies and birth. Editor N.A. Castañeda and J. J. Searcy (Toronto, ON, Canada: Demeter Press).

Gilliland, A. L. (2002). Beyond holding hands: the modern role of the professional doula. *J. Obstet. Gynecol. Neonatal Nurs.* 31 (6), 762–769.

Gruber, K. J., Cupito, S. H., and Dobson, C. F. (2013). Impact of douglas on healthy birth outcomes. *J. Perinat. Educ.* 22 (1), 49–58. doi:10.1891/1058-1243.22.1.49

Horstman, H. K., Anderson, J., and Kuehl, R. A. (2017). Communicatively making sense of doulas within the U.S. Master birth narrative: doulas as liminal characters. *Health Commun.* 32 (12), 1510–1519. doi:10.1080/10410236.2016.1234537

Hunter, C. (2012). Intimate space within institutionalized birth: women's experiences birthing with douglas. *Anthropol. Med.* 19 (3), 315–326. doi:10.1080/13648470.2012.692358

Kayne, M. A., Greulich, M. B., and Albers, L. L. (2001). Douglas: an alternative yet complementary addition to care during childbirth. *Clin. Obstet. Gynecol.* 44 (4), 692–703. doi:10.1097/00003081-200112000-00009

National Academies of Sciences Engineering and medicine (2020). "Birth settings in America: outcomes, quality, access and choice," in *Susan scrimshaw and emily P. Backes*. (Washington, DC. National Academies Press) doi:10.17226/25636

Neel, K., Goldman, R., Marte, D., Bello, G., and Nothnagle, M. B. (2019). Hospital-based maternity care practitioners' perceptions of douglas. *Birth* 46 (2), 355–361. doi:10.1111/birt.12420

Norman, B. M., and Katz Rothman, B. (2007). "The new arrival: labor douglas and the fragmentation of midwifery and caregiving." in *Laboring on: Birth in transition in the United StatesWeny simonds, bari meltzer norman and barbara Katz rothman*. Abingdon, United Kingdom: Routledge, 251–282.

Roth, L. M., Henley, M. M., Seacrist, M. J., and Morton, C. H. (2016). North American nurses' and douglas' views of each other. *J. Obstet. Gynecol. Neonatal Nurs.* 45, 790. doi:10.1016/j.jogn.2016.06.011

Sauls, D. J. (2002). Effects of labor support on mothers, babies, and birth outcomes. *J. Obstet. Gynecol. Neonatal Nurs.* 31 (6), 733–741. doi:10.1177/0884217502239209

Searcy, J. J., and Castañeda, A. N. (2020). COVID-19 and the birth of the virtual doula. *Med. Anthropol. Q.* 19. 2020 Available at: http://medanthroquarterly.org/2020/06/19/covid-19-and-the-birth-of-the-virtual-doula/.

Steel, A., Jane, F., Adams, J., and Helene, D. (2015). Trained or professional douglas in the support and care of pregnant and birthing women: a critical integrative review. *Health Soc. Care Community.* 23, 3. doi:10.1111/hsc.12112

Stevens, J., Dahlen, H., Peters, K., and Jackson, D. (2011). Midwives' and douglas' perspectives of the role of the doula in Australia: a qualitative study. *Midwifery* 27 (4), 509–516. doi:10.1016/j.midw.2010.04.002

World Health Organization (2019). Why having a companion during labour and childbirth may be better for you. https://www.who.int/reproductivehealth/companion-during-labour-childbirth/en/. (Accessed August 15, 2020).

5

Access to Maternal Health Services During the COVID-19 Pandemic: Experiences of Indigent Mothers and Health Care Providers in Kilifi County, Kenya

Stephen Okumu Ombere *

Department of Sociology and Anthropology, Maseno University, Maseno-Kisumu, Kenya

Correspondence:
Stephen Okumu Ombere
sokumu2@googlemail.com
orcid.org/0000-0002-3964-6795

COVID-19 has spread rapidly in Kenya and has not spared pregnant women. Evidence from Kenya shows that during the COVID-19 pandemic, health systems have been either stressed to their maximum capacity or are becoming overwhelmed. However, the population is advised not to attend hospital unless strictly necessary, and this advice seems to apply to all, including expectant mothers. There is a dearth of information on how poor expectant mothers with low bargaining power cope during COVID-19 in Kenya, which this study addresses for those in Kilifi County. This rapid qualitative study draws data from an extensive literature review and from interviews with 12 purposively selected mothers who were either expectant or had newborn babies during the pandemic in Kilifi County. Five matrons-in-charge of maternal health services and four traditional birth attendants were also interviewed via mobile phone. Data were analyzed thematically and are presented in a textual description. It emerged that expectant mothers feared attending hospitals for perinatal care due to the possibility of contracting COVID-19. Therefore, there was an increase in home deliveries with the assistance of traditional birth attendants (TBAs)/traditional midwives, who were also overwhelmed with women who sought their services. Since most causes of maternal morbidity and mortality can be prevented by prompt, suitable treatment by qualified health practitioners, the health officials interviewed recommended training and integration of TBAs in emergency healthcare responses to help during crises in MHS because they are trusted by their local communities. Notably, such integration of traditional midwives should be supported and should also include additional training and monetary incentives.

Keywords: coronavirus, COVID-19, Kilifi county, maternal Health Services, traditional midwives

INTRODUCTION: BACKGROUND AND CONTEXT

Maternal health remains a challenge in low-resource countries. The numbers of women dying every year from maternity-related causes have remained high in such countries despite various efforts to bring them down (World Health Organization (WHO), 2019; Otieno et al., 2020). Pregnancy, childbirth, and postnatal states are a critical period in a woman's life; her health during this phase is known as maternal health. Most potential maternal morbidity and mortality can be prevented when prompt, suitable treatment is provided by qualified health practitioners, often referred to as "skilled birth attendants" (World Health Organization (WHO), 2018). Scientists continue to investigate the coronavirus and COVID-19, but little is yet known about the maternal and fetal birth outcomes of infected women. The world population has been waiting for answers and remains alert about the pandemic's progress. COVID-19 is still relatively new to humans, and only limited scientific evidence is available to identify its impact on sexual and reproductive health (SRH) (Tang et al., 2020).

Maternal health services and other sexual and reproductive health care such as family planning, emergency contraception, treatment of sexually transmitted diseases, post-abortion care, and, where legal, safe abortion services to the full extent of the law need to remain available as core health services. Early data from the United Nations Population Fund (UNFPA) suggests a drop in facility-based care in many countries and projections of rising maternal mortality as results of COVID-19 (UNFPA, 2020). During pandemics, health systems all over the world are either stressed to their maximum capacity or anticipating becoming overwhelmed (Iyengar et al., 2015; McQuilkin et al., 2017). The COVID-19 pandemic has disrupted access to healthcare services in many countries, and states are implementing measures to curb its spread. The best ways to stop the transmission of COVID-19 infection, as other articles in this Special Issue demonstrate, are physical distancing, mask wearing, and constant washing of hands and of potentially contaminated clothing, shoes, and surfaces. In Kenya, as the government has intensified its efforts to contain the spread of the virus, particular health workers and facilities have been redirected to deal with COVID-19 cases, which means that other health services, including maternal health care, are no longer priorities as they should and must be. A recent study reported that Kenya lacks a robust pandemic emergency preparedness plan, as human and financial resources are inadequate to respond to emergencies. Although existing disaster responses and risk mitigation committees include stakeholders across different sectors, these positions are politically motivated and lack adequate technical support (Wangamati and Sundby, 2020).

Globally, the COVID-19 pandemic has had devastating effects on health care delivery systems for people of all ages, but pregnant women face particular challenges. Rocca-Ihenacho and Alonso (2020) reported that the pandemic is making it increasingly challenging to provide adequate maternity care worldwide. Even the movement of people seeking to access health care services has been restricted in many countries to prevent the spread of the virus. The pandemic has led to a complete stoppage of the import and export of many essential commodities among various countries, leading to a shortage of necessary items and affecting healthcare services badly, especially sexual and reproductive health care (Kumar, 2020). The population is advised not to attend hospital unless strictly necessary; this advice seems to apply to all, including healthy pregnant women and even those with complications (Rocca Ihenacho and Alonso 2020). Therefore, the direct and indirect effects of the COVID-19 response on pregnant women, newborn babies, young children, and adolescents are enormous.

Improvements in maternal and child health care are principal targets of the Sustainable Development Goals (SDGs) under Health Goal 3.1. This goal mainly focuses on reducing the global maternal mortality ratio (MMR—the number of maternal deaths per 100,000 live births) to less than 70/100,000 live births by 2030 (World Health Organization, 2015). Between 2000 and 2017, the MMR dropped by about 38% worldwide (World Health Organization (WHO), 2019). However, in 2017, approximately 810 women around the world died every day from preventable causes related to pregnancy and childbirth. Maternal health services (MHS), which include antenatal, labor and delivery, and postnatal care, can play a crucial role in preventing and/or treating maternal health problems (Pant et al., 2020). However, the "obstetric" population is vulnerable, as different stages of pregnancy involve multiple interactions with the healthcare system; therefore, assisting the childbearing population presents unique challenges during the coronavirus pandemic. Postpartum hemorrhage, maternal sepsis, preeclampsia, and premature rupture of the membranes are the most common COVID-19-induced adverse events reported among pregnant women (Chen et al., 2020).

The consequences of COVID-19 could even be catastrophic for maternal and newborn health (Pant et al., 2020). Before the emergence of COVID-19 in Kenya, high-quality and timely maternity healthcare services were unavailable, inaccessible, or unaffordable for millions of women around the world, most especially in low-resource countries. Now, restrictions on travel and gatherings, health facilities with limited infection prevention supplies and unreliable infection control practices, and disrupted health worker's routines threaten to exacerbate limited access to care and further negatively impact women's health.

Kenya introduced free maternity services (FMS) in all public hospitals in 2013 to encourage skilled care deliveries and provide financial risk protection and equitable access to MHS for poor and vulnerable populations. Since the introduction of FMS, Kenya has made remarkable progress towards reducing mortality rates and improving coverage of health services (Kenya National Bureau of Statistics (KNBS), 2015). Yet despite such successes, considerable inequities in health outcomes and in uptake of health services remain, disadvantaging the most vulnerable individuals (Kenya National Bureau of Statistics (KNBS), 2015). Kenya recorded an increase in the proportion of facility-based deliveries from 44% in 2008 to 61% in 2015 (Kenya National Bureau of Statistics (KNBS), 2015). This increase in skilled care deliveries has been partly attributed to the free maternity care policy introduced in June 2013 (Kenya National Bureau of Statistics (KNBS), 2015; Pyone et al., 2017).

The first case of COVID-19 was reported in Kenya on March 13, 2020 and, like many countries across the globe, the Kenyan government has implemented measures and interventions to curtail the spread of the virus and to mitigate the socio-economic effects of COVID-19 response. Some of these steps, such as the nationwide dusk-to-dawn curfew, have negatively impacted access to essential health services, particularly emergency obstetric and newborn care. The curfew has restricted people's movements, in particular by rendering all means of transport unavailable from dusk till dawn, including those of expectant mothers who need healthcare services. Moreover, many healthcare workers and facilities have been redirected to deal with COVID-19 cases; thus resources are often diverted away from maternal health care, making it increasingly challenging to provide adequate maternity care in Kenya. And studies from low resource settings have reported that limited supply of personal protective equipment (PPE) exposes healthcare providers and mothers to increased risk for infections (Strong, 2018; Karkee and Morgan, 2020), as has been the case in Kenya.

Despite the availability of free maternity services in all public health facilities, some counties in Kenya have reported high maternal and perinatal morbidities and deaths because laboring women could not access emergency transport to health facilities due to limited or no movement and fear of police during the pandemic. As one of my interlocutors (see below), a hospital matron (a nurse-midwife head of shift) stated:

> More expectant mothers could die due to complications of other ailments when we are focused on COVID-19. The government needs to direct all agencies, including the police and other law enforcing agencies to provide emergency transportation for expectant mothers.

Furthermore, fear of contracting the coronavirus has kept many women away from seeking ante- and postnatal care. Healthcare providers in Kenya have also minimized in-person contact with their patients. So far, there is reduced utilization of maternal and child health services across the country as compared to 2019. Evidence from prior outbreaks shows that this crisis could exact a massive toll on women and girls. Women are disproportionally represented in the health and social services sectors, increasing their risk of exposure to the disease (UNFPA, 2020). Therefore, there is a need to explore alternatives that women from poor resource settings may use to gain access to MHS during the COVID-19 pandemic. This article describes how indigent mothers from Kilifi County, Kenya have responded to and coped with the dramatic changes that have occurred in birth practices as a result of this pandemic, primarily by choosing perinatal care with traditional midwives.

METHODS

This article follows on from my PhD ethnographic fieldwork on local perceptions of social protection schemes in maternal health in Kenya, conducted between March–July 2016 and February–July 2017 (Ombere, 2018). "Social protection schemes" include free maternity services in all public health facilities and maternal vouchers in selected accredited public and private health facilities (These vouchers were no longer in supply during my fieldwork). After my fieldwork ended, I have occasionally been in touch with most participants, who were poor mothers, health workers, community health volunteers and traditional birth attendants (TBAs), better referred to as traditional midwives because they are regarded as such by their communities (Davis-Floyd 2018). Since March 2020, when the first case of COVID-19 was reported in Kenya, out of 40 mothers whom I followed during my ethnographic fieldwork in Kilifi County, I managed to reach 20 of them between June 13 and July 24, 2020. Data for this article were derived from the responses of 12 of these mothers who were either expectant or gave birth during the COVID-19 pandemic.

For this qualitative study, I also conducted phone interviews with five matrons (nurse-midwives who serve as department heads) in charge of maternal health services, whom I purposively selected from the two busiest health facilities that I had contact with during my initial fieldwork. And I interviewed four traditional midwives (locally called mkunga in the singular and wakunga in the plural), based on the roles they had previously played in referring expectant mothers to facilities for delivery. Most of these phone conversations were recorded and later transcribed. I teased out emerging themes for this article based on the overall objectives of this Special Issue on the impact of COVID-19 on both maternity care practices in various countries and on pregnant families' experiences of maternity care. All participants were informed about the nature of this study and only those who consented to the phone interviews participated. To maintain confidentiality and minimize the potential of identification of study participants, no identifying names have been used in reporting the study findings. Ethical approval was obtained from Maseno University Ethical Review Committee (Reference #MSU/DRPI/MUERC/00206/015). For this article, I also carried out an extensive literature review of research related to my subject matter.

FINDINGS: FEAR OF INFECTIONS, LACK OF PPE, AND AN INCREASE IN TRADITIONAL MIDWIFE-ATTENDED BIRTHS

Fear of Infections and Lack of PPE in Hospitals

> Steve, I tell you I cannot go to the hospital when I know very well I am going to get coronavirus. I know my friends who have been attending antenatal clinics who also fear going to the hospital. At least I know there is a mkunga who will assist me (Pregnant mother, expecting her seventh child)
>
> I avoided going for the clinic since corona began. I had visited the hospital once and again, going to the hospital using a motorbike is still risky because I am among the groups at risk contracting the virus and I cannot tell the virus status of those who boarded the motorcycle. I will deliver at home (Pregnant mother, expecting her third child)
>
> No need for risking. My child can miss all those clinics till that time they will say coronavirus is managed and is no longer there with us. I will just give my child healthy foods such as porridge and cow milk (A mother, supposed to go for postnatal care)

> Fear of coronavirus has affected mothers differently. It is true most pregnant mothers and those that are supposed to attend clinics have avoided coming for routine clinics (Maternity matron, public health facility 02)

The excerpts above denote the recurring theme of fear of contracting the coronavirus. Pregnant and breastfeeding mothers expressed anxiety and worry about COVID-19; thus, a majority of them avoided going to antenatal and postnatal clinics. There was a general knowledge among pregnant women that they had low immunity and thus could easily get infected by the virus. Expectant mothers expressed their confidence in delivering with the assistance of traditional midwives in their community. Mothers who had delivered would not take their babies for postnatal check-ups due to fear, resulting in missed vaccinations and other possibly essential medicines.

For their part, due to the lack of adequate protective gear, health workers also expressed fear of treating people from the community, including those who visited clinics for ante- and postnatal care. These health workers noted that even though there are government guidelines on safety measures during COVID-19, the chances were very high that poor mothers from the villages could not afford even an ordinary mask or sanitizer, and thus could expose health workers to danger. As noted above, these health facility matrons also reported that few mothers were attending maternity clinics due to fear of contagion. The matrons feared that the number of maternal deaths could increase due to pregnancy-related complications during COVID-19. Two of them stated:

> I am a human being, we don't have enough protective gear. Thus, I fear handling people from the village including the expectant mothers. I cannot know who they interacted with and how they behaved outside there. Moreover, the women around here are very poor, and some cannot even afford the face masks (Maternity matron, public health facility 01)
>
> We have few mothers reporting for the antenatal and postnatal clinics. Many children have not got their immunization. I know this is due to fear of COVID-19 (Maternity matron, public health facility 02)

Increase in Traditional Midwife-Attended Births

The traditional midwives interviewed—who tend to be older women, as few younger women want to carry on their time-honored practices—reported that there was a rapid increase in the number of women whom they assisted in delivering due to various factors, including women's fears of hospital infection and the reduction in the availability of primary healthcare services, including health facility deliveries. This increase was challenging for the traditional midwives to manage because almost all expectant mothers in the villages preferred giving birth in traditional midwives' homes, which have no beds to accommodate the expectant mothers. Usually there is a small hut for delivery in or near every traditional midwife's home. Plastic polythene is spread on the mud floor for deliveries. Poor women prefer delivering at traditional midwives' homes as those birthing spaces are often cleaner than their own homes. Another advantage is that they can pay in installments and sometimes work on the midwives' farms after they have healed by way of payment. Thus birth with a traditional midwife is often cheaper than facility birth (see below).

Two Wakunga/Community Midwives Stated

> Stephen, this virus has given me a lot of work, but again I am overwhelmed because all women from [Village Y] come to my home and you know I don't have beds here. They deliver, sit for an hour or so and their husbands collect them. I have a small hut special for assisting mothers to give birth. The floor is smeared with mud but I do spread a polythene bag then wash it after completing delivery. Women come here because I know them and they can always pay later or work on my farm after healing (Traditional midwife 002)
>
> As the mkunga, I assist women daily. Okay, some women had complications and from my records, three babies died when I was trying to help the mothers deliver. They died because two women came late when the complication was too hard for me to handle, while one was a severe complication that I could not handle. I managed to remove the baby, but it was already dead (Traditional midwife 005)

This latter statement reveals the need for training traditional midwives in how to better handle birth complications.

Concomitantly with the rise in traditional midwife-attended births, the hospital matrons noted a decrease in hospital deliveries. As previously mentioned, many health facilities were closed because the health workers were reassigned to handle COVID-19 cases, preventing mothers from delivering there. However, health workers warned that although giving birth at home was an available option—still used pre-COVID by almost 40% of pregnant women—giving birth in a hospital was nevertheless the safest way because all complications could be handled in the health facility even during the pandemic. According to two matrons:

> Women have been giving birth at home long before hospitals even existed. The problem comes in when there is a complication that needs doctors' attention; we are likely to lose the mother and the child (Hospital matron 01)
>
> It is true many health facilities were temporarily shut down and health workers reassigned duties to handle COVID-19 cases. It means that poor expectant mothers had to look for alternatives on where to deliver and definitely they went to TBAs (Hospital matron 02).

Mothers who participated in this study noted that they could not go against their husbands' advice and delivering in traditional midwives' homes was cheaper, which is why their husbands preferred this option. These mothers argued that wealthy pregnant women could go to private health facilities and also have the ability to bargain for what they want. Two mothers explained:

> It is true we are delivering at the mkunga's home during this coronavirus period. Giving birth there is cheaper because we can pay using different ways. Our husbands also have the final say, so after looking around we resort to the mkunga, which is a better option. (Mother from Village D)
>
> I cannot go to a private health facility because I don't have enough money. Private hospital is for the rich who know how to bargain and their money speaks for them, they don't beg to get services. But during this coronavirus time it is very expensive to give birth at a private health facility (A mother from Village G)

These quotes beg the question: Why don't these economically disadvantaged women use the free public hospitals for birth? The issue from these mothers' perspective is that "free" maternity services are never truly free. Poor women, who have low bargaining power, are expected to pay some money before getting some essential services in public health facilities. For examples, they have to pay for laboratory services, antenatal care, and sometimes have to purchase any medicines prescribed. Thus to them, it is expensive to give birth in even a "free" public health facility, and private health facilities are completely beyond their reach.

To avert home births during COVID-19, health workers suggested that the government could direct all agencies, including the police and other law enforcement agencies, to provide emergency transportation to health facilities to minimize maternal deaths from complications occasioned by delay in seeking care during COVID-19 due to the curfew. However, some health workers argued that traditional midwives should be better trained in how to handle complications because the community trusts them and they can help avert maternal deaths during this or other crises. For example, one matron stated:

> Traditional birth attendants have really helped many poor mothers in the villages. They are trusted by the mothers, I think there is need to always re-train these TBAs to avert maternal deaths due to complications during pandemics (Hospital matron 05).

Yet no such re-trainings have as yet been offered.

DISCUSSION AND ANALYSIS: MAKING TOUGH CHOICES THAT LEAVE WOMEN OUT, AND INCORPORATING TRADITIONAL MIDWIVES

My study findings reflect how pregnant mothers from the poor socio-economic class in Kilifi County are vulnerable during COVID-19 in Kenya. Again, sexual and reproductive health care services are essential for any community and are usually neglected and seriously affected during epidemics and pandemics, leading to long-term adverse consequences (Kumar, 2020). Evidence from other studies shows that decisions made at every level of the response to the pandemic are resulting in women being further cut off from sexual and reproductive health services, threatening sharp rises in maternal and neonatal mortality (Phumaphi et al., 2020; Pollock et al., 2020). Now, this global pandemic is making a bad situation even worse, as some countries divert resources away from other essential services (Phumaphi et al., 2020). UN Women (2020) warned that the diversion of attention and critical resources away from the provisions of sexual and reproductive health services, including maternal health care, might result in aggravated maternal mortality and morbidity. Indeed, my matron interlocutors agreed that frontline providers were forced to make tough choices about which services are most important, and women were often left out. However, even before the COVID-19 pandemic, global progress towards the 2030 Every Woman Every Child (EWEC) Global Strategy for Women's, Children's and Adolescents' Health target to save the lives of women and children was already lagging by around 20%.

Findings from this study indicate that there is a likely increase in maternal and neonatal deaths during the COVID-19 pandemic in Kenya. This increase can be attributed to the effects of the pandemic, which have led to delays in accessing life-saving procedures such as cesareans, due to staff deployment and shortages, fear, and lack of infrastructure. This concurs with recent findings from other studies that also report an increase in maternal deaths globally due to COVID-19 (Hussein, 2020; Takemoto et al., 2020). Supporting my own findings, Kimani et al. (2020) also noted for Nairobi, Kenya that fear of contracting COVID-19 likely kept many women from attending reproductive health services. Relatedly, Delamou et al. (2017) showed that fear of infection at health facilities was also reported by women in Guinea during the recent Ebola epidemic there (see also Strong and Schwartz 2016).

The results of my study show that there was a decrease in the utilization of maternal health services among the childbearers in Kilifi County, including antenatal, labor and delivery, and postnatal services. This was occasioned by fear of contracting the virus and low bargaining power for access to better health care. My findings corroborate recent findings by Pant et al. (2020), who noted that decreased access and utilization of maternal health services could have dire consequences for both women and newborns. Pregnant and postpartum women are already at high risk of nutritional deficiency during the lockdown due to decreased supply of nutritious food. On top of that, when they are unable to have regular antenatal and postnatal services, they are deprived of the micronutrient supplements that they get from the clinics. In addition, without regular checkups, there are chances of certain danger signs going unidentified, which makes them vulnerable to complications related to pregnancy and childbirth. Health workers also reported that fear of COVID-19 transmission in hospital settings was widespread because of a scarcity of proper PPE in the health facilities. A study in Nepal (Karkee and Morgan, 2020) and another in Tanzania (Strong, 2018) also confirmed that scarcity of PPE and fear were some of the factors affecting women's access to safe delivery, which is within their rights, by extending the well-known "three delays" in deciding to go to a health facility, in reaching it, and in receiving quality care once they arrive.

Although access to safe delivery care has long been acknowledged as an essential health service, many poor pregnant women in Kenya as a whole suddenly found themselves with fewer options for care as health facilities were converted into isolation wards. Wangamati and Sundby (2020) also noted that such changes led to confusion, as pregnant women and mothers did not know where to go to seek maternal health services. In this study, a majority of mothers resorted to giving birth in the homes of the traditional midwives in Kilifi, since most health facilities were temporarily shut down and health workers were reassigned to the COVID-19 crisis. It emerged that traditional midwives were valued by expectant mothers because they are well-respected, easily accessible during COVID-19, offer flexible payment modalities, understand and abide by local customs and traditions, and provide services that skilled birth attendants do not—such as pre- and postnatal massage and more compassionate care. These findings are corroborated by Byrne et al. (2016) and Ombere (2018), who reported much the same. However, the government of Kenya actively discourages TBA-supported births (Byrne et al., 2016), preferring that TBAs refer mothers to the nearest health facility. According to the health workers in this study, integration of traditional midwives during pandemics such as COVID-19 and other crises is necessary. This recommendation from the health workers concurs with findings from a recent study in Kenya by Kimani et al. (2020), who argued that integrating community health workers by expanding existing midwifery centers and creating new ones run by qualified midwives ("skilled birth attendants") that are closer to or in rural communities could be a viable long-term plan that can reduce the burden on hospitals, and minimize infections and maternal deaths during pandemics such as COVID-19.

Given that studies from the Democratic Republic of Congo (Matendo et al., 2011) and Kenya (Mannah et al., 2014; Bucher et al., 2016) indicate that training TBAs averted maternal deaths, there is a need to re-define the roles and responsibilities of traditional midwives in maternal and neonatal health care during pandemics and in more normal times. Again, viable and culturally respectful TBA training programs must be developed and widely taught, especially given that fact that around 40% of Kenyan childbearers were still choosing to birth with TBAs pre-pandemic. As my interviews showed, traditional midwives themselves admit that, despite being trusted by their communities, there are complications they do not know how to handle. There is also the problem that if TBAs are only called on during crises, and not allowed to attend births under normal conditions, they may lose any skills they have gained during trainings due to lack of practice. Thus I and others strongly suggest that traditional midwives should be fully incorporated into the Kenyan maternity care system and facilitated to attend births in all circumstances. As in other countries, such as Nigeria, Somalia and Ghana (Pyone et al., 2014; Chukwuma et al., 2019; Haruna et al., 2019), Kenya can also provide monetary incentives to the traditional midwives for maternal services referrals and for attending births. Re-training wakunga will not only enhance their knowledge and skills in maternity care and referral mechanisms, but will also lead to greater community acceptance and client satisfaction (Smith et al., 2000; Haruna et al., 2019). For example, Dynes et al. (2013) and Buffington et al. (2021) have shown how TBAs can be trained in the safe administration of Cytotec/misoprostol to stop post-partum hemorrhages and to successfully deal with other birth complications.

CONCLUSION: FUTURE RECOMMENDATIONS

The COVID-19 pandemic is an exceptional event that took the world by disbelief. It has caused the interruption of health services on a global scale, including maternal health services. COVID-19 has spread rapidly in Kenya and has not spared pregnant women. Based on my study findings, I recommend that, as governments alter their healthcare systems to deal with COVID-19 or any future pandemic, they must also act urgently to ensure that mothers and newborns are still able to get the routine and emergency care they need. This includes ensuring that funds for pandemic response go toward efforts to ensure continuity of maternity care, with adequate funding for infection prevention and control supplies and sufficient PPE for maternity care providers, including TBAs. It also includes full training and integration of these traditional midwives—who, again, still attend 40% of Kenyan births—that facilitates them to practice both in normal times and those of crisis. Full integration for TBAs should include allowing them to enter healthcare facilities with their clients and remain with them throughout labor, delivery, and the postpartum period to provide culturally safe continuity of care (see Davis-Floyd, 2003). Referral pathways and transportation must be provided for obstetric emergencies, and hospitals need to be able to properly screen, isolate, and care for infected pregnant women. Guidelines specific to reproductive age and to individual pregnant women need to be developed and effectively communicated to women and to traditional midwives in their own languages. Moreover, motivating traditional midwives using monetary incentives can increase early antenatal and postnatal care use among mothers. In conclusion, again I stress that traditional midwives should not only be utilized in times of crisis, but also under normal circumstances, forming an integral part of Kenya's maternity healthcare system. And for future research, I point to the need for longitudinal studies to explore the experiences of indigent mothers and healthcare providers around access and utilization of maternal health services during COVID-19 and other pandemics yet to come.

ETHICS STATEMENT

The studies involving human participants were reviewed and approved by the Maseno University Ethics Review Committee.

The patients/participants provided their written informed consent to participate in this study.

AUTHOR CONTRIBUTIONS

The author drafted the article, collected the data, analyzed and wrote the manuscript too.

REFERENCES

Bucher, S., Konana, O., Liechty, E., Garces, A., Gisore, P., Marete, I., et al. (2016). Self-reported practices among traditional birth attendants surveyed in western Kenya: a descriptive study. *BMC Pregnancy Childbirth* 16 (1), 1–7. doi:10.1186/s12884-016-1007-8

Buffington, S., Sibley, L., Armbruster, D., Beck, D., Lori, J., Dynes, M., et al. (2021). "Home based life saving skills: working with local leaders and families to prevent maternal and perinatal mortality," in *Birthing models on the human rights frontier: speaking truth to power*. Editors B. A. Daviss and R. Davis-Floyd (London: Routledge).

Byrne, A., Caulfield, T., Onyo, P., Nyagero, J., Morgan, A., Nduba, J., et al. (2016). Community and provider perceptions of traditional and skilled birth attendants providing maternal health care for pastoralist communities in Kenya: a qualitative study. *BMC Pregnancy Childbirth* 16 (1), 1–12. doi:10.1186/s12884-016-0828-9

Chen, D., Yang, H., Cao, Y., Cheng, W., Duan, T., Fan, C., et al. (2020). Expert consensus for managing pregnant women and neonates born to mothers with suspected or confirmed novel coronavirus (COVID-19) infection. *Int. J. Gynecol. Obstet.* 149 (2), 130–136. doi:10.1002/ijgo.13146

Chukwuma, A., Mbachu, C., McConnell, M., Bossert, T. J., and Cohen, J. (2019). The impact of monetary incentives on referrals by traditional birth attendants for postnatal care in Nigeria. *BMC Pregnancy Childbirth* 19 (1), 1–10. doi:10.1186/s12884-019-2313-8

Davis-Floyd, R. (2003). Home birth emergencies in the U.S. and Mexico: the trouble with transport. *Soc. Sci. Med.* 56 (9), 1913–1931. doi:10.1016/s0277-9536(02)00213-7

Davis-Floyd, R. (2018). "Mutual accommodation or biomedical hegemony? A brief anthropological overview of global issues in midwifery", in *Ways of knowing about birth: mothers, midwives, medicine, and birth activism by Davis-Floyd*, Editor Long, R. Grove IL: Waveland Press, p. 265–282.

Delamou, A., Ayadi, A. M. E., Sidibe, S., Delvaux, T., Camara, B. S., Sandouno, S. D., et al. (2017). Effect of ebola virus disease on maternal and child health services in Guinea: a retrospective observational cohort study. *Lancet Global Health* 5 (4), e448–e457. doi:10.1016/S2214-109X(17)30078-5

Dynes, M., Buffington, S. T., Carpenter, M., Handley, A., Kelley, M., Tadesse, L., et al. (2013). Strengthening maternal and newborn health in rural Ethiopia: early results from frontline health worker community maternal and newborn health training. *Midwifery* 29 (3), 251–259. doi:10.1016/j.midw.2012.01.006

Haruna, U., Kansanga, M. M., and Bagah, D. A. (2019). Repositioning traditional birth attendants to provide improved maternal healthcare services in rural Ghana. *Int. J. Health Plann. Mgmt.* 34 (2), e987–e994. doi:10.1002/hpm.2779

Hussein, J. (2020). COVID-19: what implications for sexual and reproductive health and rights globally? *Sex. Reprod. Health Matters* 28 (1), 1746065. doi:10.1080/26410397.2020.1746065

Iyengar, P., Kerber, K., Howe, C. J., and Dahn, B. (2015). Services for mothers and newborns during the Ebola outbreak in Liberia: the need for improvement in emergencies. *PLoS Curr.* 7 (2), 318. doi:10.1371/currents.outbreaks.4ba318308719ac86fbef91f8e56cb66f

Karkee, R., and Morgan, A. (2020). Providing maternal health services during the COVID-19 pandemic in Nepal. *Lancet Global Health* 20, 19–20. doi:10.1016/S2214-109X(20)30350-8

Kenya National Bureau of Statistics (KNBS) (2015). *Ministry of health/Kenya. National AIDS Control Council/Kenya, Kenya Medical Research Institute & National Council for Population and Development/Kenya.*

Kimani, R. W., Maina, R., Shumba, C., and Shaibu, S. (2020). Maternal and newborn care during the COVID-19 pandemic in Kenya: Re-contextualising the community midwifery model. *Hum. Resour. Health* 18 (1), 3–7. doi:10.1186/s12960-020-00518-3

Kumar, N. (2020). COVID 19 era: a beginning of upsurge in unwanted pregnancies, unmet need for contraception and other women related issues. *Eur. J. Contracept. Reprod. Health Care* 25 (4), 323–325. doi:10.1080/13625187.2020.1777398

Mannah, M. T., Warren, C., Kuria, S., and Adegoke, A. A. (2014). Opportunities and challenges in implementing community based skilled birth attendance strategy in Kenya. *BMC Pregnancy Childbirth* 14 (1), 279. doi:10.1186/1471-2393-14-279

Matendo, R., Engmann, C., Ditekemena, J., Gado, J., Tshefu, A., Kinoshita, R., et al. (2011). Reduced perinatal mortality following enhanced training of birth attendants in the democratic republic of congo: a time-dependent effect. *BMC Med.* 9, 1741. doi:10.1186/1741-7015-9-93

McQuilkin, P. A., Udhayashankar, K., Niescierenko, M., and Maranda, L. (2017). Health-care access during the ebola virus epidemic in Liberia. *Am. J. Trop. Med. Hyg.* 97 (3), 931–936. doi:10.4269/ajtmh.16-0702

Ombere, S. O. (2018). Local perceptions of social protection schemes in maternal health in Kenya : ethnography in coastal Kenya (PhD thesis). PhD Thesis. Available at: http://biblio.unibe.ch/download/eldiss/18ombere_so.pdf (Accessed July 18, 2020).

Otieno, G. A., Owenga, J. A., and Onguru, D. (2020). Determinants of maternal health care choices among women in lunga lunga sub county in kwale. *Int. J. Dev. Res.* 5, 76–85. doi:10.37118/ijdr.18779.06.2020

Pant, S., Koirala, S., and Subedi, M. (2020). Access to maternal health services during COVID-19. *Europas. J. Med. Sci.* 2 (2), 48–52. doi:10.46405/ejms.v2i2.110

Phumaphi, J., Mason, E., Alipui, N. K., Cisnero, J. R., Kidu, C., Killen, B., et al. (2020). A crisis of accountability for women's, children's, and adolescents' health. *Lancet* 396 (10246), 222–224. doi:10.1016/S0140-6736(20)31520-8

Pollock, A. M., Roderick, P., Cheng, K. K., and Pankhania, B. (2020). Covid-19: Why is the UK government ignoring WHO's advice? *BMJ* 368 (March), 1–2. doi:10.1136/bmj.m1284

Pyone, T., Adaji, S., Madaj, B., Woldetsadik, T., and Van Den Broek, N. (2014). Changing the role of the traditional birth attendant in Somaliland. *Inter. J. Gynecol. Obstet.* 127 (1), 41–46. doi:10.1016/j.ijgo.2014.04.009

Pyone, T., Smith, H., and Broek, N. V D. (2017). Implementation of the free maternity services policy and its implications for health system governance in Kenya. *BMJ Glob. Health* 2, e000249–11. doi:10.1136/bmjgh-2016-000249

Rocca-Ihenacho, L., and Alonso, C. (2020). Where do women birth during a pandemic? Changing perspectives on Safe Motherhood during the COVID-19 pandemic. *J. Glob. Health Sci.* 2 (1), 1–2. doi:10.35500/jghs.2020.2.e4

Smith, J. B., Coleman, N. A., Fortney, J. A., De-Graft Johnson, J., Blumhagen, D. W., and Grey, T. W. (2000). The impact of traditional birth attendant training on delivery complications in Ghana. *Health Policy Plan.* 15 (3), 326–331. doi:10.1093/heapol/15.3.326

Strong, A. E. (2018). Causes and effects of occupational risk for healthcare workers on the maternity ward of a Tanzanian hospital. *Human Organ.* 77 (3), 273–286. doi:10.17730/0018-7259.77.3.273

Strong, A., and Schwartz, D. (2016). Sociocultural aspects of risk to pregnant women during the 2013-2015 multinational ebola virus outbreak in West Africa. *Health Care Women Inter.* 37 (8), 922–942. doi:10.1080/07399332.2016.1167896

Takemoto, M. L. S., Menezes, M. O., Andreucci, C. B., Knobel, R., Sousa, L. A. R., Katz, L., et al. (2020). Maternal mortality and COVID-19. *J. Matern. Fetal Neonatal Med.* 5 (3), 1–7. doi:10.1080/14767058.2020.1786056

Tang, K., Gaoshan, J., Ahonsi, B., Ali, M., Bonet, M., Broutet, N., et al. (2020). Erratum: Sexual and reproductive health (SRH): A key issue in the emergency response to the coronavirus disease (COVID- 19) outbreak. *Reprod. Health* 17, 5917–5919. doi:10.1186/s12978-020-0900-9

The United Nations Population Fund (UNFPA). (2020). COVID-19 pandemic. Available at: https://www.unfpa.org/covid19 (Accessed September 14, 2020).

UNFPA. (2020). Data from: COVID-19 technical brief for maternity services. Update 1: May 2020. May, 1–55. https://www.unfpa.org/resources/covid-19-technical-brief-maternity-services.

U. N. Women. (2020). The impact of COVID-19 on women. United Nations. Available at: file:///C:/Users/camiv/Downloads/Policy-brief-the-impact-of-covid-19-on-women-en (1).pdf (Accessed April, 21 2020).

Wangamati, C. K., and Sundby, J. (2020). The ramifications of COVID-19 on maternal health in Kenya. *Sex. Reprod. Health Matters* 28 (1), 1804716. doi:10.1080/26410397.2020.1804716

World Health Organization. (2015). *WHO recommendations on health promotion interventions for maternal and newborn health 2015*, Geneva: World Health Organization, 13.

World Health Organization (WHO). (2018). Maternal health. Available at: https://www.who.int/westernpacific/health-topics/maternal-health (Accessed July 18, 2020).

World Health Organization (WHO). (2019). Maternal mortality. Available at: https://www.who.int/news-room/fact-sheets/detail/maternal-mortality (Accessed September 11, 2020).

6

Emergent Change in a Mexican Midwifery Center Organization Amidst the COVID-19 Crisis

Cristina Alonso *[*†], ***Akane Sugimoto Storey***[†], ***Ilse Fajardo***[†] ***and Hannah S. Borboleta***[†]

Luna Maya, San Cristobal de las Casas, Mexico

***Correspondence:**
Cristina Alonso
cris.alonso@gmail.com
[†]*ORCID:*
Cristina Alonso
orcid.org/0000-0002-6845-416X
Akane Sugimoto Storey
orcid.org/0000-0003-3411-1430
Ilse Fajardo
orcid.org/0000-0003-3018-5328
Hannah S. Borboleta
orcid.org/0000-0002-1545-334X

Luna Maya is a Mexican NGO that operates two full-scope midwifery centers in Mexico City and Chiapas, Mexico, providing woman-centered, culturally appropriate midwifery model maternity care on a sliding cost scale. The COVID-19 health crisis has made it necessary for Luna Maya to quickly incorporate safety protocols for out-of-hospital maternity care. Yet many of the emerging guidelines on maternity care have focused on high-income and hospital settings; there are no specific guidelines for such care in out-of-hospital settings in low- and middle-income countries. Thus we have had to create our own, based on best available and emerging evidence. In this article, we describe the guidelines and protocols we have created in response to COVID-19, the international evidence and recommendations on which we base them, and precisely how we carry them out in practice. We also present and analyze the results of qualitative interviews we conducted for this article with eight of our midwives and eight of our midwifery clients. These interviews reveal the tremendous stresses both midwives and pregnant and birthing women are experiencing as a result of the pandemic, their creative adaptations, and the structural flaws, deficiencies, and inequities of the Mexican healthcare system. The article also addresses Luna Maya's ongoing challenges in continuing to provide care completely outside of governmental support and in difficult economic times, and demonstrates the extreme need for improvements in the Mexican system of maternity care and for full integration of community-based midwives and out-of-hospital birth.

Keywords: COVID-19, out-of-hospital birth, midwifery model of care, pregnancy, birth, Mexico, Chiapas, Mexico DF

INTRODUCTION: PLACING CATASTROPHE ON TOP OF A BROKEN MATERNAL HEALTHCARE SYSTEM

The COVID-19 pandemic has highlighted health inequities and systemic gaps and failures (Bambra et al., 2020). Latin America, the most inequitable region in the world (Silva-Peñaherrera et al., 2020), is at the time of this writing (September 2020) home to some of the highest rates of cases (The Guardian, 2020). As a non-governmental and midwife-led organization, Luna Maya operates two midwifery centers (Stevens and Alonso, 2020) in San Cristobal, Chiapas and Mexico City since 2003 to bridge harmful gaps in quality of care and access to midwifery services in Mexico (Alonso et al., 2018). The Luna Maya centers provide full scope midwifery services, both gynecological and obstetric, as well as complementary medicine such as acupuncture, massage, and psychological therapy services. Luna Maya midwives are on staff and provide midwifery care assisted by midwifery students who are learning the Midwifery Model of Care through clinical apprenticeship.

Women who access Luna Maya services are Indigenous, Mestiza (mixed) and foreigners. Services are provided on a sliding scale that enables women of all socio-economic levels to access our services. Payment rates are adjusted by income and subsidized through internal and external funding sources. Women at Luna Maya can choose to birth either at home or at the midwifery center; all other care is provided in the two centers. These two Luna Maya midwifery centers are not integrated into the Mexican healthcare system and therefore rely on private purchasing of equipment and supplies. Similarly, lack of a regulatory body and standards for the practice of midwifery and midwifery centers in Mexico led Luna Maya's midwifery staff to research, apply, test and refine international protocols to protect themselves and those they serve. Midwives hired by Luna Maya have completed a course of study to follow ICM (International Confederation of Midwives) requirements. Therefore, Luna Maya midwives may also be obstetric nurses, general physicians, professional midwives, or midwives licensed in another country.

Midwives have been recognized as specialists in women's sexual and reproductive health (Sakala and Newburn, 2014) and continue to be on the frontlines of providing care during the COVID-19 pandemic, which has exacerbated existing tensions and failures in full access to safe motherhood as seen through a rights-based perspective (Jolivet et al., 2020). In addition, evidence is mounting that pregnant women and other pregnant people are increasingly seeking out-of-hospital (OOH) care out of fear of C-19 infection in hospitals and fear of violations of birthing rights (Davis-Floyd et al., 2020). Nevertheless, in many settings choices are limited and fear of home birth and lack of possibilities to pay out-of-pocket for midwifery services make this option a very complex one for most women and their families. For over 15 years, Luna Maya has provided a safe ground for women to choose safe and respectful birthing options in a country where cesarean rates exceed 50%, and over 30% of women state that they have experienced obstetric violence (Castro and Frías, 2019). Luna Maya has sustained a cesarean section rate of 15% since its inception in 2004 and has been recognized nationally and regionally as providing a safe space for women to recover their strength and power in birth and health care (Alonso et al., 2018).

As a society and as clinicians, we still lack a clear understanding of the spread and impact of the virus, and healthcare providers have been continuously adapting to ever-changing evidence and recommendations. Initial obstetric recommendations focused on in-hospital settings and high-income countries. Slowly, midwifery associations and OOH specialists have developed more relevant protocols. Luna Maya has been continuously incorporating new ways of working within the pandemic, while still providing women-centered and holistic care. With no official guidelines for OOH/community midwives, many international recommendations have been hard or impossible for them to adopt in low- and middle-income countries such as Mexico.

In this article, we explore what Luna Maya's two Mexican midwifery centers have learned, and continue to learn, about how COVID-19 affects women's decisions and wellbeing and how these impact their physiologic and psychological processes (ACNM and NACPM, 2012). We describe how the Luna Maya midwives have engaged in a continuous process of protocol adoption, testing, and revision and explore how relationships between women, their families and their midwives are being modified amidst the pandemic through the analysis of a series of qualitative interviews.

Some protocols are here to stay, at least for a while; others might change in the next few weeks, months and certainly years. Certain protocols and recommendations have been impossible or unrealistic to implement; we will describe why. This article includes reflections on changes that midwives have observed in women's birth experiences, due to the increased stress and hardship brought on by the pandemic and their impacts on women's psychological and physiologic responses. We also analyze the qualitative interviews we carried out with Luna Maya midwives and clients describing the impact of COVID-19 on their perceptions of choices and options for safe and respectful birth.

METHODS

This article is presented in two discrete sections. The first section, based on our practice experiences, describes how the Luna Maya midwives have adapted existing protocols into clinical practice. We harvested clinical guidelines and protocols from online sources, Facebook groups for midwives and email listservs where maternity care providers were discussing and sharing resources on clinical safety and adaptation during COVID. This section describes how our midwives adapted protocols emerging from high-income settings to Mexico City and Chiapas.

The second section provides insight into the experience of adapting to COVID-19 from the perspective of the midwives who work in Luna Maya and consumers of Luna Maya maternal healthcare services. Using a narrative approach, we conducted qualitative interviews to better understand the complexity of the impacts of COVID and the multi-faceted, non-linear responses to the pandemic during pregnancy and childbirth. Although protocols and clinical guidelines intend to provide frameworks for safe care, the lived experience of midwives adapting to providing care are complex and multi-layered. Similarly, women have had to make decisions based on their perceived risk of COVID-19, as well as the implications of social isolation, perception of risk of public spaces and perceptions of autonomy and control within a global pandemic. Therefore, in order to situate how these protocols and guidelines impacted the experience of birth, it was important to carry out qualitative interviews.

In May 2020, we developed two interview guides stemming from a brainstorming session carried out among the co-authors. The interview guides were revised to ensure a comparative approach between the experience of being a midwife and accessing services before and after COVID-19. Due to the semi-structured nature of the interview guides, interviews were adapted according to participant responses.

Midwives and students within Luna Maya were invited to participate through internal communication mechanisms. Participation was voluntary and one student opted out of participating. We interviewed three midwives and five midwifery students during June 2020. All interviews were carried out using Zoom and recorded.

We also carried out semi-structured qualitative interviews using Zoom with eight women who had accessed services at Luna Maya Chiapas and Mexico City during July 2020. Four women were selected because they had chosen to give birth with Luna Maya *regardless* of the COVID-19 pandemic; two had given birth and two were still pregnant. Four other women were selected because they had chosen to give birth with Luna Maya *because* of the pandemic, of whom two had already given birth and two were still pregnant. Two women are low-income, one from Chiapas and one from Mexico City. Five are middle-income women from Mexico City whose income was severely impacted by the COVID-19 pandemic, causing them to make financial adjustments to their birth plans. One interlocutor is a high-income foreigner living in Mexico City, who was already working from home prior to the pandemic and whose income was not affected by the pandemic.

These eight interlocutors were pregnant or had given birth between April and July of 2020; again, participation was voluntary. These women were selected based upon the criteria described above, including access to a telephone or the internet for a Zoom interview and availability during the interview dates. Three interviews were carried out on the phone and five via Zoom. All interviews were recorded and analyzed using an inductive approach to identify themes and conduct discourse analysis.

ADAPTING GLOBAL GUIDELINES TO COMMUNITY MIDWIFERY

COVID-19 was declared a pandemic by the World Health Organization (WHO) on March 11, 2020 (Cucinotta and Vanelli, 2020), yet in Mexico cases remained low and the severity of the outbreak was downplayed. In alignment with other Western countries (Scally et al., 2020), Mexico's strategy was slow to start and marked with inadequacies that were generated in hopes of mitigating economic impact. An international change of tone prompted Luna Maya to begin a strategy as of March 13, two days after the pandemic was declared and lockdown began in Italy, and as global concern was on the rise. Our initial strategy included measures that were concise, holistic and non-alarmist: signs to advise Luna Maya's public about COVID-19 symptoms and preventative measures, increased sanitation, a switch to paper hand towels from cloth towels, and an immune support tonic recommended to clients. Yet it quickly became clear that these measures would need upscaling. Families' economies and local supplies were affected early on. As of March 14th, many informally employed individuals were out of work and panic purchasing made it close to impossible to acquire goods such as cleaning products, sanitizers, soaps, medical supplies, protective gear and paper products; food prices were also increasing. These tendencies were exacerbated outside of Mexico City, the nation's economic and political hub where Mexico's wealth and infrastructure are concentrated. A semi-organized national strategy with stay-at-home recommendations was implemented by the end of March, with large segments of the population already struggling to make ends meet.

As members of clinical staff of Luna Maya, we co-authors have tracked and evaluated evidence-based recommendations and epidemiological trends as of mid-March to create internal guidelines. Immediate sources reviewed included a National Association of Certified Professional Midwives (NACPM) webinar (NACPM, 2020), the USA's Centers for Disease Control and Prevention (CDC) (CDC, 2020c), and scientific and news articles. Additional sources examined over the next weeks and months included items from the Royal College of Midwives (RCM, 2020), the World Health Organization (WHO, 2020a; WHO, 2020c), the International Confederation of Midwives (ICM, 2020), Open Access resources, and supplementary OOH midwifery guidelines and resources (CABC, 2020; Dar a Luz Birth and Health Center, 2020; Harper, 2020). Aside from enhanced screening and distancing, early guidance (CDC, 2020b; WHO, 2020c) did not contain precautionary measures essential for midwives, who serve as the guardians of physiologic care for healthy women and newborns (Renfrew et al., 2014), yet highlighted the importance of continued face-to face care for non-COVID-19 conditions, especially for populations at higher risk of delayed care (CDC, 2020a)—hence reinforcing the urgency of a midwifery scope of practice to keep the childbearing continuum as a normal, low risk health experience.

On March 27, the ICM, (2020) urgently called upon governments to consider midwives' needs, as lack of official guidance translated to lack of PPE allocation for midwives, resulting in otherwise healthy midwives—often with small children and families at home—becoming infected through contact at work and falling ill or dying from COVID-19. The ICM (2020) forewarned the detrimental effects the continued lack of PPE for midwives would have upon the health and wellbeing of women and newborns globally. Midwives have responded by creating their own COVID-19 protocols during the pandemic and have been on the forefront of advocating for superior guidelines that reduce community spread (Tugores and Wiseman, 2020) and include midwives. Now shifting to include midwives' safety, official guidelines (RCM, 2020; WHO, 2020a) are still oriented towards care that is hospital-based and effectively incorporated into healthcare systems, in high-income contexts. As midwifery centers are not integrated into the Mexican healthcare system (Lopez Arellano et al., 2020; Stevens and Alonso, 2020), each center has modified measures for its unique conditions. Unofficial guidelines shared by midwives and midwifery centers in higher income settings have been key in developing our strategy for Luna Maya. What measures Luna Maya has adopted and how we have implemented these measures will be examined in detail below.

Masking

Aside from additional cleaning supplies, face masks were among the first items contemplated for Luna Maya's strategy. For the Chiapas center, many items required shipment, yet it was possible to find local producers of cloth masks, ready for pickup on March 16. Still excluded from official guidance (CDC, 2020b; NACPM, 2020; WHO, 2020a), researchers, midwives, community health workers and the public were already questioning the validity of mask recommendations. Accentuating scarcities, the CDC (2020b) was recommending secured, monitored storage and restricted use of all medical masks, with N95s (WHO, 2020c) for patients with or suspected of having COVID during procedures that might put providers at risk of contact with infectious droplets—uses outside a midwifery scope of practice. Early in the pandemic in Mexico, widespread use of facemasks was undermined by a cultural preference for *not* using them—a preference that carried critical risks (WHO, 2020b).

A few of our midwives expressed unease about spending prolonged hours in close contact with laboring women and family members, prompting Luna Maya to acquire a small supply of disposable medical masks in mid-March for use at births. Even though official recommendations at the time ignored mask wearing, despite evidence gaps, the midwives were clear about the likelihood of respiratory droplet and aerosol dissemination during births and that this could be problematic for them when caring for asymptomatic carriers. Those familiar with birth can easily appreciate the degree of exertion it takes mothers to push babies out and how abundantly splashes and sprays occur with multiple kinds of fluids. In the following weeks, scientific articles began appearing advocating for wide use of non-medical cloth masks and disposable medical masks for all health workers (Abaluck et al., 2020; Greenhalgh et al., 2020; Howard et al., 2020; Tugores and Wiseman, 2020), independent of scopes of practice. By the end of March, Luna Maya was lending cloth masks acquired for midwives to clients during care, and in May began a universal policy requiring mask wearing in both centers for all who enter—despite the fact that Mexico's leading epidemiologist reiterated that this type of measure was inappropriate. Such inadequate recommendations and communications about C-19, especially for vulnerable and historically excluded sectors of the population, have added fuel to the fire of resistance and backlash in Mexico. Corruption-infused entities like national and local governments have historically obstructed participative engagement and community determination at all levels (Mills, 2017). These tendencies are accentuated in Southern areas like Chiapas, where mistrust of the government runs high due to the social and health inequities suffered by Mexico's Indigenous populations. During this crisis, multiple communities in Chiapas underserved by governments have ransacked and set fire to their local clinics, hospitals and ambulances out of fear, desperation and anger towards the incapacity of the government to respond to the pandemic and save lives (Mariscal, 2020; Redacción Animal Politico, 2020). In addition, around the country healthcare personnel have been attacked by citizens fearful of providers being contagious or enraged about loved ones who died from COVID-19 (Garcia Bermejo, 2020; Rivers and Gallon, 2020).

A systematic review and meta-analysis specific to SARS-CoV-2 and COVID-19 published in the *Lancet* (Chu et al., 2020), and a WHO change in guidelines in June, prompted a Luna Maya switch in the type of masks used at births. As community transmission escalated in Mexico, low community alignment with national recommendations, evidence on virus aerosolization through vocalization (Asadi et al., 2020; WHO, 2020d), and possibly elevated prevalence of asymptomatic carrier status during pregnancy (Bianco et al., 2020; Sutton et al., 2020) prompted us to acquire higher-filtration, N95-type masks for Luna Maya's clinical staff to wear during births.

Eye Protection

Another early measure we considered at Luna Maya was eye protection. Though early guidance was non-specific to midwifery (CDC, 2020a), homebirth COVID-19 guidelines shared among community-based midwives in Mexico and the US made casual mention of its use. Purchasing supplies for upcoming months with emergency funds acquired from Global Force for Healing, Luna Maya included protective glasses. Speculative hypotheses about fecal transmission (WHO, 2020d; Zhang et al., 2020), alongside the abundance of heavy breathing and sprays during labor and birth, prompted us at Luna Maya to recommend routine use of eye protection for our midwives during the second stage of labor, when it is challenging to avoid prolonged close contact, fluids and stool. But the initial protective glasses we obtained clouded easily in combination with facemasks, and were deemed impractical in the kind of low lighting that facilitates spontaneous birth. Midwives tested swimming goggles brought from home, also resulting in poor visibility; thus many births were attended without eye protection.

An RCM (2020) PPE infographic seen on social media by our midwives coincided with intensifying community transmission and fatalities affecting families we serve in Chiapas and Mexico City, and motivated our clinical teams to more closely examine their own PPE implementation and make improvements. Face shields were promptly acquired, resulting in better visibility and a valuable barrier from droplets and splashes. WHO research and guidelines (Chu et al., 2020; WHO, 2020a) published shortly thereafter solidified the appropriateness of this measure. As of early June, we have been recommending regular use of face shields in addition to masks while clinical teams or support staff provide care or do cleaning, administrative work, or use non-individual transportation, especially when spacing and air-exchange ventilation are poor. With local supplies now more readily available, some midwives have also acquired safety goggles.

Clothing Changes as PPE: Washing in a Middle-Income Setting

Gowns, scrubs or aprons, akin to those normally used in hospital-based care, are commonly substituted in OOH midwifery practice by clean changes of clothing and attentive personal hygiene. It is known that secretions or droplets carrying SARS-CoV-2 can be expelled from infected individuals and contaminate surfaces and objects (WHO, 2020d), creating fomites (inanimate objects or substances capable of transmitting infectious organisms from one individual to another) with viable particles present for 72 h or more (Chin et al., 2020). How long the virus lives on clothing is unknown; nonetheless our clinical teams agreed that a commonsense measure to reduce fomite transmission would be multiple changes of clothing, reducing the possibility of bringing the virus into Luna Maya or back home. Additionally, between clients bedding is changed and rooms sanitized and ventilated.

Logistics involving water can complicate these protective measures. Water quality has deteriorated after two major earthquakes in 2017 had epicenters close to both Chiapas and Mexico City. Washing machines are common, but hot water washing is not. Propane gas is expensive; thus few homes have hot water connections for laundering. In warmer climates, the families in most homes forgo water heaters altogether, or in areas of less infrastructure, use wood burning options. At Luna Maya we have adapted by using healthy doses of detergent, a disinfectant in rinse cycles, additional time for line-drying (somewhat more complicated during the rainy season) and spacing of at least five days between uses of clothing or bedding. Midwives are welcome to leave worn items inside Luna Maya's washing machines for laundering at the center or bring items home in a plastic bag, preferably sealed for 72 h prior to washing, to minimize dispersal of potentially contaminated particles. Low compliance with frequent clothing changes was becoming blatantly clear, especially at births where there is increased risk of transmission; group review of the RCM (2020) infographic of recommended PPE for obstetric and midwifery care contributed to better awareness about this measure. An additional measure to minimize fomite transmission is that midwives, staff and clients are removing shoes upon entering facilities—slippers have been placed at entrances—and it is recommended that midwives leave births with a fresh pair of shoes. Disinfectant spray is used on all items brought to births or home visits, both before and after, and when possible, washable cloth coverings are used on all surfaces of vehicles used to transport people and items.

Screening and Scheduling Adjustments

Consideration for the local context has been especially necessary for screening and scheduling adjustments. Culturally, pregnancy and birth are considered family events. Our initial screening included asking women to arrive unaccompanied to all visits, yet, since Mexican culture is extremely family-oriented, women continued arriving with partners and other family members. Luna Maya is now asking each woman to limit her companions to only those she considers essential—a single person when possible; safe physical distancing during visits is our goal. This is especially important during births when midwives spend an extended period of time in the family home, and during postpartum visits, as we know that contact has typically been made with extended family. Arriving unaccompanied has been better accepted by women needing only well-woman care. The traditional Mexican greeting with a soft kiss on the cheek and a handshake has been eliminated nationally and at Luna Maya.

At staff meetings, we continually evaluate screening measures to determine their appropriateness; we have added questions about travel, atypical symptoms and contact with suspected cases. Barriers to midwifery care are multifaceted (Lopez Arellano et al., 2020) and the WHO's (2016) optimal number of 8 prenatal visits with providers exceeds what most Luna Maya families currently receive. Reducing and spacing visit days has been more feasible than reducing in-person perinatal contacts, and also provides time to clean, sanitize and ventilate facilities and rotate clothing. This scheduling change to fewer prenatal visits also minimizes days of possible exposure of midwives and staff to clients or while commuting.

Distancing and "Telehealth"

All Luna Maya in-person classes and sessions—yoga, music for kids, childbirth preparation, and information sessions—were suspended immediately and providers offered support to continue online using a Zoom format. Middle- and upper-income families of Mexico generally have access to the internet at home, and either have laptops or smart phones for connectivity. Low income families generally do not have internet access at home but have mobile phones and frequently use WhatsApp for free communications. Therefore, video calls are available for all women seeking care at Luna Maya. We have also offered well-woman care not requiring physical assessment or evaluation online via Zoom or Whatsapp, while bodywork (massage, craniosacral treatments and any other body work), with the exception of acupuncture, has been postponed until it is safer to increase in-person visits. Virtual access has also facilitated access from other regions of Mexico and Latin America but has challenged continuity of care for those lacking a stable connection, electronic devices, or who simply prefer in-person care.

PANDEMIC STRESS: CHANGES IN BIRTH AS A PHYSIOLOGIC PROCESS

We base this section on the themes that emerged from the qualitative interviews we conducted with eight Luna Maya midwives and apprentices. These interviews revealed how our midwives are responding to the increased stress experienced by childbearers while support options remain severely limited. Several midwives expressed concern that the current lack of in-person therapeutic options to alleviate stress-related body and emotional tension added to women feeling alone and may contribute to longer, more difficult labors:

I feel further away. Some women get annoyed because of the safety measures and I try to find how to connect with them in other ways. The safety measures are there to create a barrier and keep people at a distance. They are designed to filter... to keep people out and they can be interpreted as a judgement. Midwifery is warmth, it's being with and close to women. (Luna Maya midwife, San Cristobal, Chiapas)

Both the Luna Maya clinical staff and the larger Mexican midwifery community have noted a rise in abnormal birth patterns, leading to an increase in complications and emergencies. Through social media networks such as Facebook and Instagram, midwives practicing in Mexico both independently and in other birth centers report a greater number of hemorrhages and retained placentas, second stages that last 5 h or more, more babies that need resuscitation or CPR, and stalled labors that require transfer to the hospital—the one place our clients seek most to avoid during this pandemic:

We see the [pandemic] effects before and after birth. The fact that they can´t get together with other moms makes things more difficult. Online support is fine, but the lactation consultants are not providing in-person care. In this context we see longer births, longer second stages, women fully dilated with no descent. During birth mammals need calm to release their baby. (Luna Maya midwife, Mexico City)

There are more post-term births because the babies are there, they have to be born but there is so much worry, there are blockages out of fear that things won't go well and that we have to go to a hospital. That adds more adrenaline. (Student midwife, Luna Maya Mexico City)

Midwives expressed concern that some women may be choosing home birth exclusively out of fear of COVID-19 infection in hospitals and may not be fully prepared for OOH birth. At the beginning of the pandemic, women were switching to homebirth care late in their pregnancies in a context of generalized fear and uncertainty. Our midwife interlocutors noted that all this additional stress profoundly affects women's wellbeing and undermines the foundations of midwifery care:

Some come into care at 37 weeks, so we have to hurry with visits and we don't have time for the childbirth education class, bodywork, and all of that has made it hard to establish a relationship of trust, [so] they make decisions based on fear. We had a bunch of transfers [to a hospital] in May, about 5 or so in a row. In two of them the women were 10 cm dilated... and the baby just wouldn't be born. There is so much additional uncertainty so much stress" (Student midwife, Luna Maya Mexico City)

Transfers to Hospital

During the prenatal process, women receiving care at Luna Maya decide whether they will be transferred to a public or private institution should the need arise. A vaginal or cesarean birth at a private hospital costs upwards of US$1000; thus the decision is often financial. Transfers to public hospitals often include no communication between the midwifery team and receiving medical team. Women are systematically bullied and scolded for having sought a midwife and a home birth; no support persons are allowed. Epidural for pain relief is not an option in public hospitals, where all women are placed on an oxytocin IV with no labor support from staff and are told to lie on their back with no option for movement. Most transfers to public hospitals end in cesareans. Although most such transfers are simply due to failure to progress, they are usually treated as dire emergencies by the medical staff, who often tell women their babies "were about to die" (see Davis-Floyd, 2003; Davis-Floyd, 2018).

In private hospitals, women can be accompanied by their partners and often by their midwife, who meets with the receiving obstetrician to go over case details. The outcomes of private transfers in Mexico City usually include vaginal birth with an epidural and oxytocin augmentation, whereas in Chiapas most transfers end in cesarean.

The transfers mentioned in the quote above were all due to failure to progress. One woman was transferred to a public hospital and had a cesarean birth. The remaining four were transferred to private hospitals and all but one had a cesarean. Due to COVID restrictions, only women´s partners were allowed into the birth setting after the transfer.

Further Pandemic Stressors: The Curtailing of Women's Rights, and Economic Impacts

Our interviews revealed the understanding among our Luna Maya clinical staff that the changes brought on by COVID-19 in maternity care practice are directly related to a world that does not support women and mothers in the first place and even less so during a pandemic. As has been the case during other global crises, women's rights and opportunities are often curtailed in times of instability:

We're seeing more violence against women in the home and everywhere. Families are not prioritizing a respected birth experience but are rather opting for a birth free of charge within the public health system, typically abundant with violence. Childbirth preparation class is also not a priority but covering basic living expenses and rent are. The economic constraints are very real—at the same time it seems absurd that more value is not being placed on out-of-hospital birth right now because it is a much safer option mid-pandemic. (Student midwife, Luna Maya Mexico City)

The collective feeling of stress has also taken its toll on midwives: some of our colleagues or their families have contracted COVID-19, others have anxiety and/or have trouble sleeping. More work—because of women fleeing the hospital—in a stressful situation contributes to faster provider burnout, more clinical errors, more anxiety and less sleep. Our midwives who are also mothers have additional burdens. Children are home from school and workload has increased:

There is tension sometimes. As a mom, I have more work because I spend more time with my daughter, it's a double workload for those of us who are mothers. (Student midwife, Luna Maya Chiapas)

Another important theme that emerged is the dire economic impact on families who, prior to the pandemic, were already low-income and highly vulnerable. In particular, the Chiapas center clientele is 40% Indigenous and depends mostly on informal economy systems such as selling vegetables at the market, odd jobs such as cleaning and construction, and small family agriculture. Already this cohort was unable to pay a minimum fee for services, and Luna Maya Chiapas must rely on income from the Mexico City center and external funding to subsidize services in Chiapas. Unlike some US states (see Davis-Floyd et al., 2020), Mexico has not included community midwifery as an essential service during this pandemic nor does the government subsidize midwifery care, and clients must pay out-of-pocket. Thus midwifery care remains unreachable for many women because even though Luna Maya charges on a sliding scale, many families are unable to pay even minimal fees and thus have to birth in the public hospitals they fear, where care, though often violent and abusive, is free.

WOMEN'S EXPERIENCES OF BIRTH DURING COVID-19

This section is based on our interviews with eight women who were Luna Maya clients. We asked these women about their decision to give birth at home, how COVID-19 had impacted their daily lives and their pregnancy and birth experiences, their support networks and mental health, and their perceptions of the local and national health care system and its response to COVID-19, and received responses addressing all of the above. They also discussed how COVID-19 affected their sense of family and community and what this meant during pregnancy and postpartum, and pondered on the unmet needs of pregnant women in diverse, inequitable and changing contexts and in particular in terms of the capacity of the Mexican healthcare system to meet their needs.

The Decision to Birth With Luna Maya

In the interviews, some women described that the decision to give birth with Luna Maya, at home or at the midwifery center, is often accompanied by previous knowledge of the Midwifery Model of Care and of the reality and outcomes of the Mexican healthcare system, and by the desire to avoid an unnecessary cesarean. As previously noted, Mexico holds one of the highest cesarean birth rates in Latin America, with almost 50% in public hospitals and over 80% in private institutions. Over 30% of women report having experienced obstetric violence (Castro and Frías, 2019). Our interlocutors expressed absolute clarity about their ability to give birth and the benefits of OOH birth, and about the level of safety and the professionalism of our midwives as their care providers. Women who were already suspicious of the national healthcare system confirmed that during COVID-19, their decision to birth outside of the hospital was appropriate and safe:

Birth is instinctive. When we are in favorable conditions, when we feel held, when we feel secure, we can do it. (Georgina, Mexico City)

A second pattern identified was women whose initial plan was to birth in the hospital because they felt safe there, yet sought out Luna Maya, mainly due to recommendations from other women. Learning about our model of care gave them reassurance, security and confidence, and they chose home birth so neither they nor their babies would be exposed to COVID-19 in hospitals:

When all this COVID stuff started, we were going to the Social Security system [IMSS] for care. I went to make an appointment and I saw many elderly people sitting there coughing a lot and got really scared, because I thought I was putting my two-year-old daughter, myself and my baby at risk. That was when I decided to give birth at home as a better choice...It was very valuable and comforting to find Luna Maya, that they'd listen to our particular situation and to be able to be in constant contact. They are always there to help us and they do this job from the bottom of their hearts. (Laura, Mexico City)

That is one of the things that scares me, is going to see a doctor, because you still have to go to the hospital, and they are in contact with patients and other doctors. Of course they are national heroes, but they are also objects of danger. . .I'm sure that there are hundreds of women who are comfortable having their babies in the hospital, but I decided I wasn´t. Pregnant women are a high-risk group, but my mental health was most important. (Carmen, San Cristobal)

When asked about Luna Maya´s Midwifery Model of Care, women highlighted the closeness, the welcoming feeling, the fact that they were emotionally sustained and treated well at all times. They also highlighted the importance of their partners being included, both during prenatal care and the birth and postpartum processes. In Mexico, birth partners are never permitted in public hospitals; during the pandemic, private hospitals varied on the level of accompaniment that was permitted. Women stated that they liked the attention the Luna Maya team gave to their personal circumstances, financial realities, lifestyle preferences, and adjustments due to the pandemic, and our curiosity about how they were holding up in their daily lives. One woman said:

On the day I gave birth, I forgot everything. I threw COVID out the window, I held on to the midwives that were there with me, I don't remember right now if they were wearing facemasks. During labor I experienced it as if there were no COVID, as if they didn't have any protection. They were there, there was physical embrace, there were hugs, I am very grateful for that—that they conserve and make birth possible, the most respected birth possible. (Georgina, Mexico City)

The Effects of the Pandemic

All women interviewed expressed financial hardship due to the pandemic. The most critical situations were cases where women's income depended on activities that were put on hold during lockdown and that, combined with pregnancy and birth, considerably augmented their stress, nervousness, sadness, irritability and above all, fear—a magnified fear that changed their lives radically:

I am worried about when this will end and turn into a different lifestyle—the distance between people, the isolation, the question of how to bring up my daughter in this distance. It will end or more intense things will come. (Laura, Mexico City)

The weight of financial difficulties not only affected these women's stress levels, but also led families to make important lifestyle decisions that impacted daily life and family structure:

The hardest has been the financial side. It has changed us, has altered everything, including something so simple as going to the market. I don't have a job. . . my husband's salary was cut by half. . . . It is hard to make sure that my daughter doesn't touch anything that comes from the outside. We changed as a couple, I was used to being alone and now we spend the whole day together. This family dynamic, and my daughter spending more time with her dad has its benefits, but it's only a little bit of light in the middle of so much complication. Sometimes I just feel really stressed out. (Laura, Mexico City)

Many women are living this process with a generalized unprecedented fear—of getting infected, of infecting their babies and other children, their parents—and fear because they are a vulnerable population. They are constantly questioning themselves as to whether or not the measures applied in their daily lives are enough or if they are exaggerating about avoiding contact with friends and family:

I lived through the transition [of care in Luna Maya before and during COVID]. I felt the difference. My family is far away, the only people with whom I felt understood and held were the midwives. I had a very intense pregnancy with many changes. I was relieved that I could relax and have my emotional needs taken care of. When contractions started and I encountered my midwives with masks, I felt once again that a wall had come up. I thought about the ambivalence, I had to think about being rational and taking precautions but. . . I wished that they could take it off. (Georgina, Mexico City)

Women talked about the fact of living the pregnancy and childbirth process in ways they had never imagined, feeling generally excluded, isolated and without access to a support network. These feelings contrasted with the joys of having a new baby, yet sadness about the impossibility of sharing that joy coupled with additional sadness around C-19 deaths of people close to them:

I have family members who died of COVID. We spent our moment of dreamy bliss to the opposing duality of death. That shook us deeply and filled us with fear. (Georgina, Mexico City)

The theme of individual and collective fear came up in several interviews. Women talked about how the collective situation of mass disease impacted their daily decisions. They articulated the stress caused by the uncertainty and the constant state of alarm in both identifying symptoms in others and the collective fear of each other as potential disease vectors:

I had never experienced fear like that. The first time we went out to vaccinate the baby, I came home and I changed all of my clothes because we had gone to the hospital. Just poking my head out on the street scared me so much, constantly listening to police cars, ambulances. I would get incredibly nervous. Fear was always present. . .This process has been about moving away from fear. (Georgina, Mexico City)

The women spoke of the dichotomy of having more time with their families and themselves, while at the same time feeling inadequate as mothers to protect their children and explain the situation to them. Like so many of us, they tumbled around on the emotional roller coaster of isolation, yet with the added responsibility of going through the massive life transition of welcoming a new baby:

We have a very strange psychology; we keep expecting to get it. My daughter got sick, she had a fever and sore throat, but no other symptoms. We have taken really good care of ourselves. It's really hard to explain to my daughter what is happening and that she can't play with other children. It has affected me. . .there are days where I feel really sad. And there are days where we are dancing in the living room and other days where you feel like. . . when will this day end, or you wake up with a feeling of "these four walls again." One day I wanted to buy something from the supermarket, and they wouldn't let me in. Motherhood is complicated but managing everything we are going through in addition to our pregnancy is complicated and frustrating. There is a roller coaster of feelings. We can do things together, take a [virtual] yoga class or cook. Other days feel completely useless. We have lost certain freedoms. I question everything. This has affected our emotional health as a family. (Carmen, San Cristobal)

Positive Aspects of the Pandemic: Spending Time Together

Just as was expressed in the previous quote, our interlocutors were able to identify the positive aspects of being stuck at home and spending more time with their family. In particular, pregnancy is a time when women often yearn to be more alone and at home, and some identified this as an ideal opportunity for this psychological and physiologic response.

COVID has given us the opportunity to be more connected to nature, to spend time together as a couple and process the pregnancy far from the noise and speed of the city. I would say that what really worried us was the decreased income, but even then, being outside of the city afforded us a more basic and simple lifestyle far from all the stimulus of the city. (Georgina, Mexico City)

I feel very calm. It has helped me very much to be at home. I used to work long hours at a restaurant. My routine changed very much. I can take better care of my diet and sleep. We are really enjoying this pregnancy, we have breakfast and dinner together, we share the same space. . . I've started to prepare the space [for when the baby comes]. (Damaris, San Cristobal)

Negative Aspects of the Pandemic: Isolation From Family and Friends

Mexico, as a Latinx country, relies heavily on family and social networks for meaning and ritual. Mexican women are accustomed to their mother, mother-in-law and close family members interfering, recommending, suggesting things, and caring for them during pregnancy and particularly in postpartum. It is customary for a woman´s mother or mother-in-law to move in with her during the six-week postpartum period to cook, tend to the home and other children and even prepare herbal baths and other rituals. In urban spaces, women have come to rely for support on the friendships made in childbirth education classes or in breastfeeding or childcare groups. Mexican society is highly social and highly family based, valuing the collective good over individual choice. Isolation from family, particularly elders, impacted women's experiences as it deeply challenged the meaning of the rite of passage of welcoming a new family member and the role of certain rituals for caretaking the mother:

COVID stopped us from going to visit my family, and it made me feel very disconnected from those that I love, in a time when everything is so new, during pregnancy. I had felt the calling to be a mother in a certain type of world and COVID broke that world for me, leaving me wondering what will be of tomorrow. (Samantha, Mexico City)

It has affected our access to our support network... My in-laws are high risk. That means we cannot see them because traveling would put us and them at risk. (Anabel, Mexico City)

Women described how their isolation from others affected their emotional health:

Even though I am a person who likes privacy and space, I wanted to share this process, take it outwards and make it very social. I really wanted to experience this with family and friends... I feel like I have to hold things in more, that I have to do so much more, that I'm not being sustained emotionally... it makes me very angry. (Laura, Mexico City)

At the beginning I was going to yoga and childbirth education. I believe that [sharing and] being present with other moms gave us empathy for each other, that support of just going through the same things. With COVID we haven´t been able to have those support groups. As Mexicans we need those groups. I wasn't able to keep in contact with the other moms. I can imagine they feel the same way I do, they feel isolated and we need that in-person support network. Far from feeling taken care of, I feel rejected and excluded. (Carmen, San Cristóbal)

I started to feel the need to go out, to spend time with my family. They come and visit, but they stay on the patio and we talk through the gate. That is making me depressed because we haven't hugged, and my belly is growing and I am by myself. (Damaris, San Cristóbal)

Unmet Healthcare Needs of Pregnant Women

We asked women how their experiences during the pandemic should shape maternal health policy. They agreed on the need to acknowledge and integrate the Midwifery Model of Care and midwives as care providers within the Mexican healthcare system:

[We need] the system to be more open to accepting the Midwifery Model in the healthcare system and for it to be supported with the necessary certifications and that the midwives be acknowledged. That could give us as clients the certainty to make decisions and approach the right people. (Georgina, Mexico City)

They mentioned that there should be separate settings in or out of hospitals for prenatal visits and births to avoid exposing babies and adults to infectious diseases, describing the fear of putting their families at risk by visiting hospitals—a fear that compounds their perceptions of a healthcare system that already ignores the needs of women during pregnancy and birth:

Every woman needs different care, not all women need the same thing, especially during the pandemic. Without the pandemic I think how they treat women is horrible, and during the pandemic they really should have separate spaces for women outside of the hospital, because in general it is very risky to go there. (Alondra, San Cristóbal)

Women were clear in expressing that the pandemic came to exacerbate an already deficient healthcare system that fails to put women at the center of care.

Mexico really doesn't have strategies that are adapted to our reality. They just take what they copy from elsewhere, they don't see the conditions of the majority of the population or of the groups they want to take care of. They are developed by someone who´s neither pregnant nor elderly nor at risk. (Georgina, Mexico City)

I think that more than ever we need psychological support and humanized care for pregnant women and during the postpartum. I think we have also seen that it wouldn't be a bad idea to have separate structures for providing prenatal and birth care. That way they could avoid exposing moms and babies to other risks. And I hope they didn't use this situation to keep up their cesarean section propaganda. They really need to let women have the right to choose how they birth. (Samantha, Mexico City)

Women highlighted that improved support for their pregnancies did not involve more contact or visits with physicians; rather, it centered around the provision of information, connecting with other women, and ensuring emotional support. They stressed that some women have the privilege of accessing emotional support through the internet, but that many pregnant women in Mexico lack this resource:

Especially information, sharing information that it's ok if we feel sad, tired even though I am pregnant, and this should be a happy time. Just letting us know that we might feel this way during the lockdown. Access to the internet has given me a support network to know that other women feel the same way I do. Other things like yoga, meditations... all on the internet, only that has saved us. There are women who don't have that possibility. They should share information, workshops with psychologists, doulas, that we aren't alone. (Damaris, San Cristóbal)

DISCUSSION AND CONCLUSIONS: PANDEMIC-EXACERBATED TENSIONS

As experts in physiologic birth and sexual and reproductive health, midwives understand that these processes work best when they are spontaneous and surrounded by a calm and supportive environment. With the pandemic raging and lockdown encouraged, collective psycho-emotional health has suffered and pregnant women have been forced to add another stress factor to an already complex process. Even under normal circumstances, pregnancy, birth, and the postpartum period are transformational moments and uncertainty, doubts and fear make themselves present along the way. COVID-19 has increased stress levels, worries and anxiety; these increases in stress hormones have shown their impacts on the perinatal experience.

In this article, we have attempted to highlight that in a national healthcare system that for decades has failed to provide women the support needed for a healthy pregnancy—genuine emotional and psychological support and women-centered care—the pandemic has exacerbated these tensions. Midwives and researchers have long noted that birth is more than its medical definition as the extraction of a fetus from a uterus, and that healthcare systems are designed to place attention only on surviving that act. Such systems consistently alienate women and midwives, and establish a basis of mutual fear and mistrust.

For midwives, navigating the pandemic has meant an increased burden on how they do their work and how they navigate work-life balance. Midwives with children now have to figure out childcare during births to which they used to take their children, while providing emotional support in a socially distanced way. Forced to operate outside of the healthcare system, Luna Maya must rely on a fee-for-service pay structure, meaning that with the current economic crisis, our organization is faced with significant financial deficits. Yet we carry on, doing our best to provide our clients with the humanistic, woman-centered care they need, even in the face of a pandemic and a total lack of governmental support.

The call to action brought about by the COVID-19 pandemic has been that recommendations made by public health and clinical experts must be taken seriously and implemented immediately. All over the world, as shown in the other articles in this Special Issue, we are seeing strained systems exposing their vulnerabilities. Maternity health care in Mexico serves as yet another example of exposed vulnerabilities, and places added urgency on the need to build systems that support women's health, wellbeing, community-building and evidenced based care. If the shock and catastrophe of the COVID-19 pandemic does not bring action on decades of cries for improvement and woman-centered care, we may well wonder if anything ever will. We urge all governments and maternity-care-related organizations to seize this revelatory pandemic moment to improve maternity care practices, both nationally and globally.

ETHICS STATEMENT

The studies involving human participants were reviewed and approved by Harvard Chan School of Public Health IRB. The patients/participants provided their written informed consent to participate in this study. Written informed consent was obtained from the individual(s) for the publication of any potentially identifiable images or data included in this article.

AUTHOR CONTRIBUTIONS

CA: Conceptualization, Data Analysis, wrote original draft and revisions AS: Wrote original draft and revisions IF: Conceptualization, data collection, data analysis HB: Contributed to original draft.

REFERENCES

Abaluck, J., Chevalier, J. A., Christakis, N. A., Forman, H. P., Kaplan, E. H., Ko, A., et al. (2020). The case for universal cloth mask adoption and policies to increase supply of medical masks for health workers. *Covid Economics* 5 (5), 147–159.

ACNM and NACPM. (2012). Consensus statement on physiologic birth. Avaialble at: https://mana.org/healthcare-policy/physiologic-birth (Accessed December 20, 2020).

Alonso, C., Danch, A., de López, J. M., and Tryon, J. (2018). "Lessons from Chiapas: caring for indigenous women through a femifocal model of care," in *Maternal death and pregnancy-related morbidity among indigenous women of Mexico and Central America: an anthropological, epidemiological, and biomedical approach.* Editors D. A. Schwartz, New York: Springer International Publishing, 369–384. doi:10.1007/978-3-319-71538-4_19

Asadi, S., Wexler, A., Cappa, C., Barreda, S., Bouvier, N., and Ristenpart, W. (2020). Effect of voicing and articulation manner on aerosol particle emission during human speech. *PLoS One* 15 (1), e0227699. doi:10.1371/journal.pone.0227699

Bambra, C., Riordan, R., Ford, J., and Matthews, F. (2020). The COVID-19 pandemic and health inequalities. *J. Epidemiol. Community Health* 74 (11), 964–968. doi:10.1136/jech-2020-214401

Bianco, A., Buckley, A. B., Overbey, J., Smilen, S., Wagner, B., Dinglas, C., et al. (2020). Testing of patients and support persons for coronavirus disease 2019 (COVID-19) infection before scheduled deliveries. *Obstet. Gynecol.* 136 (2), 283–287. doi:10.1097/AOG.0000000000003985

CABC (2020). Coronavirus (covid-19)—guidance for birth centers. Available at: https://cdn.ymaws.com/www.birthcenters.org/resource/resmgr/covid_resources/CABC_COVID19Guidance_March20.pdf (Accessed December 20, 2020).

Castro, R., and Frías, S. M. (2019). Obstetric violence in Mexico: results from a 2016 national household survey. *Violence Against Women* 26 (6–7), 555–572. doi:10.1177/1077801219836732

CDC (2020a). Coronavirus disease 2019 (COVID-19), healthcare facilities: strategies for optimizing the supply of eye protection, strategies to optimize PPE & equipment. Available at: https://www.cdc.gov/coronavirus/2019-ncov/hcp/ppe-strategy/eye-protection.html (Accessed December 20, 2020).

CDC (2020b). Coronavirus disease 2019 (COVID-19): strategies for optimizing the supply of facemasks. Available at: https://www.cdc.gov/coronavirus/2019-ncov/hcp/ppe-strategy/face-masks.html (Accessed December 20, 2020).

CDC (2020c). Coronavirus disease 2019 (COVID-19) in the U.S. Centers for disease control and prevention. Available at: https://www.cdc.gov/coronavirus/2019-ncov/cases-updates/cases-in-us.html (Accessed December 20, 2020).

Chin, A. W. H., Chu, J. T. S., Perera, M. R. A., Hui, K. P. Y., Yen, H.-L., Chan, M. C. W., et al. (2020). Stability of SARS-CoV-2 in different environmental conditions. *Lancet Microbe* 1 (1), e10. doi:10.1016/S2666-5247(20)30003-3

Chu, D. K., Akl, E. A., Duda, S., Solo, K., Yaacoub, S., Schünemann, H. J., et al. (2020). Physical distancing, face masks, and eye protection to prevent person-to-person transmission of SARS-CoV-2 and COVID-19: A systematic review and meta-analysis. *Lancet* 395 (10242), 1973–1987. doi:10.1016/S0140-6736(20)31142-9

Cucinotta, D., and Vanelli, M. (2020). WHO declares COVID-19 a pandemic. *Acta Biomed.: Atenei Parmensis* 91 (1), 157–160. doi:10.23750/abm.v91i1.9397

Dar a Luz birth and health center (2020). dar a Luz birth and health center position statement and policies regarding COVID-19 Dar a Luz Birth & Health Center. Available at: https://daraluzbirthcenter.org/dar-a-luz-birth-health-center-position-statement-and-policies-regarding-covid-19/ (Accessed December 20, 2020).

Davis-Floyd, R., Gutschow, K., and Schwartz, D. A. (2020). Pregnancy, birth and the COVID-19 pandemic in the United States. *Med. Anthropol.* 39 (5), 413–427. doi:10.1080/01459740.2020.1761804

Davis-Floyd, R. (2003). Home birth emergencies in the U.S. And Mexico: the trouble with transport. *Soc. Sci. Med.* 56 (9), 1911–1931. doi:10.1016/s0277-9536(02)00213-7

Davis-Floyd, R. (2018). "Home birth emergencies in the U.S. And Mexico: the trouble with transport," in *Ways of Knowing about birth: mothers, midwives, medicine, and birth activism by Robbie davis-floyd.* Long Grove IL: Waveland Press, 283–322.

Garcia Bermejo, C. (2020). Más de 200 médicos y enfermeras fueron atacados por el estigma asociado al virus en México. Salud Con Lupa. Available at: https://saludconlupa.com/noticias/mas-de-200-medicos-y-enfermeras-fueron-atacados-por-el-estigma-asociado-al-virus-en-mexico/ (Accessed December 20, 2020).

Greenhalgh, T., Schmid, M. B., Czypionka, T., Bassler, D., and Gruer, L. (2020). Face masks for the public during the covid-19 crisis. *BMJ* 369, m1435. doi:10.1136/bmj.m1435

Harper, B. (2020). *Keeping waterbirth safe during COVID-19.* Waterbirth International. Available at: https://waterbirth.org/keeping-waterbirth-safe-during-covid-19/ (Accessed December 20, 2020).

Howard, J., Huang, A., Li, Z., Tufekci, Z., Zdimal, V., Westhuizen, H.-M., et al. (2020). Face masks against COVID-19: an evidence review. Available at: https://doi.org/10.20944/preprints202004.0203.v1 (Accessed December 20, 2020).

ICM (2020). Urgent call for governments to provide personal protective equipment to Midwives. Available at: https://www.internationalmidwives.org/assets/files/news-files/2020/03/ppe-statement.pdf (Accessed December 20, 2020).

Jolivet, R., Warren, C., Sripad, P., Ateva, E., Gausman, J., Mitchell, K., et al. (2020). Upholding rights under COVID-19: the respectful maternity care charter. health and human rights journal. Available at: https://www.hhrjournal.org/2020/05/upholding-rights-under-covid-19-the-respectful-maternity-care-charter/ (Accessed December 20, 2020).

Lopez Arellano, L., Sanchez Ramirez, G., and Mendoza Cardenas, H. (2020). Professional midwives and their regulatory framework in Mexico Mexican law review. *Mexican Law Review* 12(2), 119–137. doi:10.22201/iij.24485306e.2020.2.14174

Mariscal, A. (2020). (May 29). Pobladores atacan hospital y oficinas en Chiapas; insisten en que Covid-19 "no existe." Aristegui Noticias. Available at: https://aristeguinoticias.com/2805/mexico/pobladores-atacan-hospital-y-oficinas-en-chiapas-insisten-en-que-covid-19-no-existe/ (Accessed December 20, 2020).

Mills, L.. (2017). The limits of trust. Montreal, Quebec: MQUP.

NACPM. (2020). Coronavirus: midwives on the front line. Available at: https://nacpm.org/coronavirus-midwives-on-the-front-line/ (Accessed December 20, 2020).

RCM (2020). PPE: what to wear in maternity care. Available at: https://www.rcm.org.uk/media/4084/ppe-what-to-wear-in-maternity-care.pdf (Accessed December 20, 2020).

Redacción Animal Politico (2020). Habitantes de Chiapas destrozan hospital, queman ambulancia y agreden a personal médico. Animal Político. Available at: https://www.animalpolitico.com/2020/06/destrozos-hospital-chiapas-ambulancia-agresiones-retienen-medico/ (Accessed December 20, 2020).

Renfrew, M. J., McFadden, A., Bastos, M. H., Campbell, J., Channon, A. A., Cheung, N. F., et al. (2014). Midwifery and quality care: findings from a new evidence-informed framework for maternal and newborn care. *Lancet* 384 (9948), 1129–1145. doi:10.46234/ccdcw2020.033

Rivers, M., and Gallon, N. (2020). (April 24). Docenas de trabajadores médicos han sido atacados en México en medio de temores de coronavirus. CNN En Español. Available at: https://cnnespanol.cnn.com/2020/04/24/docenas-de-trabajadores-medicos-han-sido-atacados-en-mexico-en-medio-de-temores-de-coronavirus/ (Accessed December 20, 2020).

Sakala, C., and Newburn, M. (2014). Meeting needs of childbearing women and newborn infants through strengthened midwifery. *Lancet* 384 (9948), e39–e40. doi:10.1016/S0140-6736(14)60856-4

Scally, G., Jacobson, B., and Abbasi, K. (2020). The UK's public health response to covid-19: too little, too late, too flawed. *BMJ* 369, 1–3. doi:10.1136/bmj.m1932

Silva-Peñaherrera, M., Lopez-Ruiz, M., Merino-Salazar, P., Gómez-García, A. R., and Benavides, F. G. (2020). Health inequity in workers of Latin America and the Caribbean. *Int. J. Equity Health* 19(1), 109. doi:10.1186/s12939-020-01228-x

Stevens, J. R., and Alonso, C. (2020). Commentary: creating a definition for global midwifery centers. *Midwifery* 85, 102684. doi:10.1016/j.midw.2020.102684

Sutton, D., Fuchs, K., D'Alton, M., and Goffman, D. (2020). Universal screening for SARS-CoV-2 in women admitted for delivery. *N. Engl. J. Med.* 382(22), 2163–2164. doi:10.1056/NEJMc2009316

The Guardian (2020). Global report: WHO says the Americas are centre of pandemic as cases surge. Available at: https://www.theguardian.com/world/2020/may/27/global-report-who-says-the-americas-are-centre-of-pandemic-as-cases-surge (Accessed December 20, 2020).

Tugores, L., and Wiseman, O. (2020). Should we all be wearing masks? A community midwife's view BMJ sexual and reproductive health blog. Available at: https://blogs.bmj.com/bmjsrh/2020/04/17/midwives-masks/ (Accessed December 20, 2020).

WHO (2020a). *Advice on the use of masks in the context of COVID-19: interim guidance-2, Interim guidance.* Available at: https://doi.org/WHO/2019-nCov/IPC_Masks/2020.4 (Accessed December 20, 2020).

WHO (2020b). *Advice on the use of masks in the context of COVID-19: interim guidance—6 april 2020', Interim guidance,* 5 June 2020. World Health Organization. Available at: https://apps.who.int/iris/handle/10665/332293 (Accessed January 31, 2021).

WHO (2020c). Rational use of personal protective equipment for coronavirus disease (COVID-19) and considerations during severe shortages. Available at: https://doi.org/WHO/2019-nCov/IPC_PPE_use/2020.3 (Accessed December 20, 2020).

WHO (2020d). Transmission of SARS-CoV-2: implications for infection prevention precautions. Available at: https://www.who.int/news-room/commentaries/detail/transmission-of-sars-cov-2-implications-for-infection-prevention-precautions (Accessed December 20, 2020).

Zhang, Y., Chen, C., Zhu, S., Shu, C., Wang, D., and Jingdong, S. (2020). Isolation of 2019-nCoV from a stool specimen of a laboratory-confirmed case of the coronavirus disease 2019 (COVID-19). *China CDC Weekly* 2 (8), 123–124. doi:10.46234/ccdcw2020.033

7

Transitions in Black and Latinx Community-Based Doula Work in the US During COVID-19

Mariel Rivera *†

Department of Anthropology, Syracuse University, Syracuse, NY, United States

***Correspondence:**
Mariel Rivera
mriver02@syr.edu

In response to COVID-19, many doulas, including community-based doulas (CBDs), have shifted to virtual doula work, placing aspects of doula care online. CBDs typically center Black and Brown mothers and come from the same community as their clients, granting access to doula care for many individuals who would traditionally not have access. Two partner CBD organizations in Central New York—Village Birth International and Doula 4 a Queen—transitioned to virtual doula work, continuing to center Black and Afro-Latinx people. As CBDs began to transition their work online, they had to create new ways to include both the community and doula aspects of their work. My research has captured these doulas' experiences since mid-2019 and has documented their transition from in-person doula work to virtual work. This also included their experiences of hosting doula trainings that were originally designed to be held in person. To understand this turn to virtual doula work, in this article I draw on social media engagement, online interviews, Zoom discussions, and personal experience to capture how CBD work shifted to virtual platforms can still center Black and Afro-Latinx folks in their communities and beyond.

Keywords: COVID-19, Doulas, community-based doulas, Black women, Latinx women, New York State

INTRODUCTION

COVID-19 has wholly changed the daily lives of billions of individuals worldwide. The virus carries uncertainties with it: How long will this last? Who will become infected? Will they live, or die? New terms like "social distancing" and "quarantine" have become a part of our daily lexicon as humanity figured out how to address this virus.

Updates and information about the virus and how to protect yourself from it seem to change daily. In the United States, the Center for Disease Control and Prevention (CDC) guidelines and State health departments compensated for the changes demanded by the virus by implementing new safety recommendations in all walks of life. At the beginning of the epidemic, most recommendations were to not gather in large groups, regularly wash your hands, and don't touch your face. These recommendations quickly changed to no gatherings outside of your household and only leaving home for essential items or trips. Then face masks became a necessity for engaging in essential functions outside the home. Birth, doula work, and community engagement have not been immune to the sorts of drastic changes that have come with the virus in the United States and globally.

New York State (NYS) had a rapid onset of COVID-19 cases that threatened to overwhelm the hospital system. Governor Cuomo and the State Health Department took dire measures in reaction to the virus to reduce the spread. There were significant changes in hospital-based maternity care, explicitly limiting the presence of in-person support, which directly impacted doula care. When the new maternal health policies emerged, I was in the midst of my dissertation research in Syracuse, New York, on Black and Brown community-based doulas (CBDs). Through this research, I gained an understanding of the quick adaptations doulas needed to make during a crisis to maintain their work and to express their views on the emerging policies of the local and state-level stakeholders.

Two partner CBD organizations I work with in Syracuse, New York—Village Birth International (VBI), and Doula 4 a Queen (D4Q)—transitioned to virtual doula work, continuing to center Black and Afro-Latinx folks and communities in their practice. As CBDs began to transition their work online, they had to create new ways to include both the community and individualized doula care aspects of their work. My research has captured these doulas' experiences since mid-2019 and has documented their transition from in-person doula work to virtual work. This research included their experience of hosting a virtual doula training, originally designed to be in-person, and activist-based actions related to Black Lives Matter (BLM). The doulas began to implement virtual options for care and hosted "Live" meetings on their platforms. They also extended their social media campaigns and continued their activist engagement.

This research captures how CBD work shifted to virtual work and can still center Black and Afro-Latinx folks in their communities and beyond. To understand this adaptation towards online doula care, I draw on Zoom discussions, online interviews, social media engagements, and on my participant-observation experiences as a doula and activist member of both organizations. From my research, it is evident that guaranteeing that doula care remains accessible to all community members is fundamental to CBDs for moving forward throughout this extraordinary period. However, the doulas also needed to contemplate hospital protocols, state health policies, and their overall safety and that of their clients. Thus these doulas had to negotiate their work within a myriad of elements amidst a global health pandemic.

THE BLACK DOULAS OF SYRACUSE

Doulas are non-medical support people and have historically been seen at births around the world, usually as family members or knowledgeable community members (Campbell-Voytal et al., 2011). Contemporaneously, a doula is defined as a person who delivers non-medical support to an expectant mother before, during, and after birth. The support provided can include assisting the pregnant person to create a birth plan, breastfeeding counseling, perinatal information, and constant labor encouragement (Gordon et al., 1999; Chor et al., 2016). Continuous labor support has numerous benefits physically and emotionally for birthing people (Hodnett et al., 2013; Steel et al., 2015; Bohren et al., 2017). Doula-supported birth has been proven to reduce cesarean delivery (Chor et al., 2016; Toonen, 2018); improve breastfeeding (McLeish and Redshaw, 2018); decrease the use of pain medication (Gordon et al., 1999; Jordan et al., 2008); decrease labor time (Scott et al., 2000), and increase women's overall satisfaction with their birth experiences (Thomas et al., 2017). For Black and other marginalized peoples, doulas can also help to overcome maternal health inequities and barriers while supporting a woman in having a safe and positive birth (Gruber et al., 2013; Haderman and Kozimannil, 2016). Generating more knowledge about doulas, especially doulas of color who work with Black and other marginalized peoples, is essential to understand the practice of doulas and to filling the literature gaps (Bohren et al., 2017).

Many Community-Based Doulas (CBDs) utilize a Reproductive Justice (RJ) framework within their practice, created by Black women and other women of color designed to center their lived reproductive experiences (Ross, 2017). The framework, created by Black women in the United States to talk about their reproductive experiences, goes beyond reproductive rights. The framework centers the right not to have a child, the right to have a child, and the right to parent that child, as well as sexual autonomy and gender freedom (Ross et al., 2017). In this way, RJ broadened the scope of reproductive rights. The creators of this framework wrote that RJ "created a radical shift from 'choice' to 'justice' to locate women's autonomy as a self-determination in international human rights standards and laws rather than in the constitutionally limited concepts of individuals rights and privacy" (Ross et al., 2017:18). Consequently, RJ looks past the legal paradigm of reproductive rights to eliminate all reproductive freedom barriers, from social to economic. Many CBDs are Black women or other women of color, often live in the same community as their clients, and position their work to target maternal health disparities (Ross and Solinger, 2017).

Black women in the United States confront discrimination, both implied and overt, often leading them into a birth environment in which they are vulnerable and which contributes to adverse maternal health outcomes (Adams and Thomas, 2017). Currently, Black women are three to four times more likely to die perinatally than white women and face higher instances of maternal morbidity and prematurity (Center for Disease Control and Prevention (CDC), 2020). Generally, to combat these negative maternal health outcomes, CBDs separate their work from other kinds of doulas in particular ways. CBD work includes "all of the services that private doulas offer, and adds additional home visits and a wider array of services. . .CBDs have additional training that supplements the traditional doula education curriculum. Care provided is low or no cost and is grounded in safe, dignified and respectful access to health care" (Bey et al., 2019:9). Therefore, CBDs' work maintains one-on-one support during pregnancy, birth, and the postpartum period and participates in broader community-oriented public health programming.

I work with two interrelated organizations in Syracuse—VBI, run by women of color, predominately Black women, and D4Q, a related CBD organization founded by a Black woman. These two CBD organizations employ an RJ framework and connect doulas to women who face social, economic, and medical oppression, tailoring their efforts towards Black women (Village Birth International (VBI), 2019a). Sequoia, the founder and a doula with D4Q, explained that "doula work means Black liberation. . .birth work [for us] isn't just about the nine months, or the six weeks postpartum. It's about the longevity of Black life." In this way, birth work for these doulas bring together prenatal and labor support, advocacy, and activism, demonstrating the RJ framework that is apparent in their doula practice. From my positionality as a woman of Puerto Rican and Dominican descent, I felt compelled to engage with work geared towards ensuring equity in maternal health care.

The CBDs value making doula services accessible for all, regardless of financial compensation. They have specific outreach for individuals who cannot afford doula services, such as offering sliding payment scales or “scholarships” that cover the entire cost. Parity varies: some birthing mothers have previous births, and for some, this is their first. These CBD organizations offer expectant women four prenatal meetings, birth plan counseling, uninterrupted labor support, and two postpartum visits without charge. In general, doulas practice in hospitals, birthing centers, and at home births. VBI and D4Q doulas attend births only in hospitals due to the absence of homebirth midwives in the Syracuse region. These organizations are affiliated with 10 community doulas, including myself, and are in the training process with others.

Through these organizations, women from the Syracuse community can learn about critical resources in the community, identify a doula for their own birth, and go through doula certification if they wish. Overall, CBD practice centers Black mothers and families in one-on-one care and within broader community efforts.

Community-based public health outreach is an integral part of both organizations’ work. Thus, VBI and D4Q are committed to creating programming within and for the city of Syracuse. Syracuse demonstrates similar demographics as the rest of the country; it is an urban, mid-sized city with five hospitals (Onondaga County, 2016). Historically, vast inequalities have persisted in the Black community of Syracuse. The historical legacy of this segregation marks Syracuse with patterns of low birthweight (Lane et al., 2008); gun violence (Larsen et al., 2017); disproportionate rates of incarceration for Black men (Keefe et al., 2017); and food deserts (Lane et al., 2008). Asteir, a founding doula of VBI, emphasized that the health "disparities are based in a history of oppression and racism." Due to these continued health disparities in the Black community, the CBDs place significant emphasis on broad public health work. This broader community outreach includes programs such as the Black Healing Expo, which brought Black health experts together with the community. For these doulas, to have healthy Black mothers and families, doula work needs to operate not only during pregnancy, labor, or postpartum but also throughout the broader community.

In doing this work, both VBI and D4Q have remained autonomous, relying on grant funding with some individual payments from clients and community fundraising. They do not get reimbursed by Medicaid, and were critical of the proposed NYS beyond the Medicaid-reimbursement bill and certificate policies put forth last year (New York State (NYS), 2019). The Medicaid reimbursement bill was planned to allow enrollees of Medicaid fee-for-service and Medicaid Managed Care to have their doulas paid directly through the state and included standard doula practices for each doula to follow (New York State (NYS), 2019). Moreover, Assembly Bill A364B was introduced into the New York State Senate that looked to positively sanction specific doulas based on their state-regulated certification. The bill explicitly outlined the perimeters for certified doulas, including a fee, and only permitted certified doulas to provide doula services (New York State Senate (NYSS), 2019). Governor Cuomo ultimately vetoed the bill.

The CBDs had specific objections to how doulas became recognized by the state and to what they viewed as constraints to their practice. Specifically, these constraints included licensing fees, unknown curriculum for certification, and general state regulation of doulas. VBI published an open-letter critique of the bill, which stated, "The regulation and restriction of all doulas in NY State, and implementation of certification policies without incorporating community-based doula models, erase not only this legacy but the potential to save lives and support families with the dignity and culturally sensitive reproductive care they deserve" (Village Birth International (VBI), 2019b). It is evident that the regulation and certification policies put forth by state representatives are troublesome to existing CBDs. The history of the CBDs opposing NYS doula regulation is vital to understanding how VBI and D4Q reacted to NYS health policies in response to COVID-19.

The coronavirus left much CBD work in limbo because of the necessary restrictions on face-to-face interactions. CBDs developed new concerns about Black women’s health, state regulation, and hospital policy in response to the virus’s spread. Thus, just like the rest of the world, VBI and D4Q had to form immediate responses to COVID-19, starting with their bi-annual training held during mid-March of 2020.

METHODOLOGY

I have worked with VBI and D4Q since 2018. During this time, I have attended and assisted in teaching childbirth education classes, observed client meetings with doulas, witnessed doulas’ support of laboring parents, attended births and participated in birth activism. Between March 13th and May 15th, I collected data through interviews, virtual participant-observation, and social media cataloging. The interviews were semi-structured, open-ended, and guided by three main questions: How has COVID-19 influenced doula work? How have COVID-19 hospital/public health policies impacted doula work? What do doulas need to work in person safely? Because of the rapid nature of the interviews and the limitation of COVID-19, I only interviewed six doulas for approximately 1 h each. Informed consent was previously obtained from all doulas as well as permission from the organizations to collect data during events. The virtual participant-observations took place on Zoom or FaceTime during doula planning meetings, childbirth education courses, and doula trainings. I virtually attended four trainings, three meetings, and three childbirth education classes. The social media cataloging took place on Facebook and Instagram and included engaging with ‘Live’ on the platforms. I obtained ethical approval from Syracuse University, IRB #19-231.

All qualitative data including fieldnotes, interviews and social media posts from mid-March until August was coded for thematic elements. Through coding, the themes of the doulas' immediate responses to COVID-19, public health guidelines, clients, community needs, and the future of in-person services emerged. My discussion of the findings below begins by discussing the immediate responses to COVID-19, then considers what the doulas themselves highlight as a need for re-starting in-person services. This research looks to add to the small but growing body of literature on doulas.

IMMEDIATE RESPONSE TO THE VIRUS

The onset of the coronavirus coincided with my dissertation research on these two Community-Based Doula (CBD) organizations. The beginning of March 2020 was a busy time for both organizations as there was a training planned for new doulas. During planning for the training, Asteir stressed that an essential part of becoming a doula is passing on your knowledge and creating a doula community. Every training is slightly different as new experiences occur, further information is released, and new techniques are shared. I assisted in organizing specific material for each weekend of the training, such as the Black Mamas Matter toolkit (Black Mamas Matter (BMMA), 2018), which consisted of a human rights-based approach to reproductive health for and by Black women. The training materials included discussion topics, events, films, and guest speakers. The majority of women who attended the training identified as Black, are mothers, and live in the Syracuse community. These women usually have ties to existing doulas trained by and working with VBI or D4Q doulas; some have been doula clients. Thus, many trainees come in with specific connections to doula work and reasons why they desire to become a doula in Syracuse working with Black women.

The doula training began on the first weekend the virus took hold in NYS—Friday, March 13th to Sunday, March 15th. Twelve trainees, two educators, and I spent the weekend in the community center in the Southside of Syracuse. Throughout the first cold and dark March evening, a "Welcome Dinner" took place to encourage participants to become familiar with each other. Talk about the virus sprinkled in with the usual small talk and introductions. Asteir, the lead trainer, discussed the decision to continue or postpone with the group. Most seemed adamant that they were not worried about the virus in such an intimate group and wanted to continue the training. Some cited that they could not take off more time for work if the days changed, as most had full-time jobs. At this point, we did not fully understand how the virus would alter life. So we continued for the remainder of that cold March weekend. I listened to discussions about labor stages with images that represented Black women, made rice socks with lavender (hot packs) with the trainees, and conversed about their motivations to become doulas. Attending this doula training was one of the last pre-COVID-19 experiences I had. Within a few days, the world and its outlook on the coronavirus had changed drastically. NYS had become an epicenter in the United States, and Central NY began to see cases and deaths related to the virus. Due to this situation, the doulas postponed the second weekend of training as they adapted the material virtually and rescheduled specific aspects, including planned guest speakers. Thus, this potential new cohort of doulas had to delay the completion of training and were unable to attend and support births in person.

During the beginning of COVID-19, the CBDs, like other birth workers in NYS, became worried about the state of maternal health, particularly for Black women. Some hospitals in the pandemic epicenter NYC would not allow pregnant women to bring labor support companions, forcing these women to labor alone (Davis-Floyd et al., 2020). Specifically, in mid-March 2020, New York-Presbyterian and the Mt. Sinai Hospital System briefly barred all visitors, including partners, in their labor and delivery unit after discovering that multiple pregnant and postpartum patients had COVID-19 (Hafner, 2020). Human rights and RJ advocates sounded the alarm, fearful that other hospitals would follow suit, and insisted that hospitals allow at least one support individual for birthing people. Due to the outrage, Governor Cuomo swiftly signed legislation to allow one support person for laboring women (van Syckle and Caron, 2020). However, there was a growing fear of hospital births because of possible virus exposure. Some CBDs pointed to a case in Syracuse's neighboring city, Rochester, where a man was not honest about being symptomatic so that he would be allowed to visit his wife in the maternity ward. Shortly after giving birth, his wife also began showing symptoms, and it was then that the husband admitted he was symptomatic. This incident prompted preventative protocol: all visitors must now be temperature-checked twice daily, and everyone must wear face masks (Burke, 2020).

Soon, hospital birth began to seem higher risk than a home or birth center delivery because of its unknown and invisible dangers. This potential risk of hospital delivery was particularly problematic for the Black community, who, as previously noted, already suffered from higher maternal mortality and morbidity rates than their white counterparts. The virus exacerbated an already flawed maternal health care system for Black and Brown women. Since the start of COVID-19 in NYC, the CBDs pointed to several cases where Black women or infants suffered preventable deaths. One such woman was Amber Isaac, who tweeted concerns on April 17th about her maternity care after doctors did not communicate the outcome of her bloodwork for declining platelet count (Olumhense, 2020). On April 20th, Isaac learned she had HELLP syndrome, which complicates pregnancy, was induced a month early, and ultimately passed away on April 21st following her child's cesarean delivery (Olumhense, 2020). Another woman, Chrissy Sample, lost one of her infant twins at 24 weeks because she could not get an in-person appointment (Bobrow, 2020). Sha-Asia Washington died after being pressured to receive an epidural, which was not appropriately administered (Dickson, 2020). The CBDs discussed how these examples could quickly occur in Syracuse due to the restrictions on in-person support. One Black doula noted, "I think [COVID-19] is greatly impacting [Black maternal health] because it is limiting the amount of people that can be in the laboring room. And for me, more people is more witnesses." Consequently, the CBDs noted their concern for their Black clients and overall community due to the COVID-19 regulations in NYS.

Indeed, CBDs discussed their clients' and other community members' interest in home birth or some other out-of-hospital (OOH) option. Nationally, the COVID-19 pandemic has motivated examinations into hospital birth's safety compared to OOH or "community births" at home or in freestanding birth centers (Davis-Floyd et al., 2020). On a state level, there was interest in accommodating non-hospital providers to take on more clients (New York State (NYS), 2020). However, there are few OOH options in Central New York, as only a few midwives practice outside the hospital, and those were quickly flooded with calls for their services. Sequoia, who is also in nursing school, discussed the lack of midwives in the Syracuse area, stating, "When we're thinking about COVID-19 a lot of people are like 'I want to have my babies at home...The issue is that we don't have a lot of homebirth midwives in Syracuse. We don't have *any* Black homebirth midwives in Syracuse." The lack of Black and Brown midwives, and the small number of homebirth midwives in general in Syracuse makes community birth inaccessible to most Black and Brown people.

Other concerns stemmed from the fact that Black and Brown communities have faced more financial and medical losses due to COVID-19. Many point out that such communities have poorer health outcomes in general; Asteir, who is also a mother of three, summarized her take: "[COVID-19] certainly exacerbated the crisis of mortality and illness in Black and Brown communities. But I think for Black people specifically, COVID-19 feels like something else." In other words, COVID-19 exacerbates pre-existing inequalities and health disparities in communities that already face tremendous systemic oppression, specifically within Black maternal health.

As a result of COVID-19, many doulas have turned to virtually supporting their clients to protect themselves. A CBD doula commented that "a bunch of Black doulas were like we're not that essential. Like we're not essential enough to be risking our lives." In other words, the doulas understood they had to balance their own safety with the needs of their clients during COVID-19. As Black CBDs, they acknowledge the importance of their work with the Black community and the risk of COVID-19 to that same community's health. In the midst of the pandemic, the care and treatment of Black and Brown mothers remained centralized within these organizations. Through their doula care, the CBDs not only assessed what barriers they faced in delivering their care but also the barriers of their clients, fellow doulas, and greater community.

Going Virtual

In response to hospital and state policies excluding them from the birthing room and to their own need for safety, many CBDs have begun to offer free virtual services, including prenatal, labor, and postpartum support. They have maintained activist engagement, have extended social media campaigns, and have continued dialogue online through "Live" on Facebook and Instagram to interact with followers. Another way in which the doulas reach their community and birthing clients is through free virtual childbirth courses.

Without initial approval or support from the state or hospitals to continue in-person doula care, virtual engagement became necessary. The CBDs began providing virtual doula support that ranges from being as simple as explaining specifics about infant health, or as significant as virtual labor coaching. VBI hosted a virtual training, offering guidance to many existing doulas who did not know how to provide virtual doula care. Through an Instagram post discussing the training, VBI stated:

> We must ensure that the values of birth justice and human rights in childbirth are upheld and respected in the way pregnant people and their families are treated during this pandemic...Perinatal health disparities that impact the Black community do not disappear during a pandemic. They are further illuminated.

It is evident from this statement that the training would emphasize their overall mission to support Black and other marginalized pregnant women. The Zoom-based training event taught 15 doulas various fundamentals about offering doula care and support virtually. Every doula taught can mean dozens or ultimately hundreds of women served.

An additional essential effort I witnessed was the CBDs' creation of virtual childbirth classes. They made a monthly series featuring four different topics for each class and CBD Sequoia delivered them via Zoom. The topics were the stages of labor, medicated and unmedicated comfort measures, breastfeeding, and postpartum care. During the first class, about 10 attendees joined with their partners, by themselves, with their families, in their living rooms, kitchens, bedrooms. By the end of the class, there were still topics to discuss, and many asked Sequoia to send the slides via email. Sequoia later reflected during our interview on the virtual childcare classes, stating, "I think it being online just eliminates. . . potential barriers, so more people are willing to attend." Indeed, each class that followed had a more extensive and larger presence, with about 20 individuals signing up by the final class—double the amount in the first one.

Another significant portion of the CBDs' virtual doula work focused on Black Lives Matter (BLM) and how this social movement connected to their work. This activist point of view was essential to include because it aligns with their Reproductive Justice (RJ) approach. I asked Sequoia to expand on that notion; she said, "There's been a lot of momentum around holding individual cops accountable and systems accountable. And I'm like we need this same type of energy around RJ and birth justice because we're losing too many Black moms, too many Latinx moms, too many people to preventable deaths. . . that's why we have to be thinking about how all these systems are connected." Consequently, CBDs attach great importance to advocacy and activism because these connect to Black peoples' overall endurance. Committing to this BLM movement was central to CBD work regardless of the pandemic, as this movement directly influences the Black lives of their community.

In facing the challenges generated by the pandemic, the CBDs virtually maintained this cornerstone activist component of their work. Following the police killings of George Floyd, Breonna Taylor, and Ahmaud Arbery, BLM protests of all forms sprang up throughout the nation and internationally. Both organizations posted multiple times and held campaigns in solidarity with this movement. In a social media post, D4Q captioned a photo of these three most recent victims of racism; the caption read,

"When Black parents are scared to birth Black kids into an anti-Black society, one must understand how police violence is also a reproductive justice issue. . .we will proudly proclaim that Black Lives Matter!" In other words, the CBDs view their RJ approach to doula care as tied to the BLM cause of Black liberation and equity. Therefore, creating a virtual doula practice that makes space for BLM's discussion is significant to the CBDs and how they frame their work. This inclusion of BLM is significant as it demonstrates the connection the CBDs make between their RJ-centered doula care and the larger discussions happening in their community.

THE FUTURE OF IN-PERSON DOULA CARE

After the initial virtual response to COVID-19, the CBDs were critical of how both NYS and specific hospital decisions directed the experience of birth and the CBDs' ability to care for their clients. The doulas shared apprehension that the policies to mitigate viral transmission would adversely affect maternal health experiences and outcomes for Black and other marginalized communities. I attended virtual meetings with CBDs, where there was discussion about a concern for "unnecessary inductions," "increased C-sections," and "rushed postpartum experience." Overall, the CBDs' concern was that Black women face discrimination in healthcare settings even under normal circumstances, and this was exacerbated as the pandemic placed more stress on and gave more power to medical professionals. Sequoia described the frustration with current policies: "I've heard from quite a few Black women that the doctor's office only allows *them* to go in. So their doula can't go, their partner can't go. They have to wait in the car and FaceTime. So it's limiting the amount of witnesses and support that a person can have leading up to their delivery." In other words, there is a concern that Black women, who already face adverse maternal health outcomes, will not receive the proper support, which in turn could negatively impact their birth outcomes. For many Black women, this support is crucial to achieving positive maternal health outcomes.

In April 2020, Governor Cuomo assembled a task force to create maternal health care recommendations during COVID-19 (New York State (NYS), 2020). This task force recommended permitting doulas in addition to a personal support person into the birthing room. This official acknowledgment of doulas was a significant moment for all doulas in NYS, as the language of the recommendations described doulas as "essential." While these state recommendations were certainly an improvement over the prior lack of consideration, the doulas still had apprehensions because, ultimately, the hospital had the authority to approve or decline a doula. The CBDs critically discussed the phrasing of the recommendation: "Exceptions should be made only in limited circumstances and based on clinical guidance, such as availability of [Personal Protective Equipment] PPE" (New York State (NYS), 2020). Many of the doulas view this as concerning because "decisions were in the hands of hospitals, not families." In other words, individual hospitals could have significant power in allowing or dis-allowing in-person doula care for specific patients, depending upon their ability to provide proper PPE.

Furthermore, many of the doulas criticized the contrast in the recommendations to admit doulas into maternity wards. On the one hand, the recommendations distinctly indicated that "doulas are considered an essential part of the support care team" (New York State (NYS), 2020). On the other, there was no recommendation about securing their entrance into hospitals or guaranteeing PPE. This lack of support was not unusual for the doulas, as they had long seen interest but no real commitment from local or state governments.

In discussing their specific concerns about the recommendation, the doulas were troubled by the barriers this lack of clarity may create. Asteir noted during our interview, "Why is it that in these three hospitals, doulas can't get in? Now they are saying that you need to show your certification if you show up for a birth. So I'm this person's support person and I have to validate myself with a certification that you really don't even honor." Sequoia agreed with this assessment, saying, "There is still a barrier because you have to quote 'prove' that you are a certified doula. . .it's still that barrier of regulating who is a doula." In other words, the "proof" necessary to demonstrate that they are indeed certified doulas is a barrier for CBDs because there is an implication of regulation on who is an "official" doula. Thus, this is an obstacle for CBDs because they may need to validate their position as a doula to the hospital that may decide anyway to reject or discriminate against them.

Shortly after the statewide policy changed to allow doulas in the birth room, VBI and D4Q contacted a local labor and delivery nurse to host a question-and-answer session with the CBDs. The meeting was held on Zoom with 10 local doulas, allowed the nurse to provide insight into how doulas could affect their clients during labor, and gave the doulas the ability to ask questions, such as: How does the COVID-19 policy affect the birth experience? Have any doulas been present? What can a doula do to assist virtually? It was evident during this session that the doulas were concerned about whether or not the hospital would permit the doula's presence and how they could ensure that they would be allowed to support their client. The nurse answered from her perspective, suggesting having the client inform her doctor and the maternity floor of her desire to have a doula present. The nurse emphasized the various factors that may influence the acceptance of doulas, such as the attending physician, the nurses on staff, and PPE availability. She noted that, to her knowledge, PPE was "limited but available" for doulas at her hospital.

Unfortunately, due to the limited amount of PPE at most hospitals, the doulas do not feel they can safely offer in-person care due to the close physical nature of continuous labor support. Asteir summarized the doulas' perspective, saying, "There is so much more that needs to get done if you are going to make statements like 'doulas are essential'." Sequoia echoed this response, "Where is the conversation that's matching the risk?... We need no strings attached to funding but if we're not going to get it, PPE would be great." Many doulas can provide PPE for themselves, such as face shields, gloves, and cloth or disposable face masks. However, unless provided by the hospital, the doulas do not have access to medical-grade PPE, namely 95-masks, which significantly prevents the spread of COVID-19 during close contact. For Sequoia and the other doulas, the money that the state has proposed to support the doulas carries regulations from the state and does not entrust the money to organizations that have been working towards bettering the community. Indeed, the doulas commented that this is why community support and fundraisers are crucial for their work. Their words validate the lack of structural support in NYS that these CBDs are experiencing. Both women plainly stated their need to see real investment, whether monetarily, through ensuring PPE availability, or both, in committing to in-person doula care. Of course, COVID-19 is still a risk factor. Without vital structural support, many CBDs will not operate in-person.

Two other concerns for the NYS mandate are related to the partner's attendance and the doulas' personal lives. One doula discussed the stress some expectant mothers face if their partner cannot attend the labor and birth for the entire duration. NYS and other states do not allow support people to return once they have left. This can become a major stressor for both doulas and clients. One doula said, "If their partner has to work, I know that this was one issue with a lot of people. They were like I know my partner can be there, but they might not be able to be there three, four days that I'm gonna be in the hospital." Thus, there is still a fear that Black and other marginalized women may be giving birth and experiencing the postpartum period unsupported. For doulas, personal life concerns during COVID-19 include worries about their own children. Sequoia mentioned that "with COVID-19, it's like if you are a doula who had kids, you usually can just find a babysitter and go to your birth, but now it's like, is it safe to send your kids somewhere while you go support this mom?" Gaining in-person access to hospitals still leaves doulas facing the risk of infecting themselves or their loved ones. To be willing to accept this risk, the CBDs emphasize their need to have real investment from NYS showing that its officials believe in and promote doula work. Without this kind of concrete support from the state, CBDs do not feel that they can provide in-person doula care. Instead, their doula work, from individualized birth support to activist engagement, will continue online and will monitor the ability to practice in person.

For these doulas, virtual doula care in terms of continuous labor and delivery support is complicated. Most of the doulas have noted that they provide online prenatal and postpartum support with communication during delivery through assistance from their support partner via video-calling, texting, or phone calls. Sequoia noted that for doulas "supporting labor without [physically] being there is hard because that in-person part is key." Instead, some of the doulas discussed their role during virtual labor support as guiding the support person present in the labor room. In this way, the doulas help coach the support person to fill in as a surrogate doula, give them advice on breathing methods, answer questions, or remind them of the massage techniques they had learned. Many of the doulas noted they used a smartphone to communicate with their clients during labor, but the clients did not always desire it. A doula with an upcoming birth told me that the expected "parents know to text or facetime me or whatever, when they want to talk or ask questions. . .but who wants to stay facetiming when you're having a baby?" In this vein, it is evident that continuous virtual labor support may not be convenient or wanted by the expected parent, so they will only engage with the doula when they see fit. Thus, the doulas remain flexible depending on the needs or barriers of their community, clients, hospitals, and state guidelines.

CONCLUSION

As a result of the COVID-19 pandemic, doulas have had to change their practices to keep themselves, their clients, and their communities safe. Thus, virtual doula practice has grown, with organizations like VBI, D4Q, and many more ensuring continual support. The interruption of in-person interaction did not diminish the D4Q or VBI doulas' motivation. Instead, they moved their work online and continue to provide virtual services, including monthly childbirth classes, while remaining vocal on activist issues that influence their communities and their clients. With some clients looking for out-of-hospital birth options, in the future doulas may be more able to operate outside of a hospital setting. This possibility may present new challenges but ultimately may have fewer barriers than the current hospital system under COVID-19 restrictions for CBDs. It remains to be seen how this system will change once the COVID-19 vaccine is widely available.

Despite the many barriers for CBDs in NYS, these two organizations navigated the obstacles to deliver RJ-based care that centers the need of the Black and Brown community in the city of Syracuse, specifically birthing mothers. As NYS cases of COVID-19 maintain a downward trend, CBDs may decide to re-initiate doula care in-person; yet the virus's course and the coming vaccine availability, along with local hospital and NYS restrictions, will ultimately weigh on the conclusive choice to re-start in-person doula work. Until then, VBI and D4Q will continue to reach their community and clients safely, virtually.

ETHICS STATEMENT

The studies involving human participants were reviewed and approved by the Syracuse University Institutional Review Board. The patients/participants provided their written informed consent to participate in this study.

Written informed consent was obtained from the individual(s) for the publication of any potentially identifiable images or data included in this article.

AUTHOR CONTRIBUTIONS

MR completed all research and writing with assistance from the organizations discussed.

REFERENCES

Adams, C., and Thomas, S. P. (2017). Alternative prenatal care interventions to alleviate black-white maternal/infant health disparities. *Sociol. Compass.* 12, e12549. doi:10.1111/soc4.12549

Bey, A., Brill, A., Porchia-Albert, C., Gradilla, M., and Strauss, N. (2019). *Advancing birth Justice: community-based doula models as a standard of care for ending racial disparities.* https://everymothercounts.org/wp-content/uploads/2019/03/Advancing-Birth-Justice-CBD-Models-as-Std-of-Care-3-25-19.pdf. Accessed 20 June, 2020.

Black Mamas Matter (BMMA) (2018). *Black Mamas Matter: advancing human right to safe and respectful maternal health care. The Center For Reproductive Rights.* https://blackmamasmatter.org/resources/toolkits/. Accessed 13 March, 2020.

Bobrow, E. (2020). *She was pregnant with twins during COVID. Why did only one survive?.* https://www.nytimes.com/2020/08/06/nyregion/childbirth-Covid-Black-mothers.html. Accessed 10 August, 2020.

Bohren, M. A., Hofmeyr, G. J., Sakala, C., Fukuzawa, R. K., and Cuthbert, A. (2017). Continuous support for women during childbirth. *Cochr. Database Syst. Rev.* 7 (7), CD003766. doi:10.1002/14651858.CD003766.pub6

Burke, M. (2020). *New York Man Exposed to coronavirus hid symptoms to visit wife in maternity unit of hospital.* https://www.nbcnews.com/news/us-news/new-york-man-exposed-coronavirus-hid-symptoms-visit-wife-maternity-n1173326. Accessed 15 June, 2020.

Campbell-Voytal, K., Fry McComish, J., Visger, J., Rowland, C. A., and Kelleher, J. (2011). Postpartum Doulas: motivations and perceptions of practice. *Midwifery* 27, e214–e221. doi:10.1016/j.midw.2010.09.006

Center for Disease Control and Prevention (CDC). (2020). https://www.cdc.gov/reproductivehealth/maternalinfanthealth/index.html. Accessed 23 June, 2020.

Chor, J., Lyman, P., Tusken, M., Patel, A., and Gilliam, M. (2016). Women's experiences with doula support during first-trimester surgical abortion: a qualitative study. *Contraception* 93, 244–248. doi:10.1016/j.contraception.2015.10.006

Davis-Floyd, R., Gutschow, K., and Schwartz, D. A. (2020). Pregnancy, birth and the COVID-19 pandemic in the United States. *Med. Anthropol.* 39 (5), 413–427. doi:10.1080/01459740.2020.1761804

Dickson, E. J. (2020). *Death of Sha-Asia Washington, Pregnant 26-year-Old Black Woman, Highlights Devastating trend* https://www.rollingstone.com/culture/culture-features/shaasia-washington-death-woodhull-hospital-black-maternal-mortality-rate-1026069/. Accessed 14 July, 2020.

Gordon, N., Walton, D., Mcadam, E., Derman, J., Gallitero, G., and Garrett, L. (1999). Effects of providing hospital-based doulas in health maintenance organization hospitals. *Obstet. Gynecol.* 93 (3), 422–426. doi:10.1016/s0029-7844(98)00430-x

Gruber, K. J., Cupito, S. H., and Dobson, C. F. (2013). Impact of Doulas on healthy birth outcomes. *J. Perinat Educ.* 22 (1), 49–58. doi:10.1891/1058-1243.22.1.49

Hafner, K. (2020). *'A Heart-Wrenching Thing': Hospitals Ban visits devastating families* https://www.nytimes.com/2020/03/29/health/coronavirus-hospital-visit-ban.html. Accessed 30 May, 2020.

Hardeman, R. R., and Kozhimannil, K. B. (2016). Motivations for entering the doula profession: perspectives from women of color. *J. Midwifery Womens Health* 61, 773–780. doi:10.1111/jmwh.12497

Hodnett, E. D., Gates, S., Hofmeyr, G. J., and Sakala, C.Cochrane Collaboration (2013). "Continuous support for women during childbirth," in *Cochrane database of systematic reviews* (New York: Wiley), doi:10.1002/14651858.CD003766.pub5

Jordan, E., Van Zandt, S. E., and Wright, E. (2008). Doula care: nursing students gain additional skills to define their professional practice. *J. Prof. Nurs.* 24 (2), 118–121. doi:10.1016/j.profnurs.2007.06.018

Keefe, R. H., Lane, S. D., Rubinstein, R. A., Carter, D., Bryant, T., and Thomas, M. D. (2017). African American fathers: disproportionate incarceration and the meaning of involvement. *Families Soc. J. Contemp. Social Serv.* 98 (2), 89–96. doi:10.1606/1044-3894.2017.98.13

Lane, S. D., Keefe, R. H., Rubinstein, R., Levandowski, B. A., Webster, N., Cibula, D. A., et al. (2008). Structural violence, urban retail food markets, and low birth weight. *Health Place* 14, 415–423. doi:10.1016/j.healthplace.2007.08.008

Larsen, D. A., Lane, S., Jennings-Bey, T., Haygood-El, A., Brundage, K., and Rubinstein, R. (2017). Spatio-temporal patterns of gun violence in Syracuse, New York 2009-2015. *PLoS ONE* 12 (3), e0173001. doi:10.1371/journal.pone.0173001

L. J. Ross, L. Roberts, and E. Derkas, Whitney Peoples; Pamela Bridgewater Toure (2017). in *Radical reproductive justice: foundations, theory, practice, critique.* Editors (New York, NY: The Feminist Press).

McLeish, J., and Redshaw, M. (2018). A qualitative study of volunteer doulas working alongside midwives at births in England: Mothers' and doulas' experiences. *Midwifery* 56, 53–60. doi:10.1016/j.midw.2017.10.002

New York State (NYS). (2020). *COVID-19 maternity task force: recommendations to the Governor to promote increased choice and access to safe maternity care during the COVID-19 pandemic* https://www.governor.ny.gov/sites/governor.ny.gov/files/atoms/files/042920_CMTF_Recommendations.pdf. Accessed 30 May, 2020. Accessed.

New York State (NYS). (2019). *Doula Pilot Medicaid program.* https://www.health.ny.gov/health_care/medicaid/redesign/doulapilot/index.htm. Accessed 23 June, 2020.

New York State Senate (NYSS) (2019). *Assembly bill A364B* https://www.nysenate.gov/legislation/bills/2019/a364. Accessed 23 June, 2020.

Olumhense, E. (2020). *A pregnant woman tweeted concerns about a Bronx hospital. She died Days later* https://www.thecity.nyc/health/2020/4/27/21247056/a-pregnant-woman-tweeted-concerns-about-a-bronx-hospital-she-died-days-later. Accessed 30 May, 2020.

Onondaga County (2017). http://www.ongov.net. Accessed 23 June, 2020.

Ross, L. (2017). Reproductive justice as intersectional feminist activism. *Souls: A Crit. J. Black Polit. Cult. Soc.* 19 (3), 286–314. doi:10.1080/10999949.2017.1389634

Ross, L. J., and Solinger, R. (2017). *Reproductive Justice: an introduction.* Oakland, CA: University of California Press.

Scott, K. D., Berkowitz, G., and Klaus, M. (2000). Continuous, but not intermittent, support from a doula significantly improves labor and delivery outcomes. *Evidence-Based Obstet. Gynecol.* 2, 42. doi:10.1054/ebog.2000.0142

Steel, A., Frawley, J., Adams, J., and Diezel, H. (2015). Trained or professional doulas in the support and care of pregnant and birthing women: a critical integrative review. *Health Soc. Care Commun.* 23 (3), 225–241. doi:10.1111/hsc.12112

Thomas, M. P., Ammann, G., Brazier, E., Noyes, P., and Maybank, A. (2017). Doula services within a healthy start program: increasing access for an underserved population. *Matern. Child Health J.* 21 (S1), S59–S64. doi:10.1007/s10995-017-2402-0

Toonen, D. (2018). Doula secrets revealed. *Women Birth* 30 (S1), 1–47. doi:10.1016/j.wombi.2017.08.112

Van Syckle, K., and Caron, C. (2020). *Women will not Be forced to be alone when they Give birth* https://www.nytimes.com/2020/03/28/parenting/nyc-coronavirus-hospitals-visitors-labor.html. Accessed 30 May, 2020.

Village Birth International (VBI). (2019a). Home. Available at: https://villagebirthinternational.org. Accessed 20 May, 2020.

Village Birth International (VBI). (2019b). *VBI Open Letter concerning assembly bill A364B.* https://villagebirthinternational.org/2019/06/21/vbi-open-letter-concerning-assembly-bill-a364b/. Accessed 20 June, 2020.

8

"Soldiers of the System": Maternity Care in Russia Between Bureaucratic Instructions and the Epidemiological Risks of COVID-19

Anna Ozhiganova *†

Center of Medical Anthropology, Institute of Anthropology and Ethnology (RAS), Moscow, Russia

Correspondence:
Anna Ozhiganova
anna-ozhiganova@yandex.ru
†ORCID:
Anna Ozhiganova
orcid.org/0000-0002-2283-4925

Preventive measures taken by the Russian maternity care system in response to the COVID-19 pandemic are very tough. Supporting persons (doulas and partners) are being completely excluded from the maternity hospitals. Pregnant women and newborns are distributed in different types of hospitals according to their epidemiological status (confirmed, suspected, contact, or "clear"). Severe infection control measures are introduced for women with confirmed or suspected COVID-19: separation from newborns and weeks of hospital quarantine. How do obstetricians and other perinatal specialists perceive these measures? What strategies do they choose and what new practices are being created? The study is based on interviews conducted between March and August 2020 with obstetricians-gynecologists, midwives, perinatal psychologistsdoulas, and women who gave birth during the pandemic and is focused on their subjective interpretations of COVID-related changes in maternal care. My data indicate that this pandemic with its high risks and uncertainties reveals multiple ethical and organizational conflicts among bureaucratic, managerial and professional logics in Russian health care in which mistrust has played an important role.

Keywords: COVID-19, maternity care, childbirth, obstetricians, doulas, Partner birth, mistrust, bureaucratic logic

MATERNITY CARE IN RUSSIA: BUREAUCRATIC CONTROL AND INSTITUTIONAL MISTRUST

Maternity care reforms carried out during the post-Soviet period have ambiguous and contradictory consequences. On the one hand, reforms led to the commercialization of maternity care and the emergence of paid services and private maternity hospitals. Medical care is provided free of charge to all Russian citizens in accordance with the state health insurance program. However, women from a new category of demanding and informed consumers often pay for a "birth contract" in order to receive personalized care and more comfortable conditions in the hospital (Temkina 2017). The Rule of Informed Voluntary Consent allows women to refuse unwanted medical manipulations (Federal Law No. 323, 2011). The attendance of a birth partner is also guaranteed by the law: the child's father or other family members can accompany women in the birthing room (ibid). Doulas are also allowed to accompany women in some maternity hospitals, although their status remains uncertain. In general, maternity hospitals have become more open and more focused on the needs of women and newborns than two decades ago, at least in big cities: the practice of "soft" or "natural" childbirth is becoming more widespread, the "golden hour" after childbirth is respected, and breastfeeding is encouraged (Ozhiganova 2020).

On the other hand, from Soviet times to the present day, the logic of bureaucratic control continues to play a decisive role in the Russian healthcare system and has even increased in recent years (Litvina et al., 2020). The threat of prosecution against doctors has intensified, as evidenced by several high-profile trials of obstetricians-gynecologists and neonatologists. Russian doctors do not have the same expert power and autonomy as their counterparts in Western societies, medical professional organizations do not have much influence, and the economic and political interests of doctors are largely ignored (ibid.).

Homebirth is illegal; nevertheless it exists, at least in big cities, as an expression of mistrust of obstetric practice (Ozhiganova 2019). The number of out-of-hospital births is unknown because these statistics are not kept.

Confirming Fukuyama's characterization of Russia as a "country of distrust" (Fukuyama, 1996), Russian citizens demonstrate an exceptionally high level of distrust in medicine. More than half of Russians (57%) do not consult a doctor in the case of illness, preferring self-medication; nearly a fifth of all citizens (19%) try to avoid doctors on principle (Health Mail.ru, 2019). Only 11% agree with the statement that a doctor is interested in their health (FOM 2019). The high vulnerability of doctors and the high risks of their work contribute to the fact that they themselves are not inclined to trust the system in which they work (Litvina et al., 2020).

During the coronavirus pandemic, Russian authorities have taken the infection control measures that are typical of authoritarian regimes: distortion of information, manipulation of statistics and outright disinformation; human rights violations—in particular, forced "self-" isolation; forced hospitalization of people with suspected COVID-19; and control of individuals via electronic passes containing barcodes through the Social Monitoring program, which tracks people's locations and movements (Inozemtsev 2020). Additionally, institutional gaps in healthcare management and a lack of personal protective equipment (PPE) for doctors have resulted in the punishment of medical workers for complaints and in reprisals against independent medical organizations (Vasilieva 2020).

The fight against the pandemic in Russia is taking place in a situation of a new "legal void" or "counterfeiting of legality" produced by Putin's government (Karaseva 2020: 294). Russia's authorities are not using either of two versions of emergency regimes ("an emergency situation" and "the state of emergency") provided by Russian law, but rather declared pre-emergency "high alerts," and in amendments to these decrees introduced a "regime of self-isolation," "distance work" and "quarantine"—all absent in the law. In the healthcare realm, this legal void has manifested in the mass diagnosis of "community-acquired pneumonia" instead of coronavirus infection (See, for example, the investigative journalism of Yapparova et al., 2020).

METHODS AND MATERIALS, TRUST AND MISTRUST

In recent works, Mühlfried calls for a revision of the existing social science approach to the phenomenon of mistrust "as the flip side of trust, as an annoying absence, a societal failure, or an obstacle to be overcome" (Mühlfried, 2018:7). He suggests that trust and mistrust cannot be understood as opposites: those relationships that are often attributed to mistrust in fact are examples of the coexistence of trust and mistrust that emerge in situations of uncertainty. In the case of trust, people invest in the strengthening of their relations; in the case of mistrust, in the weakening of these relations and a translocation of trust into new trust networks. In order to define "mistrust" as an empirical phenomenon, we need to ask the questions: "How does mistrust work?" and whether or not mistrust itself may be shared and create bonds (ibid: 19). According to Mühlfried, mistrust is a reasonable reaction toward all kinds of revelations and may also be the first step toward critical political engagement.

The epidemic of COVID-19 in Russia triggered many latent conflicts in which mistrust played an important role. In this article, I ask, how has maternity care responded to the challenges of the COVID-19 epidemic? Given their general mistrust of "the system," how are obstetricians reacting to the changed situation: new guidelines, anti-epidemic restrictions, and changed working conditions? What new relations and practices of trust and mistrust have emerged between perinatal professionals and women?

This article is based on interviews I conducted with 11 obstetrician-gynecologists, two midwives, two perinatal psychologists working in maternity hospitals, 6 homebirth midwives, 12 doulas, and 14 women who gave birth during the pandemic[1]. The first interviews were recorded in March, when the COVID-19 epidemic in Russia was just beginning; the last in August, when some preventive infection control measures had already been lifted. Thus it became possible to see what in the maternal health system changed initially and which changes lasted over time. Most of these recorded interviews were with perinatal specialists and women from Moscow and the Moscow region; seven were with representatives of other regions: Central, St. Petersburg, the Ural, and Siberia. I also followed the publications of an ob/gyn who blogged about his work at the Moscow COVID-19 maternity hospital on the Instagram social network (a very rare practice among Russian doctors), as well as the official pages of maternity hospitals on Facebook and Instagram.

My interviews with doctors and midwives included the following questions: How has your hospital's operating schedule changed? Has your obstetric practice changed? How do you assess the COVID-19 prevention measures in your hospital? My interviews with women included questions about whether the epidemic affected where, how and with whom the birth took place, and what factors were most influential. Since doulas usually know very well what is happening in the maternity hospitals of the city where they work, they have become valuable

[1]Ethical approval and written informed consent for participation were not required for the study of human participants in accordance with the legislation of the Russian Federation and institutional requirements. Verbal informed consent for participation in the study and for publication of the results was obtained from all participants.

interlocutors; however, the focus of my research was on doctors and their perceptions of the pandemic situation. I had several points of entry into the field: I used old contacts with doctors and midwives, but also found new interlocutors through the Association of Professional Doulas and the Center for Traditional Midwifery, which conducts training courses for obstetricians-gynecologists and midwives. It should be noted that many doctors refused to be interviewed. For those who agreed, it was extremely important that the interview was not "official," that is, they were guaranteed complete anonymity. I analyzed these interviews thematically.

In order to maintain anonymity, all personal names and names of maternity hospitals are not given. In interviews with doctors and midwives from the province, at their request, only the region is indicated, not the city, as this might make the data source potentially identifiable. Given the level of mistrust in the Russian healthcare system in general that my physician interlocutors expressed, readers may wonder why they were open enough with me as a researcher to answer my questions as frankly as they did (see below). Perhaps this openness was due not only to the anonymity I promised them, but also to my position, which I voiced before each interview: my goal is not to identify possible violations of the rules and protocols in their work, but to better understand how and in what conditions they have to work in this difficult situation of the coronavirus pandemic. It is also important to note that both in the late Soviet and post-Soviet traditions, there is a great distance between private conversation, in which people speak freely, and public speaking, in which people are generally very careful about what they say. My interlocutors perceived the interview as a private conversation.

THE MATERNITY CARE EMERGENCY RESPONSE TO THE COVID-19 PANDEMIC: DOCTORS' OPINIONS

COVID-19 Prevention Measures: Conversion of Maternity Hospitals, New Clinical Guidelines and Routing Plans

In the middle of March, the national Ministry of Health and regional Health Departments adopted a series of preventive measures in response to the COVID-19 pandemic. All maternity hospitals were divided into three groups: "clean," "infectious," and "buffer" (an intermediate zone, in which patients with an unconfirmed diagnosis are located) or respectively "green," "red," and "yellow" zones. The flows of pregnant women, women in labor, and newborns should be separated based on their COVID-19 tests, acute respiratory viral infection (ARVI) symptoms, and data on contacts with COVID-19, and directed to the appropriate hospitals according to the new routing plans. A quarantine regime was declared in all hospitals, meaning that visits to patients and partners at births were prohibited. Additional preventive measures were introduced for women with confirmed or suspected COVID-19: separation from newborns, prohibition of breastfeeding, and long-term quarantine in the hospital until negative test results are received (Guidelines 2020). Infants with neonatal disorders and COVID-19 suspected or positive should be sent to receive high-tech medical care in specialized hospitals, where special "Melzer boxes"—a completely isolated ward for infectious patients, with a gateway for staff—should be opened.

Converting Maternity Hospitals to COVID-19 Hospitals

In the beginning of the epidemic, some maternity hospitals were converted to COVID-19 hospitals, where ob/gyns do not attend births, but work as general practitioners. The doctors explained that this solution was convenient, since in Russia maternity hospitals are usually detached buildings, with a "box" system, built as infectious disease hospitals where a strict sanitary and epidemiological regime is always observed. Due to the conversion of these maternity hospitals, the remaining "clean" hospitals received sharply increased patient flows. According to some reports, the number of patients in such hospitals has more than doubled: the same number of doctors and midwives began to take over 40 deliveries per day instead of the previous 20 (Interview 1b). Some maternity hospitals specializing in treating pregnant women with chronic diseases were also closed; as a result, pregnant women with heart or kidney problems could not receive all the necessary medical care (Interview 5).

One of the largest Moscow maternity hospitals, with 210 beds, was turned into a hospital for patients with COVID-19 on March 12. This news was reported by the media as a doctors' initiative:

> The staff of the maternity hospital referred to the Moscow Department of Health with a proposal to redesign their beds for an infectious disease hospital. Doctors explain it this way: "It is our professional duty to protect citizens." (Protsenko 2020).

Dr. N., an ob/gyn of this maternity hospital, said that the decision about converting was made by this Department, and it could not be otherwise: such decisions are not made by the heads of hospitals, and still less by the staff:

> What is the initiative? This is ridiculous. Of course, it is the Department's initiative. In our country, after all, everything is so—"at the numerous requests of the working people." We all turned off instantly. Get up and go (Interview 1a).

As a result, Dr. N. and her colleagues worked for about three months as general practitioners with COVID-19 patients; the maternity hospital returned to its usual work at the end of July. Many of her colleagues were ill with COVID, and many of those ended up in intensive care. However, Dr. N. did not complain, noting that they were literally "bombarded with all sorts of benefits": provided with PPE, paid allowances, brought good food and even offered rooms in 5-star hotels. However, it was very difficult for her not to do her job, and she doubts the correctness of such a decision: "We are deprived of our work, it is awful! It seems to me that this is just some kind of ineffective use of human resources" (Interview 1a). However, she believes that nothing could be done; they could only obey. Only two doctors from the large hospital staff left the service.

Formal Cancellation of Partner Support and Informal Ways to Get Around it

Births with partners have become quite popular, especially in big cities: 30% in Moscow, and up to 70% in some maternity hospitals in Moscow and St. Petersburg. The cancellation of partnered births was painful for the women, who often searched for ways to get around it; some even decided to give birth at home. However, according to the homebirth midwives I interviewed, the pandemic did not significantly affect the number of out-of-hospital births: these were scheduled home births with a midwife.

Some maternity hospitals started to allow partners in July, but almost exclusively under contract (which actually meant that the couple had to pay for the presence of a partner) and, with rare exceptions, only fathers, not doulas. Most of the maternity hospitals, especially in the provinces, had not returned to this option by late August.

The prohibition of partnered birth has become one more manifestation of a "legal void," since it has no legal basis. According to the Ministry of Health Guidelines, "partner birth should be prohibited in probable or confirmed cases of COVID-19 to reduce the risk of infection" (Guidelines 2020: 23), but in practice it was canceled for all.

Most doctors reacted very calmly to this prohibition, since they considered it to be a routine preventive measure. Dr. A., an ob/gyn at one of the Moscow maternity hospitals, believes that it is undoubtedly correct and an "absolutely ordinary quarantine measure" that is carried out regularly, every year, during the flu and ARVI season. She emphasizes that the restrictions affected only women, and for her, as a doctor, nothing has changed dramatically: "It's just the work we do. These are the Ministry of Health's Guidelines. We are obliged to obey" (Interview 3).

Dr. E., an ob/gyn of the St. Petersburg maternity hospital, where births with partners accounted for 50% of all births, also unequivocally supports their cancellation: "This is an adequate measure: the fewer contacts, the less chance of infection." As confirmation, she told a story about an event that occurred in her maternity hospital during the swine flu epidemic in 2009: a husband visited his wife and as a result she fell ill and died. E. is convinced that women understand this prohibition: "I have not seen anyone resent it, because everyone understands that this is how the whole country lives, and no one is to blame. As a matter of fact, there is no one to make claims to" (Interview 4).

However, other doctors admit that women do not agree with the prohibition of partnered births and express their protest. Dr. V., the head of the maternity hospital in the Ural region, said that she is constantly faced with the demands of women to allow accompanying partners:

> Just recently there was a woman who was extremely negative, and I told her: contact the Ministry of Health and Rospotrebnadzor (Federal Service for Surveillance on Consumer Rights Protection and Human Wellbeing] since this is not a requirement of a maternity hospital, this is a requirement of these bodies. After that, her husband called me and said: "Yes, we turned [to them], and we were told, please, at the discretion of the maternity hospital, they can allow partners (Interview 6).

However, Dr. V. did not allow him to attend his wife's labor or birth; in her opinion, the officials were only trying to shift the responsibility to her: "These people (officials of Rosotrebnadzor] behaved unscrupulously, because if something happens, some outbreak in the hospital, then the head will answer—that is, I will answer" (Interview 6).

Partnered birth has turned into a rare and accordingly valuable service, and very quickly became the subject of all sorts of informal agreements and informal payments. Some maternity hospitals in the Moscow and St. Petersburg regions unofficially allowed partners to accompany women. Despite the order of the Health Department, a private Moscow maternity hospital continued the practice of partnered deliveries (in some cases, for one partner, and in some cases, for two) for the entire period of the epidemic in Russia. The doctor from this hospital confesses that everything remains as before but "unofficially" (Interview 2). At the same time, the contract price sharply increased, and became the reason for the joke, "In order for the coronavirus to become safe, you need to pay 350 thousand rubles; if the contract is 200 thousand or 150 thousand, then the virus is still very dangerous!" (Interview 8).

Some women decided to use a service provided by some maternity hospitals: accompaniment by a perinatal psychologist, a hospital staff member. Perinatal psychologists confirmed that the number of requests for their services increased during the epidemic. However, it turned out that not all women are satisfied with this option, since they fear that such a partner is not acting in their interests: "She will play along with the doctors, to persuade me to do something, maybe not what is best for me, but what is more convenient for a doctor, because then she will continue to work with him, and I will leave" (Interview 8). Instead, women tend to trust doulas because they are from outside the healthcare system. In such cases, women prefer online doula support over the support of a hospital psychologist.

The doulas protested the cancellation of partner births: they prepared a petition and called on women to fight for their rights. In the middle of March 2020, a doula and a lawyer, M., published on social networks a proposal to write requests to Rospotrebnadzor demanding an explanation of this measure. M. considers it illegal: since a state of emergency was not declared, the guarantees of citizens' rights established by law cannot be canceled. However, no doula initiatives received noticeable support. In some cases, partners were allowed when, on the advice of this doula, they demanded a written refusal with reference to the law. Such informal negotiations turned out to be very limited but were the only way to solve the problem of achieving partnered birth.

Maternity Hospitals for Women with COVID-19: Epidemic Expediency or Additional Risks to the Health of Women and Newborns?

Admission into a COVID-19 maternity hospital means that very harsh measures will be applied to a woman and her newborn: separation immediately after birth, and very often increased medicalization and even use of drugs that are prohibited for pregnant and lactating women: Kaletra (which is used in HIV treatment), Azithromycin, and other antibiotics. My interlocutors noted an increase in perinatal losses due to spontaneous abortions and intrauterine fetal deaths (Interview seven; Charitable Foundation "Light in Hands").

According to my interlocutors, obstetric practice has changed dramatically since the advent of COVID-19 and the number of surgical interventions in such hospitals has increased. A midwife from the Siberian region said that in her maternity hospital, designated for women with COVID-19, the number of cesarean births increased from 25% to about 60–70% because many doctors do not even give women the opportunity to enter into labor, but immediately send them to surgery (Interview 7). It should be noted that this even happened in a maternity hospital known for its support of natural birth; for example, this hospital previously allowed vaginal births after cesareans (VBACs) even if the mother had experienced two previous cesarean deliveries.

The first maternity hospital, which, in accordance with the recommendations of the Ministry of Health, was designated "to receive pregnant women with ARVI, community-acquired pneumonia and patients who are quarantined due to contact with coronavirus infection" (Guidelines 2020) began working in Moscow on March 31. It is a large 170-bed maternity hospital with more than 7,000 births per year. In April, it received a fairly large number of patients: three to four per day, some with severe symptoms of COVID-19. However, in July, an ob/gyn of this hospital wrote on his Instagram blog that they had very few patients at that time: "Honestly, there is practically nobody to treat. There are only 15 patients in the huge maternity hospital building!" (Doctor_yakunin Instagram post 3).

A 60-bed maternity hospital in a large Siberian city was assigned to work with women with COVID-19 on April 27. It accepts women from all over the city with suspected coronavirus infection, and according to midwife T., all the time there were on average about 10–12 women in all three departments. Women are tested in the admission department and placed in the "yellow" buffer zone, then based on the test results, after 3–4 days, they are transferred to the "green" or "red" zone.

Thus, those maternity hospitals that retain their status as infectious disease hospitals are only partially filled. My interlocutors say that very often women are brought to them without symptoms and with an unconfirmed diagnosis:

> An ambulance brought a woman with a screaming seven-day-old baby. The woman is worried about pain in the seam (scar) after cesarean section, which was made in an ordinary "clean" maternity hospital a week ago. After discharge, she went to her mother-in-law to pick up the older child. It turns out that this grandmother has IgG antibodies to coronavirus (he presence of these antibodies indicates the presence of an immune response, i.e. disease resistance) (Doctor_yakunin Instagram post 3).

Thus, we can see that an ambulance, by order of the Department of Health, brought women to this COVID hospital without sufficient reason (allegedly this particular woman was in contact with an infected person), just so that it would not be empty.

A similar situation has developed in the Siberian maternity hospital. By order of the regional Department of Health, it should accept women with a temperature above 37 Celsius (98.6 Fahrenheit), or with the signs of ARVI (acute respiratory viral infection), and with an obstetric pathology. However, many doctors accept pregnant women with only mild signs of a cold (Interview 7). Doctors often assess the Department's order to send women with a runny nose to an infectious maternity hospital as "absolutely absurd" and advise their patients to drip a vasoconstrictor before admission (doctor_yakunin Instagram post 1).

Doctors also understand that during childbirth, body temperature can rise due to a psycho-emotional factor, or simply because of the summer heat, or because of kidney problems, but often doctors in an ambulance do not take this into account and take the patients straight to the infectious disease hospital (Interview 7).

A woman who finds herself in a buffer ("yellow") maternity hospital (or department) also must expect a rapid cutting of the umbilical cord and separation from the child. On the official Facebook page of one of these maternity hospitals, women are told that they will have to stay in the hospital for at least two weeks during the incubation period of coronavirus infection: "We will not dismiss you if after a couple of days you feel great, because you can be a carrier of a mild illness and pass it on to others" [36roddom (maternity hospital 36) Facebook post].

Women who seek medical help due to symptoms of ARVI at any stage of pregnancy are at risk of forced admission to such a hospital. It is not surprising that some women, when they feel unwell, self-medicate and think only about hiding their symptoms from doctors. One of my interlocutors said that she and her family most likely had COVID-19 in April: for two weeks she had a fever, severe weakness and cough. She treated herself with homeopathic remedies, did not go to doctors, and in August, a month ahead of schedule, gave birth to a healthy child (Interview 9).

Doctors are ambivalent about the separation of mothers from newborns. Some believe that this measure is rational, because they believe that presently there is "too little data" on the transmission of the disease from mother to child and "it is better to be safe just in case." (Interview 3, 4). Others admit that this measure is too harsh (Interview 5), that they do not consider it reasonable either from an epidemiological or psychological point of view: "Mothers are being treated here in the hospital, either they have coronavirus, or it is an error in the analysis. We take the next analysis after 10 days, and they lie all this time, gargle, drip their nose, and cry for their babies" (Interview 7).

When asked how it is possible to obtain women's consent for such treatment, T. says that doctors always have the opportunity to intimidate, to say that it is dangerous for a child to be with his mother, that he will get sick and may die. One of my interlocutors, a woman ob/gyn who is herself an expecting mother, confirms that she not only supports the separation of mother and child, but she is ready, if necessary, to be separated from her baby immediately after the birth: "I would prefer that my child had less opportunity to get infected from me. I would rather refuse to stay together if only I understood that my child is being cared for, that he is fed and safe" (Interview 4).

The Russian Association of Natural Feeding Consultants (ANFC) opposed the practice of separating mother and child in maternity hospitals. In an open letter to the Minister of Health dated July 31, 2020, members of the Association stated that "the real risks to the health of mothers and newborns due to lack of contact and the prohibition of breastfeeding are higher than the potential risk of COVID-19 infection" and demanded that hospitals not separate COVID-positive mothers from their newborns if the mother's condition is not serious, and to ensure the right of newborns to breastfeeding in all cases, observing the antiseptic methods proposed by WHO recommendations (wearing a mask, washing hands and disinfecting surfaces) (ANFC 2020). However, the doctors did not support the initiative, and the Ministry responded with a formal refusal.

During the epidemic, many doctors found themselves in a difficult situation, especially in the provinces. According to unofficial data, the death rate of doctors from COVID-19 in Russia is much higher than in other countries (Medvestnik 2020). My interlocutors from provincial maternity hospitals confirm that disposable PPE is in short supply, so they wash and dry it in the hospital. Many doctors, midwives and nurses working with COVID-19 patients have not received the incentive payments promised to them by Presidential Decree on May 6. Midwife T. says that she was ill with COVID-19 in May but has not received any insurance payments. She said that some her colleagues are already planning to quit after the epidemic: "It is simply impossible to work; all the problems came out that we did not pay attention to before, just because we were very busy with a large flow of patients" (Interview 7). She admits that the head of the hospital always behaved very rudely with the staff and did not seek to provide the hospital with everything necessary (in particular, no needed repairs were made for a long time).

Doctors may evaluate the introduced preventive measures in different ways, but if they consider some of them not useful or even harmful and absurd, they do not declare their disagreement publicly, but simply obey bureaucratic requirements and protocols. Physicians can warn their patients and advise them how to get around restrictive measures as a part of private relations of trust. They can express their disagreement by quitting their job, but in general they cannot affect the functioning of the system.

PATIENTS AND HEALTHCARE PRACTITIONERS: PRACTICES OF SEPARATION, PROHIBITION, AND MISTRUST

This research was conducted during the "first wave" of the coronavirus pandemic (from March to August 2020) and does not cover the changes that have occurred later. The differences between central cities and the periphery and diversity in maternal care facilities that exist in a country as large and heterogeneous as Russia cannot be captured in such "quick" study. As a result, the picture turns out to be rather mosaic, however, taking into account these limitations, some preliminary conclusions can be drawn.

As demonstrated in the articles in this Special Issue, the responses of various national healthcare systems to the challenges of the COVID-19 pandemic often have a great deal in common, such as prohibiting or severely limiting visitors, doulas, birth partners, and post-birth mother-newborn contact and breastfeeding. Yet some of the measures taken in Russia are very different from those in other countries, such as the division of maternity hospitals into red, green, and yellow zones and the enforced long hospital quarantines for women and newborns "just in case." Public discussions about the risks of these prohibitions have been conducted in many countries, and in some cases, for example, in New York, they were canceled due to public protest, largely from women, midwives, and doulas (Davis-Floyd, Gutschow, and Schwartz, 2020: 7). Yet in Russia, a discussion inspired by doulas in the electronic social networks passed almost unnoticed, as the discontent of women and doulas and their proposals for humanistic improvements were not supported by the medical community and health officials.

Unlike American women who are afraid of hospitals because of the possibility of contagion, (ibid: 8), Russian women fear COVID-19 much less than the restrictive measures introduced in maternity hospitals. A sad joke appeared: "In Russia, the coronavirus is not as terrible as the fight against it." Women are afraid to go to the hospital without a partner, fearing unreasonable medical interventions, and are even more afraid of the infectious disease maternity hospitals, where they will be separated from their babies immediately after birth and for the next weeks.

The main strategy of many pregnant women in the pandemic situation is the mobilization of all resources "to insure" against possible risks: they search for reliable information about doctors and maternity hospitals; make informal agreements with doctors; commit to expensive birth contracts; and generate agreements with doulas for remote support (via video or audio communication). Thus, the pandemic situation contributes to the increase in informal relations and informal payments in maternity hospitals, and, accordingly, to the increase in inequality among different social classes, as well as between the big cities of Moscow and St. Petersburg and the provinces.

The Guidelines of the Ministry of Health and the orders of regional departments, declared to be aimed specifically at "minimizing the risks" of the spread of coronavirus infection, contradict evidence-based medicine data and international recommendations, and some of them, such as separation of mothers from newborns and prolonged hospital quarantine, cannot be considered rational medical ethics and patient's rights are viewed as irrelevant and negligible, and the principles of separation and prohibition are authoritative. The principle of prohibition as applied in Russia justifies "the system's" prohibitions as described above (see Benaglia, this issue). And according to Davis-Floyd (2003, 2018), the technocratic model of obstetrics is based on the principle of separation, in which mind is separated from body, the practitioner is separate from the patient—as in not emotionally connected to her--and, among other forms of separation, the mother is separated from both her support people and her baby. Under this ideology, it is easy to justify such separation without remorse. In contrast, the humanistic model as defined by Davis-Floyd (ibid.) is based on the principle of connection: connection of mind and body, of practitioner and patient, of the mother to her support persons, and of mother and baby. Pre-COVID, this principle of connection used to characterize maternity care in some of the more progressive Russian hospitals.

Why did the Russian system of maternity care react so harshly, canceling many progressive innovations of recent years, rejecting WHO recommendations and evidence-based medical data? My interlocutors from the older generation of doctors believe that this reaction is caused by "historical memory": in a situation of epidemic danger, health officials immediately reverted back to the old Soviet practice based on the principles of prohibition and separation, the dominance of bureaucratic logic, paternalism, and neglect of patient rights, when maternity hospitals were completely closed institutions with strict and prohibitive rules, separation of mothers and newborns, and severe sanitary and infection control measures. One obstetrician commented:

I still remember the old obstetrics. You are at war all the time. The maternity hospital is a field of military operations. Therefore, there were such strict midwives and nannies, because in fact, neither the woman nor the child was perceived as (a subject] of care. The emotional background was not taken into account. It was a very difficult psychological load, and on the staff too, because they were something like cogs of this machine (Interview 5). As my interviews show, doctors and midwives may disagree with these drastic changes, express their opposition to bureaucratic directives, and empathize with women, but they cannot state this opposition publicly. At the same time, it is clear that medical professionals are increasingly worried about their professional autonomy. In an emergency regime, which was not formally declared, the dependence of doctors on bureaucracy at various levels—from the head of the hospital to the Ministry of Health—became even more visible than in ordinary times. Russian doctors as "soldiers of the system" are obliged to follow the orders of health officials, and their professional position is regarded only as a private opinion. They cannot be sure that they will receive the necessary protection from infection and monetary compensation, nor do they have any leverage over the hospital administration and health officials. The pandemic situation reveals the fact that physicians themselves do not trust the institutions in which they work, as shown by the results of a study conducted by a group of sociologists in St. Petersburg hospitals (Borozdina and Novkunskaya, 2020). Doctors, just like patients, do not trust official information, which leads to criticism of the authorities' actions to combat the epidemic:

> To be honest, I still don't really understand what's going on. I am still in some incomprehensible state from all this, whether this is a great lie, or is it a great infection? (Interview 1b).
>
> Today I have the opinion that we are somehow very systematically prepared for the fact that the coronavirus will densely enter our lives, and we will fight with it for many, many years. They want to intimidate us so that we can endlessly fight the coronavirus (doctor_yakunin Instagram post 2).

These doctors, who themselves work in the COVID hospitals, do not deny the existence of the virus; their mistrust is a variant of Covidian dissidence—a term widely used in Russian discourse, both in media and in electronic social networks) --which should be viewed as a specific way to express mistrust toward the authorities. Such doctors may indeed be "soldiers of the system," forced labor within it and to obey its rules just as military soldiers must, but that does not mean uncritical acceptance of the system as it is nor of its rules. A new "legal void" produced by the government, lack of transparency in the actions of the authorities, and mistrust of official information about the real situation with this pandemic become reasons for reluctance and dissidence—for hesitation tinged with mistrust—to adhere to the measures of the healthcare system (Somparé and Somparé 2018: 130). Thus I argue that the pandemic as a situation with high risks and uncertainty reveals and highlights multiple latent conflicts in which mistrust has long played an important role in the Russian context. This dense tangle of problems could be untangled if both doctors and women would refuse the usual strategy of informally solving their particular problems and transition to a systematic problem-solving strategy that would involve public speaking, strengthening professional, patient, and women's organizations, and creating new practices of solidarity and trust between practitioners and patients. In such ways, doctors, with the help of women activists, could transform themselves into system changers rather than system "soldiers."

LIST OF INTERVIEWEES

1. Interview 1a. N., obstetrician-gynecologist, state maternity hospital. Moscow, March 24.
2. Interview 1b. N., obstetrician-gynecologist, state maternity hospital. Moscow, August 5.
3. Interview 2. V., obstetrician-gynecologist, private maternity hospital. Moscow, March 26.
4. Interview 3. A, obstetrician-gynecologist, state maternity hospital. Moscow, March 30.
5. Interview 4. E., obstetrician-gynecologist, state maternity hospital. St. Petersburg, July 10.
6. Interview 5. O., obstetrician-gynecologist, medical center. Moscow, July 13.
7. Interview 6. C., obstetrician-gynecologist, head of the state maternity hospital. Ural region, August 9.
8. Interview 7. T., midwife, state maternity hospital. Siberian region, August 17.
9. Interview 8a. M., doula. Moscow, Marth 20.
10. Interview 8b. M., doula. Moscow, May 8.
11. Interview 9. K., childbirth during the COVID-19 pandemic. St. Petersburg region. July 11, August 14.

INTERNET RESOURCES

1. 36 roddom [maternity hospital 36]. Coronavirus and pregnancy. Facebook, April 1. https://www.facebook.com/36roddom/posts/2909028449184940/.

2. doctor_yakunin. How to give birth to a healthy baby now? Instagram post 1, April 20. https://www.instagram.com/p/B_M5KsUAgyJ/.
3. doctor_yakunin. Instagram post 2, July 21. https://www.instagram.com/p/CC57ul5gNhh/.
4. doctor_yakunin. Instagram post 3, July 24. https://www.instagram.com/p/CDA3BpJAAqX/.

ETHICS STATEMENT

Ethical review and approval was not required for the study on human participants in accordance with the local legislation and institutional requirements. Written informed consent for participation was not required for this study in accordance with the national legislation and the institutional requirements. Verbal informed consent for participation in the study and publication of the results was obtained from all participants.

AUTHOR CONTRIBUTIONS

The author confirms being the sole contributor of this work and has approved it for publication.

REFERENCES

Association of Natural Feeding Consultants-ANFC (2020). Open letter to the Minister of health of the Russian Federation M.A. Murashko. Available at: https://m.vk.com/@akev_russia-otkrytoe-pismo-akev-ministru-zdravoohraneniya-rf-murashko-ma [in Russian].

Borozdina, E., and Novkunskaya, A. (2020). Vicious reflexes: what prevents Russian medicine from fighting the pandemic. *RosBusinessConsulting-St. Petersburg*, Available at: https://www.rbc.ru/spb_sz/20/05/2020/5ec50cf79a794713e1892347?fbclid=IwAR0NqTJiTUaiizUtV83cL8MhKMNtcZ-YnirXdUSjD0MNjqVGtmGUbcnFhFU [in Russian].

Davis-Floyd, R. (2003). *Birth as an American rite of passage.* Berkeley, CA: University of California Press.

Davis-Floyd, R., Gutschow, K., and Schwartz, D. A. (2020). Pregnancy, birth and the COVID-19 pandemic in the United States. *Med. Anthropol.* 39 (5), 413–427. doi:10.1080/01459740.2020.1761804

Davis-Floyd, R. (2018). "The technocratic, humanistic, and holistic paradigms of birth and health care," in *Ways of knowing about birth: mothers, midwives, medicine, and birth activism by Davis-Floyd R.* Long Grove, IL: Waveland Press, 3–44.

Federal Law No 323 (2011). About bases of protection of public health in the Russian Federation Available at: https://minzdrav.gov.ru/documents/7025.

FOM (2019). About doctors and the quality of medical care. How are the accessibility of medical care, the qualifications of doctors and the equipment of medical facilities? Available at: https://fom.ru/Zdorove-isport/12346 [in Russian].

Fukuyama, F. (1996). *Trust: the social virtues and the creation of prosperity.* New York, NY: The Free Press.

Guidelines of the Ministry of Health of the Russian Federation (2020). Organization of medical care for pregnant women, women in labor and newborns with a new coronavirus infection COVID-19. Available at: https://static-1.rosminzdrav.ru/system/attachments/attaches/000/050/093/original/23042020_Preg_COVID-19_1_Final.pdf [in Russian].

Health Mail.ru (2019). More than half of Russians self-medicate. Available at: https://health.mail.ru/news/bolshe_poloviny_rossiyan_zanimayutsya/, August, 23 [in Russian].

Inozemtsev, V. (2020). *Authoritarian response to the pandemic.* Virginia, Russia: Free Russia Foundation. Available at: https://www.youtube.com/watch?v=2o-FYqjeSDY, June, 18.

Karaseva, A. (2020). The legal void and COVID-19 governance. *Soc. Anthropol.* 28 (2), 294–295. doi:10.1111/1469-8676.12825

Litvina, D., Novkunskaya, A., and Temkina, A. (2020). Multiple vulnerabilities in medical settings: invisible suffering of doctors. *Societies* 10 (5), 5. doi:10.3390/soc10010005

Mühlfried, F. (2018). "Introduction. approximating mistrust," In *Mistrust: ethnographic approximations.* Editor F. Mühlfried. (Beilefeld, Germany: Transcript Verlag), 7–22.

Medvestnik (2020). Russian doctor's portal. Available at: https://medvestnik.ru/content/news/Smertnost-medikov-ot-COVID-19-v-Rossii-na-poryadok-operejaet-pokazateli-drugih-stran.html [in Russian].

Ozhiganova, A. (2020). Authoritative knowledge about childbirth and obstetrics: an analysis of the discursive practices of Russian perinatal specialists. *Popu. Eco.* 4 (4), 84–99. doi:10.3897/popecon.4.e57267

Ozhiganova, A. (2019). "What do women want": motives of refusal of maternity hospital in favor of home birth. *Monit. Public Opi.: Eco. and Soc. Chan.* 2, 263–281 [in Russian]. doi:10.14515/monitoring.2019.2.12

Protsenko, L. (2020). The staff of the maternity hospital No. 8 proposed to re-equip the beds for an infectious disease hospital.*Russian newspaper, Marth 14*, Available at: https://rg.ru/2020/03/14/reg-cfo/korpus-roddoma-v-moskve-pereoboruduiut-dlia-priema-bolnyh-s-koronavirusom.html [in Russian].

Somparé, A. W., and Somparé, E. B. (2018). "Mistrust during the Ebola epidemic in Guinea," in *Mistrust: ethnographic approximations.* Editor F. Mühlfried (Beilefeld, Germany: Transcript Verlag), 129–145.

Temkina, A. (2017). "Economy of trust" in commercial obstetric care: educated urban women as consumers and patients. *Journal of Economic Sociology* 18 (3), 14–53 [in Russian]. doi:10.17323/1726-3247-2017-3-14-53

Vasilieva, M. (2020). The Minister of Health personally complained to the police about the video of the union of doctors about the lack of protective equipment. *Open Media.* Available at: https://openmedia.io/news/n1/ministr-zdravooxraneniya-lichno-pozhalovalsya-v-policiyu-na-rolik-profsoyuza-vrachej-o-nexvatke-sredstv-zashhity/ https://openmedia.io/news/n1/ministr-zdravooxraneniya-lichno-pozhalovalsya-v-policiyu-na-rolik-profsoyuza-vrachej-o-nexvatke-sredstv-zashhity/ [in Russian]

Yapparova, L., Sarkisyan, D., and Pertsev, A. (2020). It is simply forbidden to die from coronavirus. *Meduza*, Available at: https://meduza.io/feature/2020/05/14/prosto-zapreschayut-umirat-ot-koronavirusa [in Russian].

9

Pivoting to Childbirth at Home or in Freestanding Birth Centers[1] in the US During COVID-19: Safety, Economics and Logistics

Betty-Anne Daviss[1], David A. Anderson[2] and Kenneth C. Johnson[3]*

[1]The Pauline Jewett Institute of Women's and Gender Studies, Faculty of Arts and Social Sciences, Carleton University, Ottawa, ON, Canada, [2]Centre College, Danville, KY, United States, [3]School of Epidemiology and Public Health, Faculty of Medicine, University of Ottawa, Ottawa, ON, Canada

***Correspondence:**
Betty-Anne Daviss
bettyannedaviss@gmail.com

Birth-related decisions principally center on safety; giving birth during a pandemic brings safety challenges to a new level, especially when choosing the birth setting. Amid the COVID-19 crisis, the concurrent work furloughs, business failures, and mounting public and private debt have made prudent expenditures an inescapable second concern. This article examines the intersections of safety, economic efficiency, insurance, liability and birthing persons' needs that have become critical as the pandemic has ravaged bodies and economies around the world. Those interests, and the challenges and solutions discussed in this article, remain important even in less troubled times. Our economic analysis suggests that having an additional 10% of deliveries take place in private homes or freestanding birth centers could save almost $11 billion per year in the United States without compromising safety.

Keywords: COVID-19, cost effectiveness of homebirth, safety of homebirth, ACOG statements on homebirth, freestanding birth centers, medical intervention, out-of-hospital birth

INTRODUCTION: TRYING TO STAY AT HOME FOR EVERYTHING DURING COVID: WHY WOULD YOU RISK GOING ANYWHERE ELSE FOR CHILDBIRTH?

Births at home or in a freestanding birth center were increasing in the US even before COVID-19, but since decisions around birth generally center on safety, giving birth during this pandemic has brought safety challenges to a new level. As hospitals began to apply COVID restrictions, increasing numbers of childbearers made the decision to be supported during labor by their partners in their private homes (See **Figures 1–4**), instead of facing birth alone in hospitals–in the very buildings that

---

[1]Note that some use the terms "in the community" or "community birth" to group together home birth and birth in freestanding birth centers. Others use "out-of-hospital-birth," a term that defines such births as what they are not, rather than what they are. Others think that when using the term "out of" anywhere, it is appropriate for referring to hospital births; they are "out-of-home births," as the childbearer would have had to leave home to get there, and indeed are called that in the Netherlands. In Australian literature, the term "out-of-hospital birth," also called "birth before arrival" refers to an unplanned home birth or a birth on the way to the hospital, i.e., a birth that was planned to be in hospital until circumstance got in the way. However, out of respect to the hospitals, in particular the hospitals that consider themselves to be "community hospitals," and in order to avoid any confusion, we will use the full terminologies "home birth" or "birth in private homes" and "freestanding birth centers" as much as possible throughout the article.

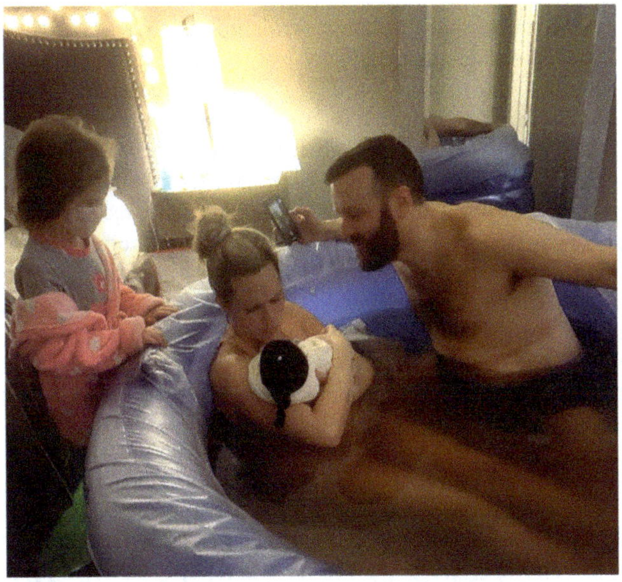

FIGURE 1 | Home birth in the time of COVID-19: Millennial father and lawyer, Robert Onley, who caught his own son in the pool in their master bedroom, puts aside his mask and iPhone momentarily, while midwives stand back for both photo-op and physical distancing and the father's real-time moment with the new baby. Midwife protocol is that the mother, Natasha Onley can birth without a mask. Daughter, Isabelle, stands by watching, still with her mask on, for the benefit of the midwives, who have to do births in other settings, and are therefore careful themselves as well to use Personal Protective Equipment (PPE). Photo by grandmother, Lori Szauter. Used with permission.

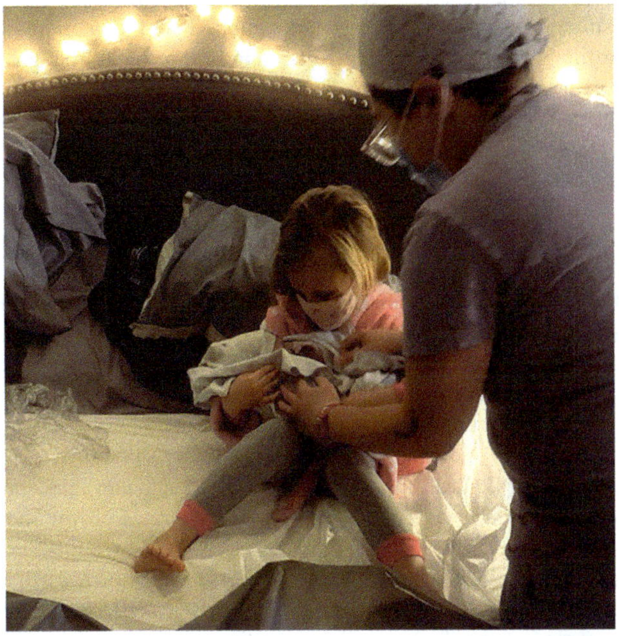

FIGURE 2 | Isabelle, age 5, one of the few children who will never ask "Where do babies come from?" cradles her new little brother, shortly after he comes out of the water. Midwife Ness Dixon, helping her, has already had both doses of the Pfizer vaccine, but both American and Canadian midwives continue to maintain caution, encouraging family members to wear masks, whether the baby is born at home or in hospital. Photo by Lorie Szauter. Used with permission.

take in the people who are sickest with this new plague (Davis-Floyd et al., 2020). While these personal safety threats to laboring people have relaxed in many areas to allow at least the partner into the hospital, and in spite of the vaccine being rolled out, it is not likely that other restrictions in hospitals, or the dangers, are going to disappear anytime soon.

Furthermore, amid the COVID-19 crisis, the concurrent work furloughs, business failures, and mounting public and private debt have made unnecessary personal and community/state expenditures an inescapable concern. For years, maternity and newborn care have constituted the largest hospital payouts from commercial insurers and state Medicaid programs, and the per-capita expenditures in the United States exceed those in every other high-resource country (Truven Health Analytics, 2013). Before COVID-19, the Committee on Assessing Health Outcomes by Birth Settings of the National Academies of Sciences, Engineering, and Medicine (NASEM, 2020: vii) clearly stated, to anyone still unaware at the beginning of 2020: "The United States spends more on childbirth than any other country in the world, with worse outcomes than other high-resource countries, and even worse outcomes for women of color."

As we will detail in this article, birthing persons have been continually achieving safe outcomes in private homes and freestanding birth centers with the assistance of midwives in the United States and abroad. Even so, there has been reluctance to include all nationally credentialed midwives in publicly funded US maternity care programs and state licensure policies. Resistance stems from beliefs that home or freestanding birth center births are riskier than hospital births[2].

COVID-19 has disrupted the perspective of actual safety because staying at home offers better protection from the pandemic for childbearers than sharing a hospital with disease-stricken patients. While freestanding birth centers, unlike hospitals, are not the settings where COVID-19 positive individuals go for treatment, they still present the risk of contamination from other patients, staff, and visitors. Yet as at hospitals, practitioners providing care in private homes and freestanding birth centers can take safety measures that include masks, sanitizing measures, and a minimized number of people at the birth (**Figure 1–2**), as other articles in this Special Issue demonstrate.

The economic analysis of public policy is usually a struggle with trade-offs. Consider a policy that increased the speed limit. It would save time, the trade-off being a predictable increase in traffic fatalities and carbon emissions. Yet in this article, we demonstrate how a public policy that expanded midwifery in the United States could save billions of dollars *without*

[2]For example, the Aetna insurance company states on its website that labor and delivery present "hazards" that "require standards for safety which are provided in the hospital setting and cannot be matched in the home situation" (Aetna, 2020).

necessitating trade-offs regarding safety. This is the first study to estimate the specific savings from public policy that increases births in private homes or freestanding birth centers by a given percentage. We intend to demonstrate that greater access to maternity care by credentialed and licensed midwives in these settings is a solution that is safe, cost effective, and increasingly popular.

For practical models, we can draw on the experiences of countries that have invested in publicly funded home and freestanding birth center births. For example, starting in the 1980s, the Canadian provincial governments charged lawyers and consultants to research a birth model that was safe, cost effective, and met the needs that childbearers were asking for. The solution: to give midwives legislative support and require the provision of a range of birth settings. Almost all provinces have implemented midwifery legislation since it was established in the province of Ontario in 1993. Now 11% of Canadian births are attended by midwives, and in the two provinces with the most midwives—B.C. and Ontario—25 and 15% of births respectively are under midwifery care (Canadian Association of Midwives, 2019). Midwives in Canada in almost all jurisdictions are required by their Colleges (their regulatory bodies) to provide both home and hospital births paid for through universal not-for-profit government agencies (**Figure 3**).

Two major breakthroughs in the last four years have occurred suggesting that former opponents to home birth and to the use of a specific group of midwives, Certified Professional Midwives (CPMs) may have softened their views:

(1) The statements on home birth during the last four years by the American College of Obstetricians and Gynecologists (ACOG, 2016) have acknowledged women's right to choose and agreed that home birth is safe in countries with well-integrated midwifery systems;
(2) Faced with the pandemic, an emergency Executive Order by Governor Cuomo of New York State permitted midwives licensed in other states or Canadian provinces, including Certified Professional Midwives, who had long been illegal in New York, to practice legally there for the initial period of major outbreak in the state (Executive Order #202.11). The timeline has continued to be extended[3].

To be clear, Certified Professional Midwives (CPMs) are the only US midwives whose educational standards require them to undergo specialized clinical training in private homes or freestanding birth centers as a condition of national certification. They are also the only US midwives who are not allowed to practice in hospitals, and they can practice legally in only 36 states, with legislation pending in others.

The pressing questions now are: Will the gaps in the US maternity care system, and the solutions generated during COVID-19 be recognized as important when the pandemic is gone? Will increasing the numbers of midwives trained to work in private homes and freestanding birth settings and fully integrating them into that system during COVID-19 finally be recognized as a paradigm shift that will serve birthing people in normal times?

In what follows, we examine the intersection of the *safety* and *economic efficiency* of birth in private homes and freestanding birth centers, which has become even more critical as the coronavirus ravages bodies and economies around the world. We contend that those interests, and the solutions of increased legislation, liability insurance, and better integration for midwives working in those settings remain important even in less troubled times.

The Pre-COVID-19 Increase in Home Births and Freestanding Birth Centers in the US

After a gradual decline from 1990 to 2004, the number of out-of-hospital births in the US increased from 35,578 in 2004 to 62,228 in 2017, so that 1 of every 62 births took place in homes and freestanding birth centers (1.61%) (Macdorman and Declercq, 2019). By 2015, there were more home births in the United States than in any other industrialized country (Martin et al., 2017)[4].

Who is available to provide births outside the hospital in the US? Certified Nurse-Midwives (CNMs) attend births primarily in hospitals; in 2018, 9,399—only 2.6% of the births that they attended were in private homes and 11,139 (5.1%) in freestanding birth centers (Martin et al., 2019). Medicaid care is mandatory in all states and most Medicaid programs reimburse CNMs at 100% of physicians' rates. The majority of states also mandate private insurance reimbursement for CNM/CM services (American College of Nurse-Midwives (ACNM), 2019).

In 2018, CPMs and other midwives who are not CNMs[5] attended 16,823 (55.7%) of their births in private homes and 7,127 (23.6%) in freestanding births centers. Clearly these groups specialize in birth in the larger community outside the hospital. Again, CPMs rarely—if ever—have hospital privileges. CPMs are not currently recognized under Medicaid at the federal level. However, as of December 2020, 14 of the states in which CPMs are legal have also opted, through a state plan amendment, to cover CPM services[6]. CPMs and families who want access to their

[3]This was an important recognition, as New York state has officially recognized only the Certified Nurse-Midwife (CNM) and Certified Midwife (CM) credentials. The CM credential is recognized in only 5 states and there are only around 120 practicing CMs, despite the fact that this credential was created by members of the American College of Nurse-Midwives (ACNM) in 1996. CMs go through the same training as CNMs (excluding the nursing component) and are certified by the same board. See May and Davis-Floyd (2006) for a full description of the creation of the CM and why it has not gone far. In contrast to the low numbers of CMs–which is also a direct-entry credential, there are around 3,000 CPMs practicing in the US.

[4]Percentage-wise, though, the rate of homebirths in the Netherlands is much higher than in the US, currently standing at 13%, while that of the US stands at under 2%. The point is that the homebirth rate is rising in the US. In seven states in 2018 it was 2.0% or above—in Idaho, Montana, Oregon, Utah, Vermont, Washington, and Wisconsin (see Table I-5 in Martin et al., 2019 at https://www.cdc.gov/nchs/data/nvsr/nvsr68/nvsr68_13_tables-508.pdf).

[5]In most US states, a non-CNM/CM midwife must first be a CPM to obtain a license, but some such midwives, once they have obtained licensure, drop their CPM certification rather than taking the trouble to renew it every 3 years.

[6]http://narm.org/pdffiles/Statechart.pdf

services are seeking federal recognition to secure Medicaid coverage in all states in which CPMs are licensed and meet certain educational requirements[7].

It is important to emphasize that births attended in private homes and freestanding birth centers require providers specifically trained to do so with proper equipment, protocols in place for transport to hospital, and back up hospitals pre-arranged. As one physician reports:

> I have served as a collaborative physician for several CNMs making the transition from hospital to home birth practice and have seen how steep the learning curve is, especially in their first year. To focus on safety in home and birth center birth, then we have to admit that it requires a different skill set than hospital birth and that providers practicing in the community setting must be trained in that skill set to maintain the safety of the environment (Personal communication, Sarita Bennett, DO, CPM).

Although many Americans have assumed that more CNMs could start doing home births if they so desired, it appears difficult for the US administrative facilities to consider something the other way around--that CPMs could work in hospitals. Because Canada deliberately chose not to create distinctions between nurse-midwives and other midwives at legislation, it is rare that Registered Midwives in Canada are also nurses. Yet all midwives in the standard Canadian model must have hospital privileges and do at least some hospital births, as well as home births.

In Canada, in the US states that have legislated and adopted insurance coverage for CPMs, and in other countries that have discovered or continued to recognize the importance of midwives who provide care in the community outside the hospital, a critical commonality has emerged. Bringing these midwives out from underground economies to have them fully integrated into what the World Health Organizations calls "the Reproductive, Maternal, Newborn and Child Health (RMNCH) Continuum of Care[8]," secures the creative strategies most adaptable and safest for families of that community, not just for pandemics but for normal times.

In the US in 2018, midwives attended 10.2% of births (Martin et al., 2019), with a home birth rate of <2%. There are no data yet available to establish how much home births and freestanding birth center births are on the rise with COVID-19, but there is ample suggestive evidence from across the country that it is: in professional journals (see Davis-Floyd et al., 2020; The Trust Project, 2020, and other articles in this Special Issue), and in a substantial increase in news media coverage about midwives[9] and the increasing numbers of US families who are seeking to give birth with midwives outside the hospital. One website called "Birth Monopoly" helps consumers track hospital policies to decide which one might have the least restrictions or whether the family feels secure enough to allow the laboring mother to go in at all[10]. Thus, investigating the efficacy and feasibility of better integrating and increasing birth in alternative settings seems timely.

EVIDENCE OF SAFETY: OUTCOMES OF BIRTH IN HOSPITAL VS. IN PRIVATE HOMES AND FREESTANDING BIRTH CENTERS

The two most recent meta-analyses examining perinatal outcomes for birthing people with low-risk pregnancies in high-income countries have demonstrated similar levels of safety for hospital and planned, midwife-attended births in private homes or freestanding birth centers. An Australian meta-analysis (Scarf et al., 2018) found no significant difference in the odds of intrapartum stillbirth or early neonatal death (0–7 days), regardless of whether the birth was planned for home, birth center, or hospital, and no difference in those odds between parous and multiparous women. That meta-analysis of four studies of planned home births also identified significantly lower odds of NICU admission than for planned hospital births, with an odds ratio (OR) of 0.71 and a 95% CI of 0.55–0.92. Scarf et al. (2018) concluded that their findings "support the expansion of birth center and home birth options for women with low-risk pregnancies."

A 2019 Canadian meta-analysis found 14 eligible international studies—representing more than 500,000 home births—which met their strict criteria for comparing planned home to planned low-risk hospital birth (Hutton et al., 2019). Stratifying their analyses by whether or not the midwives attending the home births were well integrated into the health services, they found that in jurisdictions where midwives were well integrated, perinatal and neonatal mortality summary risk estimates were essentially identical for intended home births and intended hospital births. The summary OR was 1.07 (95% CI, 0.70–1.65) for primips and 1.08 (95% CI, 0.84–1.38) for multiparous women.

In less integrated settings, Hutton et al. (2019) found that there was a possible increase in perinatal and neonatal mortality with home birth compared to hospital birth. However, because both estimates had large confidence limits due to the small numbers of deaths on which they were based, chance cannot be ruled out for the increase—the estimate on primips was based on 1 newborn death in 897 home births (The estimate for primips was OR 3.17 (95% CI, 0.73–13.76), and for multips, 1.58 (95% CI, 0.50–5.03).

[7]https://www.georgiacpm.org/certified-professional-midwives-frequently-asked-questions

[8]The "Continuum of Care" for reproductive, maternal, newborn and child health (RMNCH) includes integrated service delivery for mothers and children from pre-pregnancy to delivery, the immediate postnatal period, and childhood. Such care is provided by families and communities, through outpatient services, clinics and other health facilities. . . [It] recognizes that safe childbirth is critical to the health of both the woman and the newborn child—and that a healthy start in life is an essential step towards a sound childhood and a productive life (https://www.who.int/pmnch/about/continuum_of_care/en/).

[9]https://www.pushformidwives.org/pushheadlines

[10]https://birthmonopoly.com/covid-19/

TABLE 1 | Estimated birth costs and annual savings from an additional 10% of deliveries occurring in private homes or freestanding birth centers.

	Home birth	Birth center birth	Hospital birth	Savings from additional 10% home and freestanding birth center births (US dollars)
Estimated cost for an uncomplicated vaginal birth	$2,870[a]	$7,240[b]	$12,156[c]	
Additional 5% home births and additional 5% freestanding birth center births	$1.811 billion[d]	$959 million[e]		$2.769 billion
Lower cesarean rate for low-risk birthing people				$299 million[f]
Reduced rate of low birthweight babies				$111 million[g]
If competition brought 10% reduction in hospital birth cost				$4.267 billion[h]
Reducing cesarean rates in hospitals to 15% as WHO recommends (i)				$3.422 billion[j]
Total potential cost savings				$10.868 billion[k]

[a]*This figure is from Anderson and Anderson (1999), updated (as are all figures) to 2019 dollars using the Consumer Price Index. More recent studies of home birth costs are scarce and these costs vary widely by location. The cost for the midwife here is an estimate for the birth only, in order for it to be comparable to hospital birth. Midwives generally include prenatal and postpartum care in their fee, but this care is not included in this analysis for any of the birth locations.*

[b]*This is the mean of the total of professional and facility charges for freestanding birth center births from the Practice Profile data collected from the Perinatal Data Registry by the American Association of Birth Centers (2015).*

[c]*This is the average facility, labor, and birth charge for a vaginal hospital birth with no complications in 2011 (updated to 2019 dollars) as reported by Childbirth Connection (2013), obtained from the US Agency for Healthcare Research and Quality, available at http://hcupnet.ahrq.gov/. Published costs that are much lower than this represent a subset of the costs of birth, and perhaps only the cost of the hospital stay itself.*

[d]*Calculated as 3.9 million births × 0.05 × ($12,156 - $2,870).*

[e]*Calculated as 3.9 million births × 0.05 × ($12,156 - $7,240).*

[f]*Low risk was defined as singleton, head-down term babies when data were obtained from the NVSS system to do the calculations for the "CPM 2000" study (Johnson and Daviss, 2005a). The savings from lowering the cesarean rate were calculated as [3.9 million × 0.05 × (0.19–0.052) × $5,735] + [3.9 million × 0.05 × (0.19–0.061) × $5,735].*

[g]*Calculated as 3.9 million × 0.10 × (0.024–0.011) × $21,876.*

[h]*Calculated as 3.51 million × 0.10 × $12,156.*

[i]*See http://www.who.int/reproductivehealth/publications/maternal_perinatal_health/csstatement/en/.*

[j]*Calculated as 3.51 million × (0.32–0.15) × $5,735.*

[k]*Calculated as $1.811 billion + $959 million + $299 million + $111 million + $4.267 billion + $3.422 billion.*

Despite limited institutional support for credentialed midwives in the United States attending births in private homes and freestanding birth centers, the weight of evidence in US cohort studies indicates that births in these settings have good outcomes when the studies: 1) are based on charts rather than birth certificates, because the latter often lack accurate outcome and care details; 2) identified low-risk women; 3) are able to discern the planned place of birth, thereby avoiding counting accidental, unplanned out-of-hospital births; and 4) are conducted on a defined group of midwives with training standards. Where comparisons are possible, these US cohort studies (Murphy and Fullerton, 1998; Schlenzka, 1999; Johnson and Daviss 2005a; Stapleton et al., 2013), produced similar results for low-risk births at home, in birth centers or in hospitals, just as the international meta-analyses have found. Even where the defined group of practitioners had questionable homogeneity of education and a varying degree of integration into the US maternity care system, outcomes were similar to those in the other studies cited for low-risk birthing people (Cheyney et al., 2014).

EVIDENCE ON THE COSTS OF HOSPITAL VS. HOME AND FREESTANDING BIRTH CENTERS

Having the Safety for a Fraction of the Cost

This section demonstrates that births in homes and freestanding birth centers are far less expensive to society than hospital births. Combined with the evidence that outcomes are similar among low-risk mothers who plan their births in private homes, birth centers, or hospitals, this fact reveals a win-win situation: childbearers choosing their own home or a freestanding birth center can have the safety of hospital births at a fraction of the cost to families or insurers. The relevant discussion, then, is about whether the size of the "win" is worthwhile.

There are approximately 3.9 million births annually in the United States (Statista, 2019). The average charge by a midwife for an uncomplicated home birth is $2,870 (this and all costs are in 2019 inflation-adjusted US dollars (Anderson and Anderson, 1999). In freestanding birth centers, the average cost is $7,240 (American Association of Birth Centers, 2015). In hospitals, the average cost for an uncomplicated vaginal birth is $12,156 (Childbirth Connection, 2013).

Table 1 summarizes the potential savings from a modest increase in the use of private homes or freestanding birth centers in the United States. If an additional 5% of deliveries occurred in private homes rather than in a hospital, the savings would be $1.811 billion annually. If another 5% of deliveries occurred in freestanding birth centers rather than hospitals, the added savings would be $959 million annually. Note that about 10–20% of birthing people who plan to deliver at home or in a freestanding birth center transfer to a hospital during labor (Stapleton et al., 2013; Cheyney et al., 2014), so the number of planned out-of-hospital births would need to increase by about 6% in order for the actual increase to be 5%. For this analysis, we make the simplifying assumption that those transferred to hospital would pay the average costs associated with hospital births. **Table 1** is reproduced from Anderson et al. (2021).

Cesareans, Instrumental Deliveries, and Other Interventions: High Costs and Risks

In the Scarf meta-analysis (2018), women planning a hospital birth were nearly three times as likely to have a cesarean or instrumental (forceps or vacuum) delivery as those planning a home birth, and nearly twice as likely to have a cesarean as those planning a birth center birth. Similarly, there has been consensus across the literature for decades that planned home and birth center births in the United States entail significantly less medical intervention than planned hospital births (Johnson and Daviss 2005a; Cheyney et al., 2014; Hutton et al., 2019).

Our cost analysis of interventions focuses on cesareans because they are both the costliest intervention and the cause of numerous safety concerns. Cesareans are associated with a two-fold increase in maternal mortality, increased maternal blood loss, impaired neonatal respiratory function, increased incidence of maternal postpartum infections, increased fetal lacerations, trouble with maternal-infant interaction, extended length of stay and recovery, re-hospitalization, placenta accreta and previa, hysterectomies, transfusions of ≥4 units, maternal ICU admission, and uterine rupture (Spong, 2015). It is beyond our scope here to quantify the economic costs of a current cesarean on future pregnancies.

Although the risk of a serious problem during a typical cesarean birth is low, with almost one-third of US births being cesareans, problems occur and costs are high. The cesarean rate for planned hospital births in the United States is 32% (Martin et al., 2018), compared to 6.1% for planned birth center births (Stapleton et al., 2013) and 5.2% for planned home births (Cheyney et al., 2014). While some of the hospital births involve higher-risk childbearers with increased needs for cesareans, the majority of those cesareans are performed on those who were low-risk, begging the question, "Were they necessary?" To illustrate, data obtained from the National Vital Statistics System suggest that in 2000, when the overall US cesarean rate was 22.9%, low-risk women delivering in a hospital had a 19% cesarean rate, compared to a 3.7% rate for women who planned home deliveries with Certified Professional Midwives (Johnson and Daviss, 2005a).

A cesarean adds an average of $5,735 to the cost of a birth in the United States (International Federation of Health Plans, 2016). With the reduced likelihood of cesareans among the additional 5% home deliveries and the 5% birth center deliveries in our proposal, even if low-risk women still had only a 19% cesarean rate in hospital, the savings for families or insurance companies would be an additional $299 million annually.

The Costs of Low Birth Weight and Prematurity

When prenatal care is provided by credentialed midwives, the incidence of low birthweight decreases. For example, the rate decreased from 2.4 to 1.1% in a national study (Johnson and Daviss, 2005b) and from 2.8 to 1.8% in a study conducted in Washington State (Health Management Associates, 2007). As well, the premature birth rate at the National Institutes of Health (NIH) for non-Hispanic white births in hospital has been shown to be more than double the rate for clients cared for by Certified Professional Midwives (CPMs) at home births (Johnson and Daviss, 2005b). Low birthweight or premature birth adds an average of $21,876 to the cost of caring for an infant (Russell et al., 2007), with additional health and financial repercussions later in life. If the number of births at home and in freestanding birth centers each increased by 5%, and the decrease in the populations served reflected the prematurity rates described above, we estimate that the reduced likelihood of low birthweight alone would contribute an additional savings of $111 million.

Increased Competition for Hospitals

Competition is a moderating force for prices and an incentive for improved quality. Robinson (2011) found that hospitals with limited competition charged commercial insurers 13.0–25.1% more for specific procedures than hospitals in competitive markets. Again, CPMs can practice legally in only 36 states[11]. If legislation enables them to serve more of the 50 states and territories and join forces with the Certified Nurse-Midwives (CNMs) and Certified Midwives (CMs) who also attend births in homes and freestanding births centers, midwives can become low-cost, service-oriented hospital competitors.

The Big Push for Midwives is a national campaign in the US initiated and driven by consumers wanting to increase access to care by midwives attending births in the broader community, not just in the hospital. It focuses on increasing access to CPMs by pushing for legislation that legalizes them in the 14 holdout states and also on the need for CNMs to come out from the requirement of physician sign-off on their care:

> We like to emphasize that competition is valued as an economic concept because it reduces costs and increases access and quality of goods and services for consumers. As the Big Push for Midwives Campaign posted on social media December 30, 2020,[12] to the extent that public policy mandates hospitals or physicians to sign-off for a single visit, or that midwife-guidelines approval is granted to physicians, they have been handed the weapon they can use to limit the financial and clinical impact of competition. This is to provide clarification of the intent, and the possible negative effects, of organized medicine's involvement in out-of-hospital midwife or birth center legislation[13].

If stronger competition forced hospitals to reduce their price for an uncomplicated birth by 10%, the 3.51 million childbearers who would still deliver in the hospital under our scenario—or their insurers[14]—could save $4.267 billion. Because hospitals would still be the exclusive providers of care for complications, we assume here that only the price for an uncomplicated birth

[11]PushMap and PushChart: https://www.pushformidwives.org/what_we_do

[12]https://www.facebook.com/PushForMidwives/posts/3999886113363809

[13]https://www.facebook.com/PushForMidwives/posts/3999886113363809 in response to https://newrepublic.com/article/160706/midwives-appalachia-kentucky-maternity-care-desert

[14]In theory, it follows then, that if the insurers pay out less, they should be able to charge less.

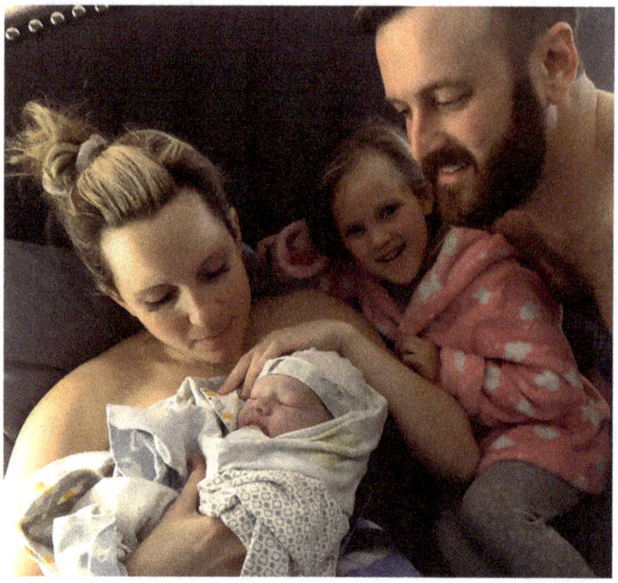

FIGURE 3 | The family gathers together in the family bed. In Canada, all births–home, hospital, or birth center–are covered through government insurance. Families can choose where they want to deliver, unhampered by considerations of cost. Midwives stand back again while the family is afforded a photo without masks, taken by grandmother, Lori Szauter. Used with permission.

would decrease. There is substantial evidence that competition also affects treatment decisions in hospitals (Gaynor et al., 2015). Intensified competition from CPM-attended home births, which have a 5.2% cesarean rate (Cheyney et al., 2014), especially when accompanied by education for families about their options, should provide a financial incentive for hospitals to bring their cesarean rates within a more acceptable range (Again, the US national cesarean rate is 32%.) If US hospitals reduced cesareans to the 15% range, as the World Health Organization (WHO) has recommended since 1985, the savings for the birthing people who would still deliver in the hospital—and especially for their insurance companies--could be an additional $3.422 billion.

The total estimated savings from increased access to births outside the hospital as we have described above amount to $10.868 billion annually. This proposal to facilitate an increase in births at home or in freestanding birth centers, if implemented, would represent a huge win for the many constituents who want access to safe and normal physiologic childbirth with fewer interventions, freedom of choice for a variety of ideological, religious, cultural, financial or personal reasons, and lower maternity care costs for American society.

OBSTETRIC AND PUBLIC HEALTH STATEMENTS ON HOME BIRTH PRIOR TO COVID-19

The successful implementation of US policy to increase rates of home and freestanding birth center births would be facilitated by at least tacit support from the national obstetric and public health communities. Some support has emerged: in 2001, the American Public Health Association (APHA) passed a resolution entitled, "Increasing Access to Out-Of-Hospital Maternity Care Services through State-Regulated and Nationally-Certified Direct-Entry Midwives,"(American Public Health Association, Maternal and Child Health Division, 2001) after they saw the methodology and preliminary data from the "CPM 2000" study on home births (Johnson and Daviss, 2005a).

A detailed description of the history and politics behind the American College of Obstetrics and Gynecology (ACOG) statements on home birth and a rationale for better integrating midwives specializing in births at home and in freestanding birth centers in the US can be found in Anderson et al. (2021). Briefly, ACOG officially opposed home birth from the 1970s on; 2011 was the first year that any evidence was quoted to support ACOG's negative statements about it, but that evidence was based on part of a meta-analysis that was later discredited (Wax et al., 2010, analyzed in; Anderson et al., 2021). To their credit, ACOG removed the Wax et al. study from their equations about perinatal and neonatal mortality in the next ACOG statement on Planned Home Birth in 2016.

However, unfortunately, ACOG has not updated its analysis to include the two new home birth meta-analyses (Scarf et al., 2018; Hutton et al., 2019) that demonstrate no difference in safety among birth settings for low-risk childbearers. Instead, Table 2 in ACOG's homebirth statements since 2016 has continued to use a single study based on birth certificates in a single state (Snowden et al., 2015) to assert that home birth "is associated with a more than twofold increased risk of perinatal death (1–2 in 1,000)[15]." The analysis in Anderson et al. (2021) questions whether such a study can be generalized to other US. In short, the Snowden et al. study was conducted in Oregon, one of only two states where licensure was not required for midwives to practice legally at that time, and where family members, naturopaths, or unlicensed midwives managed more than a third of the births.

A subsequent interview published between the principal author of the study, Jonathan Snowden, and Melissa Cheyney, the midwife in the state who happened to be the principal author of the national homebirth study of the Midwives Alliance of North America (Cheyney et al., 2014) clarified that they had several common understandings: that the absolute risk of home birth in this and other studies is low; that the risk of having a cesarean in a planned hospital compared to planned home birth in Oregon and the rest of the US is dangerously high; that one should not assume that parents choose home birth for selfish reasons without taking their baby's safety into consideration; and that

[15]In its 2017–2020 homebirth statements, the only changes that ACOG made from its 2016 statement were in Table 2(a)the addition of another sign highlighted in yellow and explanation in the footnotes about what it meant: "includes planned birth center and home birth" and(b)the switching of signs (‡ and †) that mark the Snowden et al. and Grunebaum et al. studies in the footnotes of Table 2. At first we thought they meant that the 3.9/1000 perinatal mortality figures were now being attributed to the Grunebaum study but we were mistaken. ACOG has continued to use the single study by Snowden et al. that reports 3.9/1000 perinatal deaths for planned home vs. 1.8/1000 perinatal deaths for hospital births (a "more than twofold risk") for the reporting of perinatal mortality in its statements from 2016 to 2020.

better integration and respect for midwives in Oregon as well as the rest of the US could improve outcomes (Cheyney, 2016).

By 2016, with pressure from other obstetric associations and studies that could no longer be ignored, ACOG (ACOG, 2016) accepted that home birth does occur safely in other high-resource countries and that "a characteristic common to those cohort studies reporting comparable rates of perinatal mortality" among care settings is the provision of care by midwives "well integrated into the health care system."

In their 2016–2020 statements (ACOG, 2016), ACOG also acknowledged that they would support the provision of care, not just by CNMs and CMs but by all midwives whose education and licensure meet the International Confederation of Midwives (ICM) Global Standards for Midwifery Education, which many CPMs do[16].

The other two ACOG statements on birth setting since COVID-19 will be discussed in *Then COVID-19 Struck: Highlights Even More, Need for Legislation and Health Insurance for Birth Outside Hospitals.*

WHAT EVIDENCE DO WE HAVE ABOUT WHAT CHILDBEARERS WANT?

In the *Listening to Mothers* survey carried out by the California Health Care Foundation (2018), although 99% of women in the state had a hospital birth in 2016, a substantial portion expressed interest in using a freestanding birth center or their private home for a future birth. However, only 7% of women in California in the survey used midwives as their main prenatal care providers and 9% as their birth attendant:

> Less than 1 in 10 survey participants used either midwives or labor doulas ... for their recent births. However ... over 1 in 6 women would definitely want midwives or labor doulas for a future birth. In addition, more than 1 in 3 would consider using these care team members[17].

Some of this was the result of the lack of options of available insurance providers. For example, nearly 1 in 4 Black or Latina women had their prenatal care provider assigned to them, apparently by their primary provider, compared to less than 1 in 8 white women[17].

The financial impediment may explain some of why data from the National Vital Statistics database demonstrate that white women have 2 ½ times the rate of home births as American Indian or Alaskan Native women, three times the rate of Black women, and almost four times the rate of Hispanic women

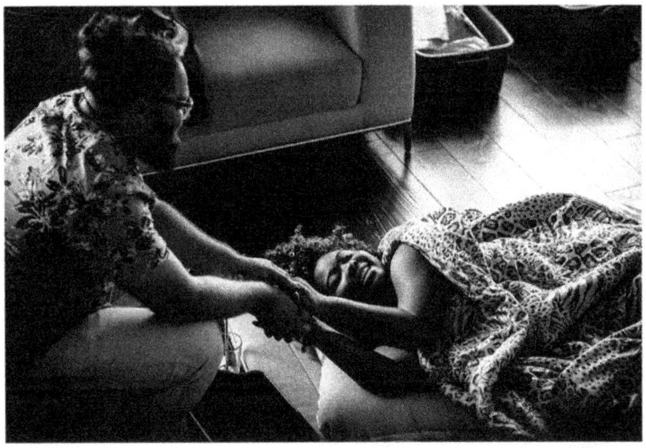

FIGURE 4 | Nicholas Richer-Brulé holds the hands of his wife, Bernadette Betchi, during a contraction. They chose a home birth because "it is a safe place where we were able to deliver our baby in the comfort of an environment that we could control. This meant even more with the unpredictability that Covid-19 has had on our surroundings. It eliminated the stresses of traveling while in labor, of being separated from each other and our children and being subjected to the hospital's restrictions and rules" (personal communication, Bernadette). Photo by Elle Odyn Breathe In Photography Ottawa Ontario. Used with permission.

(Martin et al., 2019). (See **Figures 4**, **6**, what Indigenous, Black and Latina women deserve to have offered, and **Figure 5**, how it was taken from them in the 1980s.)

The current President of the Midwives Alliance of North America, Sarita Bennett, emphasizes that there is a balancing place in US society for those not ready to choose birth in their own home but do not want to go to a hospital, especially during the pandemic:

> While we can talk about legalizing CPMs, unless we also address changing birth center legislation that is restrictive rather than evidence-based, there will still be limited options, especially for those who might accept birth center birth but aren't ready to make the leap to home birth. My birth center in a state with no birth center legislation has lots of those families who then choose home birth the next time (Sarita Bennett DO, CPM, personal communication, Jan. 2021).

Pain relief is a major concern of birthing persons, may determine where they seek care, and is related to delivery cost. In the national Listening to Mothers survey of 2013, 67% of respondents used epidural or spinal analgesia, 16% used narcotics, and 7% were given general anesthesia[18].

Some childbearers want to be more physically involved with their births and have fewer interventions. In the same survey, 17% said they used no pain medication, and 6% used nitrous oxide

[16]The complexities of which CPMs do and do not meet these ICM standards are too detailed to explain herein. For the standards themselves, see https://internationalmidwives.org/assets/files/general-files/2018/04/icm-standards-guidelines_ammended2013.pdf

[17]https://www.chcf.org/wp-content/uploads/2018/08/ListeningMothersCareTeam2018.pdf

[18]https://www.ncbi.nlm.nih.gov/pmc/articles/PMC3894594/pdf/JPE23-1_PTR_A3_009-016.pdf

(the same "laughing gas" that dentists use), which is a client-controlled and effective method of pain relief and can be made available in birth centers and at home births. It is cheaper for birthing persons to use nitrous in home or birth centers, as hospitals can take advantage of the lack of regulation to charge what they want. For example, a hospital in Wisconsin bills more than $100 for every 15 minutes that the nitrous is sitting in the room, which, for one woman, resulted in a bill of $4,836, whereas the local freestanding birth center charges only a flat fee of $100 for its use, for as long as it is needed. An epidural in the same hospital in Wisconsin costs $1,500, a third of the price of the nitrous oxide[19].

In the aforementioned 2013 *Listening to Mothers* national survey, women reported using a variety of drug-free methods to increase comfort and relieve pain, with 73% using at least one non-pharmacologic method of pain relief, led by breathing techniques (48%), position changes (40%), hands-on techniques like massage (22%), and mental strategies (e.g., relaxation methods) (21%)[18].

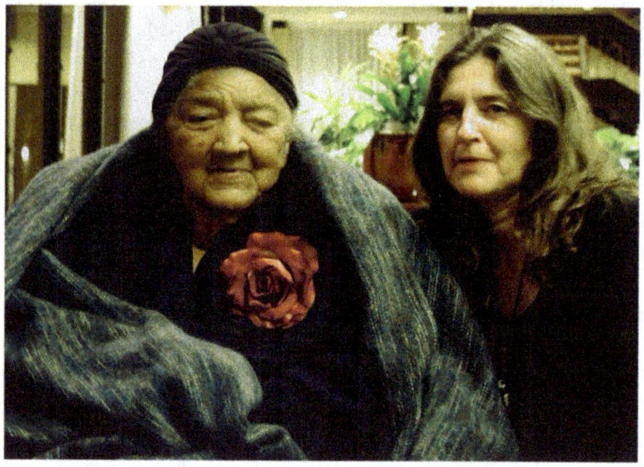

FIGURE 5 | Visiting "Miss Margaret" Charles Smith, age 98, the year she died (2004). She attended circa 3500 babies at home in Alabama, many during times when African American women were denied entry to hospitals. Betty-Anne (on the right), who attended homebrths in Alabama 1979–81, studied the statistics at that time in Russell County, Alabama, trying to understand why the "Black granny midwives"–who decided they would rather be called, the "Grand Midwives"—were having their licences revoked. She discovered their outcomes were good, but a Medicaid pay hike for physicians and the 1982 introduction of nurse-midwives had made poor African American pregnant women financially lucrative for hospital practitioners (Financial Planning Division, Alabama Medicaid 1995). Interviewing the midwives and women, Betty-Anne realized that nobody had asked the women what *they* wanted. Photo by Ken Johnson. Used with permission.

THEN COVID-19 STRUCK: THE NEED FOR LEGISLATION AND HEALTH INSURANCE FOR BIRTH OUTSIDE HOSPITALS BECOMES URGENT

A birthing person's ability to pay for a birth in their private home or at a freestanding birth center is often limited by finances because most hospital births are paid for through public or private insurance, while births not in hospital are rarely afforded the same privilege. In 2017, more than 2/3 (67.9%) of planned home births and almost 1/3 (32.2%) of birth center births were paid for by the birthing persons themselves, while only 3.4% of women self-paid for hospital births (MacDorman and Declercq, 2019).

In 2020, the report Birth Settings in America: Outcomes, Quality, and Choice concluded:

> Models for increasing access to birth settings for low-risk women that have been implemented at the state level include expanding Medicaid, Medicare, and commercial payer coverage to cover care provided at home and birth centers . . . by certified nurse midwives, certified midwives, and certified professional midwives whose education meets International Confederation of Midwives Global Standards . . . the potential impact of these state-level models is needed to inform consideration of nationwide expansion, particularly with regard to effects on reduction of racial/ethnic disparities in access, quality and outcomes of care [National Academies of Sciences, Engineering, and Medicine (NASEM) 2020:12]

Even prior to COVID-19, this report's conclusions had drawn attention to the fact that there is a "mismatch" between the care needs of the population as a whole and what is available for them, in both rural and urban areas. The NASEM researchers concluded that for most childbearers, who are largely healthy, it is unnecessary to rely primarily on "a surgical specialty" (obstetrics) for frontline care. They pointed to a growing shortage of obstetricians due to job dissatisfaction and early retirement and to the next logical step—to use the already nationally credentialed midwives as primary care providers, as most other countries do. Furthermore, the report emphasizes a need to ensure that the workforce "resembles the racial/ethnic composition of the population . . . as well as its linguistic, geographic, and socioeconomic diversity," because research demonstrates that such measures increase safety and satisfaction (National Academies of Sciences, 2020: 13). (See **Figures 5** and **6**)

Enter COVID-19. As the pandemic increased the demand for birth setting options, frustrations for childbearers wanting care in their homes also increased, as did the racial and socio-economic disparities between those who can and cannot afford choice of birth setting. Countries like Canada with universal health care coverage have removed this artificial financial barrier to home births and also established some freestanding birth centers, articulating the obvious—that births outside the hospital are cheaper and more welcoming than engagement with the

[19] https://www.npr.org/sections/health-shots/2019/05/28/726572880/bill-of-the-month-4-836-charge-for-laughing-gas-during-childbirth-is-no-joke

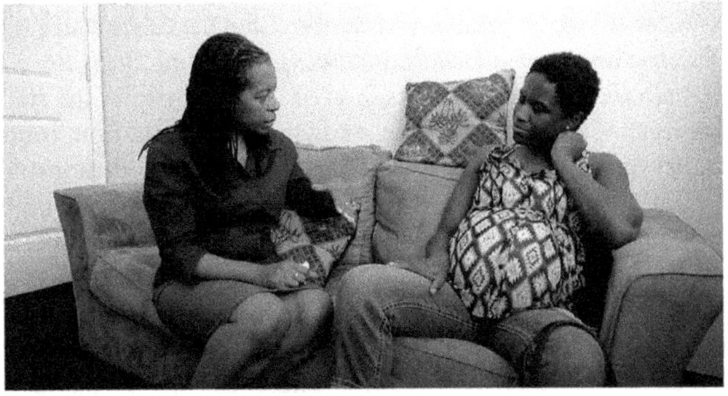

FIGURE 6 | Midwives like Jennie Joseph (left), who practices in Florida, are picking up from where Miss Margaret and the other Grand Midwives of the South have left off -because the latter are no longer permitted to practice. However, even with her Certified Professional Midwife credential and state license, and in spite of the fact that she and her team have reduced prematurity and low birth weight rates within the Black, Indigenous, and People of Color community, their attempts to get any government support from grants or other public health or civic funds have been unsuccessful. She receives a meager fee of $1500 if clients are compensated through Medicaid, but even less for the over-proportion of indigent, undocumented and uninsured who aren't on Medicaid who come to her freestanding birth center at "Commonsense Childbirth" in Orlando who receive care for free if needed, or on a sliding scale. Not supporting all pregnant women to have health care, during pregnancy or any other time of their life, is unheard of in countries like the UK where Jennie was originally trained as a midwife. These intimate moments of shared trust and respect, illustrated here between client Kristen April Brown (on the right) and Jennie, is what researchers have determined may be behind the consistently better outcomes compared to other clinics and services where women from the same demographic receive maternity care (Joseph 2021:131-144). Photo from "the American Dream," videographer Paolo Patruno, see www.birthisadream.org and https://www.youtube.com/watch?v=Si_4xUQ2MK8&t=1s. Used with permission.

hospital enterprise; almost all provincial Canadian governments now cover the birth wherever it occurs.

Canada provides a good example of how it is easier to adapt when pandemics or other challenging events occur if midwives are available who can offer a choice of birth settings[20]. Of the births being attended just by the midwives in Ontario (not the family docs or obstetricians), the planned home birth rate was 13% in March 2020, when the effects of COVID-19 were just beginning to be felt. By May 2020, with COVID-19 in full swing, the planned home birth rate among midwife-attended births in Ontario had increased from that 13–20% (Daviss et al., 2021). This increase was easily facilitated because all infrastructures—legislation, insurance coverage, quality assurance programs and integration—were already well established for homebirth providers. In March and April, clients who had formerly considered a hospital birth did not have to switch providers. They simply told their midwives that they now preferred to stay home.

The US states without adequate provisions for care at home or in freestanding birth centers even in normal times have been caught more unprepared than those that already had instituted providers for those birth options prior to COVID-19. Some jurisdictions like Washington, D.C[21]. and Kentucky[22] managed to get legislation for CPMs passed just before the pandemic struck the US. Others (like Illinois, which has had a Home Birth Safety Act that would legalize CPMs on the books for about 10 years[23]) have remained sluggish at passing such legislation, in spite of obvious need (Ayres-Brown, 2020).

In New York, the strong need for increased access to births outside the hospital prompted Governor Cuomo's Executive Order to invite midwives from outside the state of New York to come and help. This highlighted, and brought into question, the fact that in normal times, CPMs cannot legally practice there, just as they cannot in Illinois nor in the other states where they are not legal. In fact, CPMs living in New York have been persecuted for practicing rather than embraced in the state, even though the state has long allowed CNMs and CMs to attend home births (May and Davis-Floyd, 2006; Chamberlain, 2020). This is also despite the fact that New York CPMs would qualify for licenses if the state midwifery board had properly implemented the licensing statute that was approved by the state legislature in 1992[24].

Vicki Hedley, Past-President of the Midwives Alliance of North America (MANA) and Senior Advisor to NYCPM—the New York State CPM organization—thinks that COVID-19 holds hope for change but explains the complications:

> I do believe that this pandemic has potentially opened the door to legalization for CPMs in NY. More and more people are asking for our (CPM) services and wanting home birth because of the safety aspects. The problem is access. Although NY requires that licensed providers be paid by insurer's reimbursements, many insurers require liability/malpractice insurance, which many home birth midwives cannot afford and more unfortunately cannot obtain due to the lack of state licensure. We are in a Catch-22. Straight Medicaid pays about $1,300 for [full-scope] maternity care, which is far from a living wage. Of course, these issues need to be addressed in order to create the access for birthing families that is so desperately needed (Personal communication, December 5, 2020).

Meanwhile, the temporary nature of the Governor's Executive Order has caused serious problems for any CPM who does want to practice in the state to meet the increased demand by mothers and families for out-of-hospital birth options. Ida Darragh, the

[20]For examples of effective care in the immediate aftermaths of earthquakes, tsunamis and floods, see Davis-Floyd et al., 2021; Lim and Davis-Floyd, 2021

[21]https://code.dccouncil.us/dc/council/laws/23-97.html. Accessed December 17, 2020.

[22]https://newrepublic.com/article/160706/midwives-appalachia-kentucky-maternity-care-desert

[23]https://www.ilga.gov/legislation/BillStatus.asp?DocNum=1754&GAID=14&DocTypeID=SB&LegID=104736&SessionID=91&SpecSess=&Session=&GA=100

[24]PushMap and PushChart: https://www.pushformidwives.org/what_we_do

Executive Director of the North American Registry of Midwives (NARM), the organization responsible for setting standards for CPM credentialing nationally, describes the urgent need for legislation:

> There is currently a proposal for licensure of CPMs in New York being drafted by the office of Dick Gottfried, the Chair of the Assembly Health Committee. It needs some better language before being submitted and the midwives are trying to communicate with the office about it. It is the optimum time to present a bill with several months of "legal" status during the pandemic already. The executive order is renewed monthly, but that means only that midwives with a license in another state can practice legally until that expiration date. Midwives and clients need more certainty than one month of legal status! (Personal communication December 5, 2020)

This ambiguous month-to-month situation puts the CPMs currently practicing in New York in a vulnerable state: being legal for a few months, but then with the potential to have their licensure removed just when their clients are actually due to have their babies!

ACOG and ACNM recognized early on that the pandemic had created an interest in home birth, alerting them to the fact that families were nervous about institutional birth settings. They issued a joint statement in March acknowledging the pandemic but assuring the public that "Hospitals and birth centers that are both licensed and accredited *remain safe places* to give birth in the United States[25]." (italics added).

Three weeks later, on April 20, 2020, ACOG's CEO issued a further statement:

> ACOG and its members, in collaboration with the health care team, are dedicated to providing patient-centered, respectful care. Obstetrician-gynecologists see first hand the stress and uncertainty facing pregnant people, families, and their support networks during the COVID-19 pandemic, and this includes questioning the settings in which to give birth. However, even during this pandemic, *hospitals and accredited birth centers remain the safest places to give birth* [italics added]. Physicians, certified nurse-midwives and certified midwives, and the entire health care team will work to ensure that precautions are taken to make labor and delivery safe, supportive and welcoming for their patients (Phipps, 2020).

Earlier in the Phipps statement is the quote about the "more than twofold increased risk of perinatal death" of ACOG's other statements over the last four years, which from the outset was rendered questionable, since the only source for such a claim in their Table on perinatal mortality is the single Oregon study of 2015, whose generalizability is doubtful for the other states (See *Obstetric and Public Health Statements on Home Birth Prior to COVID-19* above and Anderson et al., 2021). Instead, the states that legalize nationally certified midwives can benefit from cohort studies on midwives with like certification that demonstrate similar outcomes between home and hospital births (Murphy and Fullerton, 1998; Johnson and Daviss, 2005a; Stapleton et al., 2013).

Neither the ACOG nor the ACOG/ACNM statements provide any data to demonstrate that hospitals are now safe, safer, or "remain safer" than home births under COVID-19 pandemic conditions. As far as we know, there have been no data in the US comparing outcomes of different birth settings since COVID-19 began its surge across the country. There is, on the other hand, some data to indicate that it is reasonable for families to have concerns about entering the hospital if it is not necessary. Indeed, it is not necessary--in fact, may not be advisable–if you are a low risk birthing person.

Dr. Manoj Jain, an infectious disease specialist from Memphis, TN who recognized that a patient of his had likely acquired COVID-19 from staff (Jain, 2021) provides an example of what the academic literature has brought to light about possible infection in hospital. Front-line health care workers in the US have a three times greater risk of testing positive for COVID-19 than the general community (Nguyen et al., 2020). These providers can be highly contagious if they have COVID-19 themselves, prior to having any symptoms. While obstetricians, CNMs, and obstetric nurses are not usually considered front-line workers who deal with COVID-19 patients, they are walking in and out of the hospitals where COVID-19 patients gather, and, as the physician in the Memphis story points out, eat lunch without their masks on, with other health care workers, in the lounge or cafeteria.

The true wild cards in the hospital are the anesthesiologists and nurse anesthetists who, unlike obstetric providers, cannot limit where they work to one floor of the hospital. They don and doff—and sanitize--faithfully, but they may have to quickly move from an intubation on a COVID-19 patient in one ward to doing an epidural on a pregnant patient in another section of the hospital.

COVID-19 also adds a new dimension to avoiding the reality that ACOG has admitted: that there are increased cesarean births when low risk women choose hospital birth. Even if low risk women hope to be able to manage without an epidural, their likelihood of having a cesarean increases from 3.7% with a planned home birth to 19% if they plan a hospital birth (Johnson and Daviss, 2005a)[26], which also increases their risk of exposure to more healthcare professionals in the operating room.

[25] https://www.acog.org/news/news-releases/2020/03/patient-centered-care-for-pregnant-patients-during-the-covid-19-pandemic

[26] The cesarean rate is 5.2% overall in the more recent study (Cheyney et al., 2014) but it was difficult to find the rate among low risk women in hospital for a comparison to the study. In our 2005 report we were able to obtain it.

LIABILITY

Following the first large prospective home birth study that demonstrated similar safety between home and hospital births in North America (Johnson and Daviss, 2005a), out of thousands of responses to this study, the only response to the *British Medical Journal*, which published the study, from a practicing American physician iterated that he did "not mind" women choosing home birth, but that "our pernicious legal system prevents me from ever considering the practice" (Rivera, 2005).

The present liability system can create insurmountable financial risks for practitioners that make them reticent to offer valued services that childbearers are increasingly seeking. A team of researchers concerned about the impact of the present system identified seven aims for a high-functioning liability system and studied "whether 25 strategies that have been used or proposed for improvement have met or could meet the seven aims" (Sakala et al., 2013). They concluded:

> Ten strategies seem to have potential to improve liability matters in maternity care across multiple aims. The most promising strategy--implementing rigorous maternity care quality improvement (QI) programs--has led to better quality and outcomes of care, and impressive declines in liability claims, payouts, and premium levels. A number of promising strategies warrant demonstration and evaluation at the level of states, health systems, or other appropriate entities. Rigorous QI programs have a growing track record of contributing to diverse aims of a high-functioning liability system and seem to be a win-win-win prevention strategy for childbearing families, maternity care providers, and payers. Effective strategies are also needed to assist families when women and newborns are injured.

COVID-19 raises new questions about liability for midwives who practice in private homes or freestanding birth centers. If there is a shortage of legal midwives based outside of hospital in any state, whether or not they are invited to temporarily practice as in New York state, or left without legal accommodation as in Illinois, midwives from neighboring states will inevitably come to the rescue of women in need in the state, regardless of their legal status (Ayers-Brown, 2020).

Even if midwives are legally attending births in private homes or freestanding births centers in any given state, if they don't have hospital privileges, the increased restrictions of COVID-19 can have serious implications. Ida Darragh and Vicki Hedley explain that many hospitals are now allowing the father of the baby to attend the birth, and just recently in some places, a doula (often only if she is certified by the hospital or by an organization recognized by that hospital). However, when there is a transport from a home birth, the community midwife may not be able to enter the hospital along with her own client to provide the continuity of care that is so well proven in the literature to improve outcomes (Sandall et al., 2016). Thus important information that the midwife could provide can be missed--for example, the time of rupture of the membranes, the baby's presentation, a borderline history of pre-eclampsia, or the special cultural and personal needs of a family. This could implicate both the midwife and the hospital in subsequent litigation.

Although legal reform is beyond the scope of this article, we would like to point out here that there are underutilized options to discuss and disseminate transfer and practice guidelines, to encourage swift and fair settlements in legal disputes (Anderson, 2003), and there are less litigious societies whose policies can serve as models, such as those of Sweden and Germany (Lowes, 2003).

CONCLUSION: EXPANDED ACCESS TO BIRTHS IN PRIVATE HOMES AND FREESTANDING BIRTH CENTERS IN THE US IS WARRANTED

Home and birth center births are on the rise in the US, and COVID-19 has provided a catalyst/pivotal moment that directs us to the need for increased access to nationally credentialed, licensed midwives and options for women to birth outside the hospital. Many US women have already switched to these options to avoid both hospital contagion and the forced choice of only one (or no) personal birthing companion during these Covidian times.

As we have shown above, if only 10% more US women deliver at home or in freestanding birth centers, the savings could amount to $10.868 billion per year. Outcomes are similar for low-risk mothers regardless of setting in countries where midwives are well-trained and integrated into the Reproductive, Maternal, Newborn and Child Health (RMNCH) Continuum of Care in the community[27]. The US studies on birth settings demonstrate good and similar outcomes among home, birth center, and hospital births when: 1) they are based on charts for an identified cohort rather than on birth certificates; 2) they can identify low risk women; 3) they discern the planned place of birth, thereby avoiding counting accidental, unplanned out-of-hospital births; and 4) they have studied a defined group of midwives with training standards. Cost and safety issues suggest expanded access to home and freestanding birth centers as a solution to the shortage of appropriate services and maternity-care service providers that existed even before COVID-19.

Increased access to credentialed maternity-care providers requires new legislation for CPM licensure in some states and extended public insurance for home and freestanding birth center settings in all states. While the data on the safety of home and freestanding birth centers has convinced the APHA and many state legislatures over the last two decades to promote birth in these settings, COVID-19 and pure practicality have convinced more state politicians of the importance of credentialed and licensed midwives who offer these alternatives to hospital birth.

[27]https://d3n8a8pro7vhmx.cloudfront.net/pushformidwives/pages/1144/attachments/original/1585429341/The_Big_Push_for_Midwives_Campaign_Strategic_Priorities.pdf?1585429341

There are now two other important givens that mark change: First, ACOG has admitted that safe home birth is possible in other countries where midwives are well-integrated and in accredited birth centers in the US. Second, the New York State governor has invited licensed midwives, including CPMs from other states, to help out in his state during the pandemic (Executive Order, 2020), thereby recognizing their value and essential services in a state that has had former reserve towards CPMs.

Taking two critical further steps could integrate nationally credentialed midwives into the larger US health care system and help these midwives to meet demands of birthing people. The first is to build the infrastructure of legislation, insurance, and healthy Quality Improvement programs needed to support home, freestanding birth center, and hospital maternity care providers so they can be fully integrated into their local RMNCH Continuum of Care.

The second step is to encourage a culture in which all healthcare professionals recognize and encourage each other to offer the services for which they are best suited. This would include opening rather than limiting scope of practice, eliminating physician supervision but increasing collaboration, and encouraging autonomy of midwives and clients. It would also include debunking the myths of what is "safe" and "not safe."

The first step is foreseeable and has been accomplished at least in part in about two-thirds of the United States. One would think it should be relatively easy, given the models in the other states, but of course it requires some buy-in to the second step. The second step is dependent on the first; in fact one might say the two steps are co-dependent. The second step requires visionary leaders who can turn over 100 years of conflict aside, expose the overlapping systems of self-protective competitors, and transmute the US maternity care system into a best-practice, safer and less costly model that puts the interests of the birthing population first.

Whether the primary goal is safety, reproductive justice, cost savings, avoiding infection, or increasing freedom of choice and access to birth options for birthing people, public policies that support planned, midwife-attended births in private homes and freestanding birth centers are the appropriate and long overdue response.

AUTHOR CONTRIBUTIONS

All authors listed have made a substantial, direct, and intellectual contribution to the work and approved it for publication.

REFERENCES

ACOG Committee on Obstetric Practice (2016). April 2016 Committee opinion 669 and confirmed as 697 in 2017, 2018 and 2020 with a qualification that it is an interim statement changed slightly to replace it. Available at: https://www.acog.org/Clinical-Guidance-and-Publications/Committee-Opinions/Committee-on-Obstetric-Practice/Planned-Home-Birth?IsMobileSet=false (Accessed March 6, 2019).

ACOG Committee Opinion (2011). ACOG Committee Opinion No. 476: planned home birth. *Obstet. Gynecol.* 117 (2 Pt 1), 425–428. doi:10.1097/AOG.0b013e31820eee20

Aetna (2020). Home births. Medical Clinical Policy Bulletins. Available at: http://www.aetna.com/cpb/medical/data/300_399/0329.html (Accessed December 5, 2020).

American Association of Birth Centers(2015). *Practice profile data from AABC perinatal data registry.* Perkiomenville, PA: American Association of Birth Centers.

American College of Nurse Midwives (2019). Fact sheet: essential facts about midwives. Available at: https://www.midwife.org/acnm/files/cclibraryfiles/filename/000000007531/essentialfactsaboutmidwives-updated.pdf (Accessed December 14, 2020).

American Public Health Association, Maternal and Child Health Division (2001). Increasing access to out-of-hospital maternity care services through state-regulated and nationally-certified direct-entry midwives. *Am. J. Pub. Health* 92, 453–455.

Anderson, D., Daviss, B. A., and Johnson, K. C. (2021). "What if another 10% of deliveries in the United States occurred at home or in a birth center? Safety, economics and politics," in *Birth models on the human rights' frontier.* Abingdon, England: Routledge Press, 205–228.

Anderson, D. A. (2003). "Fairness in the face of conflict: dividing environmental assets and obligations," 3:2. *Int. J. Glob. Econ. Issues* 3, 116–132. doi:10.1504/ijgenvi.2003.003860

Anderson, R., and Anderson, D. (1999). The cost effectiveness of home birth. *J. Nurse Midwifery* 44 (1), 30–355. doi:10.1016/s0091-2182(98)00072-x

Ayres-Brown, A. (2020). Illinois midwives face surge of interest in home birth during corona virus pandemic. Available at: https://www.chicagotribune.com/coronavirus/ct-coronavirus-midwives-pregnancy-home-birth-20200422-bi3wxbdgufgdhjlhv6bj2rgk6i-story.html (Accessed December 16, 2020).

California Health Care Foundation (2018). Listening to mothers in California: care team and place of birth. Available at: https://www.chcf.org/wp-content/uploads/2018/08/ListeningMothersCareTeam2018.pdf (Accessed December 1, 2020).

Canadian Association of Midwives (2019). Midwifery-led births per province and territory. Available at: https://canadianmidwives.org/wp-content/uploads/2020/11/CAM-2019-Annual-Report-Map_1920x1080_2020-10-30-E-1024x576.png (Accessed August 15, 2020).

Chamberlain, G. (2020). Second woman arrested from midwife investigation in Yates country.the chronicle-express. Available at: https://www.democratandchronicle.com/story/news/politics/albany/2020/03/09/second-woman-arrested-midwife-investigation-yates-county/5006752002/ (Accessed December 15, 2020).

Cheyney, M. (2016). Understanding recent home-birth research: an interview with Drs. Melissa Cheyney and Jonathan Snowden. *J. Perinat. Educ.* 25 (2), 80–86. doi:10.1891/1058-1243.25.2.80

Cheyney, M., Bovbjerg, M., Everson, C., Gordon, W., Hannibal, D., and Vedam, S. (2014). Outcomes of care for 16,984 planned home births in the United States: the midwives alliance of North America Statistics Project, 2004–2009. *J. Midwifery Womens Health* 59 (1), 17–27. doi:10.1111/jmwh.12172

Childbirth Connection (2013). Average facility labor and birth charge by site and method of birth, United States 2009–2011. Available at: childbirthconnection.org/wp-content/uploads/2013/06/uscharges-chart-20092011.pdf (Accessed August 31, 2019).

Davis-Floyd, R., Gutschow, K., and Schwartz, D. A. (2020). Pregnancy, birth and the COVID-19 pandemic in the United States. *Med. Anthropol.* 39 (5), 413–427. doi:10.1080/01459740.2020.1761804

Davis-Floyd, R., Lim, R., Penwell, V., and Ivry, T. (2021). "Effective maternity disaster care: low tech, skilled touch," in *Sustainable birth in disruptive times.* Editors K. Gutschow, R. Davis-Floyd, and B. A. Daviss. (New York City, New York, USA: Springer Publishing), 316.

Daviss, B. A., Roberts, T., Leblanc, C., Champet, I., and Betchi Nnomo, B. (2021). When the masks come off in Canada and Guatemala, will the realities exposed by COVID-19 provoke positive action? In the global impacts of COVID-29 on maternity care practices. *Front. Sociol.* (In Press).

Executive Order (2020). Continuing temporary suspension and modification of laws relating to the disaster emergency. Sections 6951, 6952, 6953 and 6955 of the Education Law, to the extent necessary to allow midwives licensed and in current good standing in any state in the United States, or in any province or territory of Canada, to practice in New York State without civil or criminal penalty related to lack of licensure. Available at: https://www.governor.ny.gov/news/no-20211-continuing-temporary-suspension-and-modification-laws-relating-disaster-emergency (Accessed Febuary 11, 2021).

Financial Planning/Analysis Division Alabama Medicaid Agency (1995). *A Historical Overview of the Alabama Medicaid Agency.* Originally accessed June 5, 2019 but since taken off the medicaid.alabama. gov website: https://www.medicaid.alabama.gov/documents/2.0_Newsroom/2.1_About_Medicaid/2.1_Historical_Overview.pdf.

Gaynor, M., Ho, K., and Robert, J. T. (2015). The industrial organization of HealthCare markets. *J. Econ. Lit.* 53 (2), 235–284. doi:10.1257/jel.53.2.235

Health Management Associates (2007). Midwifery licensure and discipline program in Washington state: economic costs and benefits; October 31. Available at: http://www.washingtonmidwives.org/assets/Midwifery_Cost_Study_10-31-07.pdf (Accessed August 18, 2017).

Hutton, E., Reitsma, A., Simioni, J., Brunton, G., and Kaufman, K. (2019). Perinatal or neonatal mortality among women who intend at the onset of labour to give birth at home compared to women of low obstetrical risk who intend to give birth in hospital: a systematic review and meta-analyses. *EClinicalMedicine* 14, 59–70. doi:10.1016/j.eclinm.2019.07.005

International Federation of Health Plans (2016). 2015 comparative price report: variation in medical and hospital prices by country. Available at: https://docplayer.net/48892596-2015-comparative-price-report-variation-in-medical-and-hospital-prices-by-country.html. (Accessed January 4, 2021).

Jain, M. (2021). Patients are getting infected with COVID-19 in the hospital. It happened to one of mine and killed him. Available at: https://www.washingtonpost.com/health/acquiring-covid-19-in-the-hospital/2020/12/31/8cac8b82-3a50-11eb-9276-ae0ca72729be_story.html (Accessed January 4, 2021).

Johnson, K. C., and Daviss, B. A. (2005a). Outcomes of planned home births with certified professional midwives: large prospective study in North America. *BMJ* 330, 1416. doi:10.1136/bmj.330.7505.1416

Johnson, K. C., and Daviss, B. A. (2005b). Further neonatal mortality and prematurity follow-up. Available at: http://understandingbirthbetter.com/section.php?ID=24&Lang=En&Nav=Section (Accessed June 18, 2005).

Joseph, J. (2021). "There's Something Wrong Here: African-American Pregnant Women and their Babies are at Greatest Risk in the USA," in *Birth Models on the Human Rights' Frontier*. Abingdon: Routledge Press, 131–144.

Lim, R., and Davis-Floyd, R. (2021). "Implementing the international chidbirth initiatie (ICI) in disaster zones: behi sehat's experience in Indonesia, Haiti, the Philippines, and Nepal," in *Birth models on the human rights' frontier: speaking truth to power*. Editors B. A. Daviss and R. Davis-Floyd (Abingdon, England: Routledge Press), 55–74.

Lowes, R. (2003). Malpractice: do other countries hold the key? Medical economics. Available at: https://www.medicaleconomics.com/view/malpractice-do-other-countries-hold-key (Accessed December 28, 2020).

MacDorman, M., and Declercq, E. (2019). Trends and state variations in out-of-hospital births in the United States, 2004-2017. *Birth* 46 (2), 279–288. doi:10.1111/birt.12411

Martin, J. A., Hamilton, B. E., Osterman, M. J., Driscoll, A. K., and Mathews, T. J. (2017). Births: final data for 2015. *Natl. Vital Stat. Rep.* 66 (1), 1, 2017 Available at: https://www.cdc.gov/nchs/data/nvsr/nvsr66/nvsr66_01.pdf (Accessed October 1, 2017).

Martin, J. A., Hamilton, B. E., Osterman, M. J. K., Driscoll, A. K., and Drake, P. (2018). Births: final data for 2017. *Natl. Vital Stat. Rep.* 67 (8), 1–50.

Martin, J. A., Hamilton, B. E., Osterman, M. J. K., and Driscoll, A. K. (2019). Births: final data for 2018. *Natl. Vital Stat. Rep.* 68, 1–47.

May, M., and Davis-Floyd, R. (2006). "Idealism and pragmatism in the creation of the CM: the development of midwifery in New York and the New York midwifery practice act of 1992," in *Mainstreaming midwives: the politics of change.* Editors R. Davis-Floyd and C. B. Johnson (New York, NY: Routledge), 570.

Murphy, P. A., and Fullerton, J. (1998). Outcomes of intended home births in nurse-midwifery practice: a prospective descriptive study. *Obstet. Gynecol.* 92, 461–470. doi:10.1016/s0029-7844(98)00182-3

National Academies of Sciences (2020). *Engineering, and MedicineBirth settings in America: outcomes, quality, access, and choice.* Washington, DC: The National Academies Press, 368.

Nguyen, L. H., Drew, D. A., Graham, M. S., Joshi, A. D., Guo, C. G., Ma, W., et al. (2020). Risk of COVID-19 among front-line health-care workers and the general community: a prospective cohort study. *Lancet Public Health* 5 (9), E475–E483. doi:10.1016/S2468-2667(20)30164-X

Phipps, M. (2020). ACOG statement on birth settings. Available at: https://www.acog.org/news/news-releases/2020/04/acog-statement-on-birth-settings (Accessed December 18, 2020).

Rivera, D. A. (2005). The Fly in the Ointment. Response to Johnson and Daviss, outcomes of planned home births with certified professional midwives: large prospective study in North America. *BMJ* 330, 1416. doi:10.1136/bmj.330.7505.1416

Robinson, J. C. (2011). Hospital market concentration, pricing, and profitability in orthopedic surgery and interventional cardiology. *Am. J. Manag. Care* 17 (6), e241–e248.

Russell, R. B., Green, N. S., Steiner, C. A., Meikle, S., Howse, J. L., Poschman, K., et al. (2007). Cost of hospitalization for preterm and low birth weight infants in the United States. *Pediatrics* 120, e1–e9. doi:10.1542/peds.2006-2386

Sakala, C., Yang, Y. T., and Corry, M. P. (2013). Maternity care and liability: most promising policy strategies improvement. *Womens Health Issues* 23 (1), e25–37. doi:10.1016/j.whi.2012.11.003

Sandall, J., Soltani, H., Gates, S., Shennan, A., and Devane, D. (2016). Midwife-led continuity models versus other models of care for childbearing women. *Cochrane Database Syst. Rev.* 4, CD004667. doi:10.1002/14651858.CD004667.pub5

Scarf, V., Rossiter, C., Vedam, S., Dahlen, H. G., Ellwood, D., Forster, D., et al. (2018). Maternal and perinatal outcomes by planned place of birth among women with low-risk pregnancies in high-income countries: a systematic review and meta-analysis. *Midwifery* 62, 240–255. doi:10.1016/j.midw.2018.03.024

Schlenzka, P. (1999). Safety of alternative approaches to childbirth. PhD thesis. Palo Alto, California: Stanford University.

Snowden, J. M., Tilden, E. L., Snyder, J., Quigley, B., Caughey, A. B., and Cheng, Y. W. (2015). Planned out-of-hospital birth and birth outcomes. *N. Engl. J. Med.* 373, 2642–2653. doi:10.1056/NEJMsa1501738

Spong, C. Y. (2015). Prevention of the first cesarean delivery. *Obstet. Gynecol. Clin. North. Am.* 42 (2), 377–380. doi:10.1016/j.ogc.2015.01.010

Stapleton, S. R., Osborne, C., and Illuzzi, J. (2013). Outcomes of care in birth centers: demonstration of a durable model. *J. Nurse Midwifery* 58 (1), 3–14. doi:10.1111/jmwh.12003

Statista (2019). Number of births in the United States 1990–2018. Available at: https://www.statista.com/statistics/195908/number-of-births-in-the-united-states-since-1990/ (Accessed August 29, 2020).

The Trust Project (2020). The economist: the pandemic is making America rethink its shunning of midwifer. Available at: https://www.economist.com/united-states/2020/06/18/the-pandemic-is-making-america-rethink-its-shunning-of-midwifery (Accessed December 15, 2020).

Truven Health Analytics (2013). The cost of having a baby in the United States. Available at: http://transform.childbirthconnection.org/reports/cost/ (Accessed September 9, 2019).

Wax, J. R., Lucas, F. L., Lamont, M., Pinette, M. G., Cartin, A., and Blackstone, J. (2010). Maternal and newborn outcomes in planned homebirth vs planned hospital births: a meta-analysis. *Am. J. Obstet. Gynecol.* 203, 243e1–243e8. doi:10.1016/j.ajog.2010.05.028

10

Protecting Women's and Newborns' Rights in a Public Maternity Unit During the COVID-19 Outbreak: The Case of *Dra. Eloísa Díaz - La Florida* Hospital in Santiago, Chile

Gonzalo Leiva [1,2,3]†, Michelle Sadler[3,4†], Camila López [1†], Susana Quezada[5†], Víctor Flores [1†], Cristian Sierra [1†], Susan Díaz [1†] and Christian Figueroa [1,2†]*

[1]Maternity Dra. Eloísa Díaz - La Florida Hospital, Santiago, Chile, [2]Faculty of Medicine, Pontificia Universidad Católica de Chile, Santiago, Chile, [3]Chilean Observatory of Obstetric Violence, Santiago, Chile, [4]Faculty of Liberal Arts, Universidad Adolfo Ibáñez, Santiago, Chile, [5]International Consultant, Early Childhood Development and Maternal and Child Health, Washington, DC, United States

***Correspondence:**
Gonzalo Leiva
gonzalo.leiva.rojas@gmail.com

The Maternity in Dra. Eloísa Díaz' hospital, located in the municipality of La Florida and city of Santiago, Chile, opened its doors in 2014, and has integrated a humanistic model of care called the "Safe Model of Personalized Childbirth" since 2016. With around 3,000 births per year, it has been recognized as an example of excellence in maternity care in the country. The COVID-19 outbreak presented a big challenge to this Maternity: to maintain its quality of care standards despite the health crisis. This article presents the Maternity's responses to the pandemic from March to July 2020, describing the strategies that were deployed and the obstetric outcomes achieved. Semi-structured interviews with midwives and OB-GYNs, and a retrospective review of the childbirth standards of care and outcomes of the 55 women who tested positive for SARS-CoV-2, were carried out. The results show how the Maternity's staff responded in order to avoid a significant negative impact on the rights of women and newborns. Protocols to reestablish the companion during labor and childbirth and skin-to-skin contact, which were suspended for almost three weeks at the beginning of the outbreak, and the creation of an Instagram account to communicate with the external community were some of the measures taken. After some initial weeks of adjustment, the standards of care for all women, included for those diagnosed with COVID-19, were reestablished almost to pre-pandemic levels. This case shows that quality of care can be maintained and the rights of women and newborns can be respected during health crisis such as the COVID-19 pandemic.

Keywords: humanistic childbirth, human rights in childbirth, COVID-19, public health, midwifery

INTRODUCTION

Chile and Its Healthcare System

Chile is a democratic republic located in South America, with a population of 17,574,003 inhabitants in 2017 (National Institute of Statistics, 2018). It is considered a high-income country and had a Gross Domestic Product (GDP) per capita of US$25,041 in 2019 (World Bank, 2020). During 2017, 8.6% of its population lived in poverty and 0.3% lived on less than $1.90USD per day (Ministry of Social Development and Family, 2018; World Bank, 2020). However, more than 30% of the population is economically vulnerable and income inequality remains high (World Bank, 2020). The Chilean health system has maintained the structure that was defined during the 1980s (ECLAC, 2012), which consists of both public and private sector insurance and care provision, funded through social contributions (payroll taxes), general taxes, co-payments and voluntary premiums. The total per capita health expenditure was US$2,159 in 2019, representing 9.1% of the country's GDP. Public spending represented 5.4% of GDP and out-of-pocket spending accounted for 33.9% of health expenditures (OECD, 2020). Public provision of health services is highly decentralized and is coordinated under a National Health Services System, which consists of 29 Health Services (*Servicios de Salud*), geographically distributed. Health insurance is provided by private insurers (ISAPREs) and mostly by the National Public Health Insurance Fund (FONASA), which insured 78% of the population in 2017. The public sector, unlike the private, is characterized by hospital infrastructure deficits, low privacy in patient care, impersonality in the treatment of patients, unfavorable working conditions and low wage levels (Goic, 2015). Population wise, 92% of those belonging to the lowest income decile of the population and 80.6% of women are beneficiaries of public insurance (Ministry of Social Development and Family, 2018). FONASA's beneficiaries have access to two different health care plans determined by household income and number of family members: Institutional Care Modality (MAI) and Free Choice Modality (MLE). Regarding birth, the MAI does not require any extra out-of-pocket expenditure, and the MLE does entail out-of-pocket expenditure, which in September 2020 was around US$360 (National Public Health Insurance Fund, 2020).

In 2017, 219,186 live births were registered in the country; skilled birth attendance coverage was 99.7% (National Institute of Statistics, 2019); the IMR (infant mortality ratio; infant deaths/1,000 live births) was 6/1,000 (UNICEF, 2018); and the MMR (maternal mortality ratio, maternal deaths/100,000 live births) was 13/100,000 (WHO, 2019). Although these are good maternal health indicators, they hide large gaps in access and quality of health care between private and public health facilities, disparities between territories and lack of options regarding place of birth. Only facility births are covered by insurance, and home birth, although not illegal, is discouraged and not recognized by the health system.

More than ¾ of the country's births, 77.4%, occurred in the public health sector in 2017 (Ministry of Health, 2020a). Although the quality of interpersonal care between health personnel and women is reported to be better in the private than in the public sector (OVO Chile, 2018), both health sectors exhibit alarmingly high routine obstetric interventions during childbirth, as indicated by a national cesarean birth rate of 50% in 2015 (National Institute of Human Rights, 2016). A study conducted in nine major public regional maternity hospitals with primiparous and multiparous women who were admitted in labor reported the following interventions: 91% had medically induced/augmented labors, 55% had continuous fetal intrapartum monitoring, 56% had episiotomies, and 80% delivered in the lithotomy position (Binfa et al., 2016). The rate of obstetric interventions is similarly high in private health (OVO Chile, 2018), with cesareans being 27% higher in the private than in the public sector (National Institute of Human Rights, 2016).

Chile is internationally recognized for a scaled-up flagship program for early childhood development called "Chile Grows with You" (Richter et al., 2016), which has had national coverage since 2008. An axis component of this intersectoral policy is the Biopsychosocial Development Support Program (PADB), which, among other objectives, aims to strengthen prenatal care and provide personalized care during childbirth (Ministry of Social Development and Family and World Bank, 2018). Hand-in-hand with this program, in 2008, the Ministry of Health launched the *Manual for Personalized Attention in the Reproductive Process* (Ministry of Health, 2008), with the objective of implementing a humanistic model of birth (Davis-Floyd, 2001; Davis-Floyd, 2018). Although these policies and recommendations have helped to improve some practices, mainly those that constitute indicators of PADB (such as the presence of a companion during labor and birth, and skin-to-skin contact with the newborn for 30 or more minutes immediately after birth), there has not been a profound nation-wide paradigm shift toward the humanization of care during labor and birth. Thus, the health sectoral efforts to improve maternity care during the last decade have had limited impact (Binfa et al., 2016; OVO Chile, 2018).

SARS-Cov-2 in Chile and Its Threat to Respectful Maternity Care and Birth Rights

In Chile, the first COVID-19 case was reported on March 2, 2020. Exactly two weeks later, on March 16, the Ministry of Health indicated that Chile was entering Phase 4, which corresponds to the stage of sustained community spread of the virus. That same day, schools suspended their activities throughout the national territory, and two municipalities in the Metropolitan Region declared a state of emergency: Santiago and La Florida (Municipality of La Florida, 2020). This decision was made two days before the official publication of Supreme Decree No. 104, which declared a state of constitutional exception of catastrophe, due to public calamity, in the territory of Chile (Ministry of the Interior and Public Security, 2020). On March 22, a curfew began throughout the nation for the population to remain indoors from 22:00 to 05:00. And, since March 26, "dynamic" quarantines have been implemented in territories throughout the country, defining harsher or softer measures in various regions according to their COVID-19 related indicators.

This has meant opening some communities while others remain closed, or vice versa, even when these are neighboring territories.

La Florida municipality, which is the fourth largest in the region, with a population of 402,433 and accounting for 5% of the region's inhabitants (Ministry of Health, 2020b), entered quarantine on May 15 and remained in that state until August 30, 2020, when we first submitted this article.

The Epidemiological Report N° 39, published by the Department of Epidemiology (Ministry of Health, 2020b), reported that on August 2 (5 months after the first reported case), 401,142 people had been infected and 9,968 had died from COVID-19. This placed Chile in the 8th position of diagnosed cases in the world on that date (WHO, 2020a); and as the 3rd country with the highest death rate per million inhabitants, with 53.17 deaths per million, after only the United Kingdom (70.08) and Peru (64.55) (John Hopkins University, 2020).

There was no doubt that COVID-19 would pose a challenge to healthcare systems around the world, but what its specific impact on maternity care would be was unclear. The "Guidelines for pregnant women with suspected SARS-CoV-2 infection" (Favre et al., 2020), published on March 3 suggested shortening labor to avoid exhaustion in woman with confirmed infections. Although stating that there was no evidence of vertical transmission of the virus, the authors recommended the isolation of the newborn for at least 14 days or until viral shedding cleared--time during which breastfeeding was not recommended (Favre et al., 2020). The guidelines, which could have "consequences of unpredictable magnitude in the long term" according to the authors, were translated into Spanish (Martinez-Portilla et al., 2020) and widely disseminated, despite evidence showing the harm those measures could cause (Schmid et al., 2020; Smith, 2020; Stuebe, 2020).

Up to May, according to a review of 15 articles published by 10 scientific societies, including WHO, there was no definitive evidence to suggest vertical transmission of SARS-CoV-2. Likewise, the review concluded that it is not advisable to separate mothers from newborns or to discourage breastfeeding, unless the mother is seriously ill (Narang et al., 2020). But despite the evidence, and the fact that WHO (2020b) had pointed out since early March that pregnant women should have access to specialized, respectful and woman-centered care, as the pandemic spread, voices of alert around the world expressed concern for the rights of women and newborns during childbirth (International Confederation of Midwives, 2020; Human Rights and Childbirth, 2020; Sadler et al., 2020). NGOs denounced that in many settings, women's labors were being accelerated unnecessarily (programmed induction of labor, routine Pitocin, instrumental deliveries); were given a planned cesarean as their only option for birth; were denied a partner during labor and birth; were routinely separated from their newborns; and were not allowed to breastfeed (Childbirth is Ours, 2020; OVO Chile, 2020).

In our country, the Chilean Pediatric Society published the first guidelines for mothers with COVID-19 and their newborns in mid-March. Skin-to-skin contact was not recommended in women with symptoms, regardless of the severity of the illness; early clamping of the cord was promoted; and breastfeeding was not recommended for COVID-19$^+$ mothers. In the third version of this document, published on April 2, some of these measures were revised, recommending skin-to-skin contact and breastfeeding in confirmed or suspected COVID-19 mothers, provided that their babies were full term, and that the mothers were not in serious condition (Chilean Pediatric Society, 2020). It took the Ministry of Health almost 4 months since the first reported COVID case in the country to issue guidelines on maternity care, on June 25a date until which each Health Service and maternity unit was responding to the extent of its local resources and decisions. The Chilean Obstetric Violence Observatory reported that by the end of May, 46% of public hospitals had completely suspended accompaniment during labor and birth, a situation that did not occur in any private clinic in the country (OVO Chile, 2020).

Until June 12, there were only rumors of the existence of technical documents that hadn't been officially authorized. On that date, the Ordinance N° 1891 on recommendations for postpartum women, boys and girls regarding risk factors of child morbidity and mortality and their mental health in the COVID-19 pandemic was issued, recommending the presence of a companion during birth with the adequate personal protective equipment (PPE), skin-to-skin contact after birth and breastfeeding (Ministry of Health, 2020c). It was only on June 25, after strong pressure from civil society organizations and from the National College of Midwives (Chilean College of Midwives, 2020), that the new "Guidelines for the management of SARS-CoV-2 (COVID-19) cases in pregnant and postpartum women and/or dyads" were published. The document recommends companionship in the cases of women with COVID-19, skin-to-skin contact, and breastfeeding, as the Chilean Pediatric Society had done earlier. Regarding joint sleeping, it recommends making decisions based on each institutional reality (Ministry of Heath, 2020d).

Since the onset of the pandemic, most public maternities throughout the country receded in standards of care that had gradually been improving during the last decade. But a few did not, and made huge efforts to maintain the quality of care that they had achieved. This has been the case of the Maternity of Dra. Eloísa Díaz - La Florida Hospital in Santiago, which has been operating since late 2014 and has been recognized as an example of excellence in maternal care in the country (South-East Metropolitan Healthcare Service, 2020). As a brief context, La Florida municipality had reported 13,357 COVID-19$^+$ cases by August 2 (the fourth municipality with most cases in the Metropolitan Region) and 451 deaths (second in the Region) (Ministry of Health, 2020b).

There was a great challenge ahead, the greatest in the short history of the Maternity of Dra. Eloísa Díaz – La Florida Hospital: to face the greatest threat to the populations' health of which we had a record, while maintaining the standards of care that we had achieved with hard work. And this, in one of the biggest municipalities of the country and one of the hardest hit by the pandemic.

METHODS

We approached the process of describing and systematizing the responses of Dra. Eloísa Díaz' Maternity to the COVID-19 outbreak between March and July 2020 using mixed methodologies. Qualitative semi-structured interviews were carried out to inquire about the health personnel's experiences and perceptions with eight key maternity officials: six midwives and two obstetricians. Of the midwives, five were the heads of shifts during the period studied, and one was the main supervisor of all those shifts. One obstetrician was the head of residents, and the second the head OB-GYN of the maternity. All participants signed a consent document, interviews were carried out by one of the authors through Zoom and were recorded, with an average duration of 35 min. The interview guide covered the following topics: impacts of SARS-Cov-2 on the maternity personnel and at a personal level; impacts on the standards of maternity care; opinions of the management's work and of information and communication during the outbreak; milestones or key elements identified to maintain the previous standards of care; and recommendations for future work. Additionally, four of the midwives in charge of the Maternity's newly created Instagram account responded to a short interview guide through WhatsApp calls on the following topics: the process that led to the creation of the account, the motivation to participate in the project, and the impact of the account on their work and on the Maternity's standards of care. Of these four midwives, one had also responded to the semi-structured interview, as she was head of shift and also one of the Instagram volunteers.

All interviews were transcribed verbatim, coded, and analyzed using thematic analysis--a qualitative method that enables thematic patterns to be identified from the collected data (Creswell, 2014). The first three authors transcribed the interviews, read and re-read the transcriptions to ensure accuracy with the recording, and coded the interviews. A priori codes describing broad analytical dimensions were derived from the interview guides, and inductive codes were developed as the data was examined. After the coding process, the other authors joined the following interpretation process, which occurred iteratively, reviewing interpretations and reaching final conclusions. When quoting our interlocutors throughout this article, we will follow a chronological numbering system, with (1)–(8) referring to the semi-structured interviews conducted in that order; and to (I.1)–(I.4) when alluding to the four short interviews that describe the Instagram account.

Despite our initial intention of interviewing women and families who had received care within the Maternity, we instead privileged interviews with health personnel for two main reasons: firstly, in order to gain an in-depth understanding of the decision-making process that occurred in response to the pandemic; and secondly, due to the limited availability of time to conduct research, given that most authors were themselves working as health personnel in the Maternity during the COVID outbreak. In order to include some women's experiences, the article contains a few testimonies from users posted publicly on the Maternity Instagram account. As well, and regarding the impact of the Instagram account, we carried out a quantitative analysis of the interactions on that account during its first 88 days of operation (May 4–July 31), detailing number of users and interactions, and quoting some of the posts herein.

In order to report the main obstetric outcomes of births within the Maternity, we retrieved data on all births that occurred in the Maternity during 2019 and 2020 (until July 31) from the Hospital's databases, and conducted a retrospective review of 55 pregnant women with laboratory-confirmed COVID-19 (with maternal throat swab samples that were positive for SARS-CoV-2) who were admitted to the Maternity and gave birth between May 1, 2020, and July 31, 2020. The data on COVID-19^{+} cases was collected by Maternity midwives and systematized in a table of obstetric variables based on the intrapartum set dataset extracted from the database of the American College of Nurse-Midwives (ACNM), which was modified and adapted by the researchers to the local reality and the context of the pandemic. The study protocol was approved by the Dra. Eloísa Díaz Hospital's Scientific Ethics Committee.

RESULTS

Safe Model of Personalized Childbirth in Dra. Eloísa Díaz Hospital

Hospital Dra. Eloísa Díaz is part of the South-East Metropolitan Healthcare Service and is one of the 198 hospitals of varying complexity that make up the public network in the country. The hospital provides care to women enrolled in the nine primary care centers of La Florida. Between 2016 and 2019, an average of 4,470 live births per year were registered in La Florida (Ministry of Health, 2020e), of which an average of 66% took place in the Dra. Eloísa Díaz Maternity. Between January and July 2020, 70% of all births in the municipality occurred in this Maternity (estimated by the authors from municipal data), which attends women insured under the Institutional Care Modality (MAI), which does not require extra out-of-pocket expenditures (besides the insurance program of FONASA).

The gynecobstetric unit on which this article focuses is one of the three units of the Women's Responsibility Center (henceforth referred to as "Women's CR"). The unit has four areas: a recovery room with six beds; five surgical wards where vaginal births and cesarean sections, as well as elective and emergency obstetric and gynecological surgeries, take place; a prepartum room with eight beds, where only labor takes place (in the second stage, the laboring women are transferred to a surgical ward); and four Comprehensive Childbirth Rooms inside the surgical ward, where labor and vaginal delivery take place. Women are admitted to the traditional prepartum room and gynecobstetric wards or to the Comprehensive Childbirth Rooms depending on their risk factors and room availability. The unit is organized into two teams, which are referred to as the "medical" and "non-medical" teams. The medical team is composed of 18 ob-gyns organized in groups of three that rotate every six days, being available for the three units of the Women's RC (emergency, gynecobstetric, and hospitalization). The non-medical team is composed of 103 health staff. Of the total staff, 14 work during the day, from Monday to Friday, and the rest of the team is organized into four shifts made up of: 10 nursing technicians, four service assistants, and eight midwives (called *matronas*, who in Chile follow a direct-entry (non-nursing) program of 5 years of university education). All teams rotate on day and night shifts, and then have two days off (after which the cycle repeats). The security, cleaning, food, and maintenance personnel of the unit are part of a Concessionaire Society.

Despite having opened during late 2014, the Maternity unit began working fully in 2016, when the Comprehensive Childbirth Rooms became functional and the "Safe Model of Personalized Childbirth" was implemented. This model attempts to improve women's satisfaction, reduce excessive and unnecessary interventions (including cesareans), and improve maternal, fetal, and neonatal outcomes. Since 2018, the unit's management has included a detailed, monthly analysis of births, which are analyzed according to the place of development of labor. This is done in order to promote the same standards of care of the Comprehensive Childbirth Rooms in the traditional rooms, such as the presence of a companion during labor, free movement and walking, use of non-pharmacological pain relief methods, skin-to-skin contact of 30 min or more, breastfeeding on newborn demand, and reduction of interventions such as use of Pitocin (synthetic oxytocin) and episiotomy. Between May 2016 and July 2020, 3,681 births took place in the Comprehensive Childbirth Rooms. During 2020 (until the end of July), 30% of all hospital births occurred in these rooms.

Maternity Care During the Pandemic

Anticipating the arrival of the COVID-19 pandemic in Chile, at the beginning of February, all staff at Eloísa Díaz Hospital began to be trained in 27-h courses on standard precautions for infection prevention and use of PPE such as disposable aprons, gloves, masks and face shields. The courses were focused on protecting the health personnel and their clients from infection, and not on technical issues related to pregnancy and delivery.

On March 10, the last available dates for this training were published, when the country was a week away from entering Phase 4 (of sustained spread of the virus), and La Florida of being declared in a state of emergency. By that date, there was little information on the impact of COVID-19 on pregnant and laboring women, and some of the first guidelines that had been published worldwide were recommending retreat from some standards of care that had become rights in the Maternity (companion of choice during labor, skin-to-skin contact after birth, early breastfeeding) (Favre et al., 2020).

The health staff of the maternity reported that the main feeling of those first weeks was of fear: of the unknown, of getting infected, of infecting their family members. The heads of shifts express: "The first thing that comes to my mind is fear; at first no one knew much about what we were going to face, there was a lot of fear of getting infected" (1); "It generated fear at first, because we didn't know what we were dealing with: fear of infecting ourselves, of infecting our families, our users, that a newborn could be infected" (4); "It felt like we were all very scared and that feeling was pretty strong" (5); "There was a lot of fear of the unknown, of how we were going to face this process" (6).

On Monday, March 16, the day the municipalities of Santiago and La Florida entered a state of emergency, the first email was sent by the heads of the unit to the entire team, acknowledging that the scenario was unprecedented nationally and worldwide, and listing the first measures to be implemented: suspending the regular fourth shift and moving to a 24 × 3 scheme (a 24-h shift followed by 3 days off); avoiding kissing and hand to hand greetings; prohibition of arriving to the hospital in uniform (compulsory dressing in uniform in the hospital); and suspension of vacations and training courses. One of the midwives interviewed (head of shift) points out that:

> Regarding management, I feel that my bosses understood how to be a boss, how to be a leader, with a focus on the people who worked with them, they knew how to . . . do everything possible to channel that fear. I feel they acted a bit like midwives: they took the staff, educated them, took all the precautions, so that we felt safe working. (1)

On March 17 at a meeting between the Women's CR and the staff of the Neonatology Unit, the "Measures to prevent infection by COVID-19 in pregnant women and their newborns" began to be outlined, based on the first recommendations of the Chilean Pediatric Society. At the meeting, it was clearly stated that those first measures, which were very conservative (not recommending skin-to-skin contact or breastfeeding for COVID-19$^+$ women), would be modified as more evidence became available. Two days later, the South-East Metropolitan Healthcare Service (SSMSO), which manages and coordinates three large hospitals and the primary health care corresponding to the same territory, issued recommendations for the organization of the system and the use of PPE. The WhatsApp group "COVID 19 SSMSO" was created. The midwifery care coordinator highlights the creation of this network as one of the milestones of the management process:

> Communication, not only between internal teams but also between the internal team and the extra-system: primary health care, Health Service and central level. This was essential to be able to agree on ideas and at the same time help each other. (6)

Only three days later, on March 22, we had the first COVID-19 suspicious pregnant woman at the Maternity. This case set off alarms regarding the possibility of preventive quarantines of large numbers of health staff, and made us organize the personnel in a way that would not impact the standards of care, and that at the same time would not entail too great a work overload on the teams. On that day, and coinciding with the start of a national curfew, it was decided that all visits to hospitalized users of the hospital were suspended, including the companion during labor and childbirth.

On April 3, two members of our staff announced the presence of COVID-19 symptoms and took the test in the hospital's emergency unit; it was the first time that we were forced to review the flow of personnel. Fortunately, both tests came out negative. The experience led to the creation of an executive WhatsApp group composed of the four shift leaders, the two supervisors, and the maternity coordinator (all of them midwives) as an alternative to an existing and more extensive group that included other levels of supervision.

On the following day, we decided that the use of masks was compulsory during the entire shifts and during interactions among staff and with users. Very much disliking the suspension of companionship during childbirth, we started advancing in actions to reverse this measure. From there onwards, we asked for provision of surgical masks for the entire staff, plus all women and their companions. Regarding this participatory means of management, a head of shift expresses:

> The way in which we function as a team is outstanding; I feel that every decision that has been made has always included the opinion of the shift heads and that seems good to me in terms of productivity and also because it is a matter of respect and appreciation with our work (...) Each measure that is adopted is made by a supervisor but seen by a clinical team; it makes everything easier because the collaborations are there. (3)

On the newly created WhatsApp group, we immediately began to discuss the best way to organize the staff. On April 13, three proposals were presented and the heads of the unit decided on the 24 × 4 rotary, which entailed dividing the existing four shifts and creating a fifth one. To reduce infection risk, there would be fewer personnel on each shift than before (two nursing technicians, one service assistant and one midwife less than in the previous shifts). One new midwife was hired to match these numbers, and the new organizational model was made official four days later, to begin operating on Monday April 20. The email that communicated these measures explained that "we have been working on these proposals together with the four heads of shift for more than 10 days, to be able to face in the best way possible the scenarios that we might face." Regarding these decisions, one shift head states that:

> The negotiations have been very timely; I feel that at the beginning it cost a bit to decide to make changes, there was a point where we had to jump in and make big changes, like adding a shift, and the changes that had to be made were made. From then onwards, the efforts have been super timely and assertive, and they have made things easier for us, and for the team; they have been reassuring measures. (2)

The same email insisted on the use of N-95 masks in all areas of the unit, and the shift managers and all members of the unit were asked to supervise said indication. With regards to the communication and information channels used, the shift heads point out the following:

> That the information is delivered is essential because it helps to reduce the anxiety that occurs in a context like this (...) Direct communication from the heads of shifts and heads of unit have stood out as a facilitating element to go through this period. (5)
>
> What eases the situation is the direct conversation that we have had between the five shift heads and the supervisors; I know that I have a direct line to talk and find a solution. (3)
>
> It's calming that the communication channels have always been open. Although I may not have a particular piece of information here and now, I have the peace of mind that if I need that information, I can ask; and if someone on my team doesn't know, my bosses will know; and if the bosses don't know it, I am sure they will do everything possible to have the answer. (1)

TABLE 1 | The maternity unit's health personnel in preventive quarantine and who tested positive for COVID-19 between April and July 2020; n = 103.

	COVID-19	Preventive quarantine
April	1	19
May	3	2
June	2	4
July	2	1
Total	8	26

Based on data from the Centro de Atención Integral del Funcionario (CAIF), Hospital Dra. Eloísa Díaz.

Regarding infections of staff members, between April and July we had eight COVID-19 cases, of which at least three were infected outside of the hospital (**Table 1**); these numbers are low in comparison with the other units within the hospital. The head OB-GYN explains how the unit anticipated measures:

> We have been ahead of the ministerial measures. Mainly the team of midwives and the coordinators and supervisor took the situation very seriously, and the prevention measures began much earlier than in other institutions. We started wearing a mask on a mandatory basis before the Ministry of Health said to do so. (8)

The Path From the Suspension to the Reestablishment of Standards of Care

The measure of suspending the companion for the woman during labor and birth on March 22 hit the teams hard. Two of the shift heads report:

> I feel like there is no valid justification to tell a woman she cannot have a companion; it's preaching on

> something that you deeply disagree with. I don't know how to put it into words, it was just very terrible to have to do it. (1)
>
> It was terrible because we were used to having our women being always accompanied by their loved ones during labor, delivery and their recovery. And at first, when they couldn't have this accompaniment, it was very distressing, we felt very sad because they were not accompanied. (5)

It is interesting to note the team's acknowledgment that fear played a central role in decision-making during the beginning of the pandemic. One of the shift head's expresses:

> We abused a bit of fear, and of the lack of knowledge, which led us to take exaggerated measures which perhaps were not so necessary and could have been avoided. (3)

Feelings of disapproval of the measures were expressed in the shift heads' WhatsApp group during the last days of March, which led to discussing the feasibility of developing a protocol to admit companions again. The opinions were unanimous, and on March 31, the first draft of the protocol was presented, which was finally put into operation on April 9. The unit's coordinator expresses:

> They looked for evidence, they worked in coordination and support with the neonatal unit, they reviewed the best recommendations available. (...) The hospital gave us the support and gave us all the supplies we needed to be able to comply with the protocol. It was approved in record time. It was analyzed by the midwifery and medical team, by all heads, by the neonatology unit. It went through the different areas so that everyone could give their opinion on what was better and what to incorporate. (...) It was quite positive, and it happened mainly by the impulse and desire of the team, in an aim to be always respecting women's rights. (6)

One head of shift adds:

> The team advocated for the rights of families, and on the other hand, the supervisors and heads were available to listen and see what resources were needed to make this possible. (3)

This protocol also addressed skin-to-skin contact in cases of suspected or positive COVID-19 women. The third version of the Chilean Pediatric Society's protocol (from April 2) was used as a reference; it recommended skin-to-skin contact and breastfeeding in suspected or confirmed cases, unless the newborn was premature and/or the woman's illness condition didn't make these possible. The companion during birth and skin-to-skin contact and breastfeeding were reestablished. Nevertheless, the midwives report on other negative impacts that the pandemic has had in the quality of care given, such as the effects of the use of PPE, as one midwife points out:

> There is a physical issue; we are caring for women fully covered. We are putting a physical barrier of gloves, masks, hats, plastic. It is difficult to work as we know [that supporting] a woman in labor requires touch. You know you can support her in ways that are difficult to achieve through these plastic barriers. This might sound symbolic or even poetic, but it is certainly not the same. (1)

When the Community Is Not Allowed in the Hospital, the Hospital Goes to the Community via Cellphones

The most usual form of initial contact of the Maternity with the community is through a guided tour through its premises that pregnant women and their couples take around their 36th week of pregnancy. Pre-pandemic, this tour was held every Monday, Wednesday and Friday at 11 AM: a midwife showed the facilities and explained the process of admission and care during childbirth. As a result of the pandemic, these tours were suspended, and the health team came up with the idea of conducting a "virtual guided tour" through the hospital's Instagram account. On April 22, the first guided Instagram tour was held, with great success: more than 100 people connected. The awareness of the uncertainty that the pandemic scenario generated for pregnant women led the team to request authorization to create an independent Instagram account for the entire Maternity. The medical residents' head notes: "The creativity of the midwifery team has been amazing. The virtual guided tour has distinguished us as a Maternity" (7).

On April 29, the hospital management authorized the creation of the Maternity's Instagram account, acknowledging that the initiative had been very well received in the external community, and also within the health team. A shift head points out:

> A great milestone was the creation of the Instagram account. We have been able to contact the community from wherever we are, we have carried out many activities: lives, posts, answer questions and comments, connect the maternity with primary health care, keep in touch with women after they have left the Maternity. In addition, we get more direct and continuous feedback from our patients than before, which is crucial to improve our work. (2)

On May 15, the first Instagram publication was made, and content related to the World Respected Childbirth Week began to be uploaded. In addition to a first cycle of Instagram lives around that celebration, three other cycles have been held (Perinatal Dialogues, World Breastfeeding Week, and Dialogues in Midwifery). When we were completing the first draft of this article on August 31 2020, the account @maternidaddraeloisadiaz had more than 3,240 followers, of which 92% were women and 8% men. 56% of those who followed the account were 24–35 years old, followed by the 18–24 age group. One of the midwives in charge of the project declares:

TABLE 2 | Direct messages received on the instagram account @maternidaddraeloisadiaz between May 4 and July 31, 2020.

Variable	Number	%
Number of users	228	100
La Florida	150	65.7
Other	43	18.8
Undetermined	35	15.3
Number of interactions	434	
La Florida	335	77.1
Other	61	14
Undetermined	29	6.68
NA	9	2.07
Type of interaction		
Inquiries	374	86.1
Inquiry RPO/TDP	53	
Other	321	
Congratulations	46	10.5
Complaints	5	1.1
NA	9	2.0
Average of interactions per user (all users)	1.9	
Average of interactions per user (La Florida)	2.23	
Average of daily interactions (all users)	4.9	
Average of daily interactions (La Florida)	3.8	
Responses		
Yes	423	97.5
No	11	2.5
Resolution of inter-consultations	5	1.1

> I was motivated to create links and networks with users and with other national and international health institutions, and to be able to better connect within our own South-East Service network with other hospitals and primary health care. (I.3)

A team of six volunteer midwives answer the questions of the community 24/7. Regarding their motivations, they express: "I feel that being in direct contact with the users or with their relatives makes us closer to people" (I.1); "Our aim is to reduce anxiety in pregnant women, prevent them from going out, avoid unnecessary exposure to contagion" (I.2); "As the health system is organized in such a hierarchical way, it was difficult to achieve this closeness with the population through traditional channels" (I.3); "It interested me as a channel of information, and updated information, as a way to promote changes" (I.4). This team of volunteer midwives points out the importance and positive impact that the initiative has had:

> It is super important to lower their anxiety and make them feel safe about the place where they are going to give birth; to show them that we are caring human beings, that there are no ranks or distinctions between us and them. (I.1)
>
> Women express that they feel much calmer, they know that they have an open channel, that they can communicate with us in an expeditious way, they know that we answer at night, even very late. (I.2)
>
> It makes the hospital closer to the community, it has calmed anxieties regarding COVID impressively, it has kept them much more informed. It has served to build affection toward the Maternity; they express they love the team, they love the way we work. (I.4)

Since the opening of the Instagram account on May 4 and until July 31, a total of 53 publications and 17 lives were done. In the same period, midwives answered the doubts of 228 Instagram users, in 434 interactions (dialogues of two or more messages between a user and a volunteer midwife). 77% of the interactions occurred with women from La Florida. Thus, on average, during our Instagram account's first 88 days of operation, there were 4.9 daily interactions with users, of which 3.8 were with women from La Florida (**Table 2**). Of the total number of interactions during this period, 86% corresponded to questions, and 11% to congratulations for the usefulness of the maternity's Instagram and for its work during the COVID outbreak, such as "I want to congratulate you for the page and for the information you share," posted on May 29, and "Thanks for your Instagram lives! I feel empowered and informed for my birth at my 39 weeks of pregnancy ... virtual hugs!" posted on August 14. Regarding birth experiences in the Maternity, on May 31, a new mother wrote:

> Thank you for everything. Thank you for accompanying me in this beautiful moment. Despite everything that is happening, we felt cared for as if nothing wrong was going on, we received the best care imaginable. I will never stop thanking all the support and concern for me and for my daughter.

On July 30, another woman who had recently given birth in the Maternity commented:

> Thank you very much for the tremendous work you do in the Maternity. Thanks to the midwife, to her words and her care, our daughter was born. As a couple, we saw most of the Instagram lives that the Maternity organized and they really helped us a lot to prepare for the birth. Thank you for the dedication, passion and love that you give in every birth and new life.

The Maternity's Standards of Care During the COVID-19 Outbreak

We have described our decision-making process as a maternity team since the beginning of the COVID-19 pandemic in Chile, until July 31, 2020. The first COVID-19 women were admitted to our Maternity in May 2020, after we had implemented protocols to protect the pre-pandemic standards of care. Even though the companion during birth was suspended during the last 10 days of March and first 10 days of April (a period in which we had no COVID-19^{+} women in labor), this decision had a big impact on our indicators: the 90% companionship during labor and birth (2019) dropped to 81.4% between January and July 2020—and

TABLE 3 | Main obstetric outcomes of all births in the maternity during 2019 and 2020 (until July 31st).

	2020 January–July)		2019 (January–December)	
	N	%	N	%
Total	1,518	100	3,003	100
Vaginal births	939	60.9	1975	65.7
Forceps	81	5.33	192	6.39
Cesareans	494	32.5	836	27.8
Skin to skin contact for >30′	1,064	70.9	2110	70%
Early breastfeeding	571	37.6	1,197	39.8
Companion during labor and delivery	1,236	81.4	2717	90.4
Apgar <7 at 5′	14	0.9	22	0.7

Based on monthly reports of OB/GYN Unit.

TABLE 4 | Demographic features, clinical characteristics and delivery outcomes of COVID-19⁺ women with RT-PCR (n = 55).

	(n) /[a] mean	Percentage [interval]
Nationality		
Chile	34	61%
Venezuela	8	14%
Haiti	6	11%
Colombia	2	4%
Peru	2	4%
Other: Argentina, Bolivia and Dominican Republic.	3	6%
Residence (municipality)		
La Florida	45	82%
Puente Alto	3	5%
La Granja	2	4%
La Pintana	2	4%
Other municipalities (3)	3	5%
Maternal age (years)	29.4/[a]	[15–41]
Parity		
0	21	38%
1	19	35%
2	10	18%
3 and more	5	9%
Pregnancy trimester at diagnosis		
First	0	–
Second	1	25^{+0}
Third	54	[28^{+1}–41^{+0}]
Respiratory comorbidities	2	3.6%
Symptoms		
No	41	75%
Fever	3	6%
Cough	4	7%
Dyspnea	5	9%
Other	3	6%
Route of delivery		
Vaginal	36	65.4%
C-section	15	27.3%
C-section (maternal health condition) COVID-19	4	7.3%
ICU Admission	2	3.6%
IMCU admission	2	3.6%
Gestational age at delivery (weeks)		
Extreme preterm (earlier than 28 weeks of gestation)	1	1.8%
Early preterm (earlier than 34 weeks of gestation)	2	3.6%
Late preterm (34–36 weeks of gestation)	6	10.9%
Early term (37–38 weeks of gestation)	18	32.7%
Full term (39–40 weeks of gestation)	25	45.5%
Late term (41 weeks of gestation)	3	5.5%
Post term (42 weeks of gestation and beyond)	0	–
Pregnant women who delivered within 14 days after diagnosis of COVID-19 (RT-PCR)	52	94.5%

TABLE 5 | Clinical characteristics, delivery outcomes, and standards of care of COVID-19 positive women with RT-PCR who delivered under isolation conditions (n = 29).

	Vaginal n = 14 48%	C-section n = 11 38%	C-section COVID-19 indication n = 4 14%
Maternal age (years; mean, range)	31.1 [18–40]	29.4 [22–41]	33.3 [30–36]
Symptoms (number; percentage)	2 (14%)	1 (9%)	4 (100%)
Gestational age at delivery			
Early preterm (<34 weeks)	0 (0%)	0 (0%)	2 (50%)
Late preterm (34–36 weeks)	1 (7%)	0 (0%)	2 (50%)
Term (>37 weeks)	13 (93%)	11 (100%)	0 (0%)
ICU Admission	0	0	2 (50%)
Birth weight (grams; mean, range)	3,144 [2,710 – 3,720]	3,032 [2,180 – 3,480]	2,291 [1,760 – 3,245]
Apgar score 5 min > 7	14 (100%)	11 (100%)	2 (50%)
Pregnant woman accompanied during delivery (by her partner or trusted support person)	11 (79%)	4 (36%)	0 (0%)
Skin-to-skin contact (30 min or more)	12 (86%)	3 (27%)	0 (0%)
Birth attended by midwife	12 (86%)	0 (0%)	0 (0%)

even lower, to 70%, between March and April. Another figure that stands out is the difference between cesarean births, which were 27.8% of the total births in 2019, and 32.5% during the first 7 months of 2020 (**Table 3**). The head OB-GYN of the maternity explains this increase in cesareans:

> We will have to look back at our practices. For example, cesarean sections, how it has increased, not only in our institution but in all hospitals in the Metropolitan Region, because we relaxed. We said: "People are stressed, we are not going to get so fussy about why we are conducting surgeries, we are not going to do surveillance, we are not going to audit," and that has had the impact of an increase in our cesarean section rate of 7 points. It has affected a lot. (8)

Between May and July 2020, 620 births occurred in our maternity. Fifty five (8.9%) of these women tested positive for RT-PCR SARS-CoV-2 (52/55 delivered within 14 days after diagnosis of COVID-19). Demographic features, clinical characteristics and delivery outcome of COVID-19 cases are shown in **Table 4**. Twenty one cases were migrant (39%) and 45 (82%) were residents of La Florida. Two COVID-19^{+} women had respiratory comorbidities (asthma). Fifty four infections were diagnosed in the third trimester, 41 (75%) were asymptomatic; two were admitted to IMCU (non-invasive respiratory therapy) and two were admitted to the ICU.

All women with severe COVID-19 (four cases) had a preterm delivery by cesarean and the indication was related to COVID-19 infection. Thirty six women (65.4%) with non-severe symptoms had a vaginal delivery and 15 had a cesarean birth for indications non-related to COVID-19. Although these 36 cesareans were indicated as "nonrelated" to COVID-19, we can say that the pandemic context had an impact on the criteria to perform these surgeries, as, during the pandemic, the staff became less rigorous in applying the Maternity's cesarean protocols, and in case of doubt on the physiologic progress of labor, they preferred to practice an emergency cesarean, as that provided better opportunity for the proper use of PPE.

Of the total number of 55 women with COVID-19, 29 (52.7%) were under conditions of isolation, and therefore in one of the Comprehensive Childbirth Rooms, with all the security measures established for these cases. The remaining 26 women were treated "blindly"—that is, in ignorance of the result of the RT-PCR, which began to be taken routinely on May 15th on all pregnant women who were admitted into the Maternity. Processing the exam took between 48 and 72 h, which is why in many cases, the diagnosis was only learned in the postpartum period, and therefore these women were not treated with the strictest isolation measures in a room equipped for that. The only option to enter the isolation unit was to have a known RT-PCR(+), to present symptoms, or to have referred as a COVID-19 contact. In this group, the standards that were offered can be seen in **Table 5**. Fifteen women had companions, and it stands out that from the total of 14 vaginal deliveries, of which 12 (86%) were assisted by a midwife, the skin-to-skin contact after birth for at least 30 min (which is the minimum time for contact recommended in the national protocols) reached 86%, well above the average in 2020 (70%). (Often this skin-to-skin contact lasted much longer.) The latter is accounted for by the efforts made by the health teams to promote birth rights even in these cases.

DISCUSSION

In this article, we have sought to describe the responses to the COVID-19 pandemic in the Eloísa Díaz public Maternity. As we have shown, this Maternity unit already stood out for its high standards of care since before this health crisis, implementing a humanistic model of childbirth care as described by Davis-Floyd (2001), Davis-Floyd (2018), and was able to maintain almost the same standards during the first months of the COVID outbreak (March to July).

In the La Florida Maternity, during 2019, 70% of our clients had immediate skin-to-skin contact of 30 min or more after birth, including breastfeeding, and during 2020 (until the end of July), it was 71%. Ninety percent of labors and births had a companion in

2019, which decreased to 81% in the same period of 2020 (**Table 3**). But, as we have shown, this fall reflects the ban on companionship that occurred for only 20 days, during which the Maternity's midwives pressed for protocols to reverse the measure. Once the proposals to reestablish previous standards of care were shared, all heads were supportive. This shows the strength with which a collective culture of respect for the rights of women and newborns has been instilled in the Maternity staff, as well as that of non-compliance with measures that do not have supporting evidence. As one of the midwives' head of shift expresses: "There were certain standards of care that we wouldn't compromise, such as the suspension of skin-to-skin, of a companion during birth; we were not just going to normalize it because someone told you it should be done or it 'seemed' to be adequate" (3).

One of our health team's fear was that the rate of cesarean births would rise during the pandemic, as had been reported in several countries and contexts by April. A systematic review that included 108 births of women diagnosed with COVID-19 showed that 91% had a cesarean birth (Zaigham and Andersson, 2020). A study in Spain with 82 COVID-19^{+} women showed a rate of 47% of cesareans (Martínez-Perez et al., 2020). In June, the findings from a rapid online global survey of maternal and newborn health professionals facing the COVID-19 pandemic, which included responses from 81 countries, showed that cesareans were commonly performed among women diagnosed with COVID-19, and some facilities aimed to reduce labor duration and time spent in the labor room by performing cesareans even on non-infected women (Semaan et al., 2020). In our Maternity, in contrast, the cesarean birth rate was 34.6% in the group of 55 women with COVID-19, 6.8% higher than during 2019 (**Tables 3** and **4**). Although this is an increase from our pre-pandemic standards, it is still lower than most public maternities in the country, which had a cesarean average of 41% in 2015 (National Institute of Human Rights, 2016); and the maternity's personnel has acknowledged the increase and is working on ways to reverse it.

The restrictions on in-person visits to the maternity and difficulty in accessing updated information on maternity protocols contributed to an increase in the anxiety that pregnant women and their families were already living with due to the pandemic, which motivated us to look for new ways of contact with them. As an editorial published in *Women & Birth* (Matvienko-Sikar et al., 2020) acknowledges, the COVID-19 pandemic has created the context for increased experiences of distress related to: restrictions in normal routines; concerns about the risk of infection; changes in antenatal care and in access to perinatal health care; restrictions on the presence of partners during maternity care; as well as reduced access to support networks. In this scenario, support from networks and from midwives and other healthcare professionals is critical for women's mental health during the pandemic. In our Maternity, the awareness of this increased mental health vulnerability of our community led us to the creation of an Instagram account as a communication channel and to carry out "virtual visits" to our premises. This channel was managed until the end of July by six volunteer midwives; during August, their number grew to 10. These volunteers continue to interact with the community on an ongoing basis, and we already anticipate that this communication channel must be strengthened and has great future, post-pandemic potential.

Another relevant element we must include is the creation, on July 23, of the Dra. Eloísa Díaz's Hospital "Gender Roundtable," which has begun an awareness campaign to reject any practice or conduct that violates women's rights within the hospital (Dra. Eloísa Díaz Hospital, 2020). Among the members of this unprecedented initiative are a midwife (one of our Instagram volunteers) and a woman ob-gyn from our Maternity unit.

The great awareness of women's and communities' rights to dignified healthcare has been facilitated by our staff of midwives, who are predominantly young (mostly in their 30s) and who have actively served in the social movement for greater equality and dignity for all that has mobilized Chile during the last 15 years. Many of our team's members were part of the student movement referred to as the "Penguin Revolution" of 2006, which demanded quality and free education, and of the massive social uprising of October 2019 against inequality and the unresolved needs of the population for improved education, pensions and health, as one midwife clearly expresses:

> The fact that our Maternity has young health teams right now was very, very beneficial for us. We are a generation that has faced many changes, and that has acted as a protective factor for us: the fact that we can adapt, that we are used to change, that we are a generation of changes, that we have demanded changes in our country. We are used to it, we were the generations of the "penguins," we were part of the student strikes, we have been part of the October revolt. This means we believe in our capacity to change things—not drown in problems but rather to face them and search, participate, engage, try to find creative solutions ... That is our greatest strength and what differentiates us from other institutions. (3)

Furthermore, the sense of a collective purpose has made the team grow closer and stronger. In the words of a head of shift: "This has made us become more family than we already were" (3). The OB-GYN head of residents acknowledges:

> These emergency situations consolidate work teams. Despite all the things that can happen on a daily basis, all of us have experienced the same in our working context, and we have all tried to work for the same cause. I think that is the most important thing. I have always said that we are a team, that we cannot work without midwives and technicians, and that was shown in this pandemic, that we are a team. (7)

With this devoted young team, with ease to adapt to change, with a profound gender and human rights approach that has been able to protect women and newborns' rights during the COVID-19 pandemic, we hope to lead the way for other maternities in the country and region to follow similar paths, and we are expecting to join the *International Childbirth Initiative (ICI): 12 Steps to Safe and Respectful Maternity Care* in the near future (Lalonde et al., 2019; www.internationalchildbirth.com).

Finally, an issue of great concern today is the maternity staff's mental health, which has been stressed to the maximum in the context of COVID-19, as our heads of shift express: "The whole team is subjected to a higher basal stress, and that has had repercussions especially on mental health, which will increase in the near future" (2); "An emotional drain, I think that is by far what is going to weigh the most. The stress of being in a situation in which you may not want to be, I mean the stress that everything is based on fear" (3). The concern for mental health is consistent with the preliminary results of the study "The impact of the COVID-19 pandemic on the mental health of workers in health services" in the country: of the 954 health workers interviewed throughout the country, 37.6% report lack of energy and fatigue, 38.6% lack of appetite and, most worryingly, 31.4% present moderate to high depressive symptoms (Medical College of Chile, 2020).

ETHICS STATEMENT

The studies involving human participants were reviewed and approved by Comité Etico Científico Hospital Dra. Eloísa Díaz, La Florida. The patients/participants provided their written informed consent to participate in this study.

AUTHOR CONTRIBUTIONS

GL and MS: design of the work, acquisition of data, analysis and interpretation of data, drafting the work, final approval. SQ and CL: acquisition of data, analysis and interpretation of data, drafting the work. VF: acquisition of data, design of the work, final approval. CS, SD, and CF: design of the work, final approval.

ACKNOWLEDGMENTS

Acknowledging that the mental health of our staff is one of our priorities now, we are confident that we have done and are doing everything in our power to face the COVID-19 pandemic in accordance with our principles of care. Our commitment for whatever happens next–a second wave or future pandemic–is to continue to keep the rights of women and their newborns as our *first* priority.

REFERENCES

Binfa, L., Pantoja, L., Ortiz, J., Gurovich, M., Cavada, G., and Foster, J. (2016). Assessment of the implementation of the model of integrated and humanised midwifery health services in Chile. *Midwifery* 35, 53–61. doi:10.1016/j.midw.2016.01.018

Childbirth is Ours (El Parto es Nuestro) (2020). The childbirth is ours complaint about malpractice during COVID-19. Available at: https://www.elpartoesnuestro.es/blog/2020/04/05/el-parto-es-nuestro-denuncia-mala-praxis-por-covid19 (Accessed August 9, 2020).

Chilean College of Midwives (2020). Midwives meeting health minister and raise urgent need for release a national guideline for women's health care in pandemic. Available at: https://colegiodematronas.cl/?p=2901 (Accessed August 9, 2020).

Chilean Obstetric Violence Observatory (OVO Chile) (2018). Childbirth survey Chile. Available at: https://www.researchgate.net/publication/325933924_OVO_Chile_2018_Resultados_Primera_Encuesta_sobre_el_Nacimiento_en_Chile (Accessed August 8, 2020).

Chilean Obstetric Violence Observatory (OVO Chile) (2020). Public statement about COVID-19 and childbirth in Chile. Available at: http://ovochile.cl/declaracion-publica-sobre-covid-19-y-nacimientos-en-chile/ (Accessed August 9, 2020).

Chilean Pediatric Society (2020). Guidelines to prevent COVID-19 in newborn and its clinical management during pandemic. Available at: https://sochipe.cl/v3/covid/27.pdf (Accessed August 8, 2020).

Creswell, J. (2014). *Research design: qualitative, quantitative, and mixed methods approaches.* Thousand Oaks, CA: SAGE Publications.

Davis-Floyd, R. (2001). The technocratic, humanistic, and holistic paradigms of childbirth. *Int. J. Gynaecol. Obstet.* 75 (Suppl. 1), S5–S23. doi:10.1016/S0020-7292(01)00510-0

Davis-Floyd, R. (2018). "The technocratic, humanistic, and holistic paradigms of birth and health care," in *Ways of knowing about birth: mothers, midwives, medicine, and birth activism by Robbie Davis-Floyd.* Long Grove, IL: Waveland Press, 3–44.

Dra. Eloísa Díaz Hospital (2020). Dra. Eloísa Díaz hospital gender equity round table. Available at: http://www.hospitallaflorida.cl/hospital-dra-eloisa-diaz-de-la-florida-instaura-la-mesa-de-genero/ (Accessed September 9, 2020).

Economic Commission for Latin America and the Caribbean (ECLAC) (2012). Social protection systems in Latin America and the Caribbean: Chile. Available at: https://www.cepal.org/en/publications/4031-social-protection-systems-latin-america-and-caribbean-chile (Accessed August 8, 2020).

Favre, G., Pomar, L., Qi, X., Nielsen-Saines, K., Musso, D., and Baud, D. (2020). Guidelines for pregnant women with suspected SARS-CoV-2 infection. *Lancet Infect. Dis.* 20 (6), P652–P653. doi:10.1016/S1473-3099(20)30157

Goic, A. (2015). The chilean health care system: the task ahead. *Rev. Med. Chile* 143, 774–786. doi:10.4067/S0034-98872015000600011

Human Rights in Childbirth (2020). Human rights violations in pregnancy, birth and postpartum during the COVID-19 pandemic. Available at: http://humanrightsinchildbirth.org/wp-content/uploads/2020/05/Human-Rights-in-Childbirth-Pregnancy-Birth-and-Postpartum-During-COVID19-Report-May-2020.pdf (Accessed August 9, 2020).

International Confederation of Midwives (2020). Women's rights in childbirth must be upheld during the coronavirus pandemic. Available at: https://www.internationalmidwives.org/assets/files/news-files/2020/03/icm-statement_upholding-womens-rights-during-covid19-5e83ae2ebfe59.pdf (Accessed August 9, 2020).

John Hopkins University (2020). Mortality analyses, coronavirus resource center. Available at: https://coronavirus.jhu.edu/data/mortality (Accessed August 9, 2020).

Lalonde, A., Herschderfer, K., Pascali-Bonaro, D., Hanson, C., Fuchtner, C., and Visser, G. H. A. (2019). The international childbirth initiative: 12 steps to safe and respectful motherbaby-family maternity care. *Int. J. Gynaecol. Obstet.* 146 (1), 65–73. doi:10.1002/ijgo.12844

Martínez-Perez, O., Vouga, M., Cruz Melguizo, S., Forcen, L., Panchaud, A., Chapuli, M., et al. (2020). Association between mode of delivery among pregnant women with COVID-19 and maternal and neonatal outcomes in Spain. *JAMA* 324 (3), 296–299. doi:10.1001/jama.2020.10125

Martinez-Portilla, R., Goncé, A., Hawkins-Villarreal, A., and Figueras, F. (2020). A Spanish-translated clinical algorithm for management of suspected SARS-CoV-2 infection in pregnant women. *Lancet Infect. Dis.* 20 (6), 655. doi:10.1016/S1473-3099(20)30285-1

Matvienko-Sikar, K., Meedya, S., and Ravaldi, C. (2020). Perinatal mental health during the COVID-19 pandemic. *Women Birth* 33 (4), 309–310. doi:10.1016/j.wombi.2020.04.006

Medical College of Chile (2020). The COVID-19 health care workers study. Available at: http://www.colegiomedico.cl/primer-informe-the-covid-19-health-care-workers-study-un-tercio-de-los-encuestados-presenta-sintomas-depresivos-de-caracter-moderado-a-grave/ (Accessed September 9, 2020).

Ministry of Health (2020b). Epidemiological report N° 39. SARS-CoV2 infection – COVID-19 illness. Department of Epidemiology. . Available at: https://www.minsal.cl/wp-content/uploads/2020/08/Informe-Epidemiologico-39-MINSAL-Agosto.pdf (Accessed August 9, 2020).

Ministry of Health, (2020d). Guidelines for the management of SARS-CoV-2 (COVID-19) cases in pregnant and postpartum women and/or dyads. Available at: https://colegiodematronas.cl/wp-content/uploads/2020/06/Ord.-N%C2%BA-2388.pdf (Accessed August 9, 2020).

Ministry of Health. (2008). Manual for personalized attention in the reproductive process. Available at: http://web.minsal.cl/portal/url/item/795c63caff4fde9fe04001011f014bf2.pdf (Accessed August 8, 2020).

Ministry of Health. (2020c). Ordinance N° 1891: recommendations for postpartum women, boys and girls regarding risk factors of child morbidity and mortality, and their mental health in the COVID-19. Available at: http://www.crececontigo.gob.cl/wp-content/uploads/2020/06/ORD.-N%C2%B0-1891-RECOMENDACIONES-PUERPERAS-NIN%CC%83OS-AS-RIESGO-DE-MORBIMORTALIDAD-SALUD-MENTAL-EN-PANDEMIA-COVID-19.pdf (Accessed August 9, 2020).

Ministry of Health. (2020e). Vital Statistics, Chile. Registered live births by date and municipality. Available at: https://public.tableau.com/profile/deis4231#!/vizhome/HechosVitalesdesdeel2000/NotaTcnica?publish=yes (Accessed August 8, 2020).

Ministry of Health. (2020a). Women's health program dashboard. Available at: http://www.deis.cl (Accessed August 8, 2020).

Ministry of Social Development and Family - World Bank (2018). 10 years of Chile grows with you (Chile Crece Contigo). Key components and lessons learned for the setting up of comprehensive child development support systems. Available at: http://www.crececontigo.gob.cl/wp-content/uploads/2020/08/A-10-años-Chile-Crece-Contigo-claves-y-aprendizajes-para-la-construcción-de-sistemas-comprehensivos-de-apoyo-al-desarrollo-infantil.pdf (Accessed August 9, 2020).

Ministry of Social Development and Family (MDSF) (2018). National household survey (CASEN) 2017. Available at: http://observatorio.ministeriodesarrollosocial.gob.cl/casen-multidimensional/casen/casen_2017.php (Accessed August 8, 2020).

Ministry of the Interior and Public Security (2020). Supreme decree no. 104. State of constitutional exception of catastrophe. Available at: https://www.bcn.cl/leychile/navegar?idNorma=1143580 (Accessed August 9, 2020).

Municipality of La Florida (2020). Decree No1514. Available at: https://www.laflorida.cl/sitio/wp-content/uploads/2020/07/decreto-exento-1514.pdf (Accessed August 9, 2020).

Narang, K., Ibirogba, E., Elrefaei, A., Teles, A., Theiler, R., Nomura, R., et al. (2020). SARS-CoV-2 in pregnancy: a comprehensive summary of current guidelines. *J. Clin. Med.* 9 (5), 1521. doi:10.3390/jcm9051521

National Institute of Human Rights (INDH) (2016). Situación de los derechos humanos en Chile: informe anual 2016. Available at: http://www.indh.cl/informe-anual-situacion-de-los-derechos-humanos-en-chile-2016 (Accessed August 9, 2020).

National Institute of Statistics (INE) (2018). 2017 census data. Available at: https://www.censo2017.cl/descargas/home/sintesis-de-resultados-censo2017.pdf (Accessed August 8, 2020).

National Institute of Statistics (INE) (2019). National vital statistics 2017. Available at: https://www.ine.cl/docs/default-source/nacimientos-matrimonios-y-defunciones/publicaciones-y-anuarios/anuarios-de-estad%C3%ADsticas-vitales/anuario-de-estad%C3%ADsticas-vitales-2017.pdf?sfvrsn=95e68aba_4 (Accessed August 8, 2020).

National Public Health Insurance Fund (FONASA) (2020). Income brackets 2020. Available at: https://www.fonasa.cl/sites/fonasa/conoce-fonasa (Accessed August 8, 2020).

Organization for Economic Cooperation and Development (OECD) (2020). OECD data. Health spending. Available at: https://data.oecd.org/healthres/health-spending.htm (Accessed August 8, 2020).

Richter, L., Daelmans, B., Lombardi, J., Heymann, J., Lopez Boo, F., Behrman, J., et al. (2016). Investing in the foundation of sustainable development: pathways to scale up for early childhood development. *Lancet* 389 (10064), 103–118. doi:10.1016/S0140-6736(16)31698-1

Sadler, M., Leiva, G., and Olza, I. (2020). COVID-19 as a risk factor for obstetric violence. *Sex. Reprod. Health Matters* 28, 1785379. doi:10.1080/26410397.2020.1785379

Schmid, M., Fontijn, J., Ochsenbein-Kölble, N., Berger, C., and Bassler, D. (2020). COVID-19 in pregnant women. *Lancet Infect. Dis.* 20 (6), 653. doi:10.1016/S1473-3099(20)30175-4

Semaan, A., Audet, C., Huysmans, E., Afolabi, B., Assarag, B., Banke-Thomas, A., et al. (2020). Voices from the frontline: findings from a thematic analysis of a rapid online global survey of maternal and newborn health professionals facing the COVID-19 pandemic. *BMJ Global Health* 5 (6), e002967. doi:10.1136/bmjgh-2020-002967

Smith, H. (2020). Impact of COVID-19 on neonatal health: are we causing more harm than good? *Eur J. Midwifery* 4, 9. doi:10.18332/ejm/120245

South-East Metropolitan Health Service (2020). Good practices and innovation, second meeting. Available at: https://redsalud.ssmso.cl/destacados-proyectos-de-los-establecimientos-de-salud-del-sur-oriente-fueron-premiados-en-el-2-encuentro-de-buenas-practicas-e-innovacion-del-ssmso/ (Accessed August 9, 2020).

Stuebe, A. (2020). Should infants be separated from mothers with COVID-19? First, do no harm. *Breastfeed. Med.* 15 (5), 351–352. doi:10.1089/bfm.2020.29153.ams

United Nations Children's Fund (UNICEF) (2018). Levels and trends in child mortality. Report 2018. Available at: https://www.unicef.org/publications/index_103264.html (Accessed August 8, 2020).

World Bank (2020). Data bank world development indicators. Available at: https://databank.worldbank.org/source/world-development-indicators (Accessed August 8, 2020).

World Bank (2020). The World Bank in Chile. Available at: https://www.worldbank.org/en/country/chile/overview (Accessed August 8, 2020).

World Health Organization (WHO) (2020b). Clinical management of severe acute respiratory infection (SARI) when COVID-19 disease is suspected. Available at: https://apps.who.int/iris/handle/10665/331446 (Accessed August 9, 2020).

World Health Organization (WHO) (2019). Trends in maternal mortality 2000 to 2017: estimates by WHO, UNICEF, UNFPA, World Bank Group and the United Nations Population Division. Geneva, Switzerland:WHO. Licence: CC BY-NC-SA 3.0 IGO.

World Health Organization (WHO) (2020a). WHO COVID-19 homepage. Available at: https://covid19.who.int/region/amro/country/cl (Accessed August 9, 2020).

Zaigham, M., and Andersson, O. (2020). Maternal and perinatal outcomes with COVID-19: a systematic review of 108 pregnancies. *Acta Obstet. Gynecol. Scand.* 99 (7), 823–829. doi:10.1111/aogs.13867

11

The Impacts of COVID-19 on US Maternity Care Practices

Kim Gutschow[1]* *and Robbie Davis-Floyd*[2]

[1]*Departments of Anthropology and Religion, Williams College, Williamstown, MA, United States,* [2]*Department of Anthropology, Rice University, Houston, TX, United States*

Correspondence:
Kim Gutschow
kim.gutschow@williams.edu

This article extends the findings of a rapid response article researched in April 2020 to illustrate how providers' practices and attitudes toward COVID-19 had shifted in response to better evidence, increased experience, and improved guidance on how SARS-CoV-2 and COVID-19 impacted maternity care in the United States. This article is based on a review of current labor and delivery guidelines in relation to SARS-CoV-2 and COVID-19, and on an email survey of 28 community-based and hospital-based maternity care providers in the United State, who discuss their experiences and clients' needs in response to a rapidly shifting landscape of maternity care during the COVID-19 pandemic. One-third of our respondents are obstetricians, while the other two-thirds include midwives, doulas, and labor and delivery nurses. We present these providers' frustrations and coping mechanisms in shifting their practices in relation to COVID-19. The primary lessons learned relate to improved testing and accessing PPE for providers and clients; the need for better integration between community- and hospital-based providers; and changes in restrictive protocols concerning labor support persons, rooming-in with newborns, immediate skin-to-skin contact, and breastfeeding. We conclude by suggesting that the COVID-19 pandemic offers a transformational moment to shift maternity care in the United States toward a more integrated and sustainable model that might improve provider and maternal experiences as well as maternal and newborn outcomes.

Keywords: COVID-19, SARS—CoV—2, maternity care, newborn care, midwives, community births, pregnancy, doulas

INTRODUCTION: CHANGING PRACTICES AND ATTITUDES TOWARD COVID-19 AMONG UNITED STATES MATERNITY CARE PROVIDERS

This article illuminates shifting maternity care practices and protocols among a select group of community- and hospital-based providers across the United States in response to the COVID-19 pandemic during 2020. Following up on an earlier essay (Davis-Floyd et al., 2020) that summarized provider responses about their shifting practices and attitudes early in the COVID-19 pandemic in April of 2020, we expanded our questionnaire and the set of providers we contacted to discuss how attitudes and protocols had further changed in response to new evidence and experience with SARS-CoV-2 and COVID-19 by October and November of 2020. Here, our focus is on the emergent ways in which maternity care providers—obstetricians, midwives, nurses, and doulas—reflect upon their latest adaptations to COVID-19.

Our article illustrates how and why individual providers in both community and hospital settings have shifted their practices and attitudes toward COVID-19 and the SARS-CoV-2 virus. We highlight the still-emergent knowledges and experiences for both providers and childbearers in relation to COVID-19 as well as the critical conclusions drawn during the first year of the pandemic. By the fall of 2020, the climate of fear and loss of control that had dominated the early months of the pandemic had given way to a landscape in which providers had reestablished agency by adjusting protocols to be more evidence-based, while childbearers reestablished some agency by being allowed to bring a birth partner into the labor and delivery process once again. We close by considering how the COVID-19 pandemic offers both a disruptive moment and key lessons for developing more integrated, sustainable, and resilient US maternity care system that can benefit providers, mothers, and newborns.

METHODS

Between September and December 2020, we conducted an email survey of maternity care providers about their practices and attitudes in response to COVID-19. We emailed a questionnaire (see Appendix) to a list of providers we had developed in the spring of 2020 while researching a rapid response article on COVID-19 and maternity care (Davis-Floyd et al., 2020) and used snowball sampling to enable our respondents to forward our questionnaire to other providers. We also posted our survey questions on the REPRONETWORK listserv. All of our respondents replied to our survey questions *via* email, while some briefly discussed their responses with us or replied to all providers on our list, thereby enabling those who responded later to have the benefit of prior responses. Given the constraints of a raging pandemic, most providers responded briefly. All respondents gave explicit written consent for their comments to be used, and most indicated that they wished to be identified, while a few preferred to remain anonymous.[1] Unless otherwise indicated, real names will be used for our respondents.

By November of 2020, 28 providers had responded to our survey, roughly one-third of whom were obstetricians (one was also a maternal-fetal medicine specialist), and two-thirds of whom were midwives (certified professional midwives—CPMs—and certified nurse midwives—CNMs), doulas, and a labor and delivery nurse. These providers came from Texas, Arizona, Arkansas, Virginia, North Carolina, Florida, Illinois, Idaho, Oregon, Massachusetts, and California.

We frame the provider responses within a summary of the most recent labor and delivery and newborn care guidance in response to COVID-19 and SARS-CoV-2 in the United States as of December 2020. Our literature review of this guidance drew on a repository on "COVID-19, Maternal and Child Health, and Nutrition" compiled monthly by the Johns Hopkins Center for Humanitarian Health, and keyword searches for critical terms.[2] We emphasize that evidence and provider experiences are rapidly evolving, and many systematic studies of the impacts of SARS-CoV-2 and COVID-19 on pregnancy, maternal health, and neonatal health remain to be conducted, while case studies offer only limited evidence. The views and findings described herein should be considered as provisional responses to an evolving pandemic. Our article is organized around the salient themes that emerged from our data and our questionnaire.

FINDINGS: SHIFTING ATTITUDES AND PRACTICES

Shifting Attitudes Toward Covid-19: From Fear to Action

Looking back with the hindsight of current knowledge, we cannot stress enough how disruptive and confusing the evidence around SARS-CoV-2 and COVID-19 was in the first half of 2020. The prior coronavirus epidemics of SARS and MERS, as well as experiences with Ebola and Zika viruses, compounded the trepidation around rates and routes of transmission of SARS-CoV-2, case fatality rates for COVID-19, and its specific impacts on pregnant women. Providers were responding to patient fears and misinformation, as well as to a fundamental lack of evidence with regard to how SARS-CoV-2 and COVID-19 would impact pregnancy, maternal, and newborn outcomes. In this article, we capture the shifts in their attitudes and practices from spring to fall 2020.

During the winter and spring of 2020–21, COVID-19 continued to spread rapidly and widely across the globe, often *via* asymptomatic transmission, and many regions had faced second and third waves of contagion that were even more virulent than the first. By the end of May of 2021, there were over 167 million cases and over 3.5 million deaths globally, as well as over 33 million cases and nearly 600,000 thousand deaths in the United Stated alone.[3] While the United Stated only accounts for 4.25% of the global population, it was responsible for roughly one-sixth of the global death count. With over 140 million births expected worldwide in 2020, and many pregnant women at risk for being infected with SARS-CoV-2, hospitals and institutional bodies rushed to establish protocols and guidance for labor, delivery, and postpartum care (Boelig et al., 2020a,2020b; Stephenson et al., 2020).

[1]All providers who responded to our emailed questionnaire gave written consent for their statements to be used in this article and most providers chose to be identified, while those who wished were anonymized, given a pseudonym, and all identifying details removed. Those who requested us to do so reviewed a draft before submission. Given these precautions, the Williams College IRB Chair exempted this research from IRB review.

[2]This literature repository can be found at: http://hopkinshumanitarianhealth.org/empower/advocacy/covid-19/covid-19-children-and-nutrition/.

[3]Data on global cases and deaths is from the global map at the John Hopkins University Coronavirus Resource center, at https://coronavirus.jhu.edu/map.html.

Providers' initial fears about maternal and newborn outcomes were not surprising, given the high rates of obstetric complications that pregnant women had faced during other recent coronavirus outbreaks, namely SARS and MERS (Schwartz and Dhaliwal 2020), as well as during Ebola and Zika (Strong and Schwartz 2019). While the SARS outbreak had a global case fatality rate of 11%, maternal mortality was as high as 30%, with 60% of pregnant women requiring admission to an ICU and 40% requiring intubation (Schwartz and Graham, 2020). A systematic review and meta-analysis of 19 studies analyzing pregnancy outcomes for women with confirmed SARS, MERS, or COVID-19 infections reported significantly increased rates of obstetric complications than for women without coronavirus infections (Di Mascio et al., 2020).

Rates of obstetric complication from COVID-19 were alarming (Boelig et al., 2020a), and significant increases in maternal death, stillbirths, and rates of postnatal depression were reported (Ellington et al., 2020; Chmielewska et al., 2021). For a small number of pregnant women, the most serious complications of COVID-19 included severe pneumonia, cardiomyopathy, thrombosis, and multiorgan diseases that require intensive care and mechanical ventilation (Schwartz et al., 2020b). The pooled meta-analysis of several early studies indicated the following rates of maternal and newborn complications: 41% preterm delivery before 37 weeks, 15% preterm delivery before 34 weeks, 15% preeclampsia, 19% premature rupture of membranes (PROM), 91% cesarean delivery, 7% perinatal death, 43% fetal distress, and 9% of newborns admitted to a NICU (Di Mascio et al., 2020). While miscarriages and stillbirth were rare, women who were asymptomatic during labor and delivery fared much better, and some preterm births were provider induced (Boelig et al., 2020a).

As 2020 progressed, the landscape of maternity care shifted as providers realized the significance of asymptomatic community spread and the dangers the virus posed to mother and newborns. It was estimated that 25–40% of transmissions occur before onset of symptoms and asymptomatic infections can range from 20–50% within select studies (Meyerowitz et al., 2020). The degree and rate of vertical transmission between mother and newborn, in three possible ways—intrauterine or placental transmission, intrapartum transmission, or postpartum transmission—is still being quantified, although early studies indicated that many infected newborns were asymptomatic or developed only mild cases of COVID-19 (Schwartz et al., 2020b).

Our survey respondents recognized that their clients' fears ranged widely; as obstetrician George Walters (a pseudonym), described: "We are impressed with the wide range of patient perceptions. Some remain near emotional paralysis due to fear and others are not worried at all." The most common fears about COVID-19 that our providers encountered among their clients were:

- Fear of being infected by SARS-CoV-2 or developing COVID-19
- Fear of being denied a labor support person
- Fear of having to choose between a partner and doula for labor support
- Fear of transmitting the virus to a newborn
- Fear of being separated from their newborn after delivery
- Fear of isolation during pregnancy, labor, and the postpartum period

We address all of these concerns herein, as we show how provider attitudes and practices adapted within the following areas:

- Shifting norms for PPE (personal protective equipment) and testing of both providers and childbearers
- Shifting norms about allowing support persons during labor, delivery, and the postpartum period
- Shifting norms about separating mother and newborn vs. "rooming in" in response to the shifting evidence of vertical transmission of SARS-CoV-2 from mother to newborn
- Ongoing lack of integration between community- and hospital-based providers

Our findings suggest that the changes in provider knowledge and protocols have had significant impacts on women's mental health, with downstream effects on newborn and maternal health that remain to be quantified but are just beginning to emerge. Homebirth obstetrician Stuart Fischbein of Los Angeles summarized how the hospitals in his area used COVID-19 as a pretext to abandon their "mother-baby friendly" practices in ways that compromised maternal health and agency:

> The pandemic has exposed the medical model of maternity care and clarified how they really think. The Mother-Baby Friendly moniker that they were all so proud of labeling themselves went out the window immediately. Little or no concern for the psychological well-being of the mother is clear by their separation policies...For that matter, the pandemic has exposed the fallibility of experts and trust in their judgement which I think is a good thing. The individualization of care and respect for autonomy in decision making should not go out the window because of fear.

Fischbein's comment speaks to the relatively recent humanistic changes in many United States hospitals that are termed "Mother-Baby Friendly" because they allow partners and doulas into the labor room, immediate skin-to-skin contact after birth, and newborn rooming-in. He notes how quickly these humanistic policies of connection were reversed in favor of the traditional medical model of obstetrics, which separates mothers and newborns as well as mothers from their families.

Doula Stevie Merino, cofounder of Doulas of Color Training and Birthworkers of Color Collective in California, summarizes how her experiences have improved her protocols:

> People, including providers and clients, are all operating and approaching this time with different emotions, fears, anxieties, and beliefs. I have found that there have been major bumps in the road as we are all

> navigating this unprecedented time. . .now that I have tested experience through this pandemic [I] feel more confident about best practices/protocols.

CNM Dinah Waranch, who attends birth at home and at a birth center in Texas, notes that: "Pregnant women are by definition somewhat anxious. Now some of them are more so. On the other hand, just like the country, the clientele is divided." CNM Jenny Bagg, who practices at a community health center in Florida, reflects on the risk of catching COVID-19 at her center vs. the community: "Where I am, the community is a much more likely place to catch COVID than in the hospital. Patients generally do not seem afraid of contracting COVID in the hospital." Speaking to both women's and providers' fears, obstetrician George Walters said:

> Many feared early on. But now that we know the rate of infection is low, patients are much less concerned about going to the hospital. I would not say we practitioners are afraid of catching COVID. Our entire careers have involved infection risk. We adapt and move forward. We don't like wearing masks, but we believe they help.

The notion that providers and clients no longer fear COVID-19 may not be widespread; for example, doula Stevie Merino expressed a rather different view:

> Pregnant people definitely are reporting not feeling safe and more at risk of contracting COVID-19 at hospitals which is why so many are inquiring about other options. I personally am afraid of contracting COVID-19—as a self-employed person and as a single parent, I do not have the same benefits and protections that others have during this time.

Homebirth obstetrician Fishbein explains that his clients' primary fear is not their health but hospital policies that may be driving them to pursue the "other option" of community birth that Merino alludes to; Fishbein says, "Main fear is not about health. It is about hospital restrictive policies and separation from their baby and support system." Doula Merino echoes these fears about hospitals:

> Not being able to have the support that they want because of hospital support person restrictions is the number one fear that I have heard the most. Another is the limited support options because of the fear, anxieties, risks of COVID-19 for themselves/infant(s).

Obstetrician George Walters explained why fears of COVID-19 were high but later abated:

> We are very thankful that reproductive age women are mostly unaffected by COVID. We were initially worried that it would be worse than H1N1. And we are even more grateful that newborns appear to be almost fully unaffected.

MFM specialist Charles Deena (a pseudonym) summarized the initial confusion around the major safety protocols being instituted at his large urban hospital in Illinois:

> As for safety protocols, a lot of this had to do with where COVID-positive people were allowed to labor (on L&D? In a separate unit?), how to deal with particular emergencies in a COVID+ patient (i.e., maternal code, need for intubation, need for emergency cesarean delivery or operative vaginal delivery), and contingency planning for patients who needed advanced life support (i.e., intubated on ventilator, need for ECMO).

L&D nurse Hicks from Texas explained how client fears were reduced by shifting hospital protocols around PPE and testing:

> The mothers I have worked with have expressed a generalized fear of contracting the virus in the hospital. For a lot of them, going to the hospital is one of the first times they have left their homes outside of OBGYN visits. . .The precautions taken by the facility seem to ease the fears pregnant mothers and their families have.

This range of attitudes toward COVID-19 shows both overlap and differences between community- and hospital-based providers. Overall, we found that hospital-based providers had better access to and control over PPE, testing, and restrictions on their clients than community-based providers. Many of our providers reported that the most significant changes in their protocols involved strict use of PPE, hygiene, testing, telehealth, and restrictions on support people and rooming in, which we discuss in turn below.

Labor and delivery guidance established in the United States by May 2020 included: encouraging oxytocin use at higher doses to shorten duration of labor; using amniotomies for dysfunctional or delayed labor; using prophylactic oxytocin during the third stage of labor to prevent hemorrhages; using early epidurals to minimize need for general anesthesia (which risks aerosolization of the virus); limiting the second stage of labor; performing cesareans if labor had arrested after only 4 h; limiting antenatal corticosteroids after 34 weeks; judicious use of magnesium sulfate for slowing preterm labor because it can cause respiratory suppression; avoiding aggressive fluid hydration; and limiting frequency of cervical exams (Boelig et al., 2020a; Stephenson et al., 2020). Many of these recommendations had little evidence base and overturned years of evidence in support of the more humanistic, holistic, and patient-centered care that birth activists had long fought for (Gutschow et al., 2021; Davis-Floyd, 2018).

Hasty guidance that lacked significant evidence included encouraging cesarean delivery for women who tested positive––estimated at 70% globally by April 2020 according to one systematic review (Debrandere et al., 2020); encouraging inductions and instrumental delivery; isolating newborns from mothers who tested positive; and not delaying cord clamping (Favre et al., 2020). Much of this guidance lacked evidence (Schmid et al., 2020) and some even promoted obstetric violence (Sadler et al., 2020).

The major protocols to protect risk of transmission that were reported in the literature by May 2020 included: universal PPE for providers, childbearers, and support people; universal testing of providers and pregnant women admitted to facilities; limitation to one support person for the entire labor, delivery, and postpartum period; preference for virtual labor support if possible; and no children younger than 16 permitted at any time (Boelig et al., 2020a). For out-patient visits and pregnancy consults, major recommendations included universal PPE for providers and pregnant persons; universal testing and screening before any in-patient visit; postponing elective visits if possible; telehealth for most routine prenatal consults; and keeping additional providers at home if possible (Boelig et al., 2020b). We discuss these shifting protocols and practices in turn below.

Shifting Practices: Using PPE and Incessant Sanitizing

Our first article indicated that both hospital- and community-based providers suffered severe shortages of PPE in March and April of 2020. By October of 2020, many of the PPE shortages had been resolved, although the fall wave of COVID-19 brought increased stress to hospitals and communities that had not experienced a first wave of COVID. Obstetrician Walters described the shift at his urban hospital in North Carolina:

> We were initially short of PPE. But we live in a great community. I worked for about 3 weeks in masks donated by a nail salon. A local distillery (that usually makes alcohol to drink) started cranking out hand sanitizer. You have to love American ingenuity!! We have had no supply problems in months.

Obstetrician Marco Giannotti of Texas representatively reported: "Our office staff all wear standard medical masks. Cloth masks not allowed for staff, and we provide free masks for anyone who needs one (patients and employees)," while MFM specialist Charles Deena reported that by September, his Illinois hospital had "sufficient PPE at this time." L&D nurse Hicks explained how her hospital is ensuring a steady supply of PPE for all staff:

> The major changes in the practices and protocols at the hospital I work at are geared towards protecting patients and healthcare staff from each other. . . . Our facility has enough PPE but is taking precautions to not run out. Every nurse in the emergency room and labor and delivery unit has to wear an N95 at all times, goggles during patient interactions, and face shields during deliveries, because there is always a chance that a patient will come to the unit that needs emergent care and is COVID-19 positive. All other nurses wear surgical masks at all times. The only time masks can be removed is in the designated break room. The nurses that have to wear N95 masks wear their mask until a string breaks or it gets dirty, which normally take 2 days.

CNM Bagg confirmed that her community health clinic "is doing an excellent job at protecting us as much as possible. We all have multiple N95 masks which are required to be worn at all times in the clinic." LM (licensed midwife) Jessica Willoughby, who runs a birth center in Florida, described an initial difficulty in getting masks that later resolved:

> [Now] we offer surgical masks if people do not come in with masks. We are requiring masks. We are not limiting people at visits or at births. [After initial delays] we have adequate masks. . . .K95s and surgical masks.

Doula Stevie Merino, who makes home visits and attends hospital births, described her difficulty with accessing PPE in California:

> It has been difficult for me to access sufficient PPE because I am not a medical provider. Many of the sites that I normally would purchase from are directing them understandably to medical providers/locations. Thankfully, many in my community have been great at supporting with PPE. . . . I also use continuous PPE gear when visiting homes or at births, even when clients and others have become more relaxed with it.

Community-based midwife CNM Dinah Waranch reported that at her home and birth center practice, "During labor and birth the mother is NOT masked. . . Midwives are masked. Support people . . . masked . . . . Some (clients) roll their eyes at masks." Waranch told a story about an intake visit that expresses both her own flexibility and that of the midwifery model of care concerning a client for whom she had previously served as a midwife:

> [My client] is unmasked and I make a gesture across my face for her to mask up as I am. [She] rolls her eyes, puts on a mask, and stomps into the room. "Masks are communist. They are un-American." Loudly through her mask, defiant. I am opinionated too. "Communism isn't so evil," I am smiling, teasing, but my dagger glints. Then reaching deeply for my mature, inner midwife, I say. "If you prefer not to wear a mask, let's sit outside in the park a few feet away from each other. I can do your intake history on my phone." How easy it was then to create a peace between us, to open to each other across the picnic table beside the pond; the story of her motherhood, unique but mutually understood. Our angers soften...

CPM and DO (Doctor of Osteopathy) Sarita Bennett, who runs a midwifery practice in Virginia, explained that her staff midwives "do not wear masks during the birth . . . all of our birth team members are relatively "non-social" on a good day, and do not frequent some of the higher risk areas like bars, churches or indoor group events." Homebirth obstetrician Fischbein noted:

> Science is compromised. Healthy people have little to fear. Compromised and elderly people should take precautions. We have made no major changes in our practice. We wear PPE at client request. Otherwise, my team and I are choosing to believe much of the suppressed literature that many of the recommended precautions are not evidenced based. We have a trust in our immune systems...

Fischbein alludes to a holistic belief that immune systems are critical to understanding human physiology as well as the physiology of birth. His view also reflects a broader critique of medicalized obstetrics that we have explored elsewhere (Gutschow et al., 2021). Scientists who study viruses still have many questions about why some populations or individuals are less impacted by SARS-CoV-2 and COVID-19 than others (Mukherjee, 2021; Zimmer 2021), as well as about how the evolutionary processes that created birth physiology intersect with those that produced human immunity to viruses and other pathogens.

Besides PPE, many providers reported a strong emphasis on hygiene and sanitation. Echoing other midwives, CPM Sarita Bennett instituted "a short break between clients to allow time to wipe things down and ask that children not come along to prenatal because we can't wipe down toys every time." Echoing what other community-based midwives stated, LM Willoughby reported:

> Cleaning, everything, all the time, between every patient. It. Is. Exhausting. We also have a hand sanitizer and an alcohol wipe station at the front door. . .We give isopropol alcohol wipes to the patients when they arrive to wipe down their phones. We as a staff make it a habit to wipe down our phones with those wipes several times a day and hand sanitize frequently...It was a crash course in PPE and I'm so glad I was able to connect with other birth center owners to go in on masks purchases because initially we were unable to find anything!!

She continues by placing extra stress on the drawbacks of these incessant sanitizing efforts:

> I always felt like the birth center was a sanctuary from the craziness that happens in the mainstream medical model. Now with COVID, I feel like our tranquil borders have been breached! I hate the super vigilance and paranoia I feel with the obsessive cleaning.

MFM specialist Charles Deena confirmed the benefit of increased PPE use: "Thus far, with our sufficient PPE, only a minority of clinicians have acquired COVID-19. We, luckily, have not had any colleagues die from COVID-19 exposure." By November, none of the providers who responded to our questionnaire had contracted COVID and none reported any colleagues who had died of COVID-19, although several had to self-quarantine or to quarantine staff. L&D nurse Lauren Hicks described the careful quarantine and contact tracing protocols her hospital conducted:

> Luckily, we have only had one nurse test positive. Unfortunately, she worked on the unit before she knew she was positive and had a patient that required rapid response, meaning nearly every staff member on the unit was in the room with her to help her patient. Everyone was wearing masks, so luckily no other staff member became sick. The COVID-19 positive nurse quarantined for over two weeks until her symptoms were gone. Every person that was in contact with her during the shift she worked was contacted and asked to record their symptoms for 2 weeks. We were told if symptoms started to present to contact the unit director and go to the hospital to get tested.

Shifting Practices: Testing Providers for COVID-19

In contrast to our first survey (Davis-Floyd et al., 2020), in which many providers reported that they had to beg or plead for testing, by November of 2020, there was improved access to testing for many hospital-based providers, but less for community-based providers. The early months of the pandemic had revealed the unpreparedness of United States healthcare and maternity care institutions for a pandemic. Yet many hospitals began to acquire testing capacity and to require testing for all admitted pregnant women as well as regular testing of staff. However, according to an obstetrician at a large teaching hospital in Massachusetts, the demand for testing so outstripped supply that weekly testing was initially required only for teaching staff but not for clinical staff or support staff. In contrast, CNM Jennifer Bagg, who works at a health center in Florida, reported, "The entire staff (over 200 people) are tested every other Monday." Doula Stevie Merino made a personal choice to get tested: "As a birthworker, I have made the individual choice to be tested every few weeks or more if between births. Los Angeles and Long Beach have free testing sites which I have used and found very efficient, useful."

Midwife Jessica Willoughby of VIrginia elaborated:

> We do not test our patients and staff at the birth center. Every staff member who has been sick I've made them go to the urgent care. . .to get tested. . .they've been really good to us to get our results back quick. I was sick this week and I went in and was given a rapid screen (negative) and a PCR which came back in 48 h (also negative). I have zero tolerance for people being sick. If my staff are sick, they cannot come into the birth center for 14 days unless they have a negative COVID screen.

Willoughby illustrates the value of giving all birth providers access to regular testing with rapid results in communities as well as hospitals. The irregular access to testing and frequent delays in test results for much of 2020 across the United States represent a lost opportunity. By getting tested regularly and having their results rapidly available, providers could limit inadvertent transmission, reduce fear among clients, and limit their own anxiety about attending asymptomatic clients. MFM specialist Charles Deena, who works in an urban hospital in Illinois that handles 12,000 births a year, alluded to ongoing difficulties in accessing tests for some providers: "(Testing) is a point of contention, especially given the needed resources to do universal testing. Test positive rates are pretty varied across landscapes, with the highest being in NYC, though our test positive rate. . .is (also) relatively high."

Testing in Community vs. Hospital Settings

Some of our community birth providers required their pregnant clients to be tested, while others did not. Community-based CPM Shea Childs in Arkansas notes that she would not test asymptomatic clients, but feels differently about symptomatic clients, "If they were symptomatic at 36 weeks or more, I may (test), but that has not come up." Community-based midwife Jessica Willoughby requires her staff but not her clients to get tested regularly: "We do not require COVID testing. I've never even sent a mom to get tested. If she's asymptomatic we just treat everything as normal. If she's sick we ask that she stay home, and we can do telehealth. I've never had a patient be sick in labor." Many community-based providers work with a clientele who are low risk for birth complications as well as COVID-19, and who follow social distancing and masking guidelines.

In contrast, our hospital-based providers were very serious about mandatory testing, reporting that all childbearers are routinely tested before admission to hospital for labor as well as for out-patient pregnancy consults. Yet there were difficulties, as CNM Jennifer Bagg of Florida explained: "We have started testing all pregnant patients for COVID weekly starting at 36 weeks. We do the rapid antigen tests but the whole process from start to finish takes over 30 min and severely negatively impacts our already very busy patient flow."

Hospital-based CNM Kylea Liese of Chicago said that patients in her hospital are "tested a few days prior if they have a scheduled c/s or induction." About office visits, obstetrician George Walters stated, "We prescreen with questions about symptoms and contacts every person prior to entering the building. Patients wait in their cars, not the waiting room." Texas-based obstetrician Marco Giannotti confirmed the prevalence of out-patient testing: "The biggest change has really been in screening patients before entering the office." Regarding office visits for mothers who test positive for the virus, CNM Bagg spoke representatively: "We try to make them the last appointment of the day to limit others' exposure, don full PPE and try to finish the visit as quickly as possible."

Community-based CPM/DO Sarita Bennett of Virginia described the scarcity and unreliability of testing:

> Testing has been difficult to access, unreliable in its results––we have seen some negative results that we didn't believe and treated the person as positive and been exposed to people who a week later told us they had had an asymptomatic positive test which resulted in quarantines but no further sickness. Many of our clients have no insurance or have difficulty accessing testing. Most, if not all, have protected themselves through staying out of public, masking, hand washing, etc. The testing seems the least effective way of screening at this point.

Community-based CPM Debbie Query of Arkansas adds:

> I have read the remarks from the scientist who developed the test, which is not ... considered reliable. Nor am I any more concerned about this virus than any other virus. I have always been cautious about germs and cleanliness and so my practice has pretty much stayed the same. The only change is if they or somebody in the family tests positive I will postpone their prenatal or do a "tele-med" call.

MFM specialist Deena from Illinois elaborated:

> interesting to note the differences in testing, especially the weekly testing (which seems aggressive to me) and the use of different testing platforms (i.e., rapid antigen versus PCR testing). . . .We will screen people with nasopharyngeal PCR swabs upon admission as we have a test that will produce results pretty rapidly.

These providers were alluding to the main diagnostic test for COVID-19 used in 2020, the Reverse Transcription Polymerase Chain Reaction (RT-PCR) test. This test initially extracts viral RNA from the sample, uses an enzyme to convert viral RNA into DNA, and subsequently passes through several steps to amplify viral RNA with multiple cycles. The sensitivity of this method is so great that even non-infectious fragments of viral nucleic acid can yield positive results for an asymptomatic individual (Surkova et al., 2020; Kaufman and Puopolo, 2021). We emphasize that testing positive indicates that an individual is infected with the SARS-CoV-2 virus, although such individuals are frequently labeled as "COVID-19 positive" in ordinary discourse. By February 2021, much of the medical literature we consulted distinguished between SARS-CoV-2 and COVID-19; we follow that distinction here.

A systematic review and meta-analysis of 30 population-based studies conducted in September 2020 revealed that 95% of all obstetric patients were asymptomatic (Yanes-Lane et al., 2020). In the future, careful distinctions may be made between asymptomatic but infected individuals and the smaller number of infected persons with symptomatic COVID-19. This distinction mirrors the critical distinction between being HIV positive and having a diagnosis of AIDS.

Our providers indicated a rise in telehealth, especially for doulas who reported attending to their clients virtually, using devices positioned in the sight line of the laboring person. Given that providers in the room could shut off or move the device out of range without consent of the laboring person, and that the essence of doula care is physical touch and presence, many doulas were unsatisfied with virtual support. In contrast, many providers in both hospitals and communities were comfortable using telemedicine for prenatal care. While homebirth midwives have mixed opinions about telehealth, hospital-based providers were more comfortable with this form of care. Obstetrician Lucia Gomez (pseudonym) from Texas confirmed that, "Our offices had telemedicine appts for both gyn and OB patients," yet obstetrician Marco Giannotti reported that his practice never went to telehealth. Obstetrician Marilyn Vanover had a negative opinion about telehealth, stating,

> My biggest concern is the decrease in in-person visits to assess patient needs. I am also concerned that this will become the "norm" too often once the pandemic is under control. I am concerned about the delay in diagnosis of ectopics and PID [pelvic inflammatory disease].

We will need longer-term and more systematic studies to determine whether the rise of telemedicine in maternity care continues after the pandemic passes.

Restricting Labor Support: Impacts on Maternal Mental Health and Health Equity

By mid-March and into the summer of 2020, many hospitals across the United States had begun to exclude labor support people—partners and doulas—due to fears of COVID-19 transmission (Davis-Floyd et al., 2020). In the United States, an Executive Order by New York State Governor Cuomo on March 28, 2020 explicitly allowed one support person to attend the person in labor, and other hospitals later adapted their policies around labor support people.[4] By October 2020, most of our respondents reported that their hospital or clinic allowed at least one support person, and sometimes even for women who tested positive.

CNM Diana Jolles from Arizona stated that her hospital began excluding all support people in April of 2020 but reallowed them back in September 2020. Obstetrician Walters echoed other hospital-based providers when he said, "We never excluded a support person. Our unit continues to allow one support person. That is usually the father, but other times a family member. Rarely a paid doula." Even birth centers were limiting support people, as confirmed by several of our provider respondents. CNM Dinah Waranch described more flexible limits at her birth center in Texas: "One support person only encouraged but additional support people at mother's discretion, masked. Family arriving after birth not encouraged."

Obstetrician Michael White of Texas described how the limitations on support people restricted family access during prenatal care, labor, and delivery: "We no longer allow any other family to accompany them, thus spouse and family are excluded from the prenatal care. At the hospital level it too has severely restricted family access to a delivery." Several providers reported that the situation had become quite difficult for doulas; doula Roselyn Faith from Oregon explained that:

> The local hospitals stopped allowing doula support for birthing mothers from March until now [September 2020]. They are just now opening their policies a bit, yet only for paid doulas. The volunteer program I was participating in still isn't allowed. This was a program offering birth support to all women and serving mostly low income and women of color. I'm hoping this program will be continued very soon.

Doula Stevie Merino explained how confusing these rules were, as well as how the limitations on support people put her clients and doulas in difficult situations:

> Every hospital's policies are different which has also been difficult to navigate and keep up with. . .There are very few hospitals that see doulas as an essential part of the birth team, which has allowed me and partner/support person to be present in the room. In quite a few instances, I have been chosen over a partner to be present in labor. This was an intentional and very difficult decision on all parties.

By not considering doulas as "essential personnel," hospital protocols devalued their services and limited the ability of childbearers to advocate for themselves and their newborns (Searcy and Castañeda, 2020). Even when hospitals allowed a single support person, the strict rules insisting that this support person was forbidden to leave the labor room further limited or prevented continuous support in labor, as some families cannot afford for the partner to stay the entire time. This rule can fall especially heavily on minoritized and low-income childbearers, who have been struck hardest by the virus (Obinna, 2020; Norton et al., 2020). Further, it penalizes women who already had small children at home with limited childcare, as their partners might have to choose between tending to their children or their birthing partner, who is facing increased stress and isolation (Norton et al., 2020; Almeida et al., 2020).

Speaking of his teaching hospital, MFM specialist Charles Deena described that for childbearers who tested negative, or who tested positive but were asymptomatic:

> one support person is allowed with them. Doulas are allowed, but they count as the one support person. From

[4] On March 28, 2020, Governor Cuomo of New York issued Executive Order 202.12 that explicitly allowed, "Any article 28 facility (public hospitals and nursing homes) licensed by the state, shall, as a condition of licensure permit the attendance of one support person who does not have a fever at the time of labor/delivery to be present for a patient who is giving birth." (State of New York Executive Chamber, 2020).

> my experience, most folks choose their partner. As for postpartum, if one is COVID-19 negative, you can have up to 2 people visit, although 1 can stay overnight.

Doula Merino described the lingering effects of the isolation that childbearers faced:

> Many are not having the experiences that they envisioned in terms of family, friend, community support due to social distancing recommendations. This isolation has had and will continue to have dramatic effects on postpartum people and new parents.

The restrictions denying labor support for childbearers who tested positive could indeed mean isolation and mental suffering, as MFM specialist Deena described:

> COVID-19 positive pregnant people who labor in our hospital do so in a negative pressure room on a floor above labor and delivery, have one-to-one nursing, and only one provider (no residents) at the delivery. As for the experiences of people laboring alone. . .the stories I heard from my colleagues working on the [COVID] floor is that it was heartbreaking--extremely isolating and really difficult to help people through, especially since we knew (and still know) so little about perinatal outcomes associated with the virus.

L&D nurse Hicks described the alienating scene that mothers testing positive faced:

> COVID-19 positive women. . .were not allowed to have a support person with them, and the newborn was immediately removed after delivery. Full PPE is worn while in the negative pressure room, which includes a N95, googles, face shield, gown, hair cover, and shoe covers. Nurses are encouraged to cluster care while in the patient's room. When nurses are caring for COVID positive patients, a primary nurse is allowed to go into the room while another nurse acts as a runner to get any supplies or medications the primary nurse needs.

This denial of labor support is especially critical for women of color, who have been disproportionately affected by COVID-19 and who already face formidable disparities in maternity care and obstetric outcomes (Ellington et al., 2020; Norton et al., 2020; Obinna 2020). Well before COVID-19 struck, between 2014 and 2017, the pregnancy-related mortality for non-Hispanic Black women (41 deaths/100,000 live births) was three times that of non-Hispanic white women (13.4 deaths/100,000 live births) and quadruple that of Hispanic or Latina women (11.6 deaths/100,000 live births) [Centers for Disease Control and Prevention (CDC), 2020a]. Evidence shows that the racial disparities in maternal outcomes are related to the chronic stress of structural racism as well as providers' racial bias (Bridges 2011; Eichelberger et al., 2016; Davis 2019; Valdez and Deomampo, 2019; Obinna 2020).

By defining doulas as visitors, not essential personnel, childbearers are being denied critical advocates during labor and the postpartum period when they are isolated due to COVID restrictions. A Cochrane meta-analysis of deliveries in 17 countries found that women receiving continuous labor support had shorter labors, were *more likely* to have spontaneous vaginal delivery and report positive childbirth experience, and *less likely* to have a cesarean delivery, to use any form of intrapartum analgesia, to have a baby with low (<5) Apgar score, and to have postpartum depression (Bohren et al., 2017). Yet a Canadian study (Fortier and Godwin, 2015) showed that doula presence was not viewed favorably by half of the obstetricians and one fourth of nurses in the study. Given this level of hostility to doulas, we are not surprised that the COVID-19 pandemic provided quick justification to exclude them from labor and delivery rooms, with adverse consequences for women that remain to be fully quantified.

There is evidence that laboring alone without support while sick with COVID-19 can have negative impacts on both mothers and newborns. One systematic study of 2,417 women from Massachussetts General Hospital, which compared women testing positive for SARS-CoV-2 with matched controls, found that women testing positive reported higher levels of pain during delivery, lower newborn weights, more newborn admissions to a NICU, and were 11 times more likely to have no visitors during labor and delivery (Mayopoulous et al., 2020). Further, many of these adverse effects were explicitly associated with the absence of labor support persons, proving that isolation itself (not just being seropositive) has detrimental maternal effects. Nearly half of the women who tested positive reported clinically significant acute stress symptoms (Mayopoulous et al., 2020). A Canadian study showed that after the onset of COVID-19, 37% of women had elevated depression, 46% had severely elevated anxiety, and 67% had elevated pregnancy-related anxiety, while social isolation strongly correlated with the likelihood of clinically significant depression or anxiety (Lebel et al., 2020; cited in Almeida et al., 2020).

There is some evidence that the COVID-19 pandemic has further exacerbated the pre-existing feelings of fear, stress, or loss of control and agency that women can experience during pregnancy, by adding the unknown factors about whether they or their newborns would test positive or be infected during labor, delivery, or the postpartum period, whether they would be permitted labor support, and whether having COVID-19 would further complicate their pregnancy through provider-induced preterm or cesarean delivery (Almeida et al., 2020). Shifting protocols in some hospitals began to allow labor support to women testing positive for SARS-CoV-2, as L&D nurse Lauren Hicks explained, women testing "positive are still being treated differently, but our protocols have recently improved. Now, COVID-19 positive mothers can have one companion with them, but the partner cannot leave the room during the whole hospital stay." The rule insisting that the labor partner stay for days at a time discriminates against women whose partners work or care for small children at home without access to other caregivers. We have addressed the scarcity of care in disruptive times in the conclusion to our recent volume on sustainable birth across the globe (Gutschow et al., 2021).

Shifting Practices: Mother-Newborn Separation and Transmission of SARS-CoV-2

Quite a few of our hospital-based providers reported that mothers testing positive for SARS-CoV-2 were separated from their newborns at birth, not allowed skin-to-skin contact, and discouraged from breastfeeding, based on the assumed possibility of mother-to-newborn COVID transmission. As MFM specialist Deena noted, "Some hospitals are sequestering newborns in the NICU if mothers are COVID-19 positive for up to 5 days, despite any evidence suggesting that this is beneficial."

Obstetrician Michael White and L&D nurse Hicks both confirmed that their hospitals separated mothers who tested positive from their newborns. Yet Hicks noted some improvements in protocols: "Recently at my facility they have been allowed to breastfeed and have skin-to-skin contact with their newborns...I am so glad that now my facility is treating COVID-19 positive patients almost like any other patient." Obstetrician Walters noted that his unit did not separate mothers and newborns, stating, "Babies need contact with their mom, and they need breast milk. We do allow breastfeeding and skin-to-skin, and advise hand washing and masks."

For CNM Dinah Waranch, with her low-risk client base, the protocols about separation constituted one reason not to test asymptomatic mothers before birth:

> Mothers are instructed/encouraged to test for COVID if they have symptoms or if they have a known exposure. We do not require prior to birth testing. This is partly because I do not believe my clientele would be happy to do that. It is also because I do not feel comfortable separating mother and baby after birth, which I regard as unnecessary and awful.

Returning to hospital births, unless mothers or newborns who tested positive were critically ill, they were usually sent home together within 2 days after birth even if they had been separated in the hospital. CNM Waranch responded to this paradox, stating: "No logic (to that), but then why expect logic from an illogical system?" Obstetrician Marco Giannotti added:

> When the pandemic first started, I was a big proponent of keeping positive moms with their babies and breastfeeding. There just was not any data present indicating otherwise. I received a lot of pushback from our Neonatologists and Pediatricians. Shortly afterwards--the American Academy of Pediatrics confirmed that asymptomatic COVID positive moms should not be separated from their baby, and that breastfeeding should continue as normal.

CNM Kylea Liese confirmed that her hospital separated mothers and newborns in contradiction to AAP policy:

> The rationale per peds [pediatrics] is "hospital policy" though they have acknowledged their own professional organization no longer supports this policy...the World Health Organization (WHO), Centers for Disease Control (CDC) and American Academy of Pediatrics (AAP) all recommend that mothers and babies stay together and breastfeed (if desired).

When the American Academy of Pediatrics (AAP, 2020) issued its first neonatal guidance on April 2, 2020, it recommended separating newborns from mothers who tested positive for SARS-CoV-2. Yet by September 9, 2020, the American Academy of Pediatrics (AAP, 2020) had issued new guidance recommending that "mothers and newborns may room-in according to usual center practices." The later guidance urged doctors to discuss risks and benefits of rooming in with mothers and follow the mother's choice, and also recommended delayed-cord clamping and skin-to- skin care for the mother and newborn, adding that mothers who tested positive should wear masks and practice handwashing prior to providing hands-on care for their newborns.

Nevertheless, the damage had been done. A CDC survey of 1,344 hospitals in the United States between July and August of 2020 (Perinne et al., 2020) confirmed that for mothers with suspected or confirmed COVID-19:

- Rooming in was discouraged in 38% and prohibited in 5% of hospitals
- Skin-to-skin care was discouraged in 14%, prevented in 6.5% of hospitals
- Skin-to-skin contact was only encouraged in 13% of hospitals
- Breastfeeding was discouraged in 20% of hospitals, but 17% of hospitals allowed feeding of expressed breastmilk

All of these policies were in direct contradiction to WHO, ACOG, and AAP guidance at the time, which strongly encouraged rooming-in, skin-to-skin contact, and breastfeeding for mothers with COVID-19, unless they were too ill to do so (Perinne et al., 2020). By August of 2020, the CDC had revised its guidance on rooming-in. The CDC recommended that mothers with suspected or confirmed SARS-CoV-2 infection discuss the risks and benefits of rooming in with their providers and that "healthcare providers respect maternal autonomy in the medical decision-making process." As rationale, the CDC noted that;

> Early and close contact between the mother and neonate has many well-established benefits. The ideal setting for care of a healthy, term newborn while in the hospital is in the mother's room, commonly called "rooming in." Current evidence suggests the risk of a neonate acquiring SARS-CoV-2 from its mother is low. Further, data suggests that there is no difference in risk of SARS-CoV-2 infection to the neonate whether a

neonate is cared for in a separate room or remains in the mother's room [Centers for Disease Control and Prevention (CDC), 2020b].

The guidance declared that mothers who test positive for SARS-CoV-2 should *not be considered* at risk of infecting their newborns if 10 days have passed since symptoms first appeared, at least 24 h have passed without a fever, and any other symptoms have improved [Centers for Disease Control and Prevention (CDC), 2020b]. We emphasize that these guidelines underscore our earlier point that mothers who are asymptomatic but test positive for SARS-CoV-2 are not necessarily infectious, as viral particles can be detected for days and even weeks after initial infection (Kaufman and Puopolo, 2021).

By December of 2020, further analysis of newborns whose mothers tested positive for SARS-CoV-2 revealed a low perinatal transmission rate to newborns (Schwartz et al., 2020a; Schwartz et al., 2020b; Schwartz and De Luca 2021) and supported the updated AAP and CDC guidance (Ronchi et al., 2020). A multicenter study from Lombardy, Italy of 62 newborns whose mothers tested positive for SARS-CoV-2 and who roomed-in with their mothers found that none of the newborns tested positive at birth, and after additional PCR tests at 7 and 20 days after birth, only 1.6% of newborns tested positive for the virus. Notably, nearly all newborns were breastfed (75% exclusively) and the study included newborns as young as 34 weeks (Ronchi et al., 2020).

A study of 120 newborns whose mothers tested positive for SARS-CoV-2 at a single New York City hospital also found that none of the newborns tested positive at birth (Salvatore et al., 2020). While only 68% of the newborns were followed up with a PCR test at 5–7 days of life, all newborns tested at 5–7 days and again at 14 days after birth (96% and 88% of the newborns followed up) tested negative and all were asymptomatic. Further, 83% of newborns had roomed-in with their mothers and many were breastfed or fed breastmilk by bottle (Salvatore et al., 2020). These studies (Ronchi et al., 2020; Salvatore et al., 2020) are in alignment with an AAP COVID-19 case registry that tested nearly 4,000 newborns in 2020: while 60% of the newborns roomed in with mothers, less than 2% of the newborns tested positive for SARS-CoV-2 (Kaufman and Puopolo, 2021).

The evidence on routes of newborn transmission continues to evolve. A meta-analysis of 176 newborns who tested positive for the virus in 2020 found that half of all newborns developed COVID-19 symptoms, roughly half were asymptomatic, and environmental transmission seemed more likely (70%) than intrauterine or intrapartum transmission (combined, 30%) (Raschetti et al., 2020). While unusual, transplacental transmission of SARS-CoV-2 does occur (Schwartz et al., 2020a) and the virus has been found in breastmilk (Groß et al., 2020). More studies are needed to understand the severity of COVID-19 in relation to other newborn complications, as many of the newborns who tested positive for SARS-CoV-2 were also preterm (Raschetti et al., 2020; Ronchi et al., 2020). A systematic review comparing rates of infection in newborns delivered vaginally vs. by cesarean across the globe confirmed that infection with SARS-CoV-2 is uncommon. Further, rates of infection do not differ significantly when comparing vaginal and cesarean delivery, breastfeeding or bottle-feeding, and babies rooming in vs. those separated to nurseries (Walker et al., 2020). More research is needed on the routes of vertical transmission, and on how admission to a NICU influences postnatal transmission or severity of COVID-19 in newborns.

In order to understand why hospitals moved so quickly to isolate newborns from mothers, it is important to recall that many standard obstetric practices are not evidence-based, cause harm (Miller et al., 2016), and have been analyzed as rituals that enact core technocratic values and generate a sense of safety for providers (Davis-Floyd, 2003; Davis-Floyd, 2018). This enactment of the old/new ritual of separation represents a reversion to the technocratic control that still characterizes mainstream obstetrics (Gutschow et al., 2021).

Community Birth During COVID-19

The exclusion of doulas and support people has influenced the rising demand for births at home and in freestanding birth centers. As community-based midwife Willoughby puts it: "We saw a huge jump to OOH (out-of-hospital) at first, I think, because people had already hired their doulas and didn't want to lose the support."

While our earlier survey indicated a significant increase in demand for community births (Davis-Floyd et al., 2020), the evidence was more mixed by November of 2020, with some providers reporting an increase and others seeing none. Homebirth obstetrician Fishbein did continue to see increased demand for home births in Los Angeles, and CNM Dinah Waranch of Texas noted:

> a definite greater interest in OOH births. . .my practice has always been pretty busy and at capacity, but at my state of life (64) I'm not about to hire more to increase the size of practice during COVID. There are lots of area OOH practices which are taking up the slack.

For some providers and their clients, the rise of interest in community births did not always translate to a successful homebirth for a variety of reasons, as doula Stevie Merino noted:

> I think there is definitely an increase in inquiries for home birth midwives but not an actual increase in follow through .... Many potential clients and current clients have reached out *via* email, social media, phone, and my website to ask for advice on how to find OOH options. . .Unfortunately, however many are unable to because of how far along they are in their pregnancy, insurance, cost of OOH options, high risk status, living situations, etc. I try to support however I can but also am realistic about people's access and the fact that less than 2% of people in the United States still give birth in homes.

CPM Shea Childs from Arkansas described how she adapted to the growing demand for home birth in her area by asking more pointed questions about families' motivations, and by noting that:

> All the midwives in the state have had more families interested in home birth, but in a normal year there are only 250 or so families choosing OOH in the entire state, with the licensed midwives anyway. It will be interesting to see the numbers for 2020.

Community-based CPM Marimikel Potter of Texas described her reasons for rejecting some would-be clients:

> When COVID-19 first got started, I got a bunch of calls from women wanting a home birth just because they were afraid of hospital infection. I rejected all of them because it was clear to me that they weren't actually committed to home birth, and that rarely works out well.

CPM Sarita Bennett agreed, stating:

> We didn't accept those last-minute transfers at the beginning of the pandemic because the reasons for transferring didn't give us confidence that the families were committed to our model of care and out of hospital birth. I've had several midwife friends regret that they accepted those transfers because they wound up with labor dystocias and transports way too often.

Here Bennett speaks to the notion that if a childbearing woman truly feels safer in the hospital she should deliver there, and that an ideological commitment to home birth can promote a successful outcome at home. LM Jessica Willoughby added:

> When people were terrified of COVID and wanted to now have an OOH birth with almost no understanding of the difference in models of care I was like, wait, you're afraid of COVID but what about MRSA or c-diff? What about all the other major communicable diseases that live in the hospital that you were already planning to risk exposure to when you signed up for hospital birth?

CPM Vicki Penwell, who runs a midwifery school in Boise, Idaho, saw a notable increase in demand for community births: "All the midwives all over the country that I have been speaking with recently are somehow managing to cope with client volumes of around eight births per month—twice their normal load. They are really rising to the challenge!" Yet this increased demand can add significant risks to midwives as births begin to cluster and practitioner stress and exhaustion set in. This could become a quality of care and safety issue if the demand remains high for too long; it clearly indicates the need for more community-based midwives.

Doula Stevie Merino added: "There is also an increased risk for OOH midwives who are already extremely restricted and regulated in the United States while also not being supported by most insurance options or by fair Medi-Cal reimbursements." We are curious to see whether or not the increase in demand for what Melissa Cheney (2011) has called "the systems-challenging praxis" of home birth will continue post-COVID and influence integration of care in the United States.

The Home/Hospital Divide in United States Maternity Care

Early in the pandemic, to help meet the rising demand for home births in New York, where it is illegal for CPMs to practice, Governor Cuomo issued Executive order 202.11 allowing midwives licensed anywhere in the United States and Canada to practice in New York State (Davis-Floyd et al., 2020). According to Ida Darragh, CPM and Chair of the North American Registry of Midwives (NARM), some CPMs from other states were able to work in New York, while others who had been practicing illegally in NY but licensed in another state were now able to practice legally. The governor extended this order in September 2020 with Chapter 182 of the Laws of 2020, which permitted the State Education Department to renew limited or provisional permits for midwives licensed in other states to continue practicing in New York for another 12 months.

It remains to be seen if the example set by New York State of accepting midwives licensed elsewhere will be followed by other states and whether momentum will build for more uniform acceptance of CPMs across all states, including in the 14 holdout states where they are still not allowed to practice legally. Clearly most obstetricians remain prejudiced against home births, as doula Merino described:

> Many of my clients or potential clients who have discussed [the option of community birth] with their care providers have been told outright that it is still safer to birth in hospitals and it is actually "dangerous" to birth at home. This is quite ridiculous obviously and frankly a shame that even in the face of a pandemic that some hospital-based providers still do not see OOH providers as capable or see birth beyond a medical experience.

Many of the obstetricians we surveyed flatly stated they would not support home births during the pandemic:

> Leslie Cohan: Absolutely not. Too risky. Want neo available, just in case.
>
> Melinda Yates (a pseudonym): No I do not, why when you can have the same experience in the hospital and in the event of an emergency have everything you need.
>
> Roberta Krueger: Studies show hospitals are safer than home birth.
>
> Marco Giannotti: While I of course respect any patient's decision when it comes to where she decides to deliver, I

> do feel that from a medical perspective, a hospital is *always* the safest place to deliver. Even during a pandemic. Should fetal compromise occur, the need to bring the patient to a hospital for emergent delivery takes precious time away from being able to quickly rescue a child in distress. One bad outcome is not acceptable.

Obstetrician Marilyn Vanover described community births as "risky," yet blamed her obstetric colleagues by noting that they refused to perform or had minimal training in VBACs, vaginal breech deliveries, and other evidence-based practices. MFM specialist Deena had a very different view:

> I do support OOH among people who have a trained CPM/CNM with good connections to facilitate transfer to a higher-level facility in case of issue. . .I tend to support this option more for multiparous people as adverse outcomes (e.g., need for transfer to hospital, C/S, transfusion, higher-order lacerations, need for operative vaginal delivery) are lower in this group. However, in the midst of the pandemic, I think a well-counseled person—understanding the risks and benefits of home birth—with a good care team and easy ability to access higher order care would be great as a home birth!

Deena's optimism was not shared by obstetrician Giannotti at first. Yet when we presented with evidence of CPM-attended community births showing intrapartum and neonatal mortality rates that compared favorably with the outcomes of low-risk hospital births, Giannotti agreed that community births can be safe. Obstetrician Walters responded in ways that clearly argued for maternal agency and autonomy:

> It is something of a challenge to answer this question. It is not a medical question. It is a human rights issue. . .a pregnant woman has the inalienable right to determine where she will deliver. There are risks and benefits to whichever location she chooses. Nothing is perfect.

When COVID appeared to be a serious threat to all pregnant women, Walters at first thought he might seek training in home deliveries, as he recognized that the skillset for home birth attendance was quite different from his own. He later abandoned this plan when his experience showed him that COVID did not present as much danger as initially feared:

> We see now that COVID is a minimal threat to pregnant women and newborns. So, women are not avoiding our hospital. It is pretty much the same pros vs. cons of hospital vs. home birth to be weighed by the individual mom. And then I support that decision. I offer my skills and knowledge to help her achieve her goals. But, the patient decides... [the woman] has the right to know the qualifications and training of the person who will deliver her child. There is a massive difference between an experienced home birth CNM and some other "licensed" midwives. I am not an expert in the various forms of licensing for midwifery. But the ones I have seen make simple mistakes, miss diagnoses, mismanage deliveries, etc., have consistently been non-CNMs.

These provider responses indicate that there is a long way to go in educating obstetricians about the substantial evidence that exists showing excellent outcomes for planned, CPM-attended community birth in the United States (Johnson and Daviss 2005; Armstrong, 2010; Stapleton et al., 2013; Cheyney et al., 2014; Scarf et al., 2018).

Home-to-Hospital Transfer in the Time of COVID-19

When we asked our providers if home birth transfer guidelines were being followed during home-to-hospital transport, CNM Waranch said that she is aware of the homebirth consensus transfer guidelines[5], but "It's difficult to implement them fully because the hospital is really not interested in meeting and doing that, virus or no virus." In contrast, CNM Diana Jolles noted, "We have good transfer policies, and I would like to believe we follow the guidelines—which I adore—we are home birth midwives at heart, working in a large FQHC (Federally Qualified Health Center)."

CPM Debbie Query reported two hospital transfers: "One was quite smooth as I was able to transfer the charts as well as speak to the hospital staff. One was not as smooth according to the client, and (we both) feel that was predominately because I was not allowed to be there." CPM Shea Childs saw no increase in transfers in her practice, but:

> I think the level of stress has risen for everyone in the society. We have a mother/baby friendly hospital we transfer to and the care remains consistently positive. They are allowing one person to attend those laboring and a few are allowing a doula as well with some guidelines, like having preapproval from OB, that make the midwife going in with transfers a thing of the past sadly.

Homebirth obstetrician Stuart Fischbein also deeply disapproved of not being able to accompany his transporting clients:

> Transfers are awful now! My experience is less integration. We as practitioners cannot accompany our clients in transport. It feels like forced abandonment. When we need to transport, we have to consider which facility will allow the father in the delivery or operating room. Which facility may allow the doula in. . . .Many do not allow

[5]These guidelines can be found at Best Practice Guidelines: Transfer from Planned Home Birth to Hospital|Home Birth Summit.

> doulas. Many separate the mother from the partner, and some are not letting the father of the baby or partner into the operating room. When did fathers become non-essential personnel?

When Doula Merino had to switch to virtual labor support during transport to a hospital, she found:

> that the cascade of interventions seems to increase—I can't say for fact that it is related to the limited allowance of support persons but it has definitely felt that way. . .[preventing doulas seems] ridiculous and inefficient [because] the risk also seems the same since the laboring person was with their doula/midwife/or whoever else was present at home/birthing center with them prior to transfer.

Other providers also noted the increase in interventions when doulas were not present. CPM Sarita Bennett noted that one hospital in her region is off limits to her practice because it "won't take transfers unless the person has been seen prenatally by one of the OBs on staff." She describes how she helps her clients cope with transfer, virtually:

> One client that transferred had to finally restrict entry to all those multiple pediatric residents trying to talk her into the Vitamin K and Hepatitis B injections that she had already declined. I could not physically accompany her but did the transfer by phone then stayed available by phone to the family to help them with information to advocate for themselves (like reminding her that she didn't have to put up with all those pediatric residents).

LM Jessica Willoughby appreciates the value of the fact that she and her midwifery colleagues are now allowed back. She says that, in addition to the benefits to her clients of her hospital accompaniment:

> I think that our presence at the hospital has helped with our reputation. We aren't just dumping our patients on the hospital, we are going and helping facilitate communication between the hospital and the patient. I think that the providers at the hospital appreciate that. They see that we weren't fueling this *United States vs. THEM* mentality. Listen hospital friend, we are all on the same spectrum here just different sides.

SUMMARY: LESSONS LEARNED BY PROVIDERS

Our respondents summarized the most significant lessons they learned in shifting their practices around COVID-19 as follows:

Obstetrician Marco Giannotti: The biggest lesson that we have learned (which is really an affirmation) is that patients need to be able to see their caregivers even when there is a pandemic.

Obstetrician Jeffery Wright: We are very thankful that reproductive age women are mostly unaffected by COVID. We were initially worried that it would be worse than H1N1. And we are even more grateful that newborns appear to be almost fully unaffected.

Obstetrician Michael White: For me the most significant lesson is the power and need for family support as we see the "social distancing" and elimination of the family's involvement throughout a pregnancy.

CNM Diana Jolles: Big groups of people and organizations CAN work together quickly and effectively in the interest of public health. . .[Also] there are a lot of care practices pushed on midwives and communities that aren't evidence based. . .

CNM Dinah Waranch: 1) midwife and client can listen to each other even when they have differing attitudes to the virus. This is heartwarming. and 2) I'd say we are at a point in my practice where we have our COVID system in place. . .It has been a gradual process to get clarity on the. . .guidelines and putting them into practice.... a constant state of refining.

LM Jessica Willoughby: We do not tolerate scientific ignorance in the birth center. You must wear a mask. Period.

CNM Jenny Bagg: For me personally, I learned that you can only trust yourself and what you are doing to protect yourself. You cannot rely on others to do the right thing.

CPM Shea Childs: Unfortunately, the takeaway is that folks are reluctant to take it seriously. Even though it is shared at beginning of care, many of the families seem to be shocked when I have had to relay that I have been exposed by a close contact, that I will not be seeing them for 2 weeks because of it and that if they go into labor, my back-up will be coming. . .Masking in an N95 is now second nature to me and that is the main change.

Doula Stevie Merino: Allowing some grace and patience with myself and others. I have also been more intentional about conversations with potential clients about the risks, my own work during this time, and the best practice protocols that I am practicing now. After being on call for months at a time, I finally learned that scheduled time off is important for my own overall health and wellbeing and that of my child.

CPM and DO Sarita Bennett: I believe that the lesson we should be learning is that large volume, facility birth is not sustainable and that small, community-based midwifery centers are the answer for the vast majority of pregnant people.

We highlight these responses here to show that in highly disruptive times of pandemics, United States-based providers adapt in ways that help their clients and their practice, using the lessons learned from experience. Our data has indicated that as the evidence shifts, so does practice among maternity care providers. We believe that dialogue among all kinds of providers (midwives and obstetricians, nurses, and doctors, community-based and hospital-based) promotes evidence-based care (Gutschow et al., 2021). We shift back and forth between community-based and hospital-based providers in our analysis because we believe that lessons from both settings can help shift practices most efficiently in highly disruptive times.

STUDY LIMITATIONS AND STRENGTHS

There are several limitations to this study. It is based on a snowball sample of 28 survey responses and does not presume to speak for all United States maternity care practitioners. It is not geographically representative of all United States regions, although it is slightly skewed toward the urban and coastal United States. It does not reflect the racial, ethnic, and income diversity across the United States population. Only a few of our responses were from providers of color. Yet three-fourths of our respondents were female, who remain a minoritized community among United States-based physicians.[6] Our survey represents a snapshot of time, of birth spaces, and of providers across the United States. Finally, it reflects the shifting guidance on COVID-19 that was not applied uniformly in all hospitals or by all providers.

The strengths of our study are that it illustrates in depth how some providers responded to a landscape in which much was shifting: evidence, client's needs, as well as protocols or guidance from ACOG, AAP, WHO and other institutions. Our responses reached saturation, as later responses echoed earlier ones. Our study shows a variety of protocols among a range of providers who practice in different birth settings across the United States--home, birth center, and hospital. Finally, it describes changes in provider attitudes, experiences, and practices in their own words in response to the rapidly changing landscape of maternity care during the COVID-19 pandemic.

CONCLUSION: GENERATING INTEGRATED AND SUSTAINABLE MATERNITY CARE IN DISRUPTIVE TIMES

The COVID-19 crisis represents a disruption or obstacle that is also an opportunity. It reveals the fractures in our current maternity care that might enable us to build a more sustainable and safer system of maternity care in which women can choose among multiple birth sites and multiple types of providers. We urge providers and policy makers to use these disruptive times to apply the lessons learned and work toward a leaner, more cost-effective, and *decentralized* maternity care system that integrates midwives with obstetricians and community birth providers with hospitals, while working to dismantle the systemic racism and provider bias that prevent high quality care for all (Gutschow et al., 2021; Daviss and Davis-Floyd, 2021).

There is ample evidence across the globe of sustainable models of birth that privilege midwifery models of care and provide high quality, high touch, low cost, and low-tech care (Davis-Floyd et al., 2009; Gutschow et al., 2021; Daviss and Davis-Floyd, 2021). We emphasize the teaching and transmission of midwifery skills and the midwifery model of care, which can be applied in home and hospital settings during chaotic times as well as more stable periods (Gutschow et al., 2021).

It is our hope that the fragmented maternity care system in the United States will become more integrated, by recognizing hospital- and community-based midwives and doulas as full participants in the care of mothers and newborns. In equalizing access to doulas, home birth, and freestanding birth centers through coordinated insurance schemes and subsidies, we may begin to improve health equity outcomes for minoritized populations in the United States and to de-racialize maternity care more broadly (Profit et al., 2020). We hope that community midwives can seize this pandemic moment to raise national awareness of their value, while obstetricians become more aware and accepting of the high value and cost-savings of midwifery care and community births (Daviss et al., 2021; Gutschow et al., 2021). Finally, we believe it critical that doulas be accepted as *essential* care providers, given the longstanding evidence that continuous doula support in labor reduces interventions and improves maternal and neonatal outcomes.

We hope that our maternity care system will restore humanistic strides made in facilitating normal physiologic birth and in enhancing maternal and newborn health. We hope that providers will work more collaboratively, with obstetricians recognizing midwives as colleagues rather than subordinates and doulas as essential, rather than non-essential, personnel. Finally, we believe that community midwives in the United States can achieve autonomous practice without restrictive state regulations, and thereby be empowered to practice and promote the midwifery model of care. In this way, they can continue to flexibly adapt to the next disruptions or crises that our society may face as recognized frontline providers—most especially when hospitals are overwhelmed. We hope that providers across the United States will seize the transformational moment of COVID-19 to transform the United States maternity care system to be more sustainable and more resilient in the face of future pandemics and disasters.

ETHICS STATEMENT

The studies involving human participants were reviewed and approved by the Williams College. The patients/participants provided their written informed consent to participate in this study. Written informed consent was obtained from the individual(s) for the publication of any potentially identifiable images or data included in this article.

AUTHOR CONTRIBUTIONS

All authors listed have made a substantial, direct, and intellectual contribution to the work and approved it for publication.

[6]According to the Kaiser Family Foundation, while women have outnumbered men in entering medical school since 2010, male doctors (64% of all doctors) still outnumber female doctors (36% of all doctors) in the United States today.

ACKNOWLEDGMENTS

We sincerely thank all the busy providers who responded to our email questionnaire. KG offers deep thanks to RD-F for working cooperatively and her excellent editing, and to David Schwartz for conversations on the multiple mysteries that surround our understandings of SARS-CoV-2 and COVID-19, which are still evolving. And RD-F offers thanks to KG for her deep literature dive.

REFERENCES

American Academy of Pediatrics (AAP) (2020). Frequently Asked Questions: Management of Infants Born to Mothers with Suspected or Confirmed COVID-19. Available at: https://services.aap.org/en/pages/2019-novel-coronavirus-covid-19-infections/clinical-guidance/faqs-management-of-infants-born-to-covid-19-mothers/.

Almeida, M, Shrestha, A. D., Stojanac, B., and Miller, L J. (2020). The impact of the pandemic of women's mental health. *Archives Women's Mental Health* 23 (7), 741-748. doi:10.1007/s00737-020-01092-2

Armstrong, E. M. (2010). Home Birth Matters-For All Women. *J Perinat Educ.* 19 (1), 8–11. doi:10.1624/105812410x482329

Boelig, R. C., Manuck, T., Oliver, E. A., Di Mascio, D., Saccone, G., Bellussi, F., et al. (2020a). Labor and Delivery Guidance for COVID-19. *Am. J. Obstet. Gynecol. MFM* 2 (2), 100110. doi:10.1016/j.ajogmf.2020.100110

Boelig, R. C., Saccone, G., Bellussi, F., and Berghella, V. (2020b). MFM Guidance for COVID-19. *Am. J. Obstet. Gynecol. MFM* 2 (2), 100106. doi:10.1016/j.ajogmf.2020.100106

Bohren, M. A., Hofmeyr, G. J., Sakala, C., Fukuzawa, R. K., and Cuthbert, A. (2017). Continuous Support for Women during Childbirth. *Cochrane database Syst. Rev.* 7 (7), CD003766. doi:10.1002/14651858.CD003766.pub6

Bridges, K. (2011). *Reproducing Race: An Ethnography of Pregnancy as a Site of Racialization*. Berkeley: University of California Press.

Caughey, A. B., and Cheyney, M. (2019). Home and Birth Center Birth in the United States. *Obstet. Gynecol.* 133 (5), 1033–1050. doi:10.1097/AOG.0000000000003215

Centers for Disease Control and Prevention (CDC) (2020b). Evaluation and Management Considerations for Neonates at Risk for COVID-19. August 3. Available at: https://www.cdc.gov/coronavirus/2019-ncov/hcp/caring-for-newborns.html.

Centers for Disease Control and Prevention (CDC) (2020a). Pregnancy Mortality Surveillance Program: Pregnancy-Related Deaths by Race/Ethnicity. Available at: https://www.cdc.gov/reproductivehealth/maternal-mortality/pregnancy-mortality-surveillance-system.htm (Accessed Jan 10, 2021).

Cheney, M. (2011). Homebirth as Ritual Performance. *Med. Anthropol. Quart* 25(4), 519-542. doi:10.1111/j.1548-1387.2011.01183.x

Cheyney, M., Bovbjerg, M., Everson, C., Gordon, W., Hannibal, D., and Vedam, S. (2014). Outcomes of Care for 16,924 Planned Home Births in the United States: The Midwives Alliance of North America Statistics Project, 2004 to 2009. *J. Midwifery Women's Health* 59 (1), 17–27. doi:10.1111/jmwh.12172

Chmielewska, B., Barratt, I., Townsend, R., Kalafat, E., Van der Meulen, J., Gurol-Urganci, I., et al. (2021). Effects of the COVID-19 Pandemic on Maternal and Perinatal Outcomes: a Systematic Review. *Lancet Glob. Health.* doi:10.1016/S2214-109X(21)00079-6

Davis, D. (2019). *Reproductive Injustice: Racism, Pregnancy, and Premature Birth.* New York: New York University Press.

Davis-Floyd, R., Barclay, L., Daviss, B. A., and Tritten, J. (2009). *Birth Models that Work.* Berkeley: University of California Press.

Davis-Floyd, R. (2003). *Birth as an American Rite of Passage.* Berkeley: University of California Press.

Davis-Floyd, R., Gutschow, K., and Schwartz, D. A. (2020). Pregnancy, Birth and the COVID-19 Pandemic in the United States. *Med. Anthropol.* 39 (5), 413–427. doi:10.1080/01459740.2020.1761804

Davis-Floyd, R., Lim, R., Penwell, V., and Ivry, T. (2021). "Effective Maternity Disaster Care: Low Tech, Skilled Touch," in *Sustainable Birth in Disruptive Times.* Editors K. Gutschow, R. Davis-Floyd, and B. A. Daviss (New York: Springer Nature).

Davis-Floyd, R. (2018). "The Technocratic, Humanistic, and Holistic Paradigms of Birth and Health Care," in *Ways of Knowing about Birth: Mothers, Midwives, Medicine, and Birth Activism.* Editor Davis-Floyd R. (Long Grove, IL: Waveland Press), 3–44.

Daviss, B. A., and Davis-Floyd, R. (Eds.) (2021). *Speaking Truth to Power: Birth Models on the Human Rights Frontier.* New York, NY: Routledge Press.

Daviss, B. A., Anderson, D. A., and Johnson, K. C. (2021). Pivoting to Childbirth at Home or in Freestanding Birth Centers in the US During COVID-19: Safety, Economics, and Logistics. *Front. Sociol.* 6, 618210. doi:10.3389/fsoc.2021.618210

Debrandere, M. L., Farabaugh, D. C., and Giordano, C. (2020). A Review on Mode of Delivery during COVID-19 between December 2019 and April 2020. *Am. J. Perinatol.* 38, 332-341. doi:10.1055/s-0040-1721658

Di Mascio, D., Khalil, A., Saccone, G., Rizzo, G., Buca, D., Liberati, M., et al. (2020). Outcome of Coronavirus Spectrum Infections (SARS, MERS, COVID-19) during Pregnancy: a Systematic Review and Meta-Analysis. *Am. J. Obstet. Gynecol. MFM* 2 (2), 100107. doi:10.1016/j.ajogmf.2020.100107

Eichelberger, K. Y., Doll, K., Ekpo, G. E., and Zerden, M. L. (2016). Black Lives Matter: Claiming a Space for Evidence-Based Outrage in Obstetrics and Gynecology. *Am. J. Public Health* 106 (10), 1771–1772. doi:10.2105/AJPH.2016.303313

Ellington, S., Strid, P., Tong, V. T., Woodworth, K., Galang, R. R., Zambrano, L. D., et al. (2020). Characteristics of Women of Reproductive Age with Laboratory-Confirmed SARS-CoV-2 Infection by Pregnancy Status - United States, January 22-June 7, 2020. *MMWR Morb. Mortal. Wkly. Rep.* 69, 769–775. doi:10.15585/mmwr.mm6925a1

Favre, G., Pomar, L., Qi, X., Nielsen-Saines, K., Musso, D., and Baud, D. (2020). Guidelines for Pregnant Women with Suspected SARS-CoV-2 Infection. *Lancet Infect. Dis.* 20 (6), P652–P653. doi:10.1016/S1473-3099(20)30157-2

Fortier, J. H., and Godwin, M. (2015). Doula Support Compared with Standard Care: Meta-Analysis of the Effects on the Rate of Medical Interventions during Labour for Low-Risk Women Delivering at Term. *Can. Fam. Physician* 61 (6), e284–292.

Groß, R., Conzelmann, C., Müller, J. A., Stenger, S., Steinhart, K., Kirchhoff, F., et al. (2020). Detection of SARS-CoV-2 in Human Breastmilk. *Lancet* 395 (10239), 1757–1758. doi:10.1016/S0140-6736(20)31181-8

Gutschow, K., Davis-Floyd, R., and Daviss, B. A. (Editors) (2021). *Sustainable Birth in Disruptive Times.* New York: Springer Nature.

Johnson, K. C., and Daviss, B.-A. (2005). Outcomes of Planned home Births with Certified Professional Midwives: Large Prospective Study in North America. *BMJ* 330 (7505), 1416. doi:10.1136/bmj.330.7505.1416

Kaufman, D. A., and Puopolo, K. M. (2021). Infants Born to Mothers with COVID-19-Making Room for Rooming-In. *JAMA Pediatr.* 175, 240. doi:10.1001/jamapediatrics.2020.5100

Lebel, C., MacKinnon, A., Bagshawe, M., Tomfohr-Madsen, L., and Giesbrecht, G. (2020). Elevated depression and anxiety symptoms among pregnant individuals during the COVID-19 pandemic. *J. Affect Disord.* 277, 5-13. doi:10.1016/j.jad.2020.07.126

Mayopoulos, G. A., Ein-Dor, T., Li, K. G., Chan, S. J, and Dekel, S. (2020). Giving birth under hospital visitor restrictions: Heightened acute stress in childbirth in COVID-19 positive women. *Med Rxiv.* doi:10.1101/2020.11.30.20241026

Meyerowitz, E., Richterman, A., Bogoch, I., Low, N., Cevik, M., et al. (2020). Towards an Accurate and Systematic Characterization of Persistently Asymptomatic Infection with SARS-CoV-2. *Lancet Infect. Dis.* doi:10.1016/S1473-3099(20)30837-9

Miller, S. E., Abalos, E., Chamillard, M., Chiapponi, A., Colaci, D., Comande, D., et al. (2016). Beyond Too Little, Too Late and Too Much, Too Soon: a Pathway towards Evidence-Based, Respectful Maternity Care Worldwide. *Lancet* 388, 2176–2192. doi:10.1016/S0140-6736(16)31472-6

Mukherjee, S. (2021). Why Does the Pandemic Seem to be Hitting Some Countries Harder Than Others?. *The New Yorker March* 1, 2021.

Norton, A., Wilson, T., Geller, G., and Gross, M. S. (2020). Impact of Hospital Visitor Restrictions on Racial Disparities in Obstetrics. *Health Equity* 4 (1), 505–508. doi:10.1089/heq.2020.0073

Obinna, D. N. (2020). 'Essential and Undervalued: Health Disparities of African American Women in the COVID-19 Era'. *Ethn. Health* 26, 68–79. doi:10.1080/13557858.2020.1843604

Perinne, C. G., Chiang, K. V., Anstey, E. H., Grossniklaus, D. A., Boundy, E. O., Sauber-Schatz, E. K., et al. (2020). Implementation of Hospital Practices Supportive of Breastfeeding in the Context of COVID-19—United States, July 15-August 20, 2020. *MMWR Morb Mortal Wkly Rep.* 69 (47), 1767–1770. doi:10.15585/mmwr.mm6947a3

Profit, J., Edmonds, B. T., Shah, N., and Cheyney, M. (2020). The COVID-19 Pandemic as a Catalyst for More Integrated Maternity Care. *Am. J. Public Health* 110 (11), 1663–1665. doi:10.2105/AJPH.2020.305935

Raschetti, R., Vivanti, A. J., Vauloup-Fellous, C., Loi, B., Benachi, A., and De Luca, D. (2020). Synthesis and Systematic Review of Reported Neonatal SARS-CoV-2 Infections. *Nat. Commun.* 11, 5164. doi:10.1038/s41467-020-18982-9

Ronchi, A., Pietrasanta, C., Zavattoni, M., Saruggia, M., Schena, F., Sinelli, M. T., et al. (2021). Evaluation of Rooming-In Practice for Neonates Born to Mothers with Severe Acute Respiratory Syndrome Coronavirus 2 Infection in Italy. *JAMA Pediatr.* 175, 260. doi:10.1001/jamapediatrics.2020.5086

Sadler, M., Leiva, G., and Olza, I. (2020). COVID-19 as a Risk Factor for Obstetric Violence. *Sex. Reprod. Health Matters* 28 (1), 1785379. doi:10.1080/26410397.2020.1785379

Salvatore, C. M., Han, J.-Y., Acker, K. P., Tiwari, P., Jin, J., Brandler, M., et al. (2020). Neonatal Management and Outcomes during the COVID-19 Pandemic: an Observation Cohort Study. *Lancet Child. Adolesc. Health* 4 (10), 721–727. doi:10.1016/S2352-4642(20)30235-2

Scarf, V. L., Rossiter, C., Vedam, S., Dahlen, H. G., Ellwood, D., Forster, D., et al. (2018). Maternal and Perinatal Outcomes by Planned Place of Birth Among Women with Low-Risk Pregnancies in High-Income Countries: A Systematic Review and Meta-Analysis. *Midwifery* 62, 240–255. doi:10.1016/j.midw.2018.03.024

Schmid, M. B., Fontijn, J., Ochsenbein-Kölble, N., Berger, C., Bassler, D., et al. (2020). COVID-19 in Pregnant Women. *Lancet Infect. Dis.* 20 (6), P653. doi:10.1016/S1473-3099(20)30175-4

Schwartz, D. A., Baldewijns, M., Benachi, A., Bugatti, M., Collins, R. R. J., De Luca, D., et al. (2020a). Chronic Histiocytic Intervillositis with Trophoblast Necrosis Is a Risk Factor Associated with Placental Infection from Coronavirus Disease 2019 (COVID-19) and Intrauterine Maternal-Fetal Severe Acute Respiratory Syndrome Coronavirus 2 (SARS-CoV-2) Transmission in Live-Born and Stillborn Infants. *Arch. Pathol. Lab. Med.* 145, 517–528. doi:10.5858/arpa.2020-0771-SA

Schwartz, D. A., and De Luca, D. (2021). The Public Health and Clinical Importance of Accurate Neonatal Testing for COVID-19. *Pediatrics* 147 (2), e2020036871. doi:10.1542/peds.2020-036871

Schwartz, D. A., and Dhaliwal, A. (2020). Infections in Pregnancy with COVID-19 and Other Respiratory RNA Virus Diseases Are Rarely, if Ever, Transmitted to the Fetus: Experiences with Coronaviruses, Parainfluenza, Metapneumovirus Respiratory Syncytial Virus, and Influenza. *Arch. Pathol. Lab. Med.* 144 (8), 920–928. doi:10.5858/arpa.2020-0211-SA

Schwartz, D. A., and Graham, A. L. (2020). Potential Maternal and Infant Outcomes from Coronavirus 2019-nCoV (SARS-CoV-2) Infecting Pregnant Women: Lessons from SARS, MERS, and Other Human Coronavirus Infections. *Viruses* 12 (2), 194. doi:10.3390/v12020194

Schwartz, D. A., Morotti, D., Beigi, B., Moshfegh, F., Zafaranloo, N., and Patanè, L. (2020b). Confirming Vertical Fetal Infection with Coronavirus Disease 2019: Neonatal and Pathology Criteria for Early Onset and Transplacental Transmission of Severe Acute Respiratory Syndrome Coronavirus 2 from Infected Pregnant Mothers. *Arch. Pathol. Lab. Med.* 144 (12), 1451–1456. doi:10.5858/arpa.2020-0442-SA

Searcy, J. J., and Castañeda, A. N. (2020). COVID-19 and the Birth of the Virtual Doula. Medical Anthropology Quarterly 19 June. Available at: http://medanthroquarterly.org/2020/06/19/covid-19-and-the-birth-of-the-virtual-doula/.

Stapleton, S. R., Osborne, C., and Illuzzi, J. (2013). Outcomes of Care in Birth Centers: Demonstration of a Durable Model. *J. Midwifery Women's Health* 58 (1), 3–14. doi:10.1111/jmwh.12003

State of New York Executive Chamber (2020). Executive Orders No. 202.11 & 202.12. Available at: https://www.governor.ny.gov/news/no-20211continuing-temporary-suspension-and-modification-laws-relating-disaster-emergency.

Stephens, A. J., Barton, J. R., Bentum, N.-A. A., Blackwell, S. C., and Sibai, B. M. (2020). General Guidelines in the Management of an Obstetrical Patient on the Labor and Delivery Unit during the COVID-19 Pandemic. *Am. J. Perinatol* 37 (08), 829–836. doi:10.1055/s-0040-1710308

Strong, A., and Schwartz, D. (2019). "Effects of the West Africa Ebola Epidemic on Health Care of Pregnant Women: Stigmatization with and without Infection," in *Pregnant in the Time of Ebola*. Editor D. A. Schwartz (New York: Springer Nature).

Surkova, E., Nikolayevskyy, V., and Drobniewski, F. (2020). False-positive COVID-19 Results: Hidden Problems and Costs. *Lancet Respir. Med.* 8, 1167–1168. doi:10.1016/S2213-2600(20)30453-7

Valdez, N., and Deomampo, D. (2019). Centering Race and Racism in Reproduction. *Med. Anthropol.* 38 (7), 551–559. doi:10.1080/01459740.2019.1643855

Walker, K., O'Donoghue, K., Grace, N., Dorling, J., Comeau, J., Li, W., et al. (2020). Maternal Transmission of SARS-COV-2 to the Neonate, and Possible Routes for Such Transmission: a Systematic Review and Critical Analysis. *Bjog: Int. J. Obstet. Gy.* 127, 1324–1336. doi:10.1111/1471-0528.16362

Yanes-Lane, M., Winters, N., Fregonese, F., Bastos, M., Perlman-Arrow, S., Campbell, J. R., et al. (2020). Proportion of Asymptomatic Infection Among COVID-19 Positive Persons and Their Transmission Potential: A Systematic Review and Meta-Analysis. *PLOS ONE* 15 (11), e0241536. doi:10.1371/journal.pone.0241536

Zimmer, C. (2021). The Secret Life of a Coronavirus, *New York Times*. Feb 26, 2021.

12

Creativity, Resilience and Resistance: Black Birthworkers' Responses to the COVID-19 Pandemic

Julia Chinyere Oparah [1†], Jennifer E. James [2†], Destany Barnett [3†], Linda Marie Jones [4†], Daphina Melbourne [5†], Sayida Peprah [4†] and Jessica A. Walker [4†]*

[1]Provost and dean of the faculty, Race, Gender and Sexuality Studies Department, Mills College, Oakland, CA, United States, [2]Institute for Health and Aging, University of California, San Francisco, CA, United States, [3]School of Nursing, University of California, San Diego, CA, United States, [4]Black Women Birthing Justice Collective, Oakland, CA, United States, [5]California Preterm Birth Initiative, University of California, San Francisco, CA, United States

Correspondence:
Jennifer E. James
Jennifer.James@ucsf.edu

This article documents the experiences of Black birthworkers supporting pregnant and birthing people and new mamas during the first six months of the COVID-19 pandemic. Building on the methodology and outcomes of Battling Over Birth–a Research Justice project by and for Black women about their experiences of pregnancy and childbirth–the authors utilized a "community-based sheltered-in-place research methodology" to collect the narratives of Black birthworkers, including doulas, certified nurse-midwives (CNMs), homebirth midwives, lactation consultants, community health workers and ob/gyns. The article examines the impact of restrictions put in place by hospitals and clinics, including inadequate or inconsistent care, mandatory testing, separation from newborns, and restrictions on attendance by birth support people, including doulas. Birthworkers shared the innovative approaches that they have devised to continue to offer care and the ways that they have expanded the care they offer to make sure the needs of Black birthing people and new parents are being met during this uncertain time. The article also explores the threats to health, safety, and financial security faced by Black birthworkers as a result of the pandemic, and the overt and subtle forms of racism they had to navigate. Finally, it documents the sources of strength that Black birthworkers have found to sustain them at the frontlines of a maternal health care system in crisis.

Keywords: COVID-19, maternal health, birth justice, Black women, doula care, coronavirus–COVID-19

INTRODUCTION

In March 2020, as the world grappled with the severity of the COVID-19 pandemic and daily life as we knew it changed dramatically, hospitals and medical clinics across the United States scrambled to put into place regulations and policies to protect birthing people, newborns, and staff. Across the country, non-medical birthworkers found themselves shut out of hospitals, where, for a time, some hospitals were not even allowing partners or spouses to be present for births. In this article, we explore how Black birthworkers responded to the dangers and stressors of working on the frontline of the maternal health-care system during the early days of the COVID-19 pandemic. The unfamiliar and unprecedented nature and impact of the novel coronavirus meant there was limited research about the impact of the pandemic on maternal health and health care. Initial research focused on pregnant women, revealing the heightened medical risks associated with COVID-19 infection for pregnant individuals in general, and the disproportionate impact of the COVID-19 virus on Black and Latinx pregnant women in particular (Ellington et al., 2020). These findings are consistent with research into racial disparities in maternal outcomes prior to the pandemic, which demonstrated the pervasive racialized inequities that contribute to disproportionate maternal mortality for Black pregnant persons (Oparah et al., 2018; Petersen et al., 2019; Tangel et al., 2019). However, no research to date has been published on the perspectives of Black birthworkers attending and supporting births during the pandemic. Given prior research demonstrating the positive impact of Black birthworker support in mitigating obstetric racism, this is a significant omission (Guerra-Reyes and Hamilton 2017; Oparah et al., 2018; Davis 2019). This article shares the findings of a community-based, Research Justice project into the experiences, perspectives and creative strategies of Black birthworkers during the COVID-19 pandemic. The article also describes the innovative virtual "sheltered-in-place" methodology and the Research Justice lens that facilitated data collection with a vulnerable and overworked population during a time of crisis.

This study builds on Battling Over Birth, a prior study carried out by Black Women Birthing Justice (BWBJ). BWBJ was founded after two Black mothers in Oakland, California had traumatic and coercive pregnancy and birthing experiences. The two new mothers, together with local birthworkers and advocates, formed BWBJ as a grassroots community organizing, educational and advocacy group with the vision "that every pregnant person has an empowering birth and postpartum experience, free of unnecessary medical interventions and forced separation from their child, one that honors their autonomy and maintains dignity" (BWBJ, 2020a). The group decided to find out whether and why other Black women were having similar negative experiences and to discover factors leading to positive pregnancy and birthing experience and outcomes.

Between 2011 and 2015, BWBJ conducted a participatory action research study into the perinatal experiences of 100 Black pregnant people in California. The study found a culture of fear and coercion, based on the disproportionate maternal and infant mortality facing Black communities and fueled by some medical professionals who used fear as a tool to discipline racialized birthing women, their partners and birth support individuals. For example, birthing people are often forcibly guided into unwanted interventions by the threat that failure to follow directives could make the birthing person complicit in "killing" her baby if there is a negative birth outcome. While these types of threats are used across racial groups, Black birthing people often have a heightened awareness of the potential for intervention by police or social services if their baby does not survive, or even simply for failing to comply with medical recommendations. In the context of this climate of coercion, Black pregnant people found themselves battling the very professionals whom they depended on during the vulnerable perinatal months. The study revealed the role of Black birthworkers, particularly doulas and midwives, in creating positive birthing experiences and outcomes for Black pregnant people. In keeping with the focus on action as a key part of a Research Justice approach, BWBJ launched the results of the study through a social media campaign using the hashtags #BattlingOverBirth and #LiberateBlackBirth, and employed the findings to raise awareness among Black communities, medical professionals, traditional birthworkers, media and legislators and to make recommendations for change.

BWBJ's efforts are part of a national Birth Justice movement. Seeded in the wider Reproductive Justice movement, and reflective of Black women's leadership, the Birth Justice Movement aims to "to dismantle inequalities of race, class, gender and sexuality that lead to negative birth experiences" and includes "the right to choose whether or not to carry a pregnancy, to choose when, where, how, and with whom to birth, including access to traditional and indigenous birth-workers, such as midwives and doulas, and the right to breastfeeding support" (BWBJ, 2020b). Birth Justice work is described as: "educating the community, and challenging abuses by medical personnel and overuse of medical interventions . . . (as well as) advocating for universal access to culturally appropriate, women-centered health care" (ibid).

Initially made up of grassroots organizations separated by geography and often working in isolation from one another, the Birth Justice movement gained national cohesion and visibility after the founding of the Black Mamas Matter Alliance in 2015 and the publication of Birthing Justice, an anthology of writings by scholars, birthworkers, activists and mamas that generated greater access to the stories and analyses underpinning the movement (Oparah and Bonaparte 2015). Black birthworkers have been at the forefront of this movement, working closely with pregnant and parenting people. As frontline workers who witness firsthand the "battle over birth" that often characterizes Black perinatal experiences, Black birthworkers aim to transform the conditions that lead to disproportionate Black maternal death and trauma. These efforts have led to significant gains, including the declaration of Black Maternal Health Week by Congress, the establishment of a Black Maternal Health Caucus and the development of the "Momnibus," a slate of bills that together would expand and diversify the perinatal workforce, extend postpartum care, and invest in the social determinants of health and in community based organizations serving Black pregnant persons, et alia (Black Maternal Health Caucus, 2020). At the local level, birth justice advocacy has driven greater accountability and transparency by hospitals, funding for programs to provide doulas for low-income women and women of color, and greater awareness about the rights of pregnant and birthing persons.

In March 2020, as the COVID-19 pandemic ushered in a new era, many of the gains of the Birth Justice movement were summarily eliminated, as hospitals responded to the threat of the virus with swift and strict measures. In this article we seek to answer critical questions related to race, the COVID-19 pandemic, and maternal health care. How has the pandemic impacted a community already subject to racialized birth trauma and avoidable death? How are policies adopted to safeguard community health and reduce virus transmission impacting birthworkers' ability to serve their clients? And how are Black birthworkers pushing back against rules and procedures that undermine their autonomy or negatively impact perinatal outcomes? We end our article with a call to action informed by the insights and advocacy of Black birthworkers and fueled by the urgency of the Black Lives Matter Movement.

METHODS

"By Us Not For Us": Research Justice During Covid-19

In March 2020, BWBJ began to hear stories about how the COVID-19 pandemic was impacting Black birthing people and birthworkers. As the stories streamed in—prenatal visits canceled, mothers being forced to give birth without any labor support, doulas being denied access to hospital maternity wards, laboring mothers waiting for COVID-19 test results in hospital lobbies—we decided to reconvene a community research team to document how Black maternal health care was being impacted by the pandemic. We called the research project Still Battling Over Birth to indicate a continuity between, before, and after the outbreak of the virus. For Black pregnant people, COVID-19 represents a crisis on top of a crisis: an already broken maternal health system attempting to deal with a life-threatening virus.

Given the troubled history of race and research, our research collective utilizes the "Research Justice" framework first articulated by the Oakland-based grassroots research organization Data Center in order to disrupt the inequitable racial dynamics of traditional social scientific and medical research (Assil et al., 2015; Oparah et al., 2015). Further articulated by Jolivétte (2015) in the edited collection Research Justice: Methodologies for Social Change, Research Justice builds on the principles of participatory action research (PAR), insisting on the interrelationships among theory, inquiry, reflection, and action, and re-imagining relationships between academic and community-based stakeholders in the research process.

While PAR has proven an effective tool for researchers wishing to directly engage impacted communities in the research process, it has also been critiqued for paying lip service to consulting communities while leaving traditional power dynamics and decision-making processes basically intact (Cooke and Kothari 2001). Research Justice seeks to overcome these limitations by advancing the concept of "community driven" research, whereby community members who have direct experiential knowledge and a personal stake in the problem being examined co-create the research agenda and collaboratively design the research process. Research Justice seeks to decolonize the research process by taking back power over research carried out in communities of color, eliminating hierarchies between academic and community researchers, and using research methods that honor the values and ethics of the community.

Yet, as we embarked on the project, we, the co-researchers, had to answer a number of methodological and ethical questions. How could we conduct meaningful community-based research online? How could we maintain the same ethic of care for participants as we did in person? Ultimately, we learned how to conduct what we call "community-based sheltered-in-place research" simply through the process of doing it.

TABLE 1 | Sharing circle participants.

Characteristics	N	%
Race		
Black	38	100
Location		
Alabama	2	5.3
California	19	50
Delaware	2	5
Florida	1	2.6
Georgia	1	2.6
Maryland	1	2.6
New York	5	13.2
North Carolina	2	5.3
Ontario, Canada	1	2.6
Pennsylvania	2	5.3
Texas	1	2.6
Washington	1	2.6
Profession[a]		
Community Health Worker	7	18.4
Doula	23	60.5
Lactation Consultant	2	5.3
Midwife	3	7.9
Ob/gyn	3	7.9

[a]*Many birthworkers work in several different capacities (i.e., doula and lactation consultant). We have listed the profession the birthworker indicated is her primary role.*

While we also recruited and spoke with Black pregnant and birthing people for this project, this article focuses on the experiences of Black birthworkers, who are experiencing extraordinary pandemic-related stresses due to isolation, income loss, and potentially the illness or death of loved ones, while also seeking to meet the needs of a vulnerable population. In recognition of this context and of our ethical obligations to our research participants, we aimed to make participation in the research emotionally affirming and practically supportive. This study was reviewed and approved by the Mills College Committee for the Protection of Human Subjects in July 2020 and we began to reach out to birthworkers via email, social media, personal networks, and the BWBJ Black doula locator to invite them to share and listen during a 90 min virtual "sharing circle and strategy session."

After birthworkers expressed interest in participating, they were sent an informed consent form via email. A member of our research collective reached out to review the consent form with them in detail. If participants agreed, they were offered the opportunity to participate in one of four sharing circles, held virtually over Zoom, based on their schedule and availability. Sharing circles were attended by 8-12 participants and were facilitated by two or three of the co-researchers (always including at least one birthworker). All co-researchers identify as Black women and were purposeful about creating a safe, healing space by opening the virtual circle with a spiritual, non-religious grounding, sharing group agreements, and providing caring and compassionate listening and support.

During the sharing circles, we placed a set of guiding questions in the Zoom "chat" (See Appendix A), and asked each participant to share her experience during the pandemic and/or the story of a birthing person she supported during the pandemic, with those questions in mind. Other participants were then invited to ask questions, suggest resources, or provide similar or contradictory experiences. There was also a time for group discussion, led by the interests and needs of the participants. In total, 38 birthworkers, including doulas, midwives, community health workers, and ob/gyns, participated in these sharing circles (see **Table 1**). After each circle, participating birthworkers were mailed a *Still Battling Over Birth* tote bag, designed by a local Black artist, and given three months free participation in BWBJ's Birthworker Forum, a space for mutual support and information exchange.

Sharing circles were recorded via Zoom and, first, automatically transcribed via Sonix.ai, and subsequently reviewed and corrected for accuracy by a member of our research collective. All members of our research collective read each sharing circle transcript. We met together to discuss themes that emerged to us based on the initial reading. These themes became our initial set of codes. Transcripts were analyzed using DeDoose qualitative analysis software. Three members of our team participated in coding. For each transcript, one member of TEAM would apply the pre-determined set of codes and another member would review. Any discrepancy in coding or added codes were discussed among the coders. After coding and review were complete, reports were generated of all quotes that fell under each code. These reports were reviewed by two to three members of the research collective (with at least one academic researcher trained in qualitative analysis reviewing each set of codes and quotes) for further refinement of themes. We met together to discuss this newly generated set of themes and continued to refine and analyze until we reached consensus on the most prominent themes in the data.

In the following sections, we explore the obstacles that birthworkers face as they strive to ensure Black pregnant and birthing people's wellness and autonomy, how they are seeking to push back against COVID-19-related policies and procedures that undermine the effectiveness of their work or that they believe put their clients in danger, and how racism and racialized constructions of disease and risk are shaping their clients and their own experiences during the pandemic. We also explore the challenges to the birthworkers health and safety, emotional and mental wellness, and financial security, and document the innovative approaches and strategies they have developed in order to survive and thrive.

FINDINGS

Uncertainty, Racialized Fear and Restrictions: The Impact of Pandemic-Related Policies and Procedures

Just as a baseline, the medical model wasn't meeting the needs of Black women. I mean, we already know that, right? Like before COVID... So, it went from bad to worse, essentially. (Ebony, midwife, California)

"So Many Mixed Messages": Shifting Policies and Communication Gaps

As the realities of the pandemic became clear and, as also shown in other articles in this Special Issue, hospitals instituted new policies in an attempt to mitigate the spread of the disease. These policies were in constant flux, evolving alongside knowledge of COVID-19 and ebbing and flowing as cases rose and fell in different regions of the country. For many birthworkers, it seemed that "a lot of the policies in hospitals were kind of changing every day" and birthworkers spoke of the "anxieties that come with uncertainty and not knowing what space you're going to have to adapt to" (Imani, doula, Nevada).

Birthworkers noted that the needs of Black pregnant people and new mamas became casualties to a system struggling to pivot quickly to a predominantly online modality. In this context, continuity of care was disrupted, leaving pregnant people and new mamas without clear information on how to receive support:

> [A]t least four or five people reached out to me not knowing who to contact about questions or just needing support getting visits. And that shouldn't have happened (Aliyah, ob/gyn, California)

In some cases, this lack of care resulted in neglect of medical conditions that should have received attention. One Birthworker spoke about a client who was "bleeding for no reason":

> So, she called me because she wanted me to go to the emergency room with her because they weren't listening to her. But . . . I couldn't go in with her to help advocate. So, I literally had to grab people and managers outside of the emergency room to... pretty much almost protest to get her to be heard. (Yolanda, community advocate, California)

Nia, a doula from Alabama, expressed concern for the safety of a client with a dangerous medical condition who was sent home postpartum with no immediate follow up visits; Nia said, "the problem that I'm having with this is that she's not being checked for the blood clots until six weeks after she has the baby." Given the difficulties in accessing care or receiving clear and consistent information, Birthworkers became a critical source of support for pregnant people seeking knowledge about shifting hospital practices, support in accessing health care, and strategies for navigating hospital birth during the pandemic.

"I Couldn't Really Support Her": Impact of the "Doula Ban"

When the pandemic first started, nearly all hospitals initially banned the presence of any support person, then later, due in part to community protest, began to permit a maximum of one support person to be present during birth (Davis-Floyd et al., 2020). Since most women chose their partners over their doulas, this precluded doulas from attending most hospital births in person and has been incredibly disruptive to their practices and their ability to support birthing people. Since that time, some states have passed executive orders deeming doulas essential personnel who may attend births alongside a partner; however, the majority of states at the time of writing (January 2021) continue to allow hospitals to institute a *de facto* "doula ban."

As a result, doulas have had to navigate an entirely new landscape of policies and regulations. Birthworkers reported that video calls during birth were perceived as a "liability" by medical staff and that the birthing person would have to advocate for the right to stay in touch with their doula during labor and delivery. Where doulas are allowed to physically attend births, restrictions on in-and-out privileges and the need to take turns with a partner result in unsustainable work hours and time spent in the lobby rather than the birthing room:

> I think most families need both partners in the room, because he was the one that gave her the emotional support, that love that she needed, and I was there to help her do what she needed to do. But without both of us there, it made it very hard. (Janet, doula, Delaware)

Many birthworkers are uncomfortable with the forced shift to virtual support. Physical touch is seen as a vital component of traditional birthwork in the Black community:

> [A]s the original Black auntie and the granddaughter of a midwife... touch is very important to me. So not being able to, like, reach out and touch and hug my clients, especially when you're in those formal spaces, has been very stressful. (Mariah, CNM, Delaware)

Even for those who were comfortable with offering care and support virtually, the logistics of engaging in new ways were often difficult to navigate. Teaching classes and demonstrating techniques over the computer required rethinking strategies. One birthworker spoke of attempting to offer a lactation consult over the phone to the parent of a baby in the NICU:

> I asked her if we could FaceTime, but she had explained that, well, think about it. "If I'm in the NICU, I have the baby in one hand, I have the phone in the other hand." It's really hard to do a lactation consult with no extra help in the NICU. (Deja, lactation consultant, California)

"I Want My Baby in the Room": Separation From Newborns

Several birthworkers noticed a disturbing pattern: hospitals were separating birthing people from their babies immediately after birth as a precaution, even when the new mama had not tested positive for COVID-19. As one doula, Imani, told us: "The thing that I'm most adamant about right now is the separation that I was noticing was happening. Doctor's ... haven't really been encouraging skin-to-skin or any kangaroo care." Noting that the American Academy of Pediatrics had recently revised their guidelines around newborn separation, Sienna, an ob/gyn, encouraged pregnant people to use this knowledge as an advocacy tool: "So even if the hospital policy hasn't changed, they can say, actually, your organization says that this is OK. And so, I want my baby in the room with me."

This fear of separation plays a role in birthing people's decision to consent to COVID-19 testing when they enter the hospital, as in most hospitals, a positive test would mean separation from the baby. Safiya, a community engagement coordinator from San Francisco, spoke of making this clear to her clients, saying, "yes, you have a choice not to be tested, but nobody tells you that if your baby ends up in the NICU (and you test positive), that you won't be able to be with your baby."

"These Folks are Scared for Their Lives": The Impact of COVID-19 Testing

A key tool that maternity wards deployed for pandemic mitigation was testing everyone who enters the facility for COVID-19. Yet both the process of testing and the potential results have implications for the birthing person and the birthworker. One birthworker noted that if her clients test positive, they are not allowed to have any support people attend the birth. She questioned whether this actually increased the safety of patients, providers or staff. Others echoed this concern and noted that if the birthing person tested positive, they could be separated from the baby after birth. Many birthworkers spoke of making sure their clients knew their rights and that "no one could test them against their will, because otherwise that was the pathway to seeing families separated" (Mariah, CNM, Delaware).

An unintended consequence of COVID-19 testing that frustrated several birthworkers in our study was the observation that hospital staff would not pay attention to the birthing person or her needs before they tested negative. Patricia, a doula from Philadelphia, said:

> Before that COVID-19 test was clear, it was like, "We don't care that you haven't maybe felt the baby kick . . ." Everyone was just so concerned about whether she was positive and then that was going to determine the next level of care. So, you have people sitting in triage likely by themselves waiting for a COVID-19 test to return. And meanwhile, anything could be happening to them and that's not a concern.

For some, this extended beyond the time of the COVID-19 test. Tiara, a doula from Georgia, told the story of her own family's experience with an ER visit where even after they tested negative they still felt that they were treated as carriers of the disease:

> And it was just like even though we all tested negative, it still wasn't trusted that we were actually negative. And so, it's just like even if you're doing everything that you're supposed to do and you're not having the exact symptoms of COVID, there's the underlying belief that, you know, you're still a carrier and you could still be (infecting) others.

Many birthworkers understood the fear and risk at play for hospital workers. Yet, many perceived a particularly racialized fear of Black women. Black people were assumed to be carriers of the coronavirus, based on higher rates of infection in Black communities. Patricia, a Philadelphia doula, noted:

> The media is painting us as being the carriers. Everyone in the hood is carrying it. We pass it on to each other. So, if Shaniqua come in to deliver, she got it, so y'all better step back. And Shaniqua's left to die in triage if she's complaining that something's going on, you aren't listening because you're waiting on her COVID-19 test to come back.

This racialized fear of diseased Black bodies has a long history within medicine and epidemiology. For example, Black people were considered to be tuberculosis carriers in the early 20th century, and fears of "the help" potentially infecting white children drove public health responses (Connolly and Gibson 2011). Yet, the idea that Black people are a threat to public health masks the real danger: that, due to structural racism, Black people are more likely to be exposed to the virus, and are at greater risk of serious consequences if they do contract COVID-19. As Dorothy Roberts asserted in an African American Policy Forum webinar: "It's not race that is a risk factor for COVID-19, it's racism African American Policy Forum, 2020."

"Picking Up the Slack": Creative Strategies and Adaptations

Doulas have come up with creative strategies to work around the new barriers and regulations. Participants offered more prenatal visits, extended visits beyond six weeks postpartum, and maintained closer contact via phone, texting and video calls. Hospital restrictions have changed the nature of the work doulas do with their clients. Many birthworkers shifted from direct advocacy to encouraging birthing people and their partners to be their own advocates, even without the birthworker being present. Birthworkers have also found ways to encourage their clients to take charge of their own virtual prenatal care. One doula, Sahdiah, located in New York, discussed her clients:

> I find that they're having a hard time transitioning to telehealth and so a lot of them don't know that they can get a blood pressure machine through their insurance. They don't know that they can get a scale so navigating that . . . 'Cause you know, taking your blood pressure and doing your weight is self-advocacy.

Birthworkers have also taken on new tasks not usually in their scope of work, such as helping with grocery shopping, purchasing diapers, and providing personal protective equipment. This represents both a return to traditional modes of Black birthwork, as Delaware based doula Mariah described it "the way my granny used to," and an innovation in the context of the dominant medical model:

> [E]verybody's trying to figure out telemedicine and for our clients that don't have data plans, who rely on landline phones, who don't have Internet, who don't have computers, or if they do, they have bandwidth that's dedicated to their children just being in school. The idea that somebody would pick up a bag and bring a scale and a blood pressure cuff and a Doppler and come to your home is novel.

For Black birthworkers, this holistic carework is a form of resistance to racialized medical neglect. Black birthworkers have taken the crisis of COVID-19 as an opportunity to find new ways to form community, support new parents and share Black wisdom and healing traditions.

"Who Would Take My Place?": Surviving and Thriving During the Pandemic

As Black birthworkers seek to safeguard the emotional and physical safety and wellbeing of Black mamas and infants, they themselves face significant threats to safety and wellness. Black people have a higher risk of infection and are more likely to die from the virus once infected. This is not because Black people are biologically more susceptible to the virus, but "because we are more exposed and less protected" due to overrepresentation in essential jobs, jails and homeless encampments, inadequate healthcare and higher rates of chronic conditions related to health inequities (Ford et al., 2020; Wallis 2020). Black and Latinx healthcare workers run even greater risks (Jewett 2020). A recent study found that healthcare workers were three times more likely to report a positive COVID-19 test than the general public, and healthcare workers of color were twice as likely as their white peers to test positive (Nguyen et al., 2020). Black and Latinx healthcare workers are more likely to report using inadequate or reused protective gear and to care for patients with suspected or confirmed cases of the virus. They are also more likely to serve low income communities of color, which are particularly hard hit by the virus. For Black doulas, their risk may be magnified by having to work more than one job in order to make ends meet. For example, Jayla, a reproductive consultant in California, found herself exposed to the virus in her job as a transit worker:

> When the pandemic hit, I was pregnant and considered an essential worker. I was not protected at work whatsoever... I had several passengers get on that tested positive for COVID. And when I voiced my concerns to the company as well as my health care provider, there was no care or concern about that, which I found, you know, shocking and to be honest, it was very infuriating also.

Mariah, a nurse-midwife serving Black families in Delaware, acknowledged the risk that she faces as an older Black woman in continuing to serve clients during the pandemic:

> [B]ecause I am the only Black provider in the group space where I practice, I essentially live in complete isolation when I'm not with my clients because I know that if I get COVID-19 AND get sick and even if I'm just gone for two weeks, who will care for them? And if I'm

> one of the unfortunate Black health care providers who doesn't survive COVID-19, who would take my place?

Rather than worrying about her own welfare, Mariah expressed greater concern that her clients would not get their needs met should she, as the only Black midwife in her group, succumb to the virus. This spirit of service and self-sacrifice, while motivating birthworkers to continue to support a vulnerable population during the COVID-19 crisis, can also normalize unhealthy levels of stress, isolation and risk among these essential workers.

Racial isolation was another factor impacting the birthworkers in this study. The lack of interaction with other Black doulas, midwives and peers, was mentioned by several participants:

> I'm the only Black midwife at the hospital...I do great work and I love this work. And I feel like I'm tied to my ancestors through it. But I also recognize that it is, like, physically and emotionally draining at times. And that being the "only" as many of us are, we don't always have someone to share it with. (Mariah, CNM, Delaware)

Several participants shared that the burden of navigating or speaking out against racism, and the climate of racial tension associated with reactions to the Movement for Black Lives, added to the stressors of the current moment.

"I Needed to Survive": The Financial Impact of the Pandemic

When Black healthcare employees are faced with an unsafe or racially "toxic" environment, they face the choice of leaving and potentially facing financial insecurity, or staying in an environment that is detrimental to their physical and/or emotional wellbeing. Tamika, a lactation consultant who was pregnant during the pandemic, shared this dilemma:

> I made a decision to take leave early, although I knew it would impact my family and my finances. But I needed to protect myself. I needed to survive. And I did not feel safe . . . it felt like I would for sure go into preterm labor if I had stayed in an environment that wasn't healthy or safe for me.

Unlike Tamika, most of the birthworkers who participated made the decision to continue practicing during the pandemic. Black doulas, midwives, and other birthworkers who operate independently may be faced with particularly acute financial challenges, as the pandemic causes furloughs and unemployment and simultaneously isolates women from spaces where they might otherwise have learned about independent maternal health professionals such as community midwives and doulas:

> I have five clients right now, and four of the five are all people that I'm gifting support to. They're not paying. (Asha, doula, Washington)

> [E]specially with the rise of unemployment... A lot of people aren't getting paid, so the ability for families and mothers to be able to compensate me for the services didn't really necessarily become my main goal. It was more so being able to assist in such a horrific time. (Imani, doula, Nevada)

The financial strain has been the most difficult on those birthworkers who work independently, with many noting a drop in income from either birthwork or other employment (many birthworkers also hold employment in other fields). Birthworkers working for clinics, hospitals or non-profits had a different experience and felt more stable through the first several months of the pandemic:

> We haven't been hit that much financially because if the non-profits still have their grants in place or are getting reimbursements from a few state insurance programs, we're still able to take on as many families that qualify and can't truly afford [it]. (Patricia, doula, Philadelphia)

Several participants noted a surge in demand for home birth and home-based services, resulting in an increase in income for a small proportion of respondents. However, not all pregnant women who wished to birth at home could afford the full care of a midwife. In addition, many homebirth midwives do not have access to insurance and thus cannot bill for their services. In response to their clients' financial challenges, several respondents participated in local grassroots fundraisers to pay for midwifery care for Black women who wished to give birth at home as a result of the pandemic.

"To Fight the Spiritual Battle": Birthworkers' Sources of Strength

Faced with significant financial insecurity, threats to their own health and safety, professional conflicts, racial and social isolation, and an intense sense of responsibility to serve and support Black pregnant people during the crisis, Black birthworkers are at risk of burnout or mental health challenges. Participants were conscious of the need to identify and draw on sources of strength to sustain them in their work. Nia, a doula from Alabama, found inner power by looking to a spiritual source:

> [G]oing into yourself and really reaching down for that spiritual place for yourself in this, because it's a lot . . . And there are so many negative forces around us right now in terms of COVID-19 that we don't really understand or are able to see. And so, we have to go in knowing that we do have to fight the spiritual battle, because a lot of these doctors don't have our best interest, of course.

When Black women turn to this metaphysical source, they are drawing on deep cultural wisdom that has sustained African American women's resistance against insurmountable odds from slavery through the civil rights era and beyond. This cultural wisdom is passed down through oral and written testimonies and documentaries about the Black "granny" midwives (now called "Grand Midwives") of the US South, who attended births for a century or more but were phased out of practice during the 1950s and 1960s by white doctors and health officials. Granny midwifery was considered a spiritual calling, and those called to serve could rely on a source of guidance and strength beyond their limited human resources in the context of overwhelming barriers to healthy Black births at a time when Black women were not admitted to hospitals (Smith and Linda, 1996; Susie, 2009; Turner, 2015). As we noted above, many Black birthworkers may be the only or one of only a few Black people working in maternal health in their communities. Connecting to this lineage of Black birthwork affords contemporary Birthworkers strength to carry on in the face of significant obstacles and isolation. Coming together with other Black birthworkers is another way in which participants in our study connected to this collective cultural wisdom; several participants responded to the pressure of their work by taking steps to reduce racial isolation—seeking out other Black birthworkers or participating in a Black Birthworker Forum:

> It's a beautiful space and I really just encourage everyone, especially those of you who are feeling like you're the only [one], to be a part of it. Because you're not alone. And when you know you're not alone, it makes Monday or whatever day of the week that you think of when you're walking into a space that sometimes is unwelcoming, a different energy, because you know that these women are caring and these people are carrying you as you go. (Mariah, CNM, Delaware)

DISCUSSION

Our virtual sharing circles with Black birthworkers were not only an opportunity to share and compare experiences, but also a space to strategize for the future. Birthworkers provide care on the front lines of the pandemic. They hold the joy, the pain and the fears of their clients and offer a critical view on what is needed to support Black birthing people in a time of global crisis.

Birthworkers described to us the restrictions put in place by hospitals and clinics, including inadequate or inconsistent care, mandatory testing, separation from newborns, not allowing more than one support person during birth, and, in some cases, not even allowing doulas to support their clients virtually. Birthworkers have continued to provide care despite the restrictive policies and, in fact, have offered the vital service of helping their clients to navigate new policies and procedures as they emerge. They have found innovative ways to offer care and have expanded the care they offer to make sure the needs of Black birthing people and new parents are being met during this uncertain time. Moreover, they have done so in the face of overt and subtle forms of racism, through their own pregnancies and health challenges and, at times, without financial compensation. Black birthworkers saw the needs in their communities and rose to the challenges of fulfilling those needs in innovative ways that are grounded in the traditions of birthwork as a calling in the Black community.

Yet there is more work to be done. We have heard from birthworkers about what is broken and what, from their perspective on the frontlines, needs to change. Medical providers must ensure quality prenatal care and transparency and continuity of care throughout the perinatal period. At a time when perinatal visits are limited and virtual, and when postpartum support from other community networks, such as friends and family, may be inaccessible, it is more vital than ever that doulas, midwives, lactation consultants, and other birthworkers be compensated for the critical work they are doing, and that this care is extended beyond the standard 6–8 weeks postpartum period. By providing additional care, both during and after pregnancy, in addition to essential services like bringing groceries, diapers, and personal protective equipment, they are filling a gap that is always present, but wider than ever during the pandemic.

Hospitals must adopt policies allowing doulas to support birthing people in person. Each birthing person should have the right to be supported by whomever they choose and hospitals should facilitate safety protocols to allow this. Birth should center the comfort and safety of the birthing person over risk management concerns. This includes ensuring that birthing people of any color are not separated from their babies after birth. Black birthing people need access to the latest evidence and crucial resources to make pregnancy, birth, and postpartum successful. With mixed messages and shifting policies during COVID-19, many new parents don't know where to turn or whom to trust.

Black birthworkers are providing care and serving their communities, not only in the context of a global pandemic, but also under the shadow of growing racial tension and increased focus on anti-Black state violence. All are aware of the disproportionate maternal and infant mortality rates for Black women and babies, and nearly all spoke of themselves and/or their clients experiencing racism in the course of giving or receiving care.

Restrictions and regulations in the time of COVID-19 have allowed for a resurgence of the racist and sexist policies that medicalized birth and pushed Black birthworkers to the margins. Black women's bodies have continued to be seen as risky, both for pregnancy complications and for COVID, leading to a lack of care and touch that continues to put Black birthing people in danger. As one birthworker shared with us, "We can't just look at this as 'during the pandemic' type work. This is a battle in a war we must win." While pandemic policies and regulations change, the core of the fight has stayed the same. The creative strategies and innovations proposed by Black birthworkers during the COVID-19 pandemic can be repurposed to transform birth during and beyond the pandemic. Black birthworkers are still battling over birth. Their resistance and resilience give us hope for the liberation of Black birth and for birth justice for all.

ETHICS STATEMENT

The studies involving human participants were reviewed and approved by the Mills College Committee for the Protection of Human Subjects. The participants provided their written informed consent to participate in this study.

AUTHOR CONTRIBUTIONS

The article is the result of a community based research justice project involving a collaborative research team. All listed authors are members of the research team and participated in research design, participant recruitment, data collection and analysis. The article was co-written by JO and JJ. JO and JJ contributed equally to the manuscript.

REFERENCES

African American Policy Forum (2020). Under the blacklight: the intersectional vulnerabilities that COVID lays BarePt 1. Available at: https://www.youtube.com/watch?v=OsBstnmBTaI&ab_channel=AfricanAmericanPolicyForum.

Assil, R., Kim, M., and Saba, W. (2015). An introduction to research justice. Available at: http://www.datacenter.org/new-toolkit-an-introduction-to-research-justice/.

Black Maternal Health Caucus (2020). "Black maternal health momnibus." Black maternal health Caucus. Available at: https://blackmaternalhealthcaucus-underwood.house.gov/Momnibus (Accessed March 7, 2020).

Black Women Birthing Justice (2020a). Who we are -black women birthing justice. Available at: https://www.blackwomenbirthingjustice.org/who-we-are (Accessed October 1, 2020).

Black Women Birthing Justice (2020b). What is birth justice? Available at: https://www.blackwomenbirthingjustice.com/what-is-birth-justice (Accessed January 18, 2021).

Connolly, C. A., and Gibson, M. E. (2011). The "white plague" and color: children, race, and tuberculosis in Virginia 1900-1935. *J. Pediatr. Nurs.* 26 (3), 230–238. doi:10.1016/j.pedn.2010.01.011

Cooke, B., and Kothari, U. (2001). *Participation: the new tyranny?* London, United Kingdom: Zed Books.

Davis, D.-A. (2019). Obstetric racism: the racial politics of pregnancy, labor, and birthing. *Med. Anthropol.* 38 (7), 560–573. doi:10.1080/01459740.2018.1549389

Davis-Floyd, R., Kim, G., and Schwartz, D. A. (2020). Pregnancy, birth and the COVID-19 pandemic in the United States. *Med. Anthropol.* 39 (5), 413–427. doi:10.1080/01459740.2020.1761804

Ellington, S., Strid, P., Tong, V. T., Woodworth, K., Galang, R. R., Zambrano, L. D., et al. (2020). Characteristics of women of reproductive age with laboratory-confirmed SARS-CoV-2 infection by pregnancy status - United States, January 22–June 7, 2020. *MMWR Morb. Mortal. Wkly. Rep.* 69 (25), 769–775. doi:10.15585/mmwr.mm6925a1

Ford, T., Reber, S., and Richard, V. R. (2020). "Race gaps in COVID-19 deaths are even bigger than they appear." brookings (blog). Available at: https://www.brookings.edu/blog/up-front/2020/06/16/race-gaps-in-covid-19-deaths-are-even-bigger-than-they-appear/ (Accessed June 16, 2020).

Guerra-Reyes, L., and Hamilton, L. J. (2017). Racial disparities in birth care: exploring the perceived role of african-American women providing midwifery care and birth support in the United States. *Women Birth* 30 (1), e9–e16. doi:10.1016/j.wombi.2016.06.004

Jewett, C. (2020). Healthcare workers of color nearly twice as likely to contract Covid-19–study. *The Guardian*, US news, August, 6.

Jolivétte, A. (2015). *Research justice: methodologies for social change.* Bristol, United Kingdom: Policy Press.

Nguyen, L. H., Drew, D. A., Graham, M. S., Joshi, A. D., Guo, C. G., Ma, W., et al. (2020). Risk of COVID-19 among front-line health-care workers and the general community: a prospective cohort study. *Lancet Public Health* 5 (9), e475–e483. doi:10.1016/S2468-2667(20)30164-X

Oparah, J. C., Arega, H., Hudson, D., Jones, L., and Oseguera, T. (2018). *Battling over birth: Black women and the maternal health care crisis.* 1st Edn. Amarillo, TX: Praeclarus Press.

Oparah, J. C., and Bonaparte, A. D. (2015). *Birthing justice: Black women, pregnancy, and childbirth.* New York, NY: Routledge.

Oparah, J. C., Salahuddin, F., Cato, R., Jones, L. I., Oseguera, T., and Matthews, S. (2015). By us not for us: Black women researching pregnancy and childbirth. Research justice: Methodologies for social change. Available at: https://www.academia.edu/40662223/By_Us_Not_For_Us_Black_Women_Researching_Pregnancy_and_Childbirth.

Petersen, E. E., Davis, N. L, Goodman, D., Cox, S., Syverson, C., Seed, K., et al. (2019). Racial/ethnic disparities in pregnancy-related deaths - United States, 2007-2016. *MMWR Morb. Mortal. Wkly. Rep.* 68 (35), 762–765. doi:10.15585/mmwr.mm6835a3

Smith, M. C., and Linda, J. H. (1996). *Listen to me good: the life story of an Alabama midwife.* Columbus, OH: Ohio State University Press.

Susie, D. A. (2009). *The way of our grandmothers: a cultural view of twentieth-century midwifery in Florida.* Athens, GA: University of Georgia Press.

Tangel, V., White, R. S., Nachamie, A. S., and Pick, J. S. (2019). Racial and ethnic disparities in maternal outcomes and the disadvantage of peripartum Black women: a multistate analysis, 2007-2014. *Am. J. Perinatol.* 36 (8), 835–848. doi:10.1055/s-0038-1675207

Turner, D. (2015). "Queen Elizabeth perry turner: 'granny midwife' 1931-1956," in *Birthing justice: Black women, pregnancy, and childbirth.* London, United Kingdom: Routledge.

Wallis, C. (2020). Why racism, not race, is a risk factor for dying of COVID-19. Available at: https://www.scientificamerican.com/article/why-racism-not-race-is-a-risk-factor-for-dying-of-covid-191/.

13

Pregnancy, Birthing and Postpartum Experiences During COVID-19 in the United States

Sarah E. DeYoung[1]* *and Michaela Mangum*[2]

[1]Disaster Research Center and Sociology and Criminal Justice, University of Delaware, Newark, DE, United States, [2]Disaster Research Center, Joseph R. Biden, Jr. School of Public Policy and Administration, University of Delaware, Newark, DE, United States

***Correspondence:**
Sarah E. DeYoung
sedeyoun@udel.edu

The research aims of this project were to understand the impact of the COVID-19 pandemic on pregnancy, birthing, and postpartum experiences in the United States. Our data include responses from 34 states within the US. Findings from our analyses indicate that higher perceived social support predicted higher scores of well-being, while higher scores of perceived loneliness predicted lower scores of well-being, and higher trauma predicted lower well-being measured as satisfaction with life. Qualitative data support these findings, as well as the finding that there were various sources of stress for respondents during pregnancy, birth, and the postpartum timeframe—particularly in terms of managing work/occupation obligations and childcare. Additionally, this research fills a gap in understanding infant feeding in emergencies. Respondents perceived that early release from the hospital reduced access to lactation support, and many respondents reported receiving free samples of breastmilk substitutes through a variety of sources.

Keywords: pregnancy, birthing, infant feeding, COVID-19, postpartum, post traumatic

INTRODUCTION: POST-DISASTER TRAUMAS

In disasters and humanitarian emergencies, families are vulnerable to the physical and social impacts of the hazard. They experience challenges and stress associated with evacuation and relocation (Bland et al., 1997; Lange et al., 2004; Curtis et al., 2007) and long-term psychological trauma (Boscarino and Adams, 2008). Families with small children are particularly vulnerable in disasters because they are susceptible to injury, illness, and other risks during the hazard event (Baker and Cormier, 2014). Because of the nature of lockdowns and restrictions on social gatherings during the COVID-19 pandemic, we anticipated that newly postpartum mothers and caregivers would experience more challenges with mental health, particularly postpartum stress from the burden of managing a "work-life balance". We include a brief literature review of the key issues related to birthing, pregnancy, infant feeding, and parenting in disasters and pandemics. We then present the data we collected and findings regarding decisions about infant feeding during the COVID-19 pandemic and ways in which loneliness, trauma, and social support are associated with ill- or well-being. Policy implications for this work include recommendations for improving support services for families with infants and young children during pandemics and emergencies.

Apart from the structural damage and physical harm caused by disasters and emergencies, crisis events also cause psychological and emotional distress due to economic loss, job loss, loss of family members or friends, displacement, and the overall disruption of normal routines and social networks (Osofsky and Osofsky, 2018; Dayal De Prewitt and Richards, 2019). Longer-term psychological impacts such as mental health issues and PTSD (post-traumatic stress disorder) may also impact individuals after a major disaster or emergency (Wickrama and Kaspar, 2007; Beaglehole et al., 2018). High levels of stress in families resulting from stressor events such as disasters can have significant impacts on family relations and functioning. For example, a large amount of the stress and trauma among children following a disaster can be attributed to the amount of parental stress children experience at home (Abramson et al., 2010; Pfefferbaum et al., 2016; Osofsky and Osofsky, 2018). The impact of parental stress on children can be especially important to consider when children have lost other social support systems such as schools and childcare programs (La Greca et al., 2010; Dayal De Prewitt and Richards, 2019). High family stress may also be a factor leading to other familial issues including increased family conflict and domestic violence (Wickrama and Kaspar, 2007; Pfefferbaum et al., 2016).

Post-disaster increases in partner violence and child abuse cases have been widely reported (Enarson, 1999; Weitzman and Behrman, 2016; Gearhart et al., 2018; Parkinson, 2019; Seddighi et al., 2019). Disasters can also result in increased family stress, along with other factors such as economic instability, substance abuse or a history of violence or exposure to violence that contribute to this rise in domestic violence (Goodman, 2016; Weitzman and Behrman, 2016; Seddighi et al., 2019). Sexual violence against women and girls is especially prevalent in post-disaster contexts (Weitzman and Behrman, 2016; Seddighi et al., 2019). Women and young girls may be more vulnerable post-disaster due to the loss of social support systems and protective services (Enarson, 1999; Enarson, 1999; Curtis, Miller, and Berry, 2000). Moreover, with this loss of social networks and access to protective services, many incidents of domestic violence and abuse against women and children go unreported and may be understudied (Curtis, Miller, and Berry, 2000; Parkinson, 2019; Seddighi et al., 2019).

In addition to the risks of violence and exploitation women may face after a disaster or emergency, women face many unique challenges to their mental and physical health. High levels of stress and symptoms of PTSD are likely to have a more severe impact on women, especially during pregnancy (Xiong et al., 2010; Sohrabizadeh and Khankeh, 2016). Stress can also create adverse outcomes for pregnancy and early child development. High exposure to a disaster followed by high levels of stress or PTSD while in the early stages of pregnancy could lead to higher rates of premature births and low birth weight babies (Eskenazi et al., 2007; Hamilton et al., 2009; Goodman, 2016). High levels of maternal stress experienced in the prenatal phase could also affect a child's behavioral outcomes, such as causing higher levels of anxiety during early childhood (McLean et al., 2018; Zhang et al., 2018). Overall, women's and pregnant people's health and reproductive care are at a greater risk during disasters and emergencies due to the lack of access to proper services and facilities and increased attention towards the general welfare of those impacted by the disaster or emergency, thereby limiting the availability of resources and services specifically concerned with reproductive health and care (Nour, 2011; Goodman, 2016). Disaster and emergency scenarios can lead to more adverse complications at birth and higher risks of maternal and infant mortality (Akker et al., 2011; Nour, 2011; Goodman, 2016; Mallett and Etzel, 2018; Singh et al., 2018). Unsanitary conditions and environments could cause infections or disease transmission, putting mothers and infants at increased risk of health complications and illness (Akker et al., 2011; Nour, 2011; Goodman, 2016; Mallett and Etzel, 2018; Singh et al., 2018).

Post-disaster trauma and stress are associated with an increase in premature births and low birth weight babies (Weissman et al., 1989; Eskenazi et al., 2007; Hamilton et al., 2009; Antipova and Curtis, 2015). Disasters and emergencies may likewise cause significant problems for infant feeding and nutrition. For the first six months after giving birth, infants should be exclusively breastfed and should continue to be breastfed up until the age of one or beyond (Centers for Disease Control and Prevention, 2019). Breastfeeding decreases the risk of infants contracting infections by strengthening their immune systems (Gribble et al., 2011; Hipgrave et al., 2012; DeYoung et al., 2018a; Gribble, 2018). Formula and breast milk substitutes increase a child's risk of illness and infections, especially in a disaster setting where clean water and supplies needed to sterilize bottles may not be easily accessible (Gribble et al., 2011; Hipgrave et al., 2012; DeYoung et al., 2018a; Gribble, 2018). Infant formula itself may contain bacteria or be expired (Barron and Forsythe, 2007; DeYoung et al., 2018a; Cho et al., 2019), which can lead to serious diarrheal illness that can result in an increase in infant mortality (Gribble et al., 2011; Gribble, 2018).

Despite the advantages of breastfeeding, some factors may inhibit women from breastfeeding during a disaster or emergency. These include loss of support systems, loss of lactation support services/counseling, stress from evacuation and displacement, lack of privacy, and the perception of decreased milk supply (Gribble et al., 2011; DeYoung et al., 2018a; DeYoung et al., 2018b). Another major factor that leads many mothers to resort to formula during a disaster is the excessive and imprudent distribution of infant formula by companies and humanitarian organizations as part of relief efforts (Gribble et al., 2011; Binns et al., 2012; DeYoung et al., 2018a).

In the US, the COVID-19 virus was first identified on January 20th in Seattle, Washington when a citizen returned from an international trip to Wuhan. Less than 2 weeks later, cases were reported in Illinois, California, Arizona, and Massachusetts (Jernigan, 2020). By March 1, cases had spread to Wisconsin, Oregon, Florida, Rhode Island, and New York (Lardieri, 2020). Throughout early March, cases quickly multiplied to states in the north- and south-east, eventually spreading throughout the mid- and south-west. By March 17th, every US state had confirmed cases of COVID-19, with West Virginia being the last state to confirm a case (Department of Defense, 2020). Starting in March, states began implementing stay-at-home orders and other social distancing requirements. Out of the 50 states, 42 implemented state-wide stay-at-home orders (Mervosh et al., 2020). During this time, public health facilities and hospitals began implementing strict health and safety policies to decrease risks of transmission. However, many of these policies and measures taken to reduce the spread of COVID-19 have caused additional challenges and concerns for many mothers and their infants.

Clinical research on transmission of COVID-19 in pregnant people and infants is evolving. Data from infants born in Wuhan, China indicated no evidence of vertical transmission from mother to neonate (Chen et al., 2020; Schwartz, 2020). Because of the new clinical information, healthcare systems and facilities had varied interpretations of risk for transmission to infants. After the pandemic began in the United States, guidelines from the CDC included strict recommendations about preventing infants from becoming infected (Centers for Disease Control and Prevention, 2020; Mintz, 2020). These guidelines included the separation of the mother from the infant, despite scarce evidence about transmission of COVID-19 from mother/parent to child, and scarcity of evidence that the risk of COVID-19 outweigh the benefits of breastfeeding (Tomori et al., 2020). Scholars in birthing and infant feeding research cautioned against making policy mistakes and decisions similar to those made in past outbreaks that led to adverse impacts for child and maternal health, drawing parallels between early medical guidance regarding breastfeeding, the HIV/AIDS epidemic, and COVID-19 (Gribble, et al., 2020). Another adverse impact of the pandemic on birthing families is the capacity for adequate medical care and support for birthing people and mothers due to hospitals becoming inundated with COVID-19 patients (Rocca-Ihenacho and Alonso, 2020). Another issue that emerged during the pandemic was the increase in aggressive marketing by infant formula industries (Cullinan, 2020). This is also common after disasters, yet there is less research on the social and behavioral aspects of disaster capitalism (see Klein, 2007)—specifically its impact on women, young children, and birthing and pregnant people.

RESEARCH QUESTIONS

Given the findings that COVID-19 resulted in new hospital policies, uncertainty about risk, and new efforts by formula companies to engage in aggressive marketing, the research aims of this project were to understand the following in terms of maternal and postpartum experiences:

(1) The relationships among social support, pandemic-related trauma and well-being during the pandemic.
(2) How experiences of birthing, lactation, and infant feeding are impacted by the pandemic.
(3) The impacts of managing family stress or work-life issues during the pandemic.

METHODOLOGY

In July of 2020, we launched a web-based survey to gather primary data in the United States, using Qualtrics as our survey platform. For recruitment tracking, we created a systematic list of mothering and parenting pages on social media (Facebook) from across the country. Some respondents also shared the survey in their own email listserves. We used a spreadsheet to list the names of the groups, and 30 groups per region. Specifically, we created a recruitment list of 30 groups in each region: the Northeast, Southwest, Midwest, Southeast, Central. We also sought groups in Alaska, Hawaii, Puerto Rico, The US Virgin Islands, as well as national-level groups (not tied to geographic regions). We identified the groups by searching for "parenting," "coronavirus concerns," "moms," "new moms," and key words related to infant feeding such as "breastfeeding" and "breastfeeding resources". We documented the size of each Facebook page (in followers) and whether the group was public or private. We also created a separate list of national level groups that focus on parenting, breastfeeding, birthing, and COVID-19 discussions. To respect group rules and privacy, we prioritized posting study recruitment to groups that were either listed as "public" or groups that one of us already belonged to because of her status as a parent. In our recruitment, we indicated that the study was focused on people who were pregnant or gave birth from the timeframe of Dec 2019 through the time of data collection (summer of 2020). Most of the respondents were in the postpartum timeframe when they took this survey, but some were still pregnant (see results section).

The Institutional Review Board at the University of Delaware approved this research protocol. Respondents received a $10 electronic gift card via email for their responses, and we did not match names or identifying information with quotes or responses. Our survey included 40 questions about pregnancy, birthing, infant feeding, disaster preparedness, perceived trauma, loneliness, social support, and other perceptions about experiencing the pandemic as a new parent. For pregnancy questions, we asked when they were due to give birth, where they gave birth (home, hospital, birthing center, or other), if respondents had evacuated for a hurricane or disaster in the last two years, and type of feeding for infants during the pandemic (breastmilk, breastmilk substitutes, pumped milk, solids, combination, or other). For the disaster preparedness item, we asked respondents "How prepared do you think your household is for a natural hazard event such as a hurricane, wildfire, earthquake, flood, tornado, or other event?" (Likert scale 1–5).

Scales and Data Screening

To measure potential traumatic experiences in women, we used the abbreviated PCL (PTSD Checklist) Scale by Lang et al. (2012) and Price et al. (2016). For this study, the PCL items were designed to capture the potential impacts of birthing during a pandemic. There are four items in this scale that ask for frequency of avoidance of trauma reminders, being easily startled, experiencing negative thoughts and repeated unwanted memories (Likert scale 1–5, with 1 being "least frequent" and 5 being "extremely frequent"). To measure well-being, we used the 5-item Satisfaction with Life Scale (SWLS) by Diener et al. (1985); these items include questions about perceived life satisfaction. Scale reliability using chronbach's alpha for the PCL in the current sample of respondents was $\alpha = 0.74$ and $\alpha = 0.82$ for the SWLS. The items to measure loneliness and social support were both on a 5 point Likert Scale and asked respectively: "Please rate how frequently you do/feel the following during the pandemic (from March until now) on a scale from 'never' to 'always': Feel lonely, or feel connected to a social support system." All these scales were used in the linear regression, in which the predictive variables were loneliness (Likert scale as described above), social support (Likert scale as described above), and trauma (abbreviated PCL described above). The outcome/dependent variable was well-being (SWLS).

We also included two open-ended questions at the end of the survey asking respondents: "In one to two sentences, please describe what you have been doing for self-care or would like to be doing for self-care during the pandemic (can include but not limited to: tasks for mental health, physical health, social networks, routines, creative tasks or other activities)?" and "What else would you like to share with us about your experience during the COVID-19 pandemic?" For the two open-ended questions, we asked respondents the following: 1) "In one to two sentences, please describe what you have been doing for self-care or would like to be doing for self-care during the pandemic (can include but not limited to: tasks for mental health, physical health, social networks, routines, creative tasks or other activities)?" and 2) "What else would you like to share with us about your experience during the COVID-19 pandemic?" For the self-care codes, we identified the following eight themes: 1) Physical activities (includes exercise, hiking, yoga, sleep); 2) Social strategies for coping (contact with family, friends, or partner); 3) Creative activities (includes spiritual, entertainment, cooking); 4) COVID risks preventing self-care; 5) Not able to find time; 6) Medication (antidepressants or antianxiety) or therapy; 7) Taking a break from social media; and 8) Other (response does not fall under other categories). For the "What else" item, we identified 6 code themes: 1) Concerned about partner at delivery, medical checks, and hospital policy; 2) General isolation; 3) Stress caused by job and work-life issues; 4) Breastfeeding and infant feeding concerns; 5) Positive or gratitude perceptions; and 6) Other.

All statistical analyses were conducted using SPSS 26 (IBM, 2019). To check for valid responses, we filtered out responses with a response duration of less than 120 s for response time to the entire survey or incomplete responses (i.e. if they only responded to the first item of "agree to participate," this respondent was filtered from analyses). For qualitative data, we read through the themes and agreed upon a codebook for them (Appendix A). We then independently coded one round and adapted the codes after a second round of consolidating codes and identifying additional themes (Saldaña, 2014). To check for inter-rater reliability for items described in **Qualitative Results** Section, we calculated the score agreements using the Kappa statistics in SPSS. The agreement for the coding of the question about self-care was Kappa = 0.838 and Kappa = 0.825 for the "What else would you like to share?" question. There were 210 initial responses. After filtering for complete and valid responses, we had 192 responses (caregivers and parents) available for analysis.

RESULTS

Demographics

Respondents lived in 34 different states, with the majority coming from the six following states: Delaware (51), North Carolina (26), Alabama (13), California (12), Texas (8), and Maryland (6). The majority of respondents indicated to be between the age of 26–36 (76.32%, or 145), while 7.3% (14) were age 18–25, 15.79% (30) were age 37–47, and one respondent indicated to be age 59 or older. The income of respondents varied (**Table 1**). The race of respondents skewed heavily white (88%, or 178), with 5% (10) indicating Hispanic/Latinx, 2.48% (5) Asian or Pacific Islander, one Black respondent, and 2% (4) checked "prefer not to indicate" ethnicity. For education, the sample indicated a higher education level than the general population (United States Census Bureau, 2020) (**Table 2**).

TABLE 1 | Respondents' level of reported income.

Level of income	Frequency	Percentage
10,000 or less per year	1	0.53
11,000–20,000	5	2.63
21,000–40,000	13	6.84
41,000–50,000	7	3.68
51,000–80,000	39	20.53
81,000–100,000	37	19.47
101,000–120,000	24	12.63
121,000–140,000	17	8.95
141,000–160,000	15	7.89
161,000 or higher	32	16.84
Total	190	100

One Hundred and one respondents gave birth during the pandemic, while 15 gave birth before the pandemic began or were pregnant at the time of taking the survey. Of the respondents (who had given birth), 132 reported birthing at a hospital, and 5 at a birthing center, while 3 indicated a home birth. Notably, 37.59% (53) respondents indicated complications with their pregnancy or birth. These complications ranged from gestational diabetes, HELLP syndrome (hemolysis, elevated liver enzymes, low platelet count), intrauterine growth restriction, high blood pressure, polyhydramnios, and hemorrhaging. One respondent indicated that the fetus was nonreactive after a positive maternal COVID test, resulting in an emergency cesarean. The age of infants ranged from newborn to 12 months and older (**Table 3**). Thirty eight respondents indicated receiving a variety of support services (19.79%), including the Women Infants and Children (WIC) Supplemental Nutrition Assistance Program, unemployment benefits, and pregnancy Medicaid.

Quantitative Results

For questions regarding lactation and feeding, we asked respondents if they received infant formula during the pandemic in the form of free samples (they could indicate more than one method of receiving the free sample). A total of 92 respondents (35.8%) indicated that they received a free sample of infant formula in the mail; forty-one got the free sample at the pediatrician's office (16%); and 36 (14%) received free formula at the hospital. Some respondents also indicated that they received formula from a friend or organization, or through an advertisement on social media. Sixty-five respondents (25.29%) reported "I did not receive a free sample." In response to the question, "Were you always able to get the kinds of food you wanted to feed your infant/children throughout the pandemic?" many respondents indicated "Always" (117), Frequently (40), and Sometimes (23). Two respondents indicated that they were rarely able to get the kinds of food they wanted for their children. Respondents indicated that they received postpartum telehealth care (37), in-office visits (53), a mix of both for postpartum

TABLE 2 | Respondents' level of education.

Level of education	Frequency	Percentage
Less than high school	2	1.04
High school graduate	6	3.13
Some college	18	9.38
2 years degree	6	3.13
4 years degree	56	29.17
Master's/Professional degree	58	30.21
Doctorate	46	23.96
Total	192	100

TABLE 3 | Age of infants.

Age range	Frequency	Percentage
One-two months old	72	40.22
Three-five months old	71	39.66
Six-eight months old	20	11.17
Nine-eleven months old	3	1.68
Twelve months old or older	13	7.26
Total	179	100

services (22), and some indicated that they did not request or need services (49). One respondent indicated that they were unable to afford postpartum care, and 5 indicated that they were unable to locate a provider of care for postpartum services. When asked if they received lactation support, 64.67% (97) indicated that the support they received was in the hospital or birthing center, and there were also respondents who needed lactation support but did not receive the needed services (**Table 4**).

Linear Regression

First, we conducted bivariate correlations on age, well-being, trauma, loneliness, and social support (**Table 5**). None of the variables were significantly correlated with age, which we excluded in the regression. To test for the impacts of pandemic-associated trauma, social support, and loneliness on maternal wellbeing, we conducted a linear regression analysis (see **Table 6** for descriptive statistics). The overall model was significant ($p < 0.005$) and indicated that 25% (R^2 adj = 0.23) of the variance in well-being (F (3,172) = 19.29, $p < 0.01$) was predicted by perceived loneliness $b = -0.172$ ($p = 0.27$), $t = -2.22$ (negative direction); perceived social support $b = 0.30$ ($p = 0.000$), $t = 4.10$, and trauma $b = -0.186$, ($p = 0.01$), $t = -2.60$ (negative direction) (**Table 7**). In other words, in our model, higher social support predicted higher scores of well-being, while higher scores of perceived loneliness predicted lower scores of well-being, and higher trauma predicted lower well-being.

Qualitative Results

Respondents indicated distress due to isolation, conflicting information about pregnancy and birthing and COVID-19, and stress on their families associated with the pandemic. Many respondents indicated several themes in one response.

TABLE 4 | Lactation support after giving birth.

	Frequency	Percentage
Yes, in the hospital/birthing center	97	64.67
No, even though needed support	2	1.33
Yes, after leaving hospital	16	10.67
Did not want/need support	22	14.67
Other	13	8.67
Total	152	100

For example, if a respondent indicated that they were having concerns about breastfeeding and that they felt isolated after giving birth, we coded this as "General isolation" and "Infant feeding concerns." Below we describe the themes that were most prevalent for respondents and provide example quotes from them. A major theme throughout these data were that respondents felt stressed about the isolation associated with the pandemic, despite their attempted coping mechanisms. To understand the ways in which respondents managed the isolation and stress, the self-care question and other open-ended questions provide a deeper insight to the findings from the regression analysis.

Self-Care

Respondents indicated that they engaged in self-care by doing physical activities such as walking or hiking. They also indicated keeping social connections with a small network of friends or family. Respondents also indicated that they use mental health or talk therapy, medication, and other means for managing their mental wellness. Many respondents indicated engaging in more than one form of self-care:

- *I practiced meditation and yoga throughout my pregnancy and I feel that that helped me cope well with going through the pandemic during my third trimester. . ./.. I go on socially distant walks with a few friends (who have also been socially distancing) and that has been very helpful.*
- *For self-care, my partner and I started therapy and I talk weekly to a friend and meditate.*
- *I started teletherapy and talk to my friends via text.*
- *I participate in a "Mommy Zoom" meeting every other week, chatting with my coworkers who are also on maternity leave.*
- *Going for walks, face-timing and talking to friends and family, doing puzzles, playing with my dog.../... Also, my husband has been going back to work more frequently now and I'm alone a lot. At first I enjoyed the alone time (it was self-care for me), but now I find it isolating.*

Some respondents also indicated that they do not have time for self-care or that they would like to do certain activities that they feel they cannot do because of the pandemic. For example:

- *I wish I could have more social interaction and my baby could be exposed to more close friends and family, however we are isolating.*

TABLE 5 | Bivariate correlations.

	Q_age	Sum_trauma	Sum_well-being	Q_social support	Q__lonely
Q3_age					
r	1	−0.070	−0.009	0.072	−0.067
Sig. (2-tailed)		0.343	0.898	0.334	0.367
n	190	183	185	182	181
Sum_trauma					
r	−0.070	1	−0.314[a]	−0.244[a]	0.368[a]
Sig. (2-tailed)	0.343		0.000	0.001	0.000
n	183	183	183	179	178
Sum_wellbeing					
r	−0.009	−0.314[a]	1	0.415[a]	−0.371[a]
Sig. (2-tailed)	0.898	0.000		0.000	0.000
n	185	183	185	181	180
Q_socialsupport					
r	0.072	−0.244[a]	0.415[a]	1	−0.441[a]
Sig. (2-tailed)	0.334	0.001	0.000		0.000
n	182	179	181	182	179
Q__lonely					
r	−0.067	0.368[a]	−0.371[a]	−0.441[a]	1
Sig. (2-tailed)	0.367	0.000	0.000	0.000	
n	181	178	180	179	181

[a]*Correlation is significant at the 0.01 level (2-tailed).*

TABLE 6 | Means for regression, *N* = 176.

Variable	Mean	Standard Deviation
Well-being scale	19.0909	4.01038
Q loneliness	2.6648	0.97752
Q social support	3.0341	1.07383
Trauma scale	8.4489	3.38192

- *I have not been doing enough self care. Showers, podcasts while walking with the baby, and napping are probably my main forms of care right now.*
- *I would like to be able to take some time for myself and catch up on sleep.*
- *Would like to sleep and hike more and spend time in nature, sleep, sleep and have a clean house.*

These responses are related to some of the themes that we identified for the next portion of open-ended data. In these data, respondents indicated general stress, isolation, and frustration over their experiences with being pregnant and giving birth during the pandemic. We discuss these in order of themes and in order of the pregnancy, birthing, and postpartum timeframes.

General Stress

Pregnancy was a period of uncertainty for many respondents who felt frustrated by confusing or limited guidance from their healthcare providers. They indicated receiving conflicting or confusing information about hospital protocols and other health measures:

- *Pregnancy during a pandemic was stressful in a thousand big and small ways: the lack of data on outcomes for pregnant people and fetuses of a covid infection, going to prenatal appointments alone and masked, cancelled and telehealth appointments, cancelled prenatal classes, keeping up with changing labor and delivery policies.../...the collapse of in-person support networks, weighing the risks of going in for monitoring when something felt off or the baby wasn't moving much in-utero with the risk of covid exposure, and huge uncertainties...*
- *It's been hard to go through 20 weeks of pregnancy without really seeing family or friends, and we have a lot of questions about what our delivery in November is going to look like, and the support we will have with our newborn and toddler. It's been very frustrating for me and my OB, she feels like she doesn't have enough good information to give me guidance on staying safe during my pregnancy beyond the standard "social distance, mask, etc" recommendations.*

Additionally, the general stress the respondents described was not limited to one phase of pregnancy or birth—but rather throughout all phases of pregnancy, birthing, and caring for infants and toddlers. They also lamented missing out on rituals or celebrations associated with the arrival of the new infant (i.e. baby showers or other events).

Health Protocol Concerns

Many health protocol concerns centered around respondents' hospital experiences and hospital policies related to COVID-19. In many cases, respondents had to choose between their planned support person such as a doula or their significant other or spouse. Some respondents indicated that they were worried about contracting COVID-19 before or during the timeframe of giving birth and that this might lead to separation from their newborn:

- *The hardest part of having my first baby in this was not being able to have my doula at the hospital then not being able to*

TABLE 7 | Coefficients.

Model	Unstandardized coefficients		Standardized coefficients	t	Sig.	95.0% confidence interval for B		Collinearity statistics	
	B	Std. Error	Beta			Lower bound	Upper bound	Tolerance	VIF
(Constant)	19.417	1.502		12.931	0.000	16.453	22.381		
Q_lonely	−0.705	0.317	−0.172	−2.227	0.027	−1.330	−0.080	0.730	1.370
Q_social_support	1.127	0.275	0.302	4.104	0.000	0.585	1.670	0.804	1.244
Sum_trauma	−0.221	0.085	−0.186	−2.604	0.010	−0.389	−0.054	0.849	1.177

a. Dependent Variable: Sum_WB.

safely allow for some family members to visit following the birth.

- *This is my third child. The birthing experience was different. It was hard to wear a mask during labor, I had been isolating so it felt terrifying that me or my baby could get COVID, the hospital shared that they would suggest separating Mom from baby if either tested positive (we didn't but this was also terrifying), and we were discharged exactly at the 24 h mark.*
- *The hospital birthing experience in NYC in March was scary with everything that was happening at that point. My husband and I weighed the options to deliver outside of the city or to be induced early. In the moment though, having a healthy birth and taking care of myself postpartum was most important there was little time or energy to worry about COVID in the hospital.*

Some respondents even indicated that they would not plan disclose to their healthcare providers if they experienced COVID-19 symptoms for fear of early labor inductions, separation from their infant, or some other forceful intervention. Again, some of these hesitations seemed to be related to the myriad of confusing information about birthing and hospital policies. This may also reflect a lack of trust in healthcare providers and the broader healthcare system.

Isolation

After they gave birth, many of the respondents described that their feelings of isolation made their postpartum experience more difficult. Many of their "usual" coping strategies were not possible because of the pandemic:

- *For me, having a newborn during the pandemic has been much harder than pregnancy was. We have taken social/physical distancing very seriously and have had no outside help or outsiders come (including family).../...It makes me sad that the only people who have ever held our baby or even touched her has been me and my husband and we don't know when we will feel comfortable having others interact with her safely.*
- *It's extremely hard to deal with life with a newborn without the physical support of family and friends. I feel like I am on my phone more often just to feel some sort of connection and support.*
- *Family members have not yet met my daughter and she is almost 9 weeks old. Two older relatives died of COVID-19. Two died of other causes, but we are unable to celebrate their lives with funeral services.*
- *The pandemic has caused tension and mistrust between me and family members. I feel I have to be extra cautious and question everything since I have a newborn baby.*

These quotes illustrate the combined impacts of isolation and the need to socially distance even from family members or friends that the respondents might normally see in person. Additionally, the feeling of the newborn as "fragile" seems to also be amplified because of the danger of COVID-19, which was reflected in the respondents' comments about caution, risk, and decisions about social/physical distancing to keep the family safe.

Infant Feeding

Respondents indicated that the pandemic made their infant feeding choices and efforts more complex, especially because some were unable to receive in-person lactation support after they were discharged from the hospital:

- *Getting access to services postpartum has been difficult, especially with breastfeeding help. I have struggled mentally because I feel unsupported and isolated.*
- *I do think that the pandemic/lockdown contributed to my breastfeeding journey ending quicker than I wanted it to.*
- *Also because of the pandemic I was not able to receive lactation support after we left the hospital, which I believe contributed to my inability to breastfeed. Another factor that I believe contributed is that we were not able to have any family or friend support after the birth due to social distancing, and no childcare for our toddler, so we were stretched very thin and very stressed.*

In contrast, some respondents indicated that working from home facilitated their ease of maintaining their ability to continue to breastfeed or use a breast pump:

- *It has allowed for me to breastfeed (without pumping) and spend more time than expected with my infant which has been nice.*

Next, we discuss ways in which career and work obligations collided with taking care of the newborn, older children, and struggling to maintain well-being in daily life.

Work-Life Balance

Many concerns about work-life balance were related to lack of childcare for older children, to a sense of frustration in feeling unable to provide attention to all the children at once, and to stress about focusing on work-related tasks:

- *It has been extremely difficult to work from home while having a toddler in the house. Finding that balance has not gone well. I feel like I'm failing as an employee and as a mom.*
- *It is exponentially more stressful with an infant than it would have been if i didn't have a baby. Childcare was challenging to find when I had to return to work in the office. The unknowns about the virus are terrifying and the lack of responsibility and respect from the government towards families/parents with kids is horrible.*
- *It has been stressful going from a full time working mom to a mom staying at home with 2 children and trying to juggle ongoing work responsibilities, without the option to do what I would prefer to do when spending time with the kids: taking them out to the library, playground, zoo, pool, to visit friends, etc.*

The comments about balancing childcare suggest that the pandemic creates a unique situation in which new stress is generated by the pressure to continue performing and producing at work, or to appear as though "business is going on as usual." Respondents also mentioned how normally they would include grandparents or extended family for assisting with childcare but that this was made more complex because of the pandemic.

Complex Feelings Mixed With Gratitude

Some respondents also indicated they had a lens of positivity, at least partially, for some of the new circumstances related to social distancing and being away from normal social interactions and routines. This theme does not minimize the severity of other adverse experiences, but rather reflects their attempts to cope during the pandemic:

- *I'm a pretty introverted person anyway so social distancing and quarantining isn't too hard for me to do. It helps that I love being home with my family as it is.*
- *It has been hard not being able to do things with my baby I would like to, especially holiday things. But I am also thankful for the extra time I have been able to be home (I am an elementary school teacher and never went back to work because of the pandemic, I taught online).*
- *There has been a lot of loss in this season, but we are full of gratitude for the privilege we have to be employed, supported (at a distance), and the ability to work from home full-time.*
- *It was sad not to have my family there with me to visit the baby, but there was also a strange peace about it only being my husband and I for two days we were in the hospital. I will note that the hospital staff were discharging mothers and babies as early as possible in efforts to keep people out of the environment due to the pandemic. We were out within 48 h.*

Although some respondents had a positive perspective on their experiences, many respondents indicated difficulties with coping, and this was reflected in much of the quantitative and qualitative data. Two respondents stated:

- *There is too much to include here. In short, the experience has been traumatizing.*
- *It has been incredibly frustrating to live in an area where lots of people are not taking covid19 seriously. My family has been chastised for not letting family members from outside the household visit while I was pregnant and especially now that we have a newborn at home.*

Together, these data and results suggest that most respondents experienced new challenges because of the pandemic. These challenges seemed to exacerbate the "usual" levels of stress, isolation, and other difficulties that new parents experience during the postpartum period. These findings were consistent across both the open-ended and the quantitative measures that we included for this study—particularly that social support mitigated the adverse impact of trauma.

DISCUSSION AND POLICY IMPLICATIONS

Pregnancy and birth during the pandemic were associated with anxiety and uncertainty for many of the respondents. Not being able to have their partner or support person at the hospital for birth—or having to choose between them—was a major point of concern. Respondents also indicated that release from the hospital was quick due to the new pandemic protocols. Additional research building upon these research findings should track the ways in which early release or shorter hospital stays impact outcomes for new parents and infants in a pandemic context or other major crisis event. One potential effect is that postpartum complications may go undetected—from difficulties with breastfeeding to life-threatening issues. There may also be other unanticipated mental health outcomes related to the shortened hospital stays. Some programs that carry out in-person home visits also had to adapt their protocols during the pandemic, which may have an impact on screening for postpartum depression, anxiety, and other postpartum mood disorders. Birthing in the pandemic may also increase other negative spill-over impacts related to postpartum care, because of reduced time in the hospital where many patients receive lactation and other support services.

For those respondents who felt disconnected from their social support system, the sense of isolation that many new mothers feel after the birth of their infants in normal times was exacerbated by the pandemic. Importantly, those who did feel connected to social support systems had higher levels of well-being. The postpartum period is a critical time for the new parent(s) to maintain mental health through social contact and social support systems (Tani and Castagna, 2017). However, because of the pandemic, many of the activities that the respondents wanted to do, especially attendance at social gatherings, meeting with other mothers and peers face-to-face, and other such were not possible for the parents who were self-isolating, quarantining, or adhering to guidelines put forth by health officials to mitigate the spread of COVID-19. Some respondents found creative ways to maintain social connections such as through taking outside walks or having outdoor visits with a friend or friends. However, it seems that these were not sufficient replacements for the kinds of social support and interaction that the respondents most desired.

One of our most alarming findings was that only approximately 25% of the respondents indicated that they did *not* receive a free sample of breastmilk substitutes (infant formula), while the remaining respondents did receive some form of complimentary or unsolicited infant formula sample. Often, respondents indicated that they received samples from more than one source. These sources included the mail, the hospital, the pediatrician's office, or some other source, such as through social media or from a friend or peer. In regions where food scarcity and poverty were already prevalent before the pandemic, this aggressive marketing tactic has the dangerous potential to steer families away from breastfeeding (Rosenberg et al., 2008). Breastfeeding should most especially be supported during disasters and emergencies because it is a protective mechanism for infants and for the mother or lactating parent (see e.g. Gribble, 2018; Davis-Floyd et al., 2021). While it is not surprising that aggressive formula marketing is happening in the United States during the COVID-19 pandemic, additional research is required to understand to what extent the aggressive marketing "works" or becomes more effective at recruiting infant caregivers during times of crisis, disasters, and pandemics. Such additional research should include longitudinal studies that identify factors that bolster rates of exclusive and prolonged breastfeeding. Additionally, international research is needed in this area because policies and protections for breastfeeding in emergency scenarios do vary from country to country (Hoang et al., 2020).

The work-life balance concern for caregivers has received considerable attention in mainstream media, as well as in academic research. Unsurprisingly, in the United States in particular, women left the labor market during the summer and early autumn at significantly higher rates (Hsu, 2020). While may academic and research studies may center the changes and demands of working women, pregnant people, caregivers, and parents, it is important to understand how specific mechanisms associated with pregnancy, birthing, and postpartum care are associated with potentially severe outcomes such as postpartum psychosis, intersections of mental health with parenting and work, parenting and sense of community, and changes in social support systems because of other "spillover" effects of the pandemic such as family stress due to unemployment, COVID death/s in the family, and other complexities.

Study Limitations

Our recruitment method was not a random sampling technique. However, it has been used to collect data rapidly after disasters (e.g. Mongold et al., 2020) to explore social and behavioral aspects of reactions in crisis scenarios. It is also difficult or impossible to conduct face to face interviews because of the contagious aspect of COVID-19. In future research, this systematic social media recruitment approach should be compared to other web-based recruitment techniques such as Lucid Theorem and Amazon Mechanical Turk. Partnering with a health organization or another nonprofit that has regular contact with pregnant patients and new parents would be a possibility for gathering future data, if patient/respondent privacy and autonomy is protected.

The fact that our survey sample was comprised of 88% white respondents is a serious limitation of our study. Women of color in the United States face greater health risks due to racism and discrimination in health care and lack of access to critical resources (Singh et al., 2017; Owens and Sharla, 2019). Hazards and disasters also disproportionately impact Black, Indigenous, and Hispanic populations (Davies et al., 2018). Given these aspects of vulnerability, the COVID-19 pandemic is likely to continue to adversely impact such families and result in furthering the gap between families who are thriving and families who experience barriers in accessing healthcare and support. Additional research should include measures for tracking these disparities over time and across race and ethnicity, as other scholars have already suggested (Lemke and Brown, 2020) and as other articles in this collection attempt to do.

Another limitation of this study is that the measure of the abbreviated PCL is arguably more appropriate for one event. The PCL for this study was designed to capture potential stress and trauma related to the pregnancy and birthing experience during the pandemic. The COVID-19 pandemic is a protracted crisis and not a single "point" in time. The complexity of the pandemic as an on-going event can make measurements more complicated compared to measuring stress associated with a rapid onset hazard event (such as a tsunami, earthquake, or other disaster).

CONCLUSIONS: THE ADVERSE EFFECTS OF ISOLATION AND STRESS AND THE NEED FOR THEIR MITIGATION

Our findings suggest that the isolation associated with the COVID-19 pandemic has adverse outcomes for maternal mental health, specifically psychological trauma during the postpartum time frame. This is not to say that social/physical distancing guidelines are not important, but rather that birthing and postpartum parents should be supported through social networks in new and creative ways. Many of the respondents reported that they found ways to continue socializing through virtual networks. These strategies for facilitating social interactions and social support networks should be considered by those working to provide care to families with infants and young children.

Additionally, stress associated with career and work-life balance should be mitigated through specific family-friendly policies at organizational and national levels. The United States still fails to provide adequate support for families because it does not have a national paid leave policy after birth (Nunez, 2020). The increased strain on families during the pandemic may also have adverse impacts on other indicators, such as abuse or neglect (Brown et al., 2020).

Similarly, the United States does not adhere to provisions set forth in the WHO Code, or the World Health Organization's (1981) International Code of Marketing of Breastmilk Substitutes, making it easier for companies to encroach on healthcare facilities and other spaces that target new parents—as evidenced by the fact that many respondents received free infant formula samples during the pandemic. Organizations such as WIC, community-based organizations, and hospitals can and should generate more stringent internal policies that prevent aggressive formula marketing. Overall, the COVID-19 pandemic will likely have long-lasting adverse impacts on families, and these should be mitigated through evidence-based intervention programs.

AUTHOR CONTRIBUTIONS

SD and MM designed the survey for this data collection. Both authors participated in writing the manuscript, analysing the data, and interpreting findings.

ACKNOWLEDGMENTS

We acknowledge the valuable time and perspectives of the respondents who had infants during the pandemic and faced new challenges in 2020.

REFERENCES

Abramson, D. M., Park, Y. S., and Redlener, I. (2010). Children as bellwethers of recovery: dysfunctional systems and the effects of parents, households, and neighborhoods on serious emotional disturbance in children after Hurricane Katrina. *Disaster Med. Public Health Prep.* 4 (S1), S17–S27. doi:10.1001/dmp.2010.7

Akker, T. V., de Vroome, S., Mwagomba, B., Ford, N., and van Roosmalen, J. (2011). *Peripartum infections and Associated Maternal Mortality in Rural Malawi*. http://hdl.handle.net/1887/105659.

Antipova, A., and Curtis, A. (2015). The post-disaster negative health legacy: pregnancy outcomes in Louisiana after hurricane andrew. *Disasters* 39 (4), 665–686. doi:10.1111/disa.12125

Baker, L. R., and Cormier, L. A. (2014). *Disasters and vulnerable populations: evidence-based practice for the helping professions*. (New York: Springer Publishing Company).

Barron, J. C., and Forsythe, S. J. (2007). Dry stress and survival time of Enterobacter sakazakii and other Enterobacteriaceae in dehydrated powdered infant formula. *J. Food Protect.* 70 (9), 2111–2117. doi:10.4315/0362-028x-70.9.2111

Beaglehole, B., Mulder, R., Chris, T., Frampton, M., Boden, J. M., Newton-Howes, G., Caroline, J., and Bell, S. (2018). Psychological distress and psychiatric disorder after natural disasters: systematic review and meta-analysis. *Br. J. Psychiatr.* 213 (6), 716–722. doi:10.1192/bjp.2018.210

Binns, C., Lee, M., Tang, Li., Yu, C., Hokama, T., and Lee, A. (2012). *Ethical issues in infant feeding after disasters*. http://hdl.handle.net/20.500.11937/11992. doi:10.1177/1010539512453253

Bland, S. H., ErinO'leary, S., Farinaro, E., Jossa, F., Krogh, V., Violanti, J. M., et al. (1997). Social network disturbances and psychological distress following earthquake evacuation. *J. Nerv. Ment. Dis.* 185, 188–195.

Boscarino, J. A., and Adams, R. E. (2008). Overview of findings from the World Trade Center Disaster Outcome Study: recommendations for future research after exposure to psychological trauma. *Int. J. Emerg. Ment. Health* 10 (4), 275. doi:10.1097/NMD.0b013e3182043b39

Brown, S. M., Doom, J. R., Lechuga-Peña, S., Watamura, S. E., and Koppels, T. (2020). Stress and parenting during the global COVID-19 pandemic. *Child Abuse Negl.* 10, 4699.

Centers for Disease Control and Prevention (2020). Infant and toddler nutrition. https://www.cdc.gov/nutrition/infantandtoddlernutrition/breastfeeding/recommendations-benefits.html. Accessed August 11, 2020.

Centers for Disease Control and Prevention (2019). Newborns born to mothers with suspected or confirmed COVID-19. https://www.cdc.gov/coronavirus/2019-ncov/need-extra-precautions/pregnancy-breastfeeding.html#mothers-suspected. Accessed August 13, 2020.

Chen, Y., Peng, H., Wang, L., Yin, Z., Zeng, L., Gao, H., et al. (2020). Infants born to mothers with a new coronavirus (COVID-19). *Front. Pediatr.* 8, 104. doi:10.3389/fped.2020.00104

Cho, T. J., Hwang, J. Y., Kim, H. W., Kim, Y. K., Kwon, J. I., Young, J., et al. (2019). Underestimated risks of infantile infectious disease from the caregiver's typical handling practices of infant formula. *Sci. Rep.* 9 (1), 9799–9812. doi:10.1038/s41598-019-46181-0

Cullinan, K. (2020). Infant formula companies are 'exploiting' COVID-19 pandemic. *Open Democracy*. Available at: https://www.opendemocracy.net/en/5050/infant-formula-companies-are-exploiting-covid-19-pandemic/

Curtis, A., Mills, J. W., and Leitner, M. (2007). Katrina and vulnerability: the geography of stress. *J. Health Care Poor Underserved* 18 (2), 315–330. doi:10.1353/hpu.2007.0029

Curtis, T., Miller, B. C., and Helen Berry, E. (2000). Changes in reports and incidence of child abuse following natural disasters. *Child Abuse Neglect* 24 (9), 1151–1162. doi:10.1016/S0145-2134(00)00176-9

Davies, I. P., Haugo, R. D., Robertson, J. C., and Levin, P. S. (2018). The unequal vulnerability of communities of color to wildfire. *PloS One* 13, 11e0205825.

Davis-Floyd, R., Lim, R., Penwell, V., and Ivry, T. (2021). "Effective maternity disaster care: low tech, skilled touch", in *sustainable Birth in disruptive times*, Editor R. Davis-Floyd, B. Annex, and D. G. Kim (New York: Springer Publishing).

Dayal De Prewitt, A., and Richards, T. (2019). Social and emotional support for children and their caregivers post-disasters. *J. Family Strength* 19 (1), 28.

Department of Defense. (2020). Coronavirus: DOD response timeline https://www.defense.gov/Explore/Spotlight/Coronavirus/DOD-Response-Timeline/. Accessed August 13, 2020.

DeYoung, S., Chase, J., Branco, M., and Park, B. (2018a). The effect of mass evacuation on infant feeding: the case of the 2016 fort McMurray Wildfire. *Matern. Child Health J.* 22 (12), 1826–1833. doi:10.1007/s10995-018-2585-z

DeYoung, S., Suji, M., Hannah, G., and Southall, A. (2018b). Maternal perceptions of infant feeding and health in the context of the 2015 Nepal Earthquake. *J. Hum. Lactation* 34 (2), 242–252. doi:10.1177/0890334417750144

Diener, E. D., Emmons, R. A., Randy, J., and Griffin, S. (1985). The satisfaction with life scale. *J. Pers. Assess.* 49 (1), 71–75.

Enarson, E. (1999). *Violence against women in disasters: a study of domestic violence programs in the United States and Canada* (New York: Sage Publications).

Eskenazi, B., Marks, A. R., Catalano, R., Bruckner, T., Paolo, G., and Toniolo, D. (2007). Low birthweight in New York city and upstate New York following the events of september 11th. *Hum. Reprod. (Oxf.)* 22 (11), 3013–3020. doi:10.1093/humrep/dem301

Gearhart, S., Perez-Patron, M., Hammond, T. A., Goldberg, D. W., Klein, A., Jennifer, A., and Horney, A. (2018). The impact of natural disasters on domestic violence: an analysis of reports of simple assault in Florida (1999–2007). *Violence Gend.* 5 (2), 87–92. doi:10.1089/vio.2017.0077

Goodman, A. (2016). "*Critical care obstetrics and gynecology*", in *The Aftermath of Disasters: The Impact on Women's Health*, 2–6. doi:10.21767/2471-9803.100037

Gribble, K. D., McGrath, M., MacLaine, A., and Lhotska, L. (2011). Supporting breastfeeding in emergencies: protecting Women's reproductive rights and maternal and infant health. *Disasters* 35 (4), 720–738. doi:10.1111/j.1467-7717.2010.01239.x

Gribble, K., Mathisen, R., Ververs, M., and Anna, C. (2020). Mistakes from the HIV pandemic should inform the COVID-19 response for maternal and newborn care. *Int. Breastfeed. J.* 15 (1), 1–5.

Gribble, K. (2018). Supporting the most vulnerable through appropriate infant and Young child feeding in emergencies. *J. Hum. Lactat.* 34 (1), 40–46. doi:10.1177/0890334417741469

Hamilton, B. E., Sutton, P. D., Mathews, T. J., Joyce, A., and Stephanie, J. V. (2009). The effect of hurricane Katrina: births in the U.S. Gulf coast region, before and after the storm. *Natl. Vital Stat. Rep.* 58 (2), 1. https://www.ncbi.nlm.nih.gov/pubmed/19754006.

Hipgrave, D. B., Assefa, F., Anna, W., and Sukotjo, S. (2012). Donated breast milk substitutes and incidence of diarrhoea among infants and Young children after the May 2006 Earthquake in Yogyakarta and Central Java. *Publ. Health Nutr.* 15 (2), 307–315. doi:10.1017/S1368980010003423

Hoang, D. V., Cashin, J., Gribble, K., Marinelli, K., and Mathisen, R. (2020). Misalignment of global COVID-19 breastfeeding and newborn care guidelines with World Health Organization recommendations. *BMJ Nutr. Prevent. Health* 34, 233.

Hsu, A. (2020). Why the pandemic is forcing so many Women to leave their Jobs. *National Public Radio.* https://www.npr.org/2020/11/14/935018298/why-the-pandemic-is-forcing-so-many-women-to-leave-their-jobs.

IBM Corp Released (2019). *IBM SPSS statistics for Windows, Version 26.0.* (Armonk, NY: IBM Corp).

Jernigan, D. (2020). Update: public health response to the coronavirus disease 2019 outbreak—United States, february 24, 2020. https://www.cdc.gov/mmwr/volumes/69/wr/mm6908e1.htm. Accessed August 13, 2020).

Klein, N. (2007). The shock doctrine: the rise of disaster capitalism. Macmillan.

La Greca, S., Annette, M., Silverman, W. K., Lai, B., and James, J. (2010). Hurricane-related exposure experiences and stressors, other life events, and social support: concurrent and prospective impact on children's persistent posttraumatic stress symptoms. *J. Consult. Clin. Psychol.* 78 (6), 794–805. doi:10.1037/a0020775

Lang, A. J., Kendall, W., Roy-Byrne, P. P., Golinelli, D., Chavira, D., Sherbourne, C., Raphael, D., et al. (2012). Abbreviated PTSD Checklist (PCL) as a guide to clinical response. *Gen. Hosp. Psychiatr.* 34 (4), 332–338. doi:10.1016/j.genhosppsych.2012.02.003

Lange, L. J., Toussaint, L. L., and Raymond, F. (2004). Perceptions of accident foreseeability and stress and coping during the evacuation period of technological disaster. *Environ. Behav.* 36 (5), 701–716.

Lardieri, A. (2020). Which states have reported cases of the coronavirus?. *U.S. News and World Report.* https://www.usnews.com/news/best-states/articles/2020-03-06/which-states-have-reported-cases-of-the-coronavirus.

Lemke, M. K., and Brown, K. K. (2020). Syndemic perspectives to guide Black maternal health research and prevention during the COVID-19 pandemic. *Matern. Child Health J.* 24 (9), 1093–1098.

Mallett, L. H., and Etzel, R. A. (2018). Flooding: What is the impact on pregnancy and child health?. *Disasters* 42 (3), 432–458. doi:10.1111/disa.12256

McLean, M. A., Cobham, V. E., Simcock, G., Elgbeili, G., Kildea, S., and King, S. (2018). The role of prenatal maternal stress in the development of childhood anxiety symptomatology: the QF2011 Queensland flood study. *Dev. Psychopathol.* 30 (3), 995–1007. doi:10.1017/S0954579418000408

Mervosh, S., Lu, D., and Swales, V. (2020). *See which states and cities have told residents to stay at home.* https://www.nytimes.com/interactive/2020/us/coronavirus-stay-at-home-order.html.

Mintz, J. (2020). CDC: separate moms with coronavirus from newborns. *WebMD Health News Brief* 27, 2020 https://www.webmd.com/lung/news/20200327/cdc-separate-moms-with-coronavirus-from-newborns.

Mongold, E., Davidson, R. A., Trivedi, J., DeYoung, S., Wachtendorf, T., and Anyidoho, P. (2020). Hurricane evacuation beliefs and behaviour of inland vs. coastal populations. *Environ. Haz.* 28, 1–19.

Nour, N. N. (2011). Maternal health considerations during disaster relief. *Rev. Obstetr. Gynecol.* 4, 22–27. https://www.ncbi.nlm.nih.gov/pubmed/21629495.

Nunez, A. M. (2020). The effect of paid maternity leave on maternal health and parental health Involvement within the United States. Master's thesis. https://scholarworks.gsu.edu/cgi/viewcontent.cgi?article=1092&context=sociology_theses.

Osofsky, J. D., and Osofsky, H. J. (2018). Challenges in building child and family resilience after disasters. *J. Fam. Soc. Work* 21 (2), 115–128. doi:10.1080/10522158.2018.1427644

Owens, D. C., and Sharla, M. (2019). Black maternal and infant health: historical legacies of slavery. *Am. J. Public Health* 109 (10), 1342–1345. doi:10.2105/AJPH.2019.305243

Parkinson, D. (2019). Investigating the increase in domestic violence post disaster: an Australian case study. *J. Interpers Viol.* 34 (11), 2333–2362. doi:10.1177/0886260517696876

Pfefferbaum, B., Jacobs, A., Van Horn, R., and Houston, J. (2016). Effects of displacement in children exposed to disasters. *Curr. Psychiatr. Rep.* 18 (8), 1–5. doi:10.1007/s11920-016-0714-1

Price, M., Szafranski, D. D., van Stolk-Cooke, K., and Gros, D. F. (2016). Investigation of abbreviated 4 and 8 item versions of the PTSD Checklist 5. *Psychiatr. Res.* 239, 124–130. doi:10.1016/j.psychres.2016.03.014

Rocca-Ihenacho, L., and Alonso, C. (2020). Where do women birth during a pandemic? Changing perspectives on Safe Motherhood during the COVID-19 pandemic. *J. Glob. Health Sci.* 2, e4.

Rosenberg, K. D., Carissa, A., Laurin, J., and Sandoval, A. P. (2008). Marketing infant formula through hospitals: the impact of commercial hospital discharge packs on breastfeeding. *Am. J. Public Health* 98 (2), 290–295. doi:10.2105/AJPH.2006.103218

Saldaña, J. (2014). *Coding and analysis strategies, The Oxford handbook of qualitative research.*

Schwartz, D. A. (2020). An analysis of 38 pregnant women with COVID-19, their newborn infants, and maternal-fetal transmission of SARS-CoV-2: maternal coronavirus infections and pregnancy outcomes. *Arch. Pathol. Lab Med.* 144 (7), 799–805.

Seddighi, H., Salmani, I., Javadi, M. H., and Seddighi, S. (2019). Child abuse in natural disasters and conflicts: a systematic review. *Trauma Viol. Abuse* 97, 1–10. doi:10.1177/1524838019835973

Singh, G. K., Daus, G. P., Allender, M., Ramey, C. T., Martin, E. K., Perry, C., et al. (2017). Social determinants of health in the United States: addressing major health inequality trends for the nation, 1935-2016. *Int. J. MCH AIDS* 6 (2), 139.

Singh, N. S., Aryasinghe, S., Smith, J., Khosla, R., Say, L., and Blanchet, K. (2018). A long Way to go: a systematic review to assess the utilisation of sexual and reproductive health services during humanitarian crises. *BMJ Glob. Health* 3 (2), e000682. doi:10.1136/bmjgh-2017-000682

Sohrabizadeh, S., Sogand, T., and Khankeh, H. R. (2016). Women and health consequences of natural disasters: challenge or opportunity?. *Women Health* 56 (8), 977–993. doi:10.1080/03630242.2016.1176101

Tani, F., and Castagna, V. (2017). Maternal social support, quality of birth experience, and post-partum depression in primiparous women. *J. Matern. Fetal Neonatal Med.* 30 (6), 689–692. doi:10.1080/14767058.2016.1182980

The White House (2020). Proclamation on declaring a national emergency concerning the novel coronavirus disease (COVID-19) outbreak https://www.whitehouse.gov/presidential-actions/proclamation-declaring-national-emergency-concerning-novel-coronavirus-disease-covid-19-outbreak/?utm_source=link. Accessed August 13, 2020.

Tomori, C., Gribble, K., Aunchalee, E. L., Ververs, M.-T., and Gross, M. S. (2020). When separation is not the answer: breastfeeding mothers and infants affected by COVID-19. *Maternal & Child Nutrition*, 98, e13033.

United States Census Bureau (2020). Educational attainment in the United States: 2019. https://www.census.gov/data/tables/2019/demo/educational-attainment/cps-detailed-tables.html. Accessed August 12, 2020.

Weissman, A., Siegler, E., Ran, N., Peter, J., Etan, Z., and Zimmer, A. (1989). The Influence of increased seismic activity on pregnancy outcome. *Eur. J. Obstetr. Gynecol.* 31 (3), 233–236. doi:10.1016/0028-2243(89)90158-5

Weitzman, A., and Behrman, J. (2016). Disaster, disruption to family life, and Intimate partner violence: the case of the 2010 earthquake in Haiti. *Sociol. Sci.* 3 (9), 167–189. doi:10.15195/v3.a9

Wickrama, K. A. S., and Kaspar, V. (2007). Family context of mental health risk in tsunami-exposed adolescents: findings from a pilot study in Sri Lanka. *Soc. Sci. Med.* 64 (3), 713–723. doi:10.1016/j.socscimed.2006.09.031

World Health Organization (1981). *International code of marketing of breast-milk substitutes.* World Health Organization.

Xiong, X., Harville, E. W., Mattison, D. R., Elkind-Hirsch, K., Pridjian, G., and

Buekens, P. (2010). Hurricane Katrina experience and the risk of post-traumatic stress disorder and depression among pregnant Women. *Am. J. Disaster Med.* 5 (3), 181–187. doi:10.5055/ajdm.2010.0020

Zhang, W., Rajendran, K., Ham, J., Finik, J., Buthmann, J., Davey, K., et al. (2018). Prenatal exposure to disaster-related traumatic stress and developmental trajectories of temperament in early childhood: superstorm sandy pregnancy study. *J. Affect. Disord.* 234, 335–345. doi:10.1016/j.jad.2018.02.067

14

When Maintaining Relationships and Social Connectivity Matter: The Case of New Zealand Midwives and COVID-19

Susan Crowther[1†], Robyn Maude[2†], Billie Bradford[2†], Diana Austin[2†], Andrea Gilkison[1†], Judith McAra-Couper[1†] and Jayne Krisjanous[3†]*

[1]Centre for Midwifery and Women's Health Research, Faculty of Health and Environmental Studies, AUT University, Auckland, New Zealand, [2]School of Nursing, Midwifery, and Health Practice, Te Herenga Waka Victoria University of Wellington, Wellington, New Zealand, [3]Wellington School of Business and Government, Te Herenga Waka Victoria University of Wellington, Wellington, New Zealand

***Correspondence:**
Susan Crowther
susan.crowther@aut.ac.nz

New Zealand's response to COVID-19 was go hard and go early into Level 4 lockdown on 25th March 2020. This rapid response has resulted in low rates of infection and deaths. For New Zealand midwives, the sudden changes to how they work with women and families during pregnancy, birth and postnatally, especially in the community, required unprecedented innovation and adaptation. The volume of information coming from many different sources, and the speed with which it was changing and updating, added further stress to the delivery of a midwifery model of care underpinned by partnership, collaboration, informed choice, safety and relational continuity. Despite the uncertainties, midwives continued their care for women and their families across all settings. In the rapidly changing landscape of the pandemic, news media provided a real time account of midwives' and families' challenges and experiences. This article provides background and discussion of these events and reports on a content analysis of media reporting the impact on the maternity system in New Zealand during the initial surge of the COVID-19 pandemic. We found that the New Zealand midwife was a major influencer and initiator for relational care to occur uninterrupted at the frontline throughout the COVID-19 lockdown, despite the personal risk. The initial 5-week lockdown in March 2020 involved stringent restrictions requiring all New Zealanders, other than essential workers such as midwives, to remain at home. Midwives kept women, their families and communities central to the conversation throughout lockdown whilst juggling their concerns about keeping themselves and their own families safe. Insights gained from the media analysis suggest that despite the significant stress and upheaval experienced by midwives and wāhine/women, relational continuity facilitates quality and consistent care that honors women's choices and cultural needs even during situations of national crisis.

Keywords: midwives, New Zealand, COVID-19, continuity of care, lockdown, choice, media analysis, community

INTRODUCTION: THE NEW ZEALAND RESPONSE

The New Zealand (NZ) response to the initial surge of the COVID-19 pandemic was swift and decisive, resulting in a hard early lockdown, before any deaths occurred. This approach meant that NZ achieved low rates of infections and deaths compared to other high-income countries. These low rates of infections and mortality are due to the adoption of a set of early non-pharmaceutical interventions that explicitly focused on bringing COVID-19 incidence to zero (Jefferies et al., 2020). Transmission rates were kept low by a governmental coordinated national response that interrupted transmission chains centrally and locally across the country. The highest incidences were in popular tourist areas and at large events such as weddings; these were named "clusters." The stringent early lockdowns stopped large gatherings, travel restrictions were imposed, and the geographical location of NZ enabled borders to be closed. These measures helped contain the emergence of new clusters. At the time of writing (January 2021), anyone entering NZ is required to remain 2 weeks in a managed isolation quarantine (MIQ) facility and have two negative COVID-19 tests before entering the general population. New Zealand's success in the pandemic to date stems from early decisive government-led responses including robust surveillance systems, accessible testing and quarantine processes (Robert, 2020).

However, the suddenness and extent of the response had implications for the New Zealand midwifery workforce, whose overarching principles of care are partnership, collaboration, safety and relational continuity (Pairman and McAra-Couper, 2015). These principles are at the heart of *Te Tiriti o Waitangi*, New Zealand's founding document, of *Te Ao Māori* (the Māori world) and of New Zealand midwives' commitment to cultural safety (Farry and Crowther, 2014). Choice, safety and maintaining social connectivity are core values that midwives practicing in NZ sought to ensure for all women throughout the COVID-19 response. COVID-19 represented a defining moment for the NZ midwifery workforce, placing midwives in a quickly evolving situation requiring rapid accommodation of changes to practice.

The New Zealand government developed a 4-level Alert System to communicate restrictions in relation to the level of COVID-19 risk. The most stringent restrictions were at Alert Level 4, which required all New Zealanders, other than essential workers, to remain at home. During an almost 5-week lockdown starting on 25th March 2020 (MoH, 2020a), midwives continued to provide care to women and their families across all settings. Births at home and in standalone birth centers continued, and, in some cases demand reportedly increased. Yet much of this midwifery work continued unseen, within a system where midwifery consistently finds itself under-resourced, underpaid and relatively invisible to the government (NZIER, 2020).

The situation created by the COVID-19 pandemic highlighted the relative invisibility of midwives as frontline essential workers, despite continuous efforts by the NZ College of Midwives (NZCOM) to advocate for midwives. The constantly changing guidance from myriad sources from governmental, regulatory and district health boards, and difficulties accessing personal protective equipment (PPE) for all primary care providers, especially midwives—50% of whom practice in the community—in homes, standalone birth centers, and small community hospitals—imposed further stress on an already personally stressful pandemic reality. This article discusses evidence on midwives' and childbearers' experiences, with focus on an analysis of media reports on midwives and maternity in New Zealand during the initial surge of the COVID-19 pandemic. By analyzing how the issues, challenges and experiences, as narrated by relevant voices (midwives, maternity healthcare co-ordinators, wāhine/women and their whānau/families (these are Maori terms, now commonly used across New Zealand) in a rapidly evolving situation, we further illuminate the complexity and efforts to maintain the roles and relationships with women that New Zealand midwives upheld. In particular, our analysis reveals the near-invisible work midwives do in the community and how this work is frequently undervalued by policy makers. O'Connell et al. (2020) sent out an international call for midwifery solidarity during the emerging pandemic. This show of solidarity was clearly evident in the New Zealand context through the initiatives midwives took to mitigate the consequences of lockdown, including the leadership shown to support and make sure all childbearers and midwives were safe (NZCOM, 2020b).

THE NEW ZEALAND MATERNITY CONTEXT

New Zealand has a population of 4,951,500, with 59,637 births per year (Stats NZ, 2020). At the end of 2019, 3226 midwives held practicing certificates in NZ (Midwfery Council, 2019). Midwives in NZ are educated over a 4-year degree program at five tertiary institutions (Gilkison et al., 2016). Once registered, a NZ midwife is required to renew her practicing certificate annually. Midwives practice either as "core" midwives working as employees in hospitals or standalone birth centers or as "caseload" midwives—self-employed community-based midwives providing continuity of care from early pregnancy to 6 weeks postpartum within an established and integrated maternity care system. Caseload midwives predominantly work in the community and are called Lead Maternity Carers (LMCs). Most LMCs are midwives, although they can also be family physicians and obstetricians; currently 94.2% of women choose a midwife as their LMC (MoH, 2019). Core and caseload/ community midwives attend births together in hospitals and birth centers; they also often shift between these two roles. For example, a community midwife with young children may choose to work as a core midwife on shift for the regular hours, then change back to caseload work when those children are older. This frequent role-switching helps to ensure that all midwives maintain a shared philosophy of care. All maternity care in NZ, including midwifery LMC care, is fully government-funded and free to NZ citizens and residents, unless the childbearer chooses a specialist obstetrician (Guilliland and Pairman, 2010).

The overarching premise is that women choose and know the midwife who will work with them throughout their childbearing experience. Women access midwives through word of mouth, the internet, and referral from hospitals and family physicians. LMC midwives have caseloads ranging from one to eight women each month depending on region (e.g., variation in urban/rural/remote rural). An LMC midwife caring for four to six women per month is understood as practicing full time and needs to ensure 24/7 on call by herself or an arranged backup. LMC midwives are encouraged to work in group practices to moderate the constant 24/7 on-call commitment. New Zealand maternity care is women-centered, acknowledging pregnancy and birth as normal life events (MoH, 2011). The *midwifery philosophy of partnership* is based around communication, negotiation, equality, shared responsibility and empowerment, and informed choice and consent (Guilliland and Pairman, 2010). This midwife-wāhine/whānau collaboration acknowledges a sharing of each other's knowledge, experiences, skills, and feelings. Relationships with women and their families facilitate informed decision making and are identified as an attribute of autonomous midwifery practice that motivates New Zealand midwives to advocate for women across all practice settings and circumstances (Clemons et al., 2020). Midwives' expertise in building and sustaining relationships is intrinsic to this autonomy. Relational continuity is demonstrated through communication and negotiation, thereby building a trusting relationship over time with the client, her whānau and the community; together these elements provide the safety and acceptability of midwifery services (Davies and Crowther, 2020).

New Zealand maternity services are held in great regard internationally due to their high rates of maternal satisfaction and breastfeeding initiation and lower rates of cesarean births as compared to other high income countries (Rowland et al., 2012). Infant death has decreased by 41% from 7.3 to 4.7 between 1996 and 2017 (MoH, 2020b) and there has been an impressive reduction in stillbirths between 2007 and 2015 (PMMRC, 2018). The NZ stillbirth rate of 2.3 per 1,000 was reported in the *Lancet Stillbirth Series* at 10th lowest in the world (Flenady et al., 2016).

There are, however, ongoing concerns about the economic sustainability of the NZ midwifery model of care. A recent report prepared by the NZ Institute of Economic Research (NZIER) for the NZCOM highlighted pay equity as an "underlying factor in the sustainability of improving perinatal health outcomes" (NZIER, 2020, i). In addition, problems with midwife retention and staff shortages in some sectors and regions further exacerbate issues with workforce sustainability (NZIER, 2020). However, these reports of staff shortages are at odds with figures from Midwifery Council of NZ that reveal high numbers of midwives with current annual practicing certificates and increasing numbers of graduates in 2018/2019 (MCNZ, 2019). This discrepancy might be related to the ongoing struggles of midwives for pay equity when compared with others with comparable accountability and responsibility in their professional roles, such as obstetricians and family doctors, resulting in an increasingly vocal call to value the work of midwives (Berinstein et al., 2020).

To appreciate the resentment that such discrepancy causes, it is important to note the comprehensive and autonomous role of the midwife in New Zealand maternity services. The New Zealand midwife is responsible and accountable to the public and for the care she provides to the women in her caseload, including prescribing and administering medications within her scope of practice; to order, interpret and make decisions on many diagnostic and screening tests; perform full examination of the normal neonate; and repair most cases of perineal trauma. Although midwives' maternity care may occur in conjunction with consultation and/or transfer of aspects of care to medical colleagues when complex biomedical concerns arise, for the most part, the midwife continues to coordinate care throughout a woman's maternity experience. Another point of difference compared to other regions is that New Zealand midwives cannot be sued by women in their care, although a midwife can be held to account by the Midwifery Council of New Zealand for providing a poor standard of care (MCNZ, n.d.).

A long-anticipated announcement of increased funding for maternity services, particularly primary services in the 2020 national budget did not occur, to the great disappointment of the profession. However, in June 2020, during COVID-19 lockdown, community LMC midwives were compensated with a one-time payment of NZ$2500 for extra expenses incurred during the pandemic (Herald, 2020). Better remuneration of midwives continues to be an ongoing political issue that has now moved beyond just pay equity for midwives to also highlight the need to strengthen primary and community midwifery services. With midwives providing both hospital- and community-based care to women with increasing social and medical complexities, there is recognition that investment into primary maternity services, including midwifery, will have positive long-term benefits for maternal and child wellbeing (HDSR, 2020).

Lockdown and NZ Midwifery

On March 25th, 2020 the NZ government announced a state of emergency and the country moved to Alert Level 4 full lockdown.[1] The local and national implications were an immediate move to:

- Everyone staying at home in their "bubble."
- Everyone to maintain 2 m apart when out of the home.
- Only essential personal movement (e.g., health concerns, groceries).
- Only safe recreational activity allowed in a local area.
- All travel severely limited between regions and country borders closed.

[1]Two key concepts characterized the New Zealand COVID-19 response: the national Four-Level Alert System and the "bubble" concept. Initially developed by a group of medical researchers advising New Zealand's Ministry of Health on how to protect those with disabilities from COVID-19, the bubble concept became a mainstay of communication around how New Zealanders could minimize coronavirus transmission. A person's "bubble" is essentially their household; at times of increased risk of virus transmission, New Zealanders are encouraged to "stay in your bubble" or "don't break your bubble."

- All gatherings cancelled and all public venues closed.
- Businesses closed except for essential services (e.g., supermarkets, pharmacies, clinics, petrol stations) and lifeline utilities.
- All educational facilities closed.
- Rationing of supplies and requisitioning of facilities as possible.
- Reprioritization of healthcare services.

This was a rapid, decisive response, meaning the nation had just 48 h to organize all contingencies, including the logistics of maternity care provision. With much of the government and health system focused on preparing and equipping hospitals across the country for a potential torrent of COVID-19 admissions, frontline workers such as community-based midwives struggled to be seen and heard. Yet almost 5,000 babies were born during the 4 week period at Alert Level 4.

The early stages of the lockdown created the greatest degree of overwhelm, which was highlighted through NZCOM online forums and several social media chat sites. These forums foregrounded midwives' feelings of being ignored and having their concerns not taken seriously, particularly around what midwives experienced as poorly managed policy and guidance directives and a paucity of necessary equipment such as PPE. Their unease with the unfolding countrywide lockdown was compounded by the constantly changing guidance from myriad sources, both local and international, and difficulties of access to PPE in an already stressful situation.

A significant point of difference in the New Zealand context is that a large part of funded NZ midwifery care is provided in the community, including antenatal and postnatal care, as well as primary birthing (e.g., birth at home and in standalone birth centers). The COVID-19 lockdown brought a host of very real challenges for the NZ midwifery workforce as they continued to provide continuity of care in the community, despite potential risks to themselves, colleagues and families in the context of fear about the extent of community transmission. As most New Zealanders stayed at home in their "bubbles," community-based midwifery care continued across all settings, and indeed workload increased as women avoided going to hospital unless absolutely necessary. The increased community focus was caused by more home-based prenatal care and the increased demand for community births and for early discharge from hospitals for community postnatal care. (It must be noted that exact rates of this increased community activity are still being gathered at the time of writing). Choice, safety and maintaining social connectivity were core values that midwives sought to ensure for all women in all settings. In the rapidly changing landscape of the pandemic, news media provided real-time accounts of midwives' and families' challenges and experiences.

It became evident that there was much to learn about how to better prepare for any future pandemic and how to highlight the uniqueness of the NZ model of midwifery care, which consistently prioritizes and attunes to relationships and nurturing social connectivity for women, whānau, communities and their midwives. Although this spirit of generosity has been shown to help sustain NZ midwifery practice (Hunter et al., 2016), paradoxically, in the early part of the COVID-19 lockdown, this generosity of spirit appeared to be exploited. Initially, support came from within the profession itself. What was problematic and frustrating was that the organizational structures of the healthcare system appeared not to be listening and simply did not appreciate that babies would continue to be born during a pandemic, with inevitable additional workload demands on midwives. Yet over time, media outlets and social media platforms highlighted the work and contributions of midwives and their situation became progressively recognized. Consequently, we decided as a collaboration of NZ midwifery researchers to capture and report their voices for this Special Issue on *The Global Impacts of COVID-19 on Maternity Care Practices and Childbearing Experiences.*

METHODS: MEDIA CONTENT ANALYSIS

To capture the relevant voices and discourses during the pandemic and to understand how the media reported the impact of COVID-19 on midwives and maternity care, we conducted a qualitative content analysis of NZ media articles between December 2019 and July 25, 2020. Content analysis enables meaningful insights and interpretations to be drawn from textual data and is a useful tool to explore the role of midwifery in the context of a pandemic, as it provides the opportunity to systematically analyze a broad platform of commentary and reporting of news and events as they are occurring. While online news websites and journalism are popular press media and therefore may not be as reliable as, for example, actual ethnographic research, the benefits of wide audience reach offer a compelling reason for analysis of information content disseminated during an acute event such as COVID-19. We prioritized news websites over social media, as while social media is useful to analyse sentiment, is not a medium often used as an entry-point to a news item (Vermeer et al., 2020).

New Zealand Media and Search Strategy

Within NZ, print and online news outlets are governed by a duopoly between New Zealand Media and Entertainment (NZME) (publicly owned with main brands *NZ Herald* and Newstalk ZB) and Stuff (a publicly listed company). Stuff and the *NZ Herald* dominate audience share in online news (Myllylahti and Baker, 2019). We used the Stuff (stuff.co.nz) website—NZ's largest media website—to search for relevant material. Stuff owns nine major NZ newspapers, including the *DomPost* (Wellington circulation) and *The Press* (Canterbury circulation). In electing to use the Stuff website as our data collection site, we did omit a major NZ newspaper, *The Herald*, which has an Auckland circulation as well as further online readership throughout NZ. However, given the coverage of all New Zealand regions on the Stuff website, we determined that use of this website provided a robust way of representatively capturing news that New Zealanders would have been exposed to during the search period.

Using online media sources is also appropriate given that print media (newspaper, journal and magazine) circulation and subscription are decreasing, with most newspapers also offering an online source to complement print (Myllylahti and Baker, 2019). A sweep of *The Herald* to ensure that we were not missing key items not being reported on Stuff gave us confidence that conducting analysis of the Stuff website only would give us robust qualitative insights. The comparative count and weighting of topics discussed on the *Herald* website vis a vis the Stuff website was a reassuring equivalent. We note however that we do include reference to NZ *Herald* articles (along with quotations) that we deemed useful in describing midwives' reactions to a lack of PPE and increased workload.

Additionally, we conducted a search for articles printed in popular press magazines, particularly women's lifestyle magazines (*Woman's Day NZ* and *New Zealand Women's Weekly*) using Pressreader, Te Waharoa and Ebsco databases. No print articles were retrieved for our search period. This may have been due to Bauer Media NZ closing their New Zealand business during the COVID-19 lockdown, disrupting production and publishing of these and several other New Zealand print magazines. Initial treatment of retrieved articles involved reading each online article to ensure that it was valid for our research. Of the 89 articles that we reviewed, five were rejected as they featured stories from overseas (mostly about transmission of COVID-19 to newborns in other countries). A further 12 were removed from analysis as they were considered irrelevant to the research question about COVID-19 and its effect on NZ midwives. One article was a repeat. Ultimately, a total of 71 pertinent articles were retrieved[2] for analysis.

The Analysis Process

To undertake the content analysis, we downloaded all article links to an Excel spreadsheet. Coding was undertaken by co-authors Jayne Krisjanous and Diana Austin, who also provided their spreadsheet for scrutiny and feedback to other authors. These same co-authors conducted the analysis. Both consulted each other on what they had found, and impressions gained. Final themes were derived through a consensus between these two co-authors, who again presented their findings for feedback and any reiteration to the other authors. In order to analyze the 71 articles, a systematic process was applied that incorporated first identifying major categories (first order codes), followed by a second stage that identified themes (second order codes) within each of the major categories. When identifying the general themes within the article, rather than prime or drive themes by key words, we chose any relevant discourse as it was presented to its audience. Where several themes were present within one article, we allocated these accordingly.

[2]In order to retrieve articles from the Stuff website, we posted a combination of search terms into the Stuff website search option. These included "COVID + Birth" "COVID + Pregnancy", "Corona + Birth", "Corona + pregnancy" and "midwifery/ midwives + COVID."

FINDINGS: Wāhine, Whānau, and Midwives

The major categories identified were: 1) region or location where the events in the story had occurred; 2) categories within the Stuff website to which the article was allocated (e.g., national news, lifestyle, entertainment or sports); 3) key message source of information or opinion; and 4) story topic and focus. A second stage involved breaking the major categories into themes (second order codes). Four main themes emerged as most salient: the client (women's and their whānau (family) experiences; information regarding hospital visitor and support persons and policies; and two smaller categories, one on celebrity birth and another related to health professionals and other front-line staff workforce issues (*see* **Figure 1**). Here we report on the client, visitor/ support persons and midwife findings.

Wāhine/Women's Experiences

For the wāhine/women's theme, the quoted message source was almost always the woman/client. Sometimes partners (in this case, almost always the baby's father) also "spoke," particularly about their experiences. For articles about midwives, the NZCOM was consistently quoted (apart from two articles where an individual midwife was the key source). Another body of reporting tracked the movement of changes in hospital policies and visiting hours. During the period at Alert Level 4, regulations were communicated in a stringent tone; for women this meant that just one support person could be present for the birth and was required to leave soon after. (As other articles in this collection demonstrate, New Zealand appears to be unique in never completely prohibiting the presence of at least one support person.) As the country moved to lower Alert Levels and restrictions eased, the readership was informed of changes (e.g., from a single support person at the birth only to the addition of one visitor "per day" whilst an inpatient). For articles about hospital polices, a hospital spokesperson was the message source.

The client experience theme further broke down into women's emotional responses to the upheaval, location of birth (home, small rural maternity hospital, standalone birth center, or large hospital), and the impact on fathers. Most media attention was given to women's experiences overall. Women described birth during the Alert Level 4 period as "scary," "negatively affecting mental health," and "fraught" when in hospital, due to their partner having to leave soon after the birth. Although client experience articles rarely mentioned the midwife—a community or core (hospital or birth center) midwife—it is valid to assume that a midwife would have been influential in some way to overall impressions formed through her need to provide support in the absence of others, reconfigure service delivery and cope in potentially stressful environments.

Women indeed felt the absence of support networks immensely. The Prime Minister was featured in one article asking other New Zealanders to think of mothers needing to give birth at this time (Devlin, 2020), referencing her own birth approximately two years ago and knowing "how it felt." Some women reported feeling anxious in response to suggestions that

<table>
<tr><th>Major Categories</th><th>Description</th><th>Themes across major categories</th></tr>
<tr><td>Location of the story</td><td>Specific locale, town or city</td><td rowspan="4">• Wāhine/women's experiences
• Support persons and visitors (Information regarding hospital visitor and support person and policies)
• Two sub-themes:
➤ "celebrity" birth
➤ health professionals (e.g. midwives) and other front-line staff workforce issues.</td></tr>
<tr><td>Positioning of the article</td><td>National, lifestyle, world, sport and entertainment</td></tr>
<tr><td>"Voice"- the message source</td><td>Who is telling the story, the source</td></tr>
<tr><td>Story topic and focus</td><td>Varied</td></tr>
</table>

FIGURE 1 | Themes from media analysis.

they should consider home birth when they had been planning to birth in a hospital, while others who had planned to birth at home were equally as anxious that a midwife might not be available for their planned home birth (Biddle, 2020). The NZCOM reported via the media that they were fielding many inquiries about options for home birth (NZCOM, 2020a) whilst organizations, such as Home Birth Aotearoa, providing support to parents wishing to birth at home were inundated with requests for equipment and advice (Hannagan, 2020).

Support Persons and Visitors

The experiences of fathers (and in some cases grandmothers) were also reported. For fathers, not being allowed to visit their partner or baby from soon after birth till discharge was extremely stressful. One tragic incident involved the despair one father faced when his partner was transferred to the ICU and he could visit only in the final hours prior to her death, which was presumed to be from a blood infection following cesarean section and stillbirth at 21 weeks gestation (ND, 2020). In contrast, many women reported having an enjoyable time with maternity units quiet and without the normal intensity of visitors. Two articles talked about a baby "lockdown reunion" when Level 4 restrictions were lifted and extended families could reunite, and how novel the experience would be for them to talk about in the future (Steyl, 2020). Some women were disappointed that their babies would have no photographic memories of family around them at birth, although there was good evidence that social media networks were used as a substitutes for the lack of physical contact during this phase (Shaskey, 2020; Wilson, 2020). Apart from one woman claiming that maternity hospital staff "seemed confused" about visiting hours and regulations, when women's perspectives of midwifery care (both community and core) were discussed, views were positive (Steyl, 2020).

Midwives' Experiences

The total number of news articles that focused on midwives' work during the early stages of the New Zealand Covidian experience were few compared to the focus on clients' experiences. Sixteen stories of the 71 directly addressed midwifery service. Twelve discussed midwifery workforce issues. Of these, three reported the shortage of PPE for midwives, while most of the remainder discussed how midwives were needing to change their service delivery system during lockdown to phone consultations and reduced in-person appointment times. The telephone appointments were meant to reduce the length of in-person visits when physical distancing was being advised. At times, appointments consisted of blended visits in which most of the appointment could be done by telephone consultation followed by actual physical examination, if required, done within the 15 min guideline to minimize potential exposure to the virus. Apart from the two articles that directly quoted community-based midwives—one was positive, saying "It's all plain sailing," whereas the other discussed the midwives' lack of PPE—the NZCOM was the message source. When quoted, NZCOM was supportive of both midwives and women. For example, NZCOM recommended that women consider home birth, but equally reassured them that choice was theirs, and that wherever they chose to birth, they would be supported. One story that focused on midwives providing exceptional care was in Queenstown, where a local dental clinic had been set up to provide a birth space, as the normal unit was unavailable (Jamieson, 2020). The clinic had a temporary street-side shower added, which was unacceptable, so local midwives negotiated for their clients to be accepted into a hotel to birth in more congenial surroundings. The midwives themselves paid the reduced room fee.

Extending Our Search

Although not part of our initial search strategy, several other media outlets did highlight the midwifery situation further; we determined that these outlets needed to be included in this section. Midwives' desperate pleas for basic equipment such as PPE were evident in these media, adding to the fears of an already fearful public: "Midwives have made pleas on social media for industries no longer needing face masks, gloves and other personal protective gear, to donate or sell them" (Akoorie, 2020, Para 2). This extra work was highlighted as a serious issue during COVID-19: "It's concerning the extra lengths midwives are having to go to—just to look after their new mums, or mothers-to-be" (Hawkesby, 2020, para 1). There was already public awareness of the long-term struggles of midwives to be recognized for the work they do, and a reporter suggested that the pandemic "has only made it harder to be a midwife" because midwives "constantly having to explain changes to her women, when she's still trying to get information herself, has been hard" (Writes, 2020, para 21).

Despite midwives reported to have continued to support women in both the hospital and community environments, it was acknowledged that this support came at a cost. The pandemic has exposed a midwifery workforce already under stress and not recognized for the public health services these birth workers provide, and has potentially been "a tipping point for midwives" (Burrows, 2020, para 29). The style and content of reporting of midwifery services in the media during this period reflected the current context in which they are situated in the health system. Their limited visibility as a public health service fostering the wellbeing of families and the wider community resulted in a slow Ministry of Health and District Health Boards engagement with the profession to enable this core service to continue safely.

DISCUSSION: BIRTH CHOICES AND MIDWIFERY PRACTICE

The overall impressions of the media responses analyzed herein reveal the shaping of the New Zealand-generated public media discourse around birth during the most acute period of COVID-19 in NZ at the time of initial writing (September 2020). Our media content analysis has provided evidence of what news and commentaries the New Zealand public had available to them via the media that enabled them to construct their own perceptions. The greatest number of relevant articles appeared from February 2020 to April 2020. By May 2020, there were very few such articles appearing in the media sources we analyzed. It is fair to say that while media focus valued the experience and voice of the midwifery client and chose to foreground this in the main, any successes or difficulties midwives themselves were experiencing were communicated only through NZCOM, with few exceptions.

Birth Choices

The array of choices of birth place—home, primary small community hospitals, standalone birth centers, large hospitals—continued to be supported as safe, accessible and acceptable options, and were actively promoted throughout lockdown by NZCOM, midwifery leaders, the Royal Australia and New Zealand College of Obstetricians and Gynaecologists (RANZCOG) and many LMC midwives, and were reflected in the related media coverage. In addition, in NZ breastfeeding was at no time discouraged and all efforts were made to ensure that immediate mother-baby skin-to-skin contact and breastfeeding were supported, even for mothers who tested COVID-positive (Lowe and Bopp, 2020). Some midwives have reported up to a quarter of their wāhine/women birthing at home during Alert Level 4 (Bathgate, 2020; Biddle, 2020; personal communication from NZCOM Wellington regional meetings). We know that in the pre-COVID context, most New Zealand wāhine gave birth at a secondary facility—a hospital with special care for neonates (40.5%) or a tertiary maternity facility (which includes more extensive neonatal services and additional specialist services for inpatients) (45.5%); 10.5% of wāhine gave birth in a primary facility such as a standalone birth center or small community hospital; and 3.6% of wāhine had home births. These rates have been stable over the last 10 years (MoH, 2018). At the time of this writing, data for the COVID-19 period is not yet available and even anecdotal evidence seems unclear, so no conclusions about trends and differences in rates of out-of-hospital births can be made with confidence.

Initially there were some restrictions on birth partners', support persons' and others' (friends and whānau) attendance at hospital births (Brookes, 2020; Moore, 2020)[3]. There have been anecdotal stories from women of all ethnicities of feeling isolated, lonely and even traumatized by the visitor restrictions, particularly when partners were sent away so quickly after the birth. Some women chose to birth at home as a way of having their partner with them and avoiding breaking their bubble. Likewise, there have been reports of women choosing to go home from hospitals sooner than they would have liked. There was regional variation on how this aspect of postnatal care materialized. For example, one rural standalone birth center north of Auckland reported an increase in postnatal stays of women birthing elsewhere, then immediately transferring to the birth center so partners could be directly involved (personal communication, WWBC directors)[4]. The impacts on women and whānau of having restrictions around the presence of partners and support people during maternity admissions need to be more fully explored to avoid unnecessary harm (For such explorations, see the articles by Thayer and Gildner, Rivera, DeYoung and Mangum, Reyes, Rudrum, and Ozhiganova in this Special Issue).

Having significant others near at birth is a particularly culturally sensitive aspect for Indigenous Māori/Pasifika communities, for whom being with extended family is part of birthing culture. Despite many reports of positive experiences, some women did get separated from partners, whānau and significant others, with yet unknown negative cultural, spiritual and psychosocial consequences—especially for Māori and Pasifika childbearers, who perhaps felt less empowered to

[3]Doulas are not part of New Zealand maternity culture, partly due to the emphasise on midwives providing continuity of carer across jurisdictions and providing the relational continuity that doulas have been shown to provide in other regions.

[4]This refers to the Warkworth Birth Center, which has a unique setup, and thus may give the impression that all women can have this type of postpartum of care in New Zealand, which is unfortunately untrue. The NZ government does not provide resources for all families to experience this level of postnatal care provision. We mention it here to illustrate the extent of regional differences apparent across New Zealand.

speak out or exercise their choices, or lacked the resources to ensure that their needs were addressed in the context of the prevailing Eurocentric medical and political responses to the pandemic.

Foregrounding Midwifery Practice in a Pandemic

Our study has clearly demonstrated a resilient primary maternity service in which midwives have continued to provide partnership-oriented midwifery care, both in the community and in hospitals in the face of an emerging pandemic. Midwives' responses were characterized by a commitment to continue providing their services, underpinned by strong interactional and relational components, in both the hospital and community environments, whilst also trying to protect themselves and their clients. In New Zealand and elsewhere, midwives' efforts, passion, commitment, and skills required to maintain the best possible quality service in a uniquely challenging situation must not be forgotten or minimized in the complex milieu of pandemic health system responses. The extent of the embeddedness of the NZ maternity care system in the community is likely to be a contributing factor to this resilience. Yet it is imperative that added stress to midwives' workloads be acknowledged, as they were often the only health provider in contact with families throughout lockdown. Moreover, it has been highlighted elsewhere (including in most of the articles in this Special Issue) that the pandemic has hit women harder, partly because essential workers (such as midwives) are mostly female (Lim, 2020). Ensuring ongoing sustainability of maternity care during the pandemic requires the additional workloads of midwives during a pandemic to be resourced appropriately—for example with adequate PPE and payment equity.

Disputes around the value of women's work and its relative invisibility are historical and ongoing. For example, the "indeterminate" work of French women professionals has suggested that understanding occupational knowledge is a balance between indeterminacy and technicality (Jamous and Peloille, 1970). Jamous and Peloille described "technicality" as explicit knowledge using rules, protocols and taught skills (e.g., how to do an abdominal palpation to determine fetal growth and position), whereas "indeterminate knowledge" refers to tacit and private knowledge that resists rule-based protocols and measurable descriptions (e.g., forming relationships over time to build trust and safety, as midwives do). Comparing the pandemic responses of family physicians and midwives illustrates this point. The New Zealand government provided immediate funding of NZ $30 million ($19 million USD) for family physicians and pharmacists on the 2nd of April, yet the cost of the increased workload for midwives was not acknowledged until after the initial lockdown. Although family physicians of course are both male and female, the general perception of the medical profession in NZ is one of male domination, inferring ways of knowing and skills that are quite different from those of midwives, who are almost all women. Jamous and Peloille's seminal work reveals how women's work can be caught in a relentless, self-perpetuating system that fails to acknowledge women's professionalism and sees their work as less important than men's.

Arguably, much has changed for women and midwives over the last 50 years, yet many of these issues continue. Kirkham (2015) study of midwives in the UK showed that midwifery is often at best misunderstood and at worst exploited, leading to adversarial conditions for the professional midwife. Kirkham argued that midwifery work is often not prioritized because relationships and care are not counted as measurable commodities and therefore get afforded less value and are overlooked by economic and political systems. This focus undervalues midwives' significant emotional work of building and maintaining relationships. Yet it is well-established that relationships built and sustained over time enable intuitional ways of knowing that facilitate trust and safety (Davis-Floyd and Elizabeth, 1996; Crowther and Smythe, 2016). Furthermore, it is these relationships with women and families that support and sustain midwives' professional autonomy and their resultant enjoyment of practice (Clemons et al., 2020).

In the context of the pandemic, midwives are caught in a competitive fiscal environment that does not prioritize the significance of relationships, despite their obvious centrality to women's experiences as described in the media. Accepting that the core NZ midwifery value is *partnership*—the embeddedness of relationships with women, families and communities—suggests that any attempt to quantify in monetary terms the significance and value of this relational work could be detrimental (Davies et al., 2019). Yet it is vital that this relational work be afforded monetary value for midwives to be paid appropriately. The COVID-19 lockdown highlighted how midwives, women and communities are invested in these relationships despite the fiscal constraints caused by insufficient governmental investment in midwifery. The NZ midwife is proving to be a major influencer and initiator for relational care to occur uninterrupted at the frontline throughout the COVID-19 lockdown, despite the personal risk. Midwives kept women, their families and communities central to the conversation throughout lockdown, whilst juggling concerns about keeping themselves and their own families safe.

Women were at no point required to be COVID tested before birth. Everyone accessing healthcare is routinely asked screening questions, and staff apply PPE or test accordingly. This may relate to the fact that community transmission of the virus has been well-controlled in NZ. New Zealand midwives were not required to wear full PPE at home and in birth centers unless the wāhine or their whānau were either positive for COVID or been exposed and were awaiting test results. In these situations, women were advised to birth in the hospital. The recommendation for home and birth center settings was to provide care as normal using PPE as appropriate and to maintain physical distancing from other members of the whānau and support persons as much as is feasible in these primary settings. Each midwife determined the risk and donned PPE accordingly as the professional guidance evolved over time. Yet in the early phase of the pandemic, the ambiguous and changing guidance and lack of available PPE caused anxiety for many midwives.

With multiple job losses related to the pandemic for many workers, midwifery was able to establish itself more visibly as a core service and a secure career prospect. This positive Covidian outcome is offset by stress, low pay and midwives departing the workforce for these reasons—a factor that has a significant impact on recruitment to undergraduate midwifery programs. However, there could be a shift in that image, as a momentous boost to the maternity system was announced as we were finalizing this article: NZ maternity services will receive an extra NZ $180 million ($118 million USD), including a pay raise for midwives and particular consideration towards rural midwifery and the rising complexities related to birth. This is very good news for midwives and for the entire NZ maternity care system.

It is essential that NZ women, families and communities continue to receive quality equitable care across all regions. Therefore, attracting new midwives to the profession will be necessary to enable the workforce to strengthen and replace those for whom "enough was enough." Although COVID-19 brought heightened vigilance for personal safety and served to magnify midwives' employment conditions and pay inequities, there was never any doubt that women would be left without their midwives or be coerced into childbirth choices they did not want.

Despite the sudden challenges imposed by COVID-related lockdowns, midwives across NZ provided high quality, individualized care with passion and commitment, and continued to facilitate choice to the best of their capability within the imposed restrictions and resource concerns—which at times may have come at personal and professional costs. Ongoing informal communications about clinical practice concerns and how to ensure continuity of care whilst keeping the whānau/families they serve, themselves and their own whānau safe have been continuously highlighted in the NZ media. What was apparent when examining multiple media sources was lack of preparedness and an avalanche of changing guidance, leaving midwives vulnerable. This was set against a backdrop of a workforce that often already felt marginalized and unappreciated by policy makers and politicians, in which idiosyncratic midwifery relational knowing continues to be subjugated by dominant gender, neoliberal and biomedical discourses.

STRENGTHS AND LIMITATIONS

The strength of our study is that it has been conducted close to the phenomena being explored both in context and time. At the initial time of writing (September 2020), a further regional lockdown was occurring, highlighting the significance of this genre of work to ensure that voices and learnings are not lost. We note again the limitation of excluding *The Herald* database in our counting of articles for the media content analysis. We do believe that by doing this we have avoided any potential error confounded by duplication. Another limitation is our application of Western research methods, theoretical concepts, knowing and paradigms. These do not privilege *Te Tiriti o Waitangi* nor Indigenous knowledge; as New Zealand researchers we must acknowledge this as a limitation to our exploration. Media content analysis is a valuable and insightful telling of various stories, but the degree to which this also reflects the true lived experiences of midwifery practice, or indeed the cultural diversity of NZ, cannot be validated and requires further examination.

CONCLUSION: THE NEED FOR FULL RECOGNITION OF MIDWIVES' CONTRIBUTIONS

Whilst the world continues to grapple with the COVID-19 pandemic, NZ is now in the fortunate position of low infections and deaths relative to many other high-income countries. At the final time of writing (January 2021), we have continued to experience regional lockdowns, so conclusions about changes to outcomes or/and variation of choices of care can only be tentative. The premise of our article was to illuminate the complexity and efforts of New Zealand midwives during lockdown; however, based on the discussion points raised in combination with the content analysis of contemporaneous experiences reported in the media, an array of future related research is warranted. It is clear that midwives must be fully recognized for their contributions to society and for how their work influences the very warp and weave of NZ's social fabric—especially in a national crisis. Our media content analysis has contributed to foregrounding midwives' contributions. As Davies et al. (2019: 245) conclude:

> [The] continuity of care model works on the premise that the underlying philosophy of the midwifery profession supports a community based primary health service that strengthens family relationships and promotes normal birth...[this] supports the principles of social sustainability such as equity, social justice, community capacity...[and meets] the cultural and spiritual needs of women, their babies and families.

It is this social connectivity that enables women and their families to extend beyond prior expectations of childbirth and to flourish even in profoundly disruptive times of crisis. The COVID-19 disruptions further reveal what midwives in NZ aspire to do—which is to ignite the power that already and always rests with women through relationship-focused care. To be clear, women and midwives need not be empowered—they already and always have been empowered; they just need the circumstances for their power to emerge and flourish. Midwives have continued to provide their clients with exemplary and creative solutions to the unrelenting pandemic-imposed challenges throughout COVID-19 in NZ.

Irrespective of the global fear-based rhetoric and misinformation concerning maternity care, it is clear that NZ midwives, like the Puerto Rican, US, Canadian, Mexican, Chilean, Kenyan, Pakistani, and Guatemalan midwives described in other articles in this issue, showed fortitude during the worst of COVID-19 in NZ. Our media content analysis has revealed how NZ midwives have continued to the best of their ability in times of adversity to provide evidence based relational care that places women, their families and communities at the center of all care decisions. Long-term insights from this media analysis suggest that relational continuity facilitates quality and consistent care that honors women's choices, cultural needs, and human rights even during situations of national crisis. The healthcare needs of women, especially childbearing women, must remain priorities during pandemics and other disasters. The dedication of frontline midwives deserves our praise and appreciation. Midwives need to be heard, seen, understood, and treasured by policy makers and politicians. Only then can our midwifery colleagues receive the strong governmental mandate needed to continue to undertake their powerful and valuable work for society, including in times of crisis.

AUTHOR CONTRIBUTIONS

All authors have contributed to the conceptual framework of this article, data gathering and analysis as well as a final write up and agreed version now uploaded.

REFERENCES

Akoorie, N. (2020). Midwives have made please on social media for industries no longer needing face masks, gloves and other personal protective gear, to donate or sell them. *NZ Herald* (Accessed March 25, 2020).

Bathgate, B. (2020). Coronavirus: new life, and new birthing procedures, amidst the lockdown. *Stuff* Available at: https://www.stuff.co.nz/national/health/coronavirus/120792144/coronavirus-new-life-and-new-birthing-procedures-amidst-the-lockdown (Accessed April 5, 2020).

Berinstein, J., Ellen, B., and Guilliand, K. (2020). Valuing the labour of midwives in Ontario, Canada and New Zealand. *Sustainability, Midwifery and Birth* 64–80. doi:10.4324/9780429290558-4

Biddle, D.-L. (2020). Coronavirus: lack of protective gear means women may be forced to birth alone. *Stuff* (Accessed March 31, 2020).

Brookes, E. (2020). Lockdown birth: no visitors, epidural in doubt. *Stuff* (Accessed March 28, 2020).

Burrows, M. (2020). Coronavirus: midwives leaving their jobs 'in droves' as COVID-19 exposes culture of overwork, stress, poor pay. *Newshub* (Accessed May 13, 2020).

Clemons, J. H., Gilkison, A., Mharapara, T. L., Dixon, L., and McAra-Couper, J. (2020). Midwifery job autonomy in New Zealand: i do it all the time. *Women and Birth* 34, 30–37. doi:10.1016/j.wombi.2020.09.004

Crowther, S., and Smythe, L. (2016). Open, trusting relationships underpin safety in rural maternity a hermeneutic phenomenology study. *BMC Pregnancy Childbirth* 16 (370), 370. doi:10.1186/s12884-016-1164-9 Available at: http://rdcu.be/m0cN.

Davies, L., Crowther, S., and Hunter, B. (2019). "Midwifery continuity of care: theorising towards sustainability," in *Midwifery continuity of care*. Editors C. Homer, P. Brodie, and J. Sandall (Melbourne, Australia: Elsevier), 231–248.

Davies, L., and Crowther, S. (2020). The midwife as social connector. *Sustainability, Midwifery and Birth*, 83–98. doi:10.4324/9780429290558-5

Davis-Floyd, R., and Elizabeth, D. (1996). Intuition as authoritative knowledge in midwifery and home birth. *Med. Anthropol. Q.* 10 (2), 237–269. doi:10.1525/maq.1996.10.2.02a00080

Devlin, C. (2020). Coronavirus: Prime Minister Jacinda Ardern urges people be mindful of new mums. *Stuff* (Accessed March 29, 2020).

Farry, A., and Crowther, S. (2014). Cultural safety in New Zealand midwifery practice. Part 2. *Pract. Midwife* 17 (7), 30–33.

Flenady, V., Aleena, M., Middleton, P., Ellwood, D., Erwich, J. J., Coory, M., and et al. (2016). Stillbirths: recall to action in high-income countries. *The Lancet* 387 (10019), 691–702. doi:10.1016/S0140-6736(15)01020-X

Gilkison, A., Pairman, S., McAra-Couper, J., Kensington, M., and James, L. (2016). Midwifery education in New Zealand: education, practice and autonomy. *Midwifery* 33, 31–33. doi:10.1016/j.midw.2015.12.001

Guilliland, K., and Pairman, S. (2010). *The midwifery partnership*. 2nd Edn. Christchurch, New Zealand: New Zealand College of Midwives.

Hannagan, S. (2020). What Covid-19 means for women giving birth in Aotearoa: home birth aotearoa. Available at: https://homebirth.org.nz/what-covid-19-means-for-women-giving-birth-in-aotearoa/ (Accessed March 30, 2020).

Hawkesby, K. (2020). Midwives in crisis during Covid 19 coronovirus pandemic. *NZ Herald* (Accessed April 6, 2020).

HDSR (2020). Final report - Pūrongo Whakamutunga: health and disability system review. Available at: https://systemreview.health.govt.nz/assets/Uploads/hdsr/health-disability-system-review-final-report.pdf (Wellington).

Herald, N. Z (2020). Covid 19 coronavirus: cash injection brings relief but anxiety over long-term funding remains. *NZ Herald* (Accessed June 30, 2020).

Hunter, M., Crowther, S., McAra-Couper, J., Gilkison, A., MacGregor, D., and Gunn, J. (2016). Generosity of spirit sustains caseloading Lead Maternity Carer midwives in New Zealand. *New Zealand College of Midwives* 52, 50–55. doi:10.12784/nzcomjnl52.2016.8.50-55

Jamieson, D. (2020). Coronavirus: Queenstown lockdown baby born in a four-star hotel. *Stuff* (Accessed April 6, 2020).

Jamous, H., and Peloille, B. (1970). "Professions or selfperpetuating systems?' Changes in the French university-hospital system," in *Professions and Professionalisation*. Editor J. A. Jackson (Cambridge, UK: Cambridge University Press).

Jefferies, S., French, N., Gilkison, C., Graham, G., Hope, V., Marshall, J., et al. (2020). COVID-19 in New Zealand and the impact of the national response: a descriptive epidemiological study. *Lancet Public Health* 5 (11), e612–e623. doi:10.1016/S2468-2667(20)30225-5

Kirkham, M. (2015). Commodification around birth: sociology for midwives. Cambridge, UK: Polity Press.

Lim, E. (2020). COVID-19 BRIEF: impact on women and girls. *US Global Leadership Coalition* (Accessed August 10, 2020).

Lowe, B., and Bopp, B. (2020). COVID-19 vaginal delivery–a case report. *Aust. N. Z. J. Obstet. Gynaecol.* 60, 465–466. doi:10.1111/ajo.13173

MCNZ (2019). Annual report of the midwifery Council of New Zealand. Wellington, NZ: Midwifery Council Te Tatau o te Whare Kahu. Available at: https://www.midwiferycouncil.health.nz/common/Uploaded%20files/Annual%20reports/Midwifery%20Council%20Annual%20Report%202019.pdf.(Wellington).

MCNZ (n.d.). Concerns about a midwife Wellington. Wellington, NZ: Midwifery Council of New Zealand. Available at: https://www.midwiferycouncil.health.nz/ (Accessed December 2020).

Midwfery Council (2019). 2019 Midwifery workforce survey. Wellington, NZ: MCNZ

MoH (2020a). COVID-19 (novel coronavirus). Available at: https://www.health.govt.nz/our-work/diseases-and-conditions/covid-19-novel-coronavirus (Accessed August 8, 2020). Ministry of Health.

MoH (2020b). Fetal and infant deaths web tool. Wellington, NZ: Ministry of Health.

MoH (2011). New Zealand Maternity Standards: a set of standards to guide the planning, funding and monitoring of maternity services by the Ministry of Health and District Health Boards. Wellington, NZ: Ministry of Health.

MOH (2018). Report on maternity (2016). Wellington: Ministry of Health.

MoH (2019). Report on maternity 2017. Wellington, NZ: Ministry of Health.

Moore, R. (2020). Coronavirus: a Manawatu dad is separated from his premature baby in Wellington Hospital. *Stuff* (Accessed April 5, 2020).

Myllylahti, M., and Baker, S. (2019). JMAD (Journalism, Media and Democracy) New Zealand Media Ownership Report 2019. Auckland: AUT.

ND. (2020). Auckland DHB investigating after increase in maternal deaths. *Stuff* (Accessed May 30, 2020).

NZCOM (2020a). *Media release: midwives baffled and disappointed by lack of govt financial support.* Aotearoa, NZ: New Zealand College of midwives. Available at: https://www.midwife.org.nz/news/midwives-baffled-and-disappointed-by-lack-of-govt-financial-support/ (Accessed April 21, 2020).

NZCOM (2020b). *Special Covid-19 online edition.* Aotearoa, NZ: Midwife Aotearoa New Zealand. (Accessed June, 2020).

NZIER (2020). *Sustainable midwifery: supporting improved wellbeing and greater equity.* Christchurch, New Zealand: NZCOM.

O'Connell, M., Crowther, S., Ravaldi, C., and Homer, C. (2020). Midwives in a pandemic: a call for solidarity and compassion. *Women and birth* 33 (3), 205–206. doi:10.1016/j.wombi.2020.03.008

Pairman, S., and McAra-Couper, J. (2015). "Theoretical framewworks for midwifery practice," in *Midwifery: preparation for practice.* Editors S. Pairman, J. Pincombe, C. Thorogood, and S. K. Tracy, (Elsevier Health Sciences APAC), 386–411.

PMMRC (2018). Twelfth annual report of the perinatal and maternal mortality review committee: reporting mortality 2016. Wellington: Health Quality & Safety Commission.

Robert, A. (2020). Lessons from New Zealand's COVID-19 outbreak response. *Lancet Public Health* 5 (11), e569–e570. doi:10.1016/S2468-2667(20)30237-1

Rowland, T., McLeod, D., and Froese-Burns, N. (2012). *Comparative study of maternity systems.* Wellington, NZ: Malatest International consultant and advisory services.

Shaskey, T.(2020). Coronavirus: 'Scary and uncertain time' for mothers and midwives. *Stuff* Available at: https://www.stuff.co.nz/taranaki-daily-news/news/120847610/coronavirus-scary-and-uncertain-time-for-mothers-and-midwives (Accessed April 13, 2020).

Stats, N. Z (2020). Stats NZ Tatauranga Aotearoa. *Population.* Available at: https://www.stats.govt.nz/topics/population (Accessed August 5, 2020).

Steyl, L. (2020). Fond memories for parents of lockdown babies. *Stuff* Available at: https://www.stuff.co.nz/life-style/121933230/fond-memories-for-parents-of-lockdown-babies. (Accessed June 25, 2020).

Vermeer, S., Trilling, D., Kruikemeier, S., and de Vreese, C. (2020). Online news user journeys: the role of social media, news websites, and topics. *Digital Journalism* 8 (9), 1114–1141.

Wilson, L. (2020). Baby Anahera made her entrance just before lockdown, providing 'good news in a stink time. *Stuff* Available at: https://www.stuff.co.nz/life-style/parenting/baby/120651826/baby-anahera-made-her-entrance-just-before-lockdown-providing-good-news-in-a-stink-time.

Writes, E. (2020). Covid-19 has only made it harder to be a midwife. *Spinoff* (Accessed May 5, 2020).

15

When the Masks Come Off in Canada and Guatemala: Will the Realities of Racism and Marginalization of Midwives Finally be Addressed?

Betty-Anne Daviss[1,2*], *Tammy Roberts*[3], *Candace Leblanc*[4], *Iris Champet*[5], *Bernadette Betchi*[6], *Angela Ashawasegai*[4] *and Laura Gamez*[7]

[1] *The Pauline Jewett Institute of Women's and Gender Studies, Faculty of Arts and Social Sciences, Carleton University, Ottawa, ON, Canada,* [2] *l'Hôpital Montfort and The Ottawa Hospital, Midwifery Divisions, Ottawa, ON, Canada,* [3] *Independent Researcher, Elliot Lake, ON, Canada,* [4] *Independent Researcher, Ottawa, ON, Canada,* [5] *Asociación para la Promoción, Investigación y Educación en salud en el Occidente de Guatemala (PIES), Quetzaltenango, Guatemala,* [6] *Algonquin College, Ottawa, ON, Canada,* [7] *Independent Researcher, Hamilton, ON, Canada*

Correspondence:
Betty-Anne Daviss
bettyannedaviss@gmail.com

This article addresses the effects of COVID-19 in Eastern and Northern Ontario, Canada, with a comparative glimpse at the small province of Totonicapán, Guatemala, with which Canadians have been involved in obstetric and midwifery care in particular over the last 5 years. With universal health care coverage since 1966 and well-integrated midwifery, Canada's system would be considered relatively well set up to deal with a disaster like COVID-19 compared to low resource countries like Guatemala or countries without universal health care insurance (like the USA). However, the epidemic has uncovered the fact that in Ontario, Indigenous, Black, and People of Color (IBPOC), as elsewhere, may have been hardest hit, often not by actually contracting COVID-19, but by suffering secondary consequences. While COVID-19 could be an issue through which health care professionals can come together, there are signs that the medical hierarchies in many hospitals in both Ontario and Totonicapán are taking advantage of COVID-19 to increase interventive measures in childbirth and reduce midwives' involvement in hospitals. Meanwhile, home births are on the rise in both jurisdictions. Stories from a Jamaican Muslim woman in Ottawa, an Indigenous midwifery practice in Northern Ontario, registered midwives in Eastern Ontario, and about the traditional midwives in Guatemala reveal similar as well as unique problems resulting from the lockdowns. While this article is not intended to constitute an exhaustive analysis of social justice and human rights issues in Canada and Guatemala, we do take this opportunity to demonstrate where COVID-19 has become a catalyst that challenges the standard narrative, exposing the old ruts and blind spots of inequality and discrimination that our hierarchies and inadequate data collection—until the epidemic—were managing to ignore. As health advocates, we see signs that this pandemic is resulting in more open debate, which we hope will last long after it is over in both our countries.

Keywords: Canada, COVID-19, Guatemala, IBPOC, racism, social justice, midwifery

INTRODUCTION: A GLIMPSE AT SOME OF THE SOCIAL JUSTICE ISSUES IN ONTARIO AND TOTONICAPÁN, GUATEMALA

I was up late dealing with two births, exhausted, and developed a fever of 38.1 Celsius (100.6 Fahrenheit). I knew that I would have to go to the local hockey arena—the setting designated as the COVID testing site in Ottawa, Canada. I thought, how great a thing to have it in an ice hockey arena, where everybody should feel at home because they are familiar with the setting. Indigenous, Asian, Somali, Lebanese, Punjabi, and White families alike can take advantage of our Rideau Canal when it freezes over in winter—"the longest skating rink in the world"—winding through and connecting various parts of the city and the many ice hockey arenas. It was a sight to behold. There at Brewer's Arena, everybody lined up like good sports, no ethnicity, race, class, profession, or gender being given priority—except kids, who, with their parents, were afforded a private entrance up to the bleachers where they got to wait until their turn came and to pretend that they were watching a game down on the rink.

The rink—bereft of ice—was now covered with us would-be "game contestants" sitting dutifully on the edges of our fold-up black chairs, all neatly lined up a hockey stick apart (i.e. 6 ft). After each of our OHIP[1] cards had been checked, we had to give the history about why were there: we were phoned by a friend that they had COVID, we had traveled, or we had symptoms. As the "Head Coach" on the microphone called out our names, we were instructed politely to turn our chair around as we rose so that the chair cleaners could easily identify those needing to have any COVID cooties whisked away with disinfectant. From there we got to get our poke in the nose.

Yet while we were all treated equally during this testing process, I knew that we were not all going home to equitable housing. We were not all returning to secure jobs, the same ability to social distance or feed our kids and grandkids during this time. And aware that women of color are one of the hardest groups hit with COVID, especially those working in nursing homes, I thought that they were the ones who actually should *be given priority in the lines. And then I began to google hockey and racism, and was struck by the trouble on our hockey rinks, where immigrants send their kids, knowing it will help them blend into the social fabric in small towns, Ottawa, and Montreal—but where they are subjected to racial slurs. Who knows but maybe one of those little boys or girls were reliving their first incident of racism in this very arena as they sat up there in the bleachers? Canadians may have a society that prides itself on trying to be fair, but COVID-19 is providing us ample opportunity to re-evaluate our concept of ourselves.*

-Betty-Anne, reflections from the COVID testing arena, 2020

A comparison about pandemic effects between a province in a high resource country (Canada) and one in a low resource country (Guatemala) might seem unfair, like comparing apples with oranges. In 2017, maternal mortality in Guatemala was 95/100,000[2] and in Canada was 10/100,000 births[3]. Guatemala has the sixth-highest rate of chronic malnutrition (stunting or low height-for-age) in the world—at 47% percent—with the prevalence reaching around 70% in Totonicapán[4]—the Guatemalan province we wanted to compare with the province of Ontario, Canada.

Despite these large differences, comparisons can expose the good and the bad of any health care system, and this article reveals some surprising similarities between our two countries. Both countries at least profess to have universal health care, but the Indigenous populations in both countries suffer more from malnutrition, poverty, education, and health care disparities than others. Canada boasts well-integrated midwifery services and complete government funding for birth at home, birth center, or hospital. Guatemala has midwifery services, but they are unsupported by the government. As in other countries, COVID-19 has exposed the inequities in the Canadian social/health and welfare system. In this article, we present an overview of how, with some success, we have dealt with COVID-19 in the province of Ontario, but also how it has negatively affected populations with health and economic disparities, in particular IBPOC[5] people, forcing, among other measures, racial/ethnic data retrieval to become a priority.

This Introduction is providing an overview and will explain how we came up with our methodology for the comparison. A brief review of historical events demonstrating the prevalence of racism in both countries provides some context to understand what has led to inequities in the health care systems.

The section, The Effects of COVID-19: Which Populations Are Suffering Most? will compare COVD-19 cases and death rates in Canada and Guatemala and what ethnicities/races are most affected. It becomes evident that while racism has manifest as violent genocide and unbridled femicide in Guatemala, in Ontario, attempts to address subtle racism have been predominantly performative and symbolic.

Section Childbirth in Ontario under the Strain of COVID-19: Information Dissemination and Canadian Compliance explains the backdrop of compliance among Ontario citizens with COVID-19 followed by intimate first-hand accounts about the lockdown from:

1. a solo Registered midwife in Northern Ontario who describes the effect on her work among Indigenous communities, Amish and Mennonite communities (Section Northern Ontario Narrative);
2. midwives in Eastern Ontario who describe both increased collaboration and increased tension among the professions as a result of COVID-19 and
3. a Jamaican Muslim woman who describes an experience of subtle racism in hospital in Ottawa (Section How COVID-19 Has Affected Maternity Care In Eastern Ontario).

[1]OHIP: Ontario Health Insurance Card which all Ontario residents are entitled to and which pays for all of their health care, including all perinatal care, excluding only dentistry, pharmaceuticals, and extraordinary luxuries like *in-vitro* fertilization.

[2]https://www.indexmundi.com/guatemala/maternal_mortality_rate.html

[3]https://www.indexmundi.com/canada/maternal_mortality_rate.html

[4]https://www.usaid.gov/sites/default/files/documents/1864/Guatemala-Nutrition-Profile-Mar2018-508.pdf

[5]IBPOC: Indigenous, Black, and People of Color.

In the section, How COVID-19 Has Affected Maternity Care In Eastern Ontario data is presented on the socio economic status of Ontario midwife clients and how their choice for home birth increased quickly with the onset of COVID-19.

The section on Guatemala: Experiences Among the Traditional Midwives of Guatemala, provides narratives about the traditional Indigenous midwives' experience in Totonicapán, revealing similar as well as unique problems compared to Ontario midwives from the pandemic lockdowns.

We offer this work as a means to understand the problems and articulate how to improve those systems that are inherently racist, colonialist, sexist, white cisnormative, and biased toward a medical hegemony. Midwives, nurses, and physicians working with these populations often see (but do not always work on rectifying) the inequities, the biases, and the vulnerabilities. They also fall prey to trying to mitigate a system that can either become increasingly abusive or more forgiving during a pandemic—or both—as we will describe below.

Methodology

This article was first conceived when a Vancouver, B.C. midwifery practice and Betty-Anne Daviss, a cisgender white midwife who began her midwifery career 45 years ago working with traditional midwives in Guatemala and now works in Ontario, jointly approached the National Aboriginal Council of Midwives (NACM) to solicit their engagement in a national article about COVID-19.

Betty-Anne also contacted the co-ordinators of the "Maternal, Newborn, and Child Health (MNCH) Project: Reducing Gaps for Indigenous Peoples in Totonicapán, Guatemala," a project, which started in 2016 and will end in 2021, implemented by Horizons of Friendship (Horizons), a Canadian international development organization, and the Association for Health Promotion, Research and Education in the Western highlands of Guatemala (PIES de Occidente) working in Totonicapán. The exchanges between Betty-Anne and the staff at Horizons and PIES facilitated insights on how COVID-19 was affecting the people in the region[6].

It was difficult to interview individual Maya K'iche' traditional midwives—called *comadronas*—in a "department" (province/state) where Spanish is the second language, where the high school literacy rate is 17.6%[7], and where internet access is intermittent or limited. Some comadronas have email but the answers are not always forthcoming, or are very short. We decided to use the synopsis of what is happening in Totonicapán from the coordinator of the MNCH project at PIES, Dr. Iris Champet. Laura Gamez, who currently manages the Horizons of Friendship' MNCH project and has worked in other programs in Central America and Mexico, on conflict resolution, peacebuilding, policy development, and the delivery of humanitarian aid for forcibly displaced populations, provided invaluable commentary and edits on the situation in Guatemala.

While NACM thought the project important, their board cautioned that they did "not have the capacity to research and write a piece at this time. Indigenous midwives should be the ones doing this research and writing, from their own perspectives, but we cannot do this now." Soon after, the Vancouver midwives dropped out of the project because of difficulties in accommodating to COVID-19 life/work challenges with their young families.

The focus was then narrowed to address the effects of COVID-19 in Eastern and Northern Ontario, Canada, to compare it with the department (province) of Totonicapán, Guatemala. Betty-Anne sent out an email with open and closed questions, to all midwives in the Eastern region of Ontario (approximately 50), about how COVID-19 has affected their practice and their clients. At first she received little response, she assumed, because of all the extra COVID-19 updates, complicated briefs, new rules, multiple types of PPE to try, and the feeling that danger was lurking everywhere, and the midwives were "COVIDed-out." But the answers of the three who did respond were very enlightening, and she had other means through which to pry—occasional face-to-face workshops and online meetings, with follow-up clarifications via email.

Two Indigenous midwife practices in Eastern Ontario and three in Northern Ontario were approached. One Indigenous practice in each of the regions immediately responded with interest, one saying they would approach Six Nations as well to offer the story from their viewpoint about what was transpiring. A sign of the times, only one came through—Tammy Roberts, a midwife working with four Indigenous communities as well as non-Indigenous communities around Elliot Lake.

Betty-Anne then approached two midwifery clients who are activists in the IBPOC community: Candace Leblanc, who has been both a doula and a La Leche League Leader in Ottawa; and Bernadette Betchi, born in Cameroon, who grew up in Canada, worked as Sophie Gregoire Trudeau's Communications specialist and press secretary and then chose to leave for a job with the Human Rights Commission of Canada (see **Figure 1**). Both were instrumental in helping the article take shape with their perspectives as members of the IBPOC community.

We sought data regarding disparities among socio-economic groups and ethnicities and to study whether choice of birth settings changed following the pandemic. We solicited narratives from both clients and midwives to bring forward concerns and experiences navigating the pandemic—stories that cannot be told through any database. The questionnaire for both Indigenous and white settler practices asked:

1. Whether or not they had had any COVID-19 cases and how those were dealt with, clinically, logistically, and emotionally; what the compliance of clients and midwives was to the use of PPE (personal protective equipment) and lockdown procedures.
2. Whether dealing with the constraints of COVID-19 may have improved relations and unified forces at the hospital but also

[6]As part of the project, an initiative funded by Global Affairs Canada, Canada-Guatemala knowledge exchanges were set up by PIES de Occidente (The Association for Health Promotion, Research, and Education) and Horizons of Friendship, a Canadian international development organization.

[7]http://www.thedialogue.org/wp-content/uploads/2017/02/Educational-Challenges-in-Guatemala-and-Consequences-for-Human-Capital-and-Development.pdf

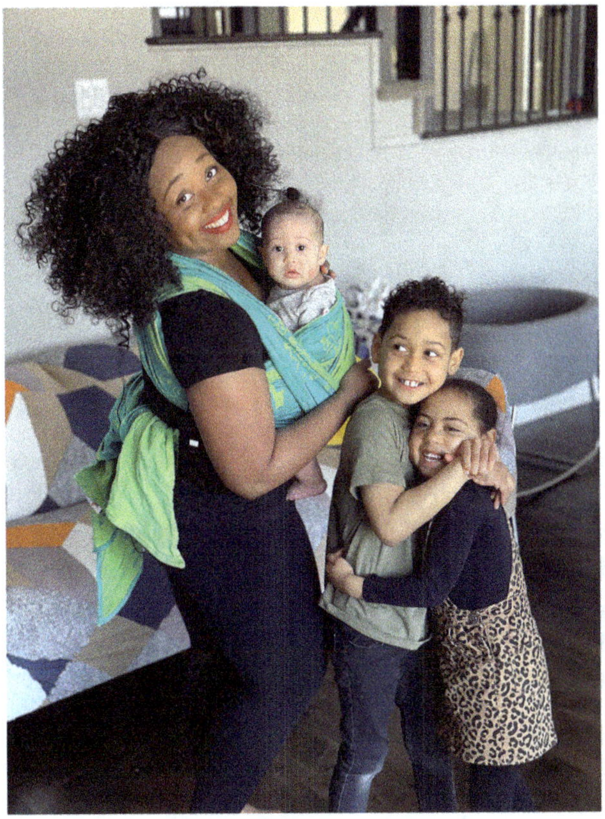

FIGURE 1 | Bernadette Betchi recently joined in the Black Class Action Lawsuit in the Federal Court of Canada. She is employed by the Canadian Human Rights Commission. Her career with the Public Service began at the Canada Revenue Agency. "My experience working there was emotionally and physically draining. I moved from team to team, was bridged in as a term employee, while my white counterparts were all given permanent and higher positions right away." She is seeking concrete, permanent solutions to undo the damage that has already been done, but looking ahead, for her children and their children, so they don't ever have to go through what her family is going through.

how the situation may have laid bare the limitations of the health care infrastructure.

3. Whether COVID-19 changes had improved or exacerbated structural inequalities for marginalized communities.
4. What other experiences indicated strengths or weaknesses, in the model of care around childbirth in their jurisdiction.

Ontario, Canada: Some Good Health and Social Safety Nets Yet Colonialism and Racism Still Intact

Canadians have generally prided themselves on using government in positive ways. In fact, Canadians of all ethnicities have generally come to expect their government to ensure basic social programs—universal health care, unemployment insurance, education, social assistance, and human rights. Even if racism abounds, many Canadians are programmed at least to *believe* that everyone deserves to have the resources they need.

Because social programs express guarantees of human rights and commitments by governments to redistribute resources and to intervene in the market and the family to create equality, we are criticized by our US neighbors for harboring "socialism," a branding which, hopefully, most of us wear proudly. However, over the last 15 years, a series of declarations and national truth commissions have exposed and shaken our foundation of pride in our system, exposing white privilege in Canada, starting first with regard to Indigenous rights:

1. The United Nations Declaration on the Rights of Indigenous Peoples (UNDRIP, United Nations Press Briefing, 1999) was adopted by the UN on September 13, 2007 to enshrine the rights that "constitute the minimum standards for the survival, dignity and well-being of the indigenous peoples," which Canada shamefully at first did not agree to endorse.
2. The Canadian Truth and Reconciliation Commission (TRC) exposed the crimes of the Fathers of Confederation in establishing the residential school system, now acknowledged as a "cultural genocide" agenda to strategically take over Indigenous lands by eliminating Indigenous peoples' governments, language, and culture, by "killing the Indian in the child" in these schools (Truth and Reconciliation Commission in Canada, 2015, p. 1).
3. The Final Report of the National Inquiry into Missing and Murdered Indigenous Women and Girls (MMIWG) revealed that persistent and deliberate human and Indigenous rights violations and abuses are the root causes of Canada's staggering rates of violence against Indigenous women, girls and 2SLGBTQQIA people[8].
4. The Sixties Scoop Settlement Agreement of 2018 was the result of winning a 9-year court case brought against the federal government by Indigenous people who suffered the loss of cultural identity when placed in white adoption and foster homes starting in the 1950s (https://sixtiesscoopsettlement.info). The principle of the financial settlement is a step in the right direction to begin the healing journey for their loss of cultural identity. But in the words of one of our authors, Angela Ashawesegai, it goes deeper: "I want closure for the historical abuse trauma. I was a child household slave and abused mentally, physically, and/or sexually on a daily basis. I'm still living with the haunting psychological impacts. We've only gone halfway with reconciliation with Canada." (see upcoming book Lost Between Two Worlds: A 60's Scoop Adoptee's Search for Belonging forthcoming, 2020) (see **Figure 2**).

These events have somewhat shifted Canadian cultural understandings in a positive way toward expressed common goals. Since they transpired, grants for Indigenous midwifery in Canada have increased and a small but important exchange with Guatemalan health care providers included acknowledgment and respect for their traditional midwives because of their Indigenous rights. The latter is a milestone, as it is in direct

[8]2SLGBTQQIA stands for 2Spirit, Lesbian, Gay, Bisexual, Transgender, Queer, Questioning, Intersex, and Asexual. Available online at: https://www.mmiwg-ffada.ca/wp-content/uploads/2019/06/Final_Report_Vol_1a-1.pdf.

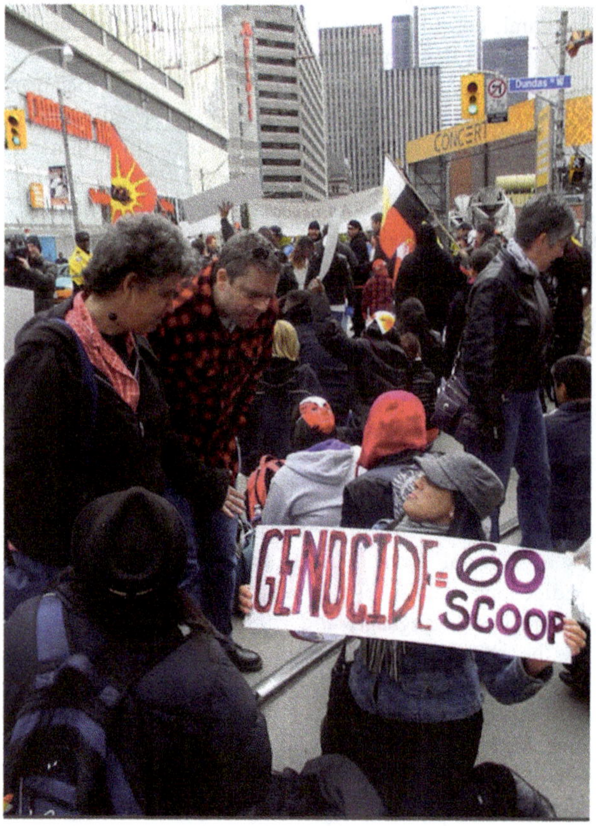

FIGURE 2 | Two sympathetic passers-by stop to talk with 60s Scoop survivor, Angela Ashawasegai, at a rally in Toronto in 2011. Like most Canadians, they had never heard of the 60's Scoop or of the historical abuses of Indigenous children at the hands of White adoption and foster families until rallies and news media started drawing attention to it. Angela is now a certified trauma therapist, specializing in 60's Scoop trauma & Complex PTSD.

opposition to the WHO/FIGO/ICM[9] decision to instead stop the funding of traditional midwives, with little consideration of the negative effects on their communities (WHO, 2004).

Meanwhile, Black Lives Matter and other groups are finally gaining more attention to their persistent message of many years—that racism is very much alive in Canada, just as in the US, yet not the national priority it is becoming there (DasGupta et al., 2020; Desmond, 2020).

One of our authors, Bernadette Betchi, made a decision, along with over 600 other Black federal employees, that the time was rife in 2020 to finally launch a class action suit-long time coming– against the various federal departments in which they work[10]. They want to draw attention to the racism they find evident in so many parts of their lives, with intersections not even considered, starting with the very institutions that should be safeguarding human rights (see **Figure 1**).

Racism is rooted in a system that has been intentionally created in a way to benefit a very specific demographic. While COVID-19 and the uprisings following the George Floyd and Breonna Taylor killings were not the reason to launch the class action suit, the confluence of these events created a world that is now watching and listening, even in Canada. We suggest that the work done thus far by all political parties has been predominantly performative and symbolic in Canada. It will take some serious changes and a shift of mindset to dismantle the system of oppressions in which we live and that benefit some Canadians more than others.

Totonicapán, Guatemala: Following Genocide Attempts, Indigenous Groups Are Gaining Some Recognition of Their Own Systems and Values

The Mayan K'iche', Mam, Kakchiquel, Kekchi, and other Indigenous groups have become more politically successful since the widely publicized exposure of the genocide carried out on their peoples by a succession of national military governments supported by the US (United Nations Press Briefing, 1999). The 36-year civil war saw the genocide of more than 160,000 Indigenous people (Horizons, 2018). One report says that the Mayan Quiché, living in the departments of Quiché, Huehuetenango, and Totonicapan (the department we are studying), were the victims of 80% of the massacres, "the worst hit of all the indigenous groups in Guatemala during the war [and which] remains the most discriminated against because of its past" (Research Directorate, 1998). Another report says that Totonicapán itself was less affected than some of the other communities, priding itself on being able to strongly protect its ancestral rights[11]; 98% of its population identify as Indigenous (Guatemalan Census, 2008).

Besides the historical and ongoing discrimination and marginalization of the Mayan Kiche' people as a whole, as more than 100,000 Indigenous women were victims of mass rape and forced into sexual slavery for the military (Horizons, 2018), women face an additional risk *because they are women.* Guatemala has the third highest femicide rate[12] in the world. In spite of the fact that Guatemala championed a decree about femicide in its constitution in 2008[13], 685 women were assassinated in Guatemala in 2010, compared to 213 in 2000

[9]The World Health Organization, International Confederation of Midwives, and International Federation of Gynecology and Obstetrics describe a *skilled attendant* is an accredited health professional—such as a midwife, doctor, or nurse—who has been educated and trained to proficiency in the skills needed to manage normal (uncomplicated) pregnancies, childbirth, and the immediate postnatal period, and in the identification, management and referral of complications in women and newborns (World Bank, 2018 p. 1). This definition excludes traditional midwives. In Daviss and Davis-Floyd (2021) we seek acknowledgment of the tireless and fearless expertise they often provide for their communities, and of the need to integrate them into health care services instead of eliminating them.

[10]https://www.blackclassaction.ca/plaintiffs

[11]https://d2071andvip0wj.cloudfront.net/totonicapan-tension-in-guatemalas-indigenous-hinterland.pdf

[12]The murder of women, committed by men, for the simple reason of their being women (http://www.oea.org/es/mesecvi/docs/DeclaracionFemicidio-EN.pdf).

[13]https://www.theguardian.com/healthcare-network/2018/mar/07/health-workers-stop-thousand-women-killed-guatemala-femicide and https://www.insightcrime.org/news/analysis/why-does-latin-america-have-the-world-s-highest-female-murder-rates/.

(Nobel Women's Initiative, 2012). Between 2000 and 2019, more than 11,594 women were victims of violence[14].

The Nobel Women's Initiative also says that more than 95% of crimes against women are never even investigated by authorities because of the "machismo" that prevails in Mexico, Honduras, and Guatemala. This has normalized the violence and provided excuses for it.

More than 80% of the Maya K'iche' live below the poverty line. A large percentage of the population also lacks access to basic services like healthcare, education, clean water, and sufficient food (Horizons, 2018). Protests over mining and hydroelectric projects, educational reform, and access to land and public utilities[15], and evangelical Christians wanting to impose their religion on Indigenous Mayan tradition[16], occur in tandem with increased community demand that the traditional midwives become acknowledged and receive at least a token financial contribution from their government (Daviss, 2021).

Following amnesty after the war, a universal health care system was established, at least on paper (Pena, 2013). However, it has been hard to guarantee due to limited government resources and other problems regarding access. Studies from foreign goodwill ambassadors continue to lament the fact that Indigenous peoples in Guatemala do not often access modern reproductive health care (Ishida et al., 2012). However, PIES de Occidente chooses not to limit the definition of "good care" to one exclusively viewed through a modern medical lens, since it is well-known that the medical approach to birth conducts unnecessary inductions, forceps, and cesareans at high cost financially and to women's bodies (Anderson et al., 2021). As a result, the Canadian/Guatemalan exchanges strategically emphasize that the Canadians have been invited to "share" how they attend births, while the comadronas have in turn shared with the foreign health care professionals what they have in their bag of interventions, including the use of herbs and sauna sweats. This has both validated and entrenched the importance of their cultural nuances in an effort to reduce any attempts by the Canadians to impose *their* cultural norms during knowledge exchanges.

Contrasting Ontario and Totonicapán Midwives

Ontario and Totonicapán midwives share with midwives around the world, the oppression of a medical hegemony that is threatening normal birth (Daviss, 2021). As Ontario midwives are required to fulfill a quota for the number of homebirths they do, and Indigenous midwives in Canada do not always choose to work within the confines of the mainstream Colleges (regulatory bodies)[17], thus exclusively and legally serving Indigenous communities out of hospital, all Ontario midwives share the home birth experience with their traditional midwife counterparts in Totonicapán.

Unlike traditional midwives, Registered Midwives (RMs) in Ontario remain the primary care providers in hospital, unless major intervention like forceps or cesareans are necessary, when they transport from a home birth because they all have hospital privileges. Accommodations are also being worked out for non-registered Indigenous midwives in Ontario[18]. Prior to COVID-19, the traditional Indigenous midwives in Totonicapán were also permitted to attend their clients at the hospital and catch the baby in the birth position of the mother's choice. The PIES program implemented this acceptance of comadronas into the hospital to encourage, rather than discourage, them from bringing birthing persons to hospital if circumstances required medical surveillance or intervention. This program has demonstrated better collaboration, when supportive physicians admit that the traditional midwives have something to offer and treat them as part of their team.

THE EFFECTS OF COVID-19: WHICH POPULATIONS ARE SUFFERING MOST?

Comparison of Cases and Deaths

As is seen in **Figure 3** from the European Center for Disease Control, both Canada and Guatemala have boasted relatively low to moderate figures with respect to confirmed deaths from COVID-19 per million people. The approximate number of deaths per million in Guatemala at this time was under 400 and in Canada, under 600 per million. After a relative "leveling of the curve" that started in June 2020, by late September 2020, Canada was beginning to see a rise again in deaths per million people, while the numbers of cases in Guatemala have just continued to steadily rise.

There are multiple reasons why there is a relatively moderate number of cases in the two countries of Guatemala and Canada, but a fascinating one may be explained through the work of cultural psychologist Michele Gelfand, an expert on "tightness–looseness theory," which explains variations in the strength of social norms and punishments across human groups (Gelfand et al., 2011). Her research indicates that "individuals in tight societies are more prevention focused, have higher self-regulation strength and have higher needs for order and self-monitoring abilities than individuals in loose societies." They help people "to adapt to the level of constraint, or latitude, in their cultural context, at the same time, reinforce it[19]."

The United States is described as having a "loose cultures" (Gelfand et al., 2011; Gelfand, 2021) and Mexico is described as tight in 2011 but by 2021 as "loose." The category suggests interesting consequences:

[14]http://ggm.org.gt/wp-content/uploads/2019/06/Estad%C3%ADsticas-mayo-y-acumulado-2019-CAIMUS-GGM.pdf

[15]https://d2071andvip0wj.cloudfront.net/totonicapan-tension-in-guatemalas-indigenous-hinterland.pdf

[16]https://briarpatchmagazine.com/articles/view/reviving-indigenous-authorities-in-guatemala

[17]https://www.ontariomidwives.ca/indigenous-midwifery

[18]https://www.ontariomidwives.ca/self-determination-key-improved-outcomes-midwifery-care-within-torontos-indigenous-community

[19]https://outlookseries.com/A0996/Science/3989_Michele_Gelfand_University_Maryland_Understanding_Tight_Versus_Loose_Cultures_Critical_Interdependent_World_Michele_Gelfand.htm (accessed February 13, 2021).

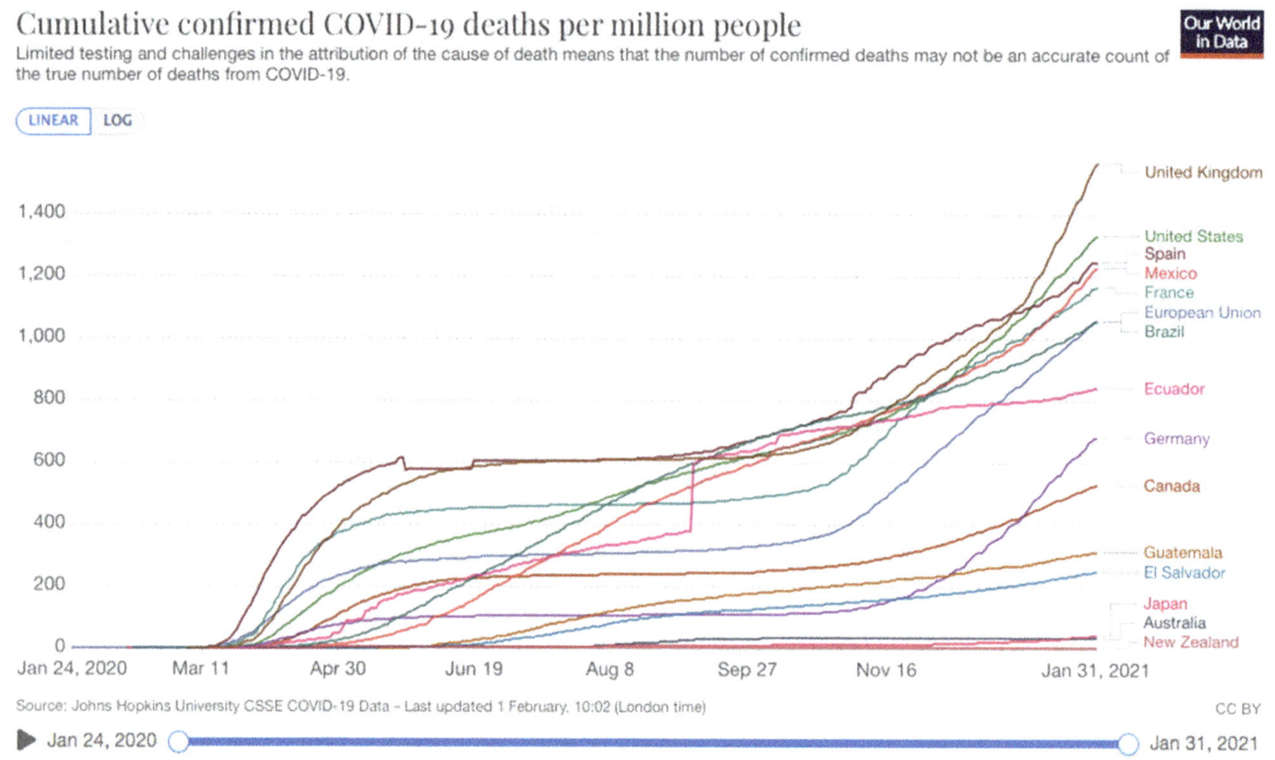

FIGURE 3 | Our World in Data from the European Center for Disease Control January 31, 2021; https://www.ecdc.europa.eu/en.

people in loose cultures had far less fear of the Covid-19 virus throughout 2020, even as cases skyrocketed. In tight nations, 70% of people were very scared of catching the virus. In loose cultures, only 49% were. Reality never bit in these populations in part because people in cultures that are adapted to low levels of danger didn't respond as swiftly to the "threat signal" embodied by the pandemic when it came (Gelfand, 2021).

Notice in **Figure 3** which of these countries has more deaths per million people. Mexico and the US sit high on the graph, with their respective neighbors, Guatemala and Canada, far lower for the number of deaths reported per million. Although not assessed by Gelfand, it appears that the Guatemalan and Canadian cultures have some commonalities around being more "tight"—Guatemala possibly because it has learned to live a protective life following a 36-year civil war, Canada because it has a moderate culture which has had to develop community to withstand cold temperatures and its imposing American neighbor. One of the jokes describing polite, compliant, Canadian culture is, "How do you get 50 people out of the pool?" Answer: "Just say, 'Everybody out of the pool.'"

Table 1 takes a point in time in September 2020 to compare the effects of COVID-19 on the two less-loose countries.

Questions always arise about outcome accuracies in a country with low resources for data collection such as Guatemala. It is difficult to trust census data in a country with rugged mountain terrain and with Indigenous peoples of various dialects, not all of whom register their babies' births. But at least in Totonicapán, groups like PIES, for which physician Iris Champet is coordinating the MNCH project, are becoming more serious about accurately collecting and understanding the data, working in partnership with Indigenous midwives, and supporting their advocacy efforts to be officially recognized and paid a living wage (Daviss, 2021).

Considering the reservations from Laura Gamez and Betty-Anne's own thesis from the 1980s on Guatemala, namely that getting demographics in Guatemala is extremely difficult (Daviss, 1981), the available data on Guatemala may not be correct. The data suggest that in Canada we appear to have fewer cases per 100,000 of COVID-19 (472.3 cases in Guatemala vs. 357.27 in Canada) but continue to have more deaths per million people (17. 2 in Guatemala vs. 24.47 in Canada).

If the numbers are close to accurate, why would a high resource country have more deaths than a low resource country? Heart researchers suggest that Canada has seen higher COVID-19 deaths than many countries with fewer health care resources because more Canadians live longer with chronic heart disease, putting them at greater risk of dying from COVID-19 (Botley et al., 2020; Szklarski, 2020). In other words, because the Canadian health care system is pretty good and keeps people alive longer, it is the ones already sick or 65 or older who have been provided with good health care—the ones who might have already died in under-resourced nations like Guatemala before COVID-19—who are now dying instead in Canada as a result of

TABLE 1 | Guatemalan and Canadian COVID-19 data September 9, 2020.

Data obtained from national reports	
Guatemala	**Canada**
79,622 accumulated registered cases*	134,294 accumulated registered cases**
68,308 estimated cases that have recuperated*	118, 000 that have recuperated***
2,897 cases that failed to register*	Not available
472.3 cases per 100,000 inhabitants*	357.27 cases per 100, 000 people**
2,897 deaths	9,223 deaths
17.2 died per 100,000 inhabitants*	24.47 per 100,000 inhabitants**
Life expectancy 2018, 74.06****	Life expectancy 2018, 81.95****
COVID-19 cases started slowly in March, grew in July, and continued to rise.	Cases started in March, with the first death March 9. Cases peaked by the beginning of May, and leveled off by the beginning of July, but a rise started in late September as schools began to open and people were becoming less vigilant.
Cases in the "Departmento" (province) of Totonicapan*	**Cases in the province of Ontario**
874/100,000 people, 8th in place for number of cases, but 4th for number of deaths.	301/100,000, while neighboring Quebec is at 757.15/100,000 people
Dependent on testing; it is not clear how well that is being done.	By September, testing was ramped up.

**Ministerio de Salud Pública y Asistencia Social (2020).*
***Canadian Broadcasting Company (CBC) (2020).*
****Corona Disease Canada (2020).*
*****World Bank (2018).*
**~Laura Gamez at Horizons states: "Totonicapan up to October was in red alert as one of the highest case counts in the country with a case fatality rate of 6.4, almost double the national rate. The Guatemalan national registry of persons has seen an increase of deaths across the country, though most are not categorized as COVID-19 because they did not get tested. Dr. Iris Champet in communication with Horizons has shared that in many cases, COVID testing is not available in the communities; likewise, many community members do not get tested since there is a stigma surrounding testing positive. Only cases that have extreme complications and which are referred to the hospital are reflected here".*

COVID-19. Canada certainly has a higher life expectancy rate in non-pandemic times compared to Guatemala (see **Table 1**).

Effects of COVID-19 on Indigenous Communities and People of Different Ethnicities

It is not clear how much more Indigenous populations are being affected by COVID-19 compared to white populations or Asian ancestries in Ontario. The narrative in Section Northern Ontario Narrative is set in the Algoma District in Northern Ontario, where about 20% of the population characterize themselves as Aboriginal (Cuddy and Moazzami, 2017), and data is very exacting as to how many fall into Metis, Inuit, First Nations, one, or all those categories (Statistics Canada, 2016). Then there is a weekly count of how many COVID cases are recorded at the Algoma health department[20]. But these databases do not connect and COVID-19 cases do not appear to be categorized by ethnicity—yet.

Another tactic in Ontario to find out who has been affected has been to try to obtain data from neighborhoods with high and low levels of "ethnic concentration" achieved through the Canadian census. Public Health Ontario has found that "ethno-culturally diverse neighborhoods in Ontario, primarily those concentrated in large urban areas, are experiencing disproportionately higher rates of COVID-19 and related deaths compared to neighborhoods that are the less diverse[21]."

This difficulty in locating data on ethnicities is similar in Guatemala. It is clear, however, that the Guatemalan Health Ministry in 2017 found that the Guatemalan government was spending less per capita on health services in largely Indigenous departments than in departments with a majority of non-Indigenous communities[22]. This means that these rural areas are not prepared for the protection, prevention, and treatment that are required for COVID-19. Note that in Totonicapán, our comparison province, there were by September nearly double the cases per 100,000 than in the rest of Guatemala (see **Table 1**). Totonicapán was 8th in line in the departments for number of cases of COVID-19, but 4th in line for the number of deaths—and almost triple the cases of Ontario. It is possible that this is a result of the fact that Indigenous people constitute 98% of the population, with clean water, health care, and even PPE resources more difficult to come by.

With regard to Indigenous women in Canada, results of a survey and two consultations done by the Native Women's Association have revealed a spike in the number of Indigenous women facing more violent incidents since the pandemic began, suggesting that "more of these women are concerned about domestic violence in the midst of this pandemic than they are about the virus" (Wright, 2020). In Guatemala, it is understood

[20]http://www.algomapublichealth.com/disease-and-illness/infectious-diseases/novel-coronavirus/current-status-covid-19/#NO

[21]https://www.publichealthontario.ca/-/media/documents/ncov/epi/2020/06/covid-19-epi-diversity.pdf?la=en

[22]https://www.aljazeera.com/news/2020/4/16/fears-grip-guatemalas-indigenous-groups-as-coronavirus-sets-in

that while COVID-19 exacerbates the problem of violence, presently there are suspicions that Guatemalan women are too afraid to call police on partners with whom they are locked down (Erum, 2020).

The Elephant in the Room in Ontario

Bernadette Betchi and Betty-Anne Daviss

While health care professionals and the media in Ontario have been concentrating on specific groups at risk based on age and co-morbidities, a large Elephant in the room was asking in April, 2020, why, when Black Americans continue to experience the highest COVID-19 mortality rates in the US—more than twice as high as the rate for whites and Asians, who have the lowest actual rates (American Public Media (APM) Lab, 2020)—the Canadian government was not even collecting such data (Nasser, 2020)? Data reports cannot report what they do not collect. Yet by June 2020, with racial focus becoming mandatory because of uprisings in the US, Ontario changed course and now mandates data collection around race, income, household size and language when following up with people infected with COVID-19 (Farooqui, 2020). We still see little on the radar about 2SLGBTQQIA people.

No doubt concerned by the void in knowledge of racial disparities in Canada, a partnership between the African-Canadian Civic Engagement Council (ACCEC) and the Innovative Research Group (INNOVATIVE) produced a report from a survey posted on their website (ACCEC INNOVATIVE, 2020). It revealed that:

- Black Canadians are more likely to report COVID-19 symptoms, in either themselves or someone they know, more likely to say they sought treatment for COVID-19, and nearly three times as likely (21 to 8%) to report knowing someone who has died due to the virus.
- Black Canadians are more likely to report that their job requires them to work with people face-to-face (Net: +41 vs. +25 national average).
- Black Canadians are more likely to feel that no matter what steps they take, their day-to-day routine puts them at an uncomfortably high risk of catching the virus (Net: −2 vs. −17% national average).
- Black commuters are much more likely than the national average to report symptoms, to seek medical treatment, and to admit themselves or know someone admitted to the hospital, and twice as likely as average Canadian workers to say their commute is unsafe (24 vs. 12%). Black Canadians who commute to their work are also twice as likely to use public transit as other Canadians (25 vs. 12%).
- Black Canadians report much worse financial impact from COVID-19 than other Canadians (2020).

One reporter used the continually updated ECDC graph (**Figure 3**) to calculate during the first week of September that "If the US had Canada's Covid-19 death rate, 100,000 more Americans would likely be alive today" (Lopez, 2020). However, comparing ourselves to the country that has the most cases in the world gives Canadians a superficial sense of satisfaction that perpetuates the myth that we care more about our marginalized and racialized communities. This false sense of superiority has been maintained and perpetuated for so long that Canadians have a difficult time analyzing their history and acknowledging their faults. Although Canadians have universal health care insurance, they can't, like US citizens, access National Health Institute data to understand where their disparities lie.

In sum, until January 2021, we see that the approximate number of deaths per million in Guatemala is under 400 and in Canadians under 600 per million. It is difficult to obtain data on Indigenous groups in either jurisdiction but it is suspected that at least in Totonicapán, the Indigenous population is at increased risk both from COVID-19 as well as violence. In Ontario, it is clear that communities that have more ethno-culturally diverse populations have increased number of COVID-19 cases and two NGOs have demonstrated that the Black population is at increased risk.

CHILDBIRTH IN ONTARIO UNDER THE STRAIN OF COVID-19: INFORMATION DISSEMINATION AND CANADIAN COMPLIANCE

The "tighter culture" and pool analogy may explain why Canadians are relatively compliant, and COVID-19 restrictions were met with obedience, especially at the beginning during the COVID lockdown.

Like everyone else, midwives in Ontario were thrown into a difficult situation, with rules and regulations—best practices based on uncertain data—changing weekly, sometimes daily. The Provincial Council for Maternal and Child Health (PCMCH) was tasked by the Ministry of Health to put together an expert group to address practice changes regarding maternal-neonatal health in relation to COVID-19[23]. It included representatives from nursing, midwifery, obstetrics, family practice, pediatrics, neonatology, infectious diseases, and microbiology. They created guidelines and continue to update practitioners about best care. The committee recommended that obstetric interventions be based on obstetric indication rather than COVID-19 status. That is, if a blood pressure looks bad, or a baby is in distress during labor, appropriate interventions are used, but it is not assumed—as it has been in other countries—that inductions or cesareans are better for the mother or baby based on a COVID-19 diagnosis alone. In this respect, Ontario guidelines resonate with the recommendations of the International Federation of Gynecology and Obstetrics (FIGO Safe Motherhood and COVID-19, 2020).

Following this committee's recommendations, there was general agreement and understanding by mid-March in Ontario that only one support person would be permitted at hospital, birth center, and home births alike, as the home setting in Ontario is treated like any other institution. Most clients have been compliant with this restriction, in keeping with the community

[23]https://www.obgyn.utoronto.ca/sites/default/files/jon_barrett.pdf

spirit of protecting the healthcare practitioner as well as the parents. While everybody wanted to have doulas and other friends and family attend their births, general accounts, in particular in the first months, suggest that clients did not feel overly oppressed by this limitation, knowing that many in our neighboring country (the US) were not permitted even to have their spouses attend.

NORTHERN ONTARIO NARRATIVE

Tammy Roberts

We respectfully begin the narratives with a candid reality piece from a Registered Midwife, Tammy Roberts, whose practice in a rural Indigenous community, like the others, is "locked down," submitted August 31, 2020. Tammy Roberts has mixed Aboriginal/white background and grew up in Northern Ontario. She answered our questionnaire orally and then edited the transcript, focusing on issues of compliance and how her relations with the hospital and the community changed as a result of COVID-19 and the hoops she found most difficult to jump through.

The National Aboriginal Council of Midwives (NACM) would like us to clarify that the perspective being shared is that of the registered midwife. Indigenous Midwives are the only midwives not required to register with the College of Midwives to legally practice in Ontario; they are exempt as stated in the Midwifery Act. Tammy chose to become registered to serve both the Indigenous and non-Indigenous population in her community.

The Lockdown in a Northern First Nations Community

I work as a midwife along the North Channel of Lake Huron. My catchment area includes four First Nations communities: Serpent River, Sagamok, Mississauga, and Thessalon. To date there have been no reported cases in these communities, and only three reported cases within my catchment area. The surrounding areas of Sudbury and the Sault have had just over 120 reported cases combined (This was written in August; cases shot up from 5 to 38, 3 days after Christmas).

In March, every First Nations community within my catchment imposed a lockdown, banning visitors and monitoring community members' travel. Each community dealt with things a little differently. One community initiated a pass system, allowing only one trip per week outside of the community. As the restrictions eased, it became twice a week. In other communities, people were encouraged, but not mandated, to limit travel.

In order to access the communities, I had to be added to the list of essential workers each community had developed. When I communicated with the Chief in one community, I was advised that their essential worker list was generated by community members identifying who would be attending at their residence, and I was instructed to have clients reach out to the person in charge of the essential worker list to have my name added. If a client doesn't want someone to know of the pregnancy, they can advise the list coordinator that they are receiving regular visits from an essential worker and that the Chief is "aware," of the confidential situation.

Blockades were installed at each entrance to each community and access was allowed only at the main entrance. Yet the monitoring was inconsistent. Some communities had 24/7 monitoring; others had unmanned blockades but a police presence in the community monitoring for non-community members. For instance, when I arrived at the barricade of one very strict community, I had to identify myself as a midwife working in the community. They wanted to know whom I am visiting, but due to confidentiality I could not say. Referring to PHIPA (the Personal Health Information Protection Act), has worked to grant access.

One of my clients had a family member working at the Band office. The client had a history of precipitous birth and the family had some anxiety about whether I would arrive before the baby, once labor started. My client's family member took measures to ensure I would have quick access and be able to avoid the screening measures and the lineup at the blockade. On the day of the labor, things were progressing quickly as expected. The family member called and advised the border attendants that I was on my way and that I would just wave on my way by, which I did. I arrived at the client's home just in time to have a listen to the baby's heart rate and set up my equipment before the baby arrived!

Compliance in My Community

All my prenatal and postpartum visits are done in clients homes. My clients and their families have been good about self-isolating. In March and April, I had clients who had been sent home from work with pay for as long as 3 weeks to wait things out and see if it was safe for them to return to work. Many have taken early maternity leave or sick leave. Highway traffic has been very sparse and in town, pedestrian and vehicle traffic also very minimal—proof that people have been taking the recommendation to stay home very seriously. The mask wearing rate in our immediate area is quite good; it is rare to see someone in public without a mask.

The Amish and Mennonite communities that I serve received visits from public health personnel with updates on the guidelines. Initially they were permitted to continue holding church services, but as the allowable numbers for gatherings diminished, church services were eventually discontinued. Once the numbers for gatherings increased again, church services resumed, sometimes in creative ways such as outdoor services held in fields, with each family staying in their own buggy to align with physical distancing guidelines. Due to the limited number of school-aged children in one community, they were able to continue holding classes until the numbers for gatherings fell below ten. Most of the young children were from the same family, so they were allowed to continue having classes. For the older children from other families, the teacher would drop lessons off weekly at the house.

The Chief of Obstetrics for St. Joseph's General Hospital in Elliot Lake became the COVID point person for our area. She stayed abreast of the most current guidelines and research and disseminated that information throughout the area. We have a radio station and formal and informal online news sources, which she contributed to regularly.

Did Relations Change at the Hospital?

Relations have indeed changed at St. Joseph's General Hospital in Elliot Lake since COVID struck. Mostly, existing relationships were reinforced, but our Chief of Obstetrics was very keen to limit unnecessary hospital visits. Early discharge was actively encouraged, and home birth was recognized as a good option. As things progressed, issues I would normally consult for in person or send somebody into the hospital for, like postpartum hypertension, were dealt with outside of hospital over the telephone if possible and reasonable. I give the history, prescriptions are sent to the pharmacy, and I follow up with the client as per the physician's advice, limiting hospital visits and personal contact.

Our COVID assessment is quite unique. The Family Health Team swabs people at their home. If a swab is required, a nurse calls to advise when she is on her way, the patient waits at the front door, the nurse dons her PPE at her vehicle, and then performs the swab. She had an assistant to help with donning, doffing, and sanitizing.

Blind River is about 40 min from Elliot Lake. Normally clients in that area of the catchment will have outpatient lab work and ultrasound done in Blind River; however, all non-urgent investigations have been postponed indefinitely. The definition for "urgent" is very limited and does not apply to routine pregnancy, so even clients needing repeat screens and RhIg (Rh Immune globulin) have traveled to Elliot Lake rather than having it done in their own community. Transportation is a challenge for many people in our area, so that has added hardship for some.

Biggest Problems: Isolation and Endless Emails

As a solo midwife, with only a part-time administrator, one of my biggest challenges has been keeping up with the volume of COVID-related information. With the degree of concern related to COVID, I felt that I had to stay on top of all of the emerging information and recommendations. That meant reading endless e-mails, watching the news, and checking public health websites. Add in the administrative work of sourcing PPE and mandated responses to surveys regarding PPE stock and usage—it is all quite onerous for one person. Making contingency plans for who would take over should I get COVID-19 and just getting help to cover myself once in a while to get rest has been onerous.

Summary of the North Channel

In Tammy's account, we observe the brutal reality of living a life as an isolated midwife in a rural area without backup, worsened by the pandemic. There is evidence of compliance with PPE, as is in keeping with the Canadian "tight" culture. At least for the most part, this rural midwife feels supported by those whom she serves, the hospital, and the community border patrol. She feels her credentials and the confidentiality of her clients are respected. Her main problem is her feeling of isolation as a single midwife in a practice in a province where urban practices boast 8–20 midwives, with one or two people able to take the load of figuring out where to find the PPE, how to put it on, where to keep it, how to keep the clinics safe, and how to follow each new recommendation. To examine how other midwives reacted to pandemic regulations, in Ontario we turn to narratives from Eastern Ontario.

HOW COVID-19 HAS AFFECTED MATERNITY CARE IN EASTERN ONTARIO

Betty-Anne Daviss

When I became engaged in this article, I saw COVID-19 in our hospital as a juncture that was offering an important unifying issue through which all parties were coming together to sort out the best ethical care for childbearers. I watched with great relief at how well physicians, nurses, and midwives rallied around the COVID-19 issue at the Montfort Hospital.

I sent out the survey to 50 midwives, being particularly interested in knowing whether or not my hunch was correct and other midwives were feeling the same way I did about COVID-19 being a *boost* to relations among hospital staff, but also about how they were feeling it was affecting clients.

Compliance

At first not all midwives and nurses providing frontline care were provided with masks, due to supply demands. Midwives ended up being supplied with bonnets, drapes, and masks homemade by clients, dentists and dental hygienists, and even by Tim Horton's (a fast-food restaurant chain). Visors were made by an innovative midwife with a 3-D printer. Following provincial recommendations, by May 2020, all mothers in Ontario hospitals were required to wear masks even in pushing stage, but this was not enforced with all births outside the hospital in our area (at home birth and the Ottawa Birth and Wellness Center), as mask wearing during pushing makes it much harder to breathe. While most clients have adopted to not having their spouses at visits, but permitted to at least have them at the birth, clients in our area have threatened to birth unassisted, and some have done so because of the restrictions both in hospitals and in birth centers regarding the number of support people allowed. Two practices have reported that even some who are at higher obstetric risk, yet fear the virus or the restrictions more, have given birth unassisted. While those numbers are not determinable, preliminary data suggested an increase in home births among the midwives (see **Table 2**).

How Relationships Have Been Affected at the Hospitals in Eastern Ontario

At the Montfort Hospital, my home hospital, the difficult tight rope in protecting the baby from the mother who has tested COVID-19 positive, yet still affording the baby breast milk and maternal/infant bonding, were sorted out based on informed choice and safety standards. It has been established among pediatrics and the obstetric/nursing/midwifery team, based on the Task Force recommendations, which did not—like the CDC in the US, and in other jurisdictions like China and India—recommend that COVID+ mothers be separated from their babies.

I was awestruck at how thoughtful the letter was from our Head of Pediatrics to all staff at our hospital:

> Parents have the legal and ethical right to make these decisions for their babies. At NO time do we have the right to remove a baby from its parents unless we have a legal order from the CAS [Children'Aid Society], or if ethically the health care professional is concerned for the baby's well-being with the decisions made by the parent....in our recommendations to parents who are either suspects or COVID positive, it is very important to present the facts and known risks to their newborn baby so far. Since we have no evidence of harm to the baby if the mother wishes skin-to-skin or to breastfeed (with the precautions mentioned in the pandemic plan), **we cannot refuse this.**
> We cannot separate the baby from the mother without her consent (again implicitly if the baby is not sick after birth).
> If the baby needs admission to NICU care, he will be separated from mom—like other non-COVID-19 babies who require that care. The difference now is the protection of the unit and our staff, as well as other patients. Parents cannot visit their babies at NICU if they are suspected or positive for COVID-19—as this puts the well-being of many people at risk....It is important to continue to practice with empathy, because what these parents are going through is also extremely difficult for them.
> -Julie Nault, Head of Pediatrics, Montfort Hospital, April 24, 2020

This is only part of Dr. Nault's statement, but paragraph after paragraph were laid out passionately, delicately, clearly, and on high moral ground. The context is that we had been through several years of hostile meetings over whether and how to attend breech births (see Daviss and Bisits, 2021) and over issues around whether or not midwives should be consulting for labor induction. Informed choice, on which our midwifery profession is based, has been a hard sell at times with the other health professionals at the hospital, who do not always think our clients make wise choices or that we bring them to their senses enough to follow the rules. But when it came to COVID-19, the Head of Pediatrics stated what we could all be on board with.

In other hospitals, however, after only three midwives answered the initial email request, negative comments began to trickle in verbally and at meetings. Few wanted to express via email their sadness and frustration with a medically-dominated system which, they felt, was using the COVID crisis to lay down rules of exclusion, and which, they intuited, the physicians had always wanted. Midwives with privileges at several other hospitals were being rendered non-essential for cesarean sections, whereas before, they could be there to receive the baby, remaining the "baby doctor" after the cesarean. At one hospital, this restriction was enforced almost until the end of the 2020, when it was lifted.

At the Almonte Hospital, about 45 min from Ottawa, the physicians had decided to request (originally interpreted as "require") that all birthing patients have an epidural on admission as there was fear about being able to don the PPE in convenient time. The midwives and their clients protested, and it was then clarified that the epidural imposition was not mandatory. But it *was* an indication that physicians and hospital administration can impose control and make decisions based on their own convenience—unless someone blows the whistle.

Then at the second hospital where I have privileges (but not to do vaginal breeches as I can at the Montfort), I was frustrated that the development of an interdisciplinary breech squad had been put off yet again. As a result, there has been an increase in women being designated to a cesarean for breech among midwifery clients through the required physician consult at that hospital.

Vulnerable Populations in Eastern Ontario

Among the most egregious concerns discussed by the midwives have been the effects of COVID on vulnerable populations. For families needing child protective services, access visits to see children have been canceled. Northern Inuit women who come South for their births to Ottawa have to quarantine for 2 weeks with their babies under security guard before flying back home.

The first report about our numbers came out in June 2020 through the "BORN" system, a database capturing all of the births of registered practitioners in the province[24]. From March 1 to May 29, 2020, there were only 36 COVID-19 cases in pregnant clients that had actually been reported from the participating practices across the entire province[25]. However, by April 23, 2021, with pregnant women accounting for 30% of the patients in the ICU in at least one Toronto hospital, possibly more vulnerable to the new variants new COVID-19 variants (Johnson, 2021), they were placed in the top priority group to receive the vaccine. The extent to which groups are affected—not just by COVID but with regard to their socio/economic/racial/gender distinctions—is currently being missed in our obstetric database. It is complicated but it is starting to be addressed (see BORN, 2016).

Moses and the Basket: My Positive and Negative Experiences of Hospital Care During COVID-19 by Candace LeBlanc, a Mother, Doula and La Leche League Leader in Ottawa, Eastern Ontario

I am a Canadian-born woman who was raised in rural Jamaica. I returned to Canada when I was 15 years old, so even though my English has no trace of an accent, I can easily identify what it means to be new to a country and have to learn to understand its culture and customs, in the way that new immigrants do. I also became Muslim when I was 19 and this has also colored the way in which I view and interact with the world. I live with these three ways of life intertwined. I wear a hijab, which I know affects the way people see me. Usually when people hear the name Candace LeBlanc, the last person they expect to see is an English and non-French-speaking hijab-wearing Jamaican Muslim.

I had my first three babies at home with a wonderful Ottawa midwife. The problems with my fourth pregnancy started during COVID lockdown. Living in a low-income neighborhood means that people are extremely fearful and paranoid. I got very ill during the first two trimesters of pregnancy and my children often had the police called on them for riding their bikes outside—an activity that absolutely follows social distancing guidelines, but still police will show up if they are called. So my

[24]Midwives cannot get paid unless they turn in their data on the births they attend, and to add in their COVID cases would not be too much of a stretch.

[25]https://www.bornontario.ca/en/index.aspx

children had to stay inside all the time because I was not well enough to supervise them outdoors.

During the pregnancy, for circumstances outside my control, I also had to start divorce proceedings and made a decision to initiate a consultation with CAS (Children's Aid Society) to get advice regarding protection for my circumstances. In addition to all this, the children and I got runny noses and because of COVID-19 rules, I couldn't go to my regular midwife visits or get the last blood and urine tests I should have had at the end of the second trimester. I had to wait for several weeks until my and my children's symptoms cleared completely. The day that I could finally go and get the lab tests also happened to be the day that I noticed that my eyes were yellow and I had itchiness all over my body. My midwife asked me about the color of my urine as well. I told her that yes, in fact, my urine had been dark the week before. To my surprise, she said that I should meet her at the hospital right away! Fortunately, I was able to drop the kids off with the community members of my masjid (mosque community) on the way to the hospital.

At the hospital, they found that I had elevated liver enzymes, and recommended that I come in every few days for tests to monitor my levels. A few days later, they found protein in my urine and I was admitted. Thankfully, my mosque community was incredibly supportive and my three children were very well taken care of by many different "aunties"; even groceries were provided. I attribute this to the vision of our masjid, which is not simply to establish another house of worship, but to build a healthy community. It takes a village to raise a child, and my family needed this village more than ever.

Required to remain in hospital for monitoring my high liver enzymes, due to the COVID measures in place at the hospital I was not allowed to have any visitors at all or leave my room for a walk or fresh air. All food or belongings brought for me had to be left downstairs at hospital reception and staff were responsible for bringing them to my room—when and if they had the chance. During two long weeks in the hospital, with nursing all that I had for support, I was struck by the importance of the quality of care. Three nurses stand out who were incredible: a French-Canadian nurse, who also happened to volunteer with La Leche League, a Vietnamese nurse, and a Haitian nurse.

The human touch of *friendship* that these three offered to their professional relationship with me made all the difference. I believe that ethnic background plays a role in this. Other (white) nurses would say, "People cannot drop off food for you because of COVID rules." Those ever-confusing and evolving rules were applied differently: sometimes my food would show up to my room 3 h later and sometimes it would never come at all. Many nurses refused to heat up my food for me or bring me hot water for tea, citing vague COVID regulations, while my three friendly nurses would take the 5 min to bring my food upstairs, boil me some water for tea, or heat up some food for me—small kindnesses, humanity, when you can't leave your room and really need companionship and empathy. I was thrilled when one of the three ended up being there for the birth—indeed, eternally grateful.

It took two religious communities to help this eventful birth unfold. My grandmother, a white Catholic woman, called upon her church to pray for me and the baby, as did my own masjid community. Through two inductions of my premature baby and 40 h of labor combined, I leaned heavily into these communities for support. Sometimes, it takes a village to *birth* a child.

The Montfort staff were generally respectful of my choices and listened when I explained what I wanted and what my concerns were; they patiently answered my questions and actively engaged with me in my care. This is unique because I have not seen my doula clients treated in this way when birthing in other hospitals across Ottawa. It is possible that this was because, as a doula and a La Leche League leader, and having already given birth myself three times, I am more familiar with birth than the average patient and that the Montfort hospital stands out as actively working with midwives and their clients. And the obstetric/nursing staff there appear more experienced (and therefore receptive) when it comes to an informed choice model of care.

I told my birthing team I wanted to do late cord clamping and allow the baby to hear the Muslim prayers that are traditionally done right after the birth. I had the prayers recorded by my Shaykh on my phone. My doctor, midwife, and nurse allowed me to let my baby listen to them right after the birth and my son was totally calm, breathing well, and resting on my belly. After the prayers, the doctor said, "OK it has been 10 minutes" and my baby was whisked to the warmer. I later learned that the Neonatal Resuscitation Program that all the health professionals in obstetrics take requires transport of the premature baby to the warmer within 30 s, so I was even more grateful and overjoyed that the birthing team had complied with my wishes.

After my son was taken to the nursery, he had breathing issues. This is where things started going awry. A decision was made to send my baby to the Children's Hospital of Eastern Ontario (CHEO) through a rule that dictates that a transfer to the NICU there must be done if the baby is on CPAP >24 h; I was not invited to be a part of this decision, only suddenly informed that the baby would be transported—in the next 30 min. I was told not to worry: although I couldn't travel with him in the ambulance, there would be a bed for me beside him once I arrived at CHEO. I quickly went to my room and packed up all of my belongings and hurriedly got discharged (Thanks again to one of my three heroine nurses!).

When I got back to the nursery, the staff were suddenly acting very strange and whispering to each other. To my surprise, the paper they handed me said that we were going to another NICU at a totally different hospital! They informed me that I was rerouted; later I found out that this rerouting was due to a COVID-19 scare at CHEO. I do wonder whether or not I would have been treated differently if I were white—that is, given more of an explanation as to what was happening with my child.

At the new hospital I was informed, rather dryly, that not only was there no bed for me to stay by my son's side, but if I fell asleep in the chair beside his incubator, I would be asked to leave the NICU. Less than 48 h after giving birth, I had to choose between sleeping and being by my son's side. I could only last for 18 h. I was faced with the decision to place my baby, proverbially, in a basket on the river Nile, and wait for God to bring him back to me, eventually. This is what it felt like to leave my baby in the hospital, alone—or should I say, in the House of Pharaoh—to me, a foreign place, unnatural in its design and oppressive in its rules, a place that was governed by liability, not empathy, a place with too much "head" and not enough "heart." This was my Red Sea to cross.

After a few days of going back and forth to the hospital, I realized, having used the early labor lounge as a doula, that it was available; I dragged my stuff in there and fell asleep. However, when the staff found out, they locked it so that I couldn't use it, even though it was not being used by anyone else. After 6 long, exhausting days, my son had been off CPAP for a few days and could take a bottle. I therefore felt he was well enough to come home. First, I phoned my midwife to ask her whether she could come and follow up on the baby's health at home if I signed out Against Medical Advice (AMA). We had a discussion about my perception of how I was being treated as a racialized woman and she agreed to support me in doing whatever was best for the baby. Then, I asked the resident whether or not I could take out the baby AMA. The resident told me she would go and call the doctor so that I could consult with him. I waited patiently, but she didn't return for nearly 2 h. Eventually she informed me that she had reported me to CAS, without consulting me first. I felt that she did this because I was Black. I had not even consulted with the doctor yet, nor been told they were calling CAS, which—I checked—is the first step before getting CAS involved.

I called my midwife to ask her to advocate for me to the NICU staff, and when she realized that the nurse manager had been informed by the resident that I already had a CAS file opened up on me, my midwife made sure to inform them, "This is a file that *Candace* opened herself three weeks ago. She is an educated, well-informed La Leche League Leader, and actually, Jamaican and from a group that tend to know their rights and how to manage the system—hence her pro-active opening of the CAS file, to protect her and her family."

My goal was to do what was best for the baby, whether it was to keep him in or take him out of the hospital. The CAS file was closed and, a day or so later, they agreed to move me to CHEO. It was heaven; I could finally have a bed next to my baby.

Unfortunately, my first night at CHEO, my baby and I shared a room with a young mother with only a curtain between us. Thus, I overheard that she also wanted to take her baby out of the hospital AMA. Late into the night she could be heard yelling at the doctors and nurses and being extremely disrespectful to them. I overheard her say to her partner on the phone that she had a previous police record, was not legally allowed to be within a certain distance of her current partner, and worried that the police would charge her for that offense if they were to be seen together. She made disturbing jokes about her infant falling off the couch while she was on the phone but insisted to the doctors she "just didn't know" what had happened to her son. Her baby had a broken humerus and CAS suspected child abuse. But she told her CAS worker that she wanted to leave the hospital that night.

"There is no way she is leaving tonight" I thought to myself.

As she continued her rude behavior toward the staff, I learned her baby was exactly the same age as mine, 2 weeks old. The staff weakly tried to convince her to stay overnight. She flatly refused and signed her baby out AMA. She left with her baby that night. She was white.

I crossed the Red Sea of racism and inconsistent protocols and got to take my son out of hospital and bring him home to meet his sisters 2½ weeks after his birth. I was permitted under the proviso that my midwife visit me a couple of times a week, which she did faithfully. He is now a healthy growing boy who indeed came back to his people in a blessed way, just like Moses (see **Figure 4**).

Summary and Analysis of Candace's Story

While Candace has a low economic status—in particular because she married young and now is a single mother with four children—she has some university education, has a white father, and is well aware of white middle class biases and people's unknown or unspoken attitudes. We would therefore be hard-pressed to suggest she is of the proverbial "low" socio-economic class, which inherently also can infer less education. In her story, she perceives the subtle racism so frequently spoken about among the IBPOC population—how she was treated differently by the nurses who respected her in one hospital and by a staff in a different hospital, following her desperate situation with nowhere to sleep. Ironically, a staff member injudiciously called CAS prematurely, without telling her or honoring her wishes to speak with the physician, making assumptions until they found out that it was Candace who had opened up her own file. And the final blow: how she could only interpret the treatment of a white woman, acting irresponsibly yet being discharged anyway, as a sign of white privilege.

In the next section, we explore some inherent gaps in the population that midwives serve in Ontario, looking at the demographics of midwifery clients by socio-economic classes designated by neighborhood.

Data on Socio Economic Status of Midwives' Clients

While COVID-19 was waging, a retrospective cohort study emerged in our national midwifery journal about a sobering concern that has troubled the midwifery profession in Ontario.

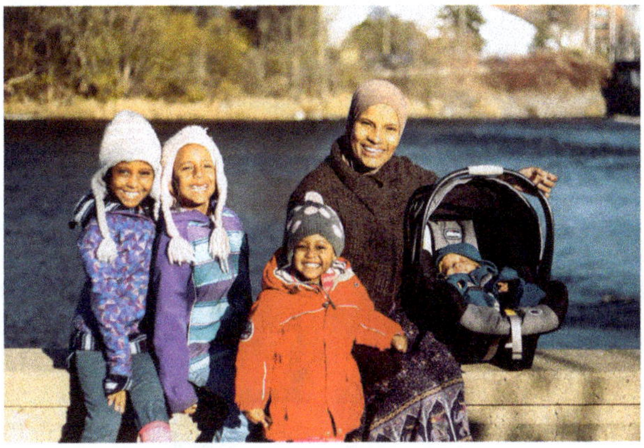

FIGURE 4 | Candace and her family after crossing over the hospital Red Sea of tape. Photo by Kamal Abdulhakim. Used with permission.

Prior to midwifery legislation in Ontario in 1993, because Canadian health insurance covered only hospital births with physicians and the far North, largely only people who could afford the full cost of midwives hired them. Many midwives would take refugees, immigrants, lower income clients, and those living rurally at a reduced rate, or barter for lambs, plants, pottery, bread, carpentry, and child care. For many midwives, the impetus for legislation was to be able to serve the population that could not afford midwives (Daviss, 1999).

Fast forward, a new study based on neighborhood-level maternity care 2006–2017 demonstrates that one or two decades after legislation, childbearers of low socio-economic status in Ontario are less likely to receive midwifery care than those of high socio-economic status. The researchers were careful to say that ethnicity was not part of their study (Darling et al., 2020). Fortunately, the rest of the articles in this edition of the *Canadian Journal of Midwifery* provide models that are stepping up to the plate to change the situation.

Given Candace's example, we have some difficulty in assumptions made about what is meant by the term "low socio-economic class," since Candace, living in a low-income neighborhood, would have been classified as such in this study, not particularly accurately. On reflection, she suggests that it invites assumptions—evident in the hospital staff's attitudes toward her—as "uneducated, ignorant reactive and uninformed," in her case, she felt, because she was Black and wearing a hijab. The fact that midwives do not well serve the populations living in those neighborhoods is disturbing, but the stereotyping can also serve to revictimize the people living there.

Data Demonstrating an Increase in Home Births in Ontario With COVID-19

The data in **Table 2** were taken from the BORN database [BORN (Birth Outcomes Registry Network) Ontario, 2020], but preliminary because the data were not all yet incorporated into the database for the 2020 months at the time of retrieval, November 8, 2020. It shows that in 2019, the planned hospital birth rate among midwifery clients each month was approximately 80–82%, and the planned homebirth rate was 13–14%. By May of 2020, the trend for this preliminary data indicated that the planned hospital birth rate had dropped to 74.4%, and the planned home birth rate had climbed to 20.0%[26].

TABLE 2 | Planned place of birth for Ontario Midwifery Clients, March to May, 2019 and 2020.

Month and Year	Hospital	Home	Birth Center	Midwifery Clinic	Total
March 2019	1517	260	86	14	1877
	(80.8%)	(13.9%)	(4.6%)	(.7%)	(100%)
March 2020	1073	173	79	19	1344
	(79.8%)	(12.9%)	(5.9%)	(1.4%)	(100%)
April 2019	1555	245	82	17	1899
	(81.9%)	(12.9%)	(4.3%)	(0.9%)	(100%)
April 2020	1028	235	51	29	1343
	(76.5%)	(17.5%)	(3.8%)	(2.2%)	(100%)
May 2019	1509	266	106	16	1897
	(79.5%)	(14.0%)	(5.6%)	(0.8%)	(100%)
May 2020	934	252	48	21	1255
	(74.4%)	(20.0%)	(3.8%)	(1.7%)	(100%)

Summary Section How COVID-19 Has Affected Maternity Care in Eastern Ontario

This section has demonstrated the stressors faced by the midwives as a result of COVID-19. It has revealed some goodwill, responsibilities and ethics both of the midwives and hospital management, but it has also exposed some of the opportunistic reactions of care providers and authorities. It raises the concerns about the subtle racism and the reality that childbearers of low socio-economic status in Ontario are less likely to receive midwifery care than those of high socio-economic status.

We move next to the story of Guatemala, where Indigenous oppression is not quite so subtle and professed universal health care not as readily available.

GUATEMALA: EXPERIENCES AMONG THE TRADITIONAL MIDWIVES OF GUATEMALA

Stepping Up to the Plate on Gender Equality

Working with the healthcare providers in Totonicapán, the MNCH program implemented by Horizons and PIES was very careful to include programs that engaged the larger issues of lack of resources and violence in the communities they were serving prior to COVID-19. They carried out workshops not just on midwifery skill sharing and childbirth but also on gender equality. In addition, they have been able to provide personal counseling sessions for both women and men in that regard. One of the stories, told through a midwife's eyes, demonstrates how cultural attitudes devalue women, and may affect long-term health outcomes:

> Valenzuela grew up watching her father violently assault her mother. His attacks were both verbal and physical, often telling Valenzuela and her mother that they were useless women. This violence resulted in Valenzuela's mother experiencing several miscarriages. It was seeing her mother experience this loss at the hands of her father that marked her for life. This story captures how gender-based violence has resulted in significant consequences for the well-being of women and their children in Totonicapán (Horizons, 2018).

However, today, Valenzuela Cos Matul is a *comadrona,* has become a leader in her community and, has helped train other midwives on best practices for providing maternal and child health care (see **Figure 5**). As part of the project, more than 940 midwives received training in safe birthing practices and care,

[26]The interpretation and conclusions contained herein do not necessarily represent those of BORN Ontario.

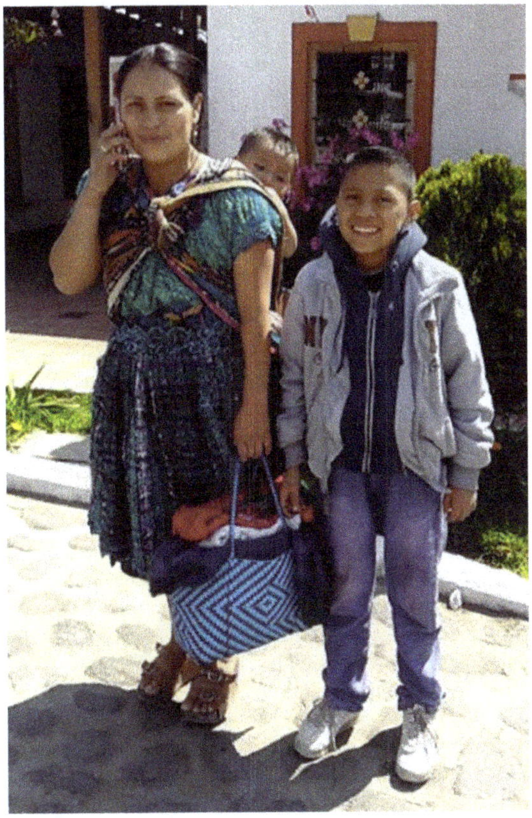

FIGURE 5 | Valenzuela Cos Matul on her cellphone, her children in tow, representing the new generation of comadronas, teaching best practices of maternal child health, the rights of women, and the impacts of gender-based violence. Photo by Betty-Anne Daviss in Totonicapán, 2017. Used with permission.

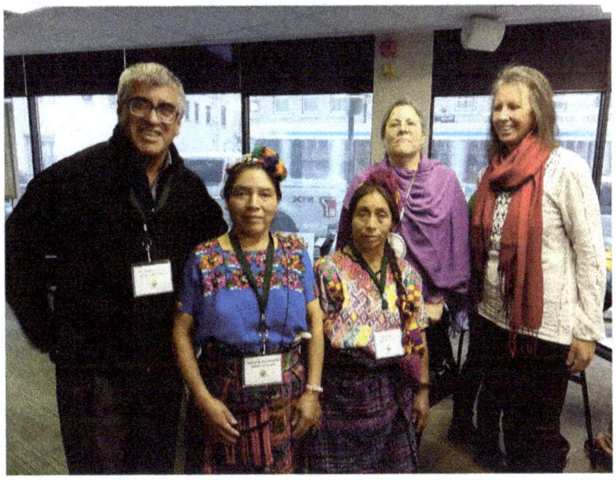

FIGURE 6 | From left to right: Dr. Diaz, Angela Antonietta Perez Vicente and Nazaria Ajamel Xiloj from Momostenango, Guatemala, with Dorothy Green from Kenhte:ke Midwives Tyendinaga Mohawk Territory (in purple shawl) and Lynn Brant, nurse practitioner and community advocate—two Mohawk women offering support for traditional Indigenous knowledge exchange. Photo in Kingston, Ontario provided by the Horizons' Office (2017), used with permission.

and also on the impact of gender-based violence and the need to respect and recognize the rights of women.

How COVID-19 Affected the Midwives in Totonicapán

Introducing Iris Champet

Dr. Iris Champet was born and raised in Totonicapán, educated as a primary school teacher, physician, and surgeon, and has worked for approximately 10 years supporting the work of midwives, health promoters, health commissions, and community leaders. She coordinates the MNCH project for PIES. She and Betty-Anne met in Guatemala in 2017 when the first contingency of Canadian health care providers—doctors, nurses, and midwives—was sent to Guatemala for the PIES/HORIZONS project. Betty-Anne requested that PIES/HORIZONS create a chapter for a book she was writing, Birthing Models on the Human Rights Frontier. Although it did not transpire, Dr. Champet provided some details for the book about the work the comadronas were doing to seek remuneration for their work. That is, although a bill to compensate them had been passed by Congress it was vetoed by the President of Guatemala (Daviss, 2021). For this current article, Dr. Champet sent the following account in Spanish, which Betty-Anne translated. See **Figure 6** for a photo of the Guatemalan team meeting with the Indigenous team in Kingston, Ontario.

COVID-10 in Totonicapán

The COVID 19 pandemic affected all of us. In particular, the traditional midwives, called *comadronas,* found themselves in need of making changes in their personal and family lives and in the development of their activities as midwives. On March 13, 2020, the first positive case was detected in Guatemala, and since then, various directives have been given by the President. There were no longer knowledge-exchange meetings with the comadronas, because crowds had to be avoided. Then a "curfew" was decreed, a restriction of mobility from 4:00 p.m. to 4:00 a.m. every day. If you circulated during these restricted hours, there was a fine to pay.

With the curfew, it was not clarified whether or not one was allowed out to deal with emergencies. This made it difficult for the midwives to work, because as is well known, the greatest number of deliveries are attended at night. Thus, several comadronas chose to commute to their patient's home at permitted times to avoid paying the fine; if the labor did not develop, they returned to their homes in the morning and returned again to the pregnant woman's house in the afternoon until she went into labor.

Another downside was that in the health services, there was so much attention paid to COVID-19 that the midwives had less support. Pre-COVID, the comadronas were allowed to go to the hospital with their mothers in labor, explain the reason for the transfer, and usually even do the delivery. (Others were not permitted to accompany the mothers). Currently, the comadronas are not permitted to enter nor attend the deliveries because of the protocols that exist for the prevention of COVID-19.

Yet another change is that women are choosing not to go to hospitals for fear of getting infected. This has meant an increase in the care of pregnant, parturient and puerperal women by traditional midwives, both in Totonicapán and at the national level. This has posed difficulties with births that are complicated and *need* referral. The comadronas have been trained to identify danger signs, but have found that women and their families do not always accept referrals in these cases, both for fear of hospital contagion and because misinformation abounds in the community; there are rumors that you have to get swabbed for COVID-19 if you go to the hospital, when in fact that is only if you have signs and symptoms. The mothers are also afraid that if they test positive, their baby will be taken away from them.

On many occasions, the comadronas have increased expenses, because they have to depend on their own resources as they try to figure out how to return to their homes. They are not permitted to be in the hospital with their patients, and the cars that take the patients do not wait for the midwives. *There is no public transportation, and the comadronas do not own their own cars.* Even before COVID-19, these midwives lacked appropriate equipment for the care of women and their families. They have cloth masks, donated by the Maternal and Neonatal Health Project, but they are not N95s. And they do have direct contact with people.

At the beginning of the restrictions, as the directive was to "stay at home," the community authorities were very demanding during hospital transports: the midwives had to be duly identified with their midwives' card, and sometimes they had to pass through review of their documents by authorities up to five times on the way to the hospital.

Another difficulty has been figuring out a system by which to make the restrictions known. After identifying some of the problems, the President of Guatemala clarified that maternal and vaccination care should continue on a regular basis. In addition, the Indigenous Peoples' Unit issued a circular, which was sent up to the authorities, indicating that the mobilization restriction did not apply to midwives and that they should be supported in their work. This strong level of support gave them more confidence.

Within the MNCH Project, funded through Horizons of Friendship and the Government of Canada, liquid soap, cloth masks, waterproof coats, protective glasses, hats, towels, and gloves, among others, were donated to the midwives; they have been a tremendous support. The MSPAS (Ministerio de Salud Pública y Asistencia Social, 2020) has donated some supplies that have been distributed to some midwives; it has not been possible to reach all of them. These comadronas are very afraid of becoming infected, because they do not know who is and who is not infected with COVID 19, as little testing is available.

Ishim Yac

Ishim Yac, a young woman who has been involved with the comadronas, works for the Guatemalan Stove Project, an NGO in a Neighboring area to Totonicapán—Quetzaltenango. She sent us the information below about the general situation across the region in February 2021 (translated by Betty-Anne):

> COVID-19 has demonstrated how precarious our health and education system are, as well as our entire infrastructure. When COVID-19 hit our country, the country was closed. This included markets, public transport, schools, and businesses, etc. as a form of restraint, following the installation of temporary hospitals for COVID-19. Unfortunately, there was no equipment, human resources, and above all, unoccupied space or beds to care for COVID-19 patients.
>
> The closure of the country definitely affected the poor population, mostly Indigenous people. In Totonicapán, the women mostly deal with middlemen who sell their *huipiles* (colorful embroidered blouses) in the market, but with the market closed, they were unable to work. This has affected the economy. . . People have chosen to cure themselves of COVID-19 with natural treatments such as eucalyptus, ginger, lemon, and chamomile rather than go to hospital.
>
> COVID-19 cases in rural areas are very low compared to large cities, such as Guatemala and Quetzaltenango, where the numbers are high. As for education, children can't attend school and distance education has become much more complicated in an environment where parents can't read and write. You can imagine how complicated it is where virtual education is almost impossible, and children don't have a device to zoom in on, meet teachers or each other, to receive classes.
>
> Strong hugs from afar.

Summary of Section Guatemala: Experiences Among the Traditional Midwives of Guatemala on Totonicapán, Making Some Comparisons With Ontario

The Guatemalan comadronas demonstrate through this scenario how resilient and flexible they are. Aggravated by the recent breakdown of the economy, they are so dedicated and responsible to the mothers with whom they work that they sleep overnight at women's houses to make sure they are not caught by the curfew. No doubt they were stopped many times on the road by police because of their Indigenous status. Unlike Ontario, where people of lower socio-economic status (SES) are less likely to receive midwifery care than people of higher SES, in Guatemala, indigenous women are served by midwives from their communities, who are in the same SES group. Tammy in Northern Ontario, serving the Amish/Indigenous population, echoes the feeling of isolation of the traditional midwives during COVID-19 but appears to feel more appreciated and supported by authorities for her situation.

In both countries, midwives' roles in hospital or with local authorities, and thus client care, appeared to suffer with COVID-19 as better systems were being worked out. The Canadian midwives could learn from the PIES program about how to face gender-based violence. The upside in both countries is that midwives are clearly becoming the link for seeking choice in their communities, and childbearers are increasingly discovering the benefits of staying home for their births. It was a positive development that midwives in both Ontario and Guatemala were granted the right to have a vaccination in the first phase of vaccinations in March, 2021, a recognition of their vulnerability. In Guatemala, the comadronas were slated for their vaccination ahead of the firemen and paramedics[27].

With increased clientele because of COVID-19, and recognition of their roles by the government through the vaccination program, one would think that the comadronas' contribution and faithfulness to their community could be rewarded by the small wage for they are asking, from their national government.

CONCLUSIONS: PEELING OFF THE MASKS

We can now state that a comparison about pandemic effects between a province in a high resource country (Canada) and a low resource country (Guatemala) reveals similar problems and similar solutions. The first outstanding similarity is that Indigenous populations suffer marginalization in both Totonicapán and Ontario. The femicide problem is of increased concern in both countries for Indigenous peoples during COVID-19, with violence proven to be spiking in Canada, with suspicions of the same thing happening in Guatemala, although the problem is clearly affecting women across Guatemala as a whole. The health conditions of people on the Indigenous reservations in Ontario, with contaminated or threatened water supplies, now additionally suffering under lockdown, are also somewhat similar to those in Guatemala.

As a result of COVID itself or the fear of restrictions and interventions, home births are on the rise—even with those who are higher risk and need to be in hospital—in both jurisdictions. The obvious upside in Ontario is that first, midwives get paid, and second, the Federal government has increased funding to Indigenous midwives. In Totonicapán, where PIES is recognizing more than ever the fortitude and value of their traditional midwives, the national government should now find it harder to ignore the will of the people who are increasingly demanding these midwives' services. Whether or not the government will be fair about it and agree to pay them—thereby reducing the strain on the hospital system—remains to be seen.

Just as the white privileged US population tends to have polarized attitudes toward its IBPOC population, Guatemalan authorities and *Ladino* (non-Indigenous people of mixed origin, similar to the *mestizos* of Mexico) peoples have had an historically polarized dissonance toward their Indigenous peoples. In Canada, despite our national identity of making sure that "nobody is left behind" because the vulnerable are part of "us," the issues of racialized people have still been largely rendered invisible, ethnically diverse neighborhoods have been hit harder by COVID-19, with substantial proof from the Black population. Subtle racism continues in health care. Indigenous, 2SLGBTQQIA and women's communities continue to struggle.

Midwives, nurses, and physicians working with vulnerable populations may see, but do not always work on, rectifying the inequities, the biases, and the oversights. Midwives also fall prey to being abused themselves, as they try to mitigate a medical system that does not always share their values of informed choice. This can become more abusive as higher echelons take advantage of the pandemic to impose restrictions they have often wanted even in non-COVID times. However, seeing inequities laid bare and how far authoritarianism can go without whistle blowers can be turned into an opportunity. The mirror that is held up during these times gives authorities a chance to consider rights, such as they did with regard to rights of babies in the nursery at the Montfort, and they did admit being "wrong" in phoning CAS on a Jamaican hijab-wearing patient a little too quickly—before telling her.

When hospitals excuse themselves for not stepping up to other reforms, such as making the change to allow vaginal breeches attended by midwives, "because of COVID-19," the pandemic becomes a crutch to beg forgiveness, rather than a tool to make the changes needed.

We offer this work as a means to understand the problems and articulate how to improve our systems that are inherently racist, colonialist, sexist, white cisnormative, and biased toward a medical hegemony. We suggest that one way to make our health care systems safer and more culturally appropriate would be to enhance community-based midwifery practices and collaborative models (Daviss, 2021).

If we ever get to take off our COVID-19 masks, it would be good to peel off the larger whitewashed masks that have been rendering the issues of racism and marginalization of midwives not an issue that is supposed to be discussed in Canada. As with activists in other arenas such as the environment, as Ontario health care advocates, we hold up hope that COVID-19 can be the catalyst that challenges the standard narrative, exposing and then eliminating the old ruts and blind spots of inequality and discrimination that until COVID-19, our obstetric and hospital and health care system hierarchies and our white citizens were managing to put on the backburner.

ETHICS STATEMENT

Ethical review and approval was not required for the study on human participants in accordance with the local legislation and institutional requirements. The patients/participants provided their written informed consent to participate in this study. Written informed consent was obtained from the individual(s) for the publication of any potentially identifiable images or data included in this article.

[27]https://www.mspas.gob.gt/noticias/noticias-ultimas/5-noticias-mspas/1214-inicia-distribución-de-vacuna-covid19-astrazeneca-covishield-a-las-29-áreas-de-salud.html; https://covid-19.ontario.ca/getting-covid-19-vaccine-ontario

AUTHOR CONTRIBUTIONS

B-AD oversaw the development of the article and encouraged community input. TR wrote her experience in her Indigenous registered midwife practice in Northern Canada. CL wrote the section about her first birth in hospital and the subte racism she felt. IC wrote the section on Guatemala. BB advised B-AD during the development of the paper, provided useful input, and editing throughout. LG provided insight and facilitated the exchange on the situation on Guatemala during COVID-19. AA wrote part of and consulted over the Indigenous history in Canada. All authors contributed to the article and approved the submitted version.

REFERENCES

ACCEC and INNOVATIVE (2020). *Impact of COVID Black Canadian Perspectives.* Released September 2. African-Canadian Civic Engagement Council (ACCEC) and Innovative Research Group (INNOVATIVE). Available online at: https://innovativeresearch.ca/wp-content/uploads/2020/09/ACCEC01-Release-Deck.pdf (accessed October 1 2020).

American Public Media (APM) Lab (2020). *The Color of Coronavirus: COVID-19 Deaths by Race and Ethnicity in the U.S.* Available online at: https://www.apmresearchlab.org/covid/deaths-by-race (accessed September 2 2020).

Anderson, D., Daviss, B. A., and Johnson, K. C. (2021). "What if another 10% of deliveries in the united states occurred at home or in a birth center? Safety, economics and politics," in *Birthing Models on the Human Rights Frontier: Speaking Truth to Power,* eds B. A. Daviss and R. Davis-Floyd (Abingdon: Routledge Press), 205–228.

BORN (2016). *BORN Engagement With Indigenous Stakeholders: 2012-2013.* For BORN Users and Stakeholders. Available online at: https://www.bornontario.ca/en/publications/resources/Documents/Indigenous/Indigenous-Stakeholder-Feedback-to-BORN-Report_2016-Final_accessible.pdf (accessed April 1, 2021).

BORN (Birth Outcomes Registry and Network) Ontario (2020). Available online at: https://www.bornontario.ca/en/index.aspx

Botley, L., Martin-Rhee, M., Kasiban, A., Swartz, R. H., Mulvagh, S. L., Lindsay, M. P., et al. (2020). COVID-19 pandemic: global impact and potential implications for cardiovascular disease in Canada. *Canad. Cardiovasc. Soc.* 2, 265–272. doi: 10.1016/j.cjco.2020.06.003

Canadian Broadcasting Company (CBC) (2020). *Evolution of COVID.* Available online at: https://ici.radio-canada.ca/info/2020/coronavirus-covid-19-pandemie-cas-carte-maladie-symptomes-propagation/index-en.html (accessed September 9, 2020).

Corona Disease Canada (2020). Available online at: https://www.google.com/search?client=safari&rls=en&q=active+cases+of+COVID+in+CAnada&ie=UTF-8&oe=UTF-8 (accessed September 9, 2020).

Cuddy, J., and Moazzami, B. (2017). *Northern Projections Human Capital Series—Algoma District.* Research Paper No 17. April. Available online at: https://www.northernpolicy.ca/upload/documents/publications/reports-new/hcs_algoma-en.pdf (accessed February 10, 2021).

Darling, E. K., Murray-Davis, B., Ahmed, R., and Vanstone, M. (2020). Access to Ontario midwifery care by neighbourhood-level material deprivation quintile, 2006–2017: a Retrospective Cohort Study. *Canad. J. Midwifery Fall* 19, 8–23.

DasGupta, N., Shandal, V., Shadd, D., Segal, A., and in conjunction with CivicAction. (2020). *The Pervasive Reality of Anti-Black Racism in Canada:The Current State, and What to do About It.* December 14, 2020. Available online at: https://www.bcg.com/en-ca/publications/2020/reality-of-anti-black-racism-in-canada (accessed February 9, 2020).

Daviss, B. A. (1981). *The Guatemalan Factor.* Thesis submitted to the Department of Journalism as part of completion of a Bachelor of Journalism, Carleton University.

Daviss, B. A. (1999). *From Social Movement to Professional Midwifery Project: Are We Throwing the Baby Out with the Bathwater?* A thesis submitted to the Faculty of Graduate Studies and Research in partial fulfillment for the degree of Master of Arts in Canadian Studies. Ottawa: Carleton University. Available online at: https://curve.carleton.ca/f0c4023d-182a-4a3d-a49b-a51f4458acbe (accessed February 28, 2021).

Daviss, B. A. (2021). "Introduction: Speaking truth to power for social justice in pregnancy and childbirth; Chapter 6: How did she think she could win in court?; and Conclusions: Speaking truth to power individually and collectively will redistribute the power," in *Birthing Models on the Human Rights Frontier: Speaking Truth to Power,* eds B. A. Daviss and R. Davis-Floyd (Abingdon: Routledge Press), 1–52; 184–204; 403–446.

Daviss, B. A., and Bisits, A. (2021). "Bringing back breech: dismantling hierarchies and re-skilling practitioners," in eds. *Birthing Models on the Human Rights Frontier: Speaking Truth to Power,* eds B. A. Daviss and R. Davis-Floyd (Abingdon: Routledge Press), 145–183.

Daviss, B. A., and Davis-Floyd, R. (2021). *Birthing Models on the Human Rights Frontier: Speaking Truth to Power.* Abingdon: Routledge Press.

Desmond, C. (2020). *The Skin We're In: A Year of Black Resistance and Power.* Toronto, ON: Penguin Random House. Doubleday.

Erum, M. (2020). The impact of covid-19 on gender-based violence and femicide cases in Guatemala. *Central America, The Organization for World Peace.* Available online at: https://theowp.org/the-impact-of-covid-19-on-gender-based-violence-and-femicide-cases-in-guatemala/ (accessed November 16, 2020).

Farooqui, S. (2020). *University of Toronto Research to Explore Racism in Health Care During Epidemic.* The Canadian Press, August 25, 2020 01:40 PM. Available online at: https://toronto.ctvnews.ca/university-of-toronto-research-to-explore-racism-in-health-care-during-pandemic-1.5078884

FIGO Safe Motherhood and COVID-19 (2020). Available online at: https://www.figo.org/safe-motherhood-and-covid-19 (accessed October 3, 2020).

Gelfand, M. (2021). Why countries with 'loose', rule-breaking cultures have been hit harder by Covid. *The Guardian.* Available online at: https://www.theguardian.com/world/commentisfree/2021/feb/01/loose-rule-breaking-culture-covid-deaths-societies-pandemic?utm_term=799656106019e8fa390f61c6b09e5acdandutm_campaign=BestOfGuardianOpinionUSandutm_source=espandutm_medium=EmailandCMP=opinionus_email (accessed Februaary 1, 2021).

Gelfand, M., Raver, J. L., Nichi, L.,Leslie, L. M., Lun, J., Lim, B., et al. (2011). differences between tight and loose cultures a 33-nation study. *Science* 332, 1100–1104 doi: 10.1126/science.1197754

Guatemalan Census (2008). Available online at: https://www.censopoblacion.gt/

Horizons (2018). *Guatemala: Two Women Killed Every Day.* Available online at: https://www.horizons.ca/blog/2018/1/3/guatemala (accessed January 31, 2021).

Ishida, K., Stupp, P., Turcios-Ruiz, R., William, D., and Espinoza, E. (2012). Ethnic inequality in Guatemalan women's use of modern reproductive health care. Int. Perspect. Sexual Reprod. Health 38, 99–108, doi: 10.1363/3809912

Johnson, N. (2021). Toronto Hospital Reports Alarming Number of Pregnant Patients in COVID-19 ICU. Available online at: https://toronto.ctvnews.ca/toronto-hospital-reports-alarming-number-of-pregnant-patients-in-covid-19-icu-1.5393855

Lopez, G. (2020). *If the US had Canada's Covid-19 Death Rate, 100,000 More Americans Would Likely be Alive Today.* Washington, DC: Vox.

Ministerio de Salud Pública y Asistencia Social (2020). *Gobierno de Guatemala. Situactión de COVID-19 en Guatemala.* Available onlone at: https://tablerocovid.mspas.gob.gt (accessed September 9, 2020 and for the department September 11, 2020).

Nasser, S. (2020). Early signs suggest race matters when it comes to COVID-19. So why isn't Canada collecting race-based data? *CBC News.* Posted on April 17, 2020 Available onlone at: https://www.cbc.ca/news/canada/toronto/race-coronavirus-canada-1.5536168 (accessed May 6, 2020).

Nobel Women's Initiative (2012). *From Survivors to Defenders: Women Confronting Violence in Mexico, Honduras, and Guatemala.* Available online at: http://nobelwomensinitiative.org/wp-content/uploads/2012/06/Report_AmericasDelgation-2012.pdf

Pena, C. (2013). *Improving Access to Health Care Services through the Expansion of Coverage Program (PEC): The Case of Guatemala.* UNICO Studies Series; No. 19. World Bank, Washington DC.

Research Directorate, Immigration and Refugee Board, Canada (1998). *Guatemala: The Quiché Maya Indigenous Group and Whether Its Situation is Comparable to or Distinguishable From the Other Indigenous Groups in Guatemala, and Whether there are Reports of its Mistreatment by Government Agents.* Immigration and Refugee Board of Canada, May 1 1998, GTM29321.E. Available online at: https://www.refworld.org/docid/3ae6acb45f.html (accessed September 14, 2020).

Statistics Canada (2016). *Aboriginal Population Profile, 2016 Census Algoma, District [Census division], Ontario.* Available online at: https://www12.statcan.gc.ca/census-recensement/2016/dp-pd/abpopprof/details/page.cfm?Lang=EandGeo1=CDandCode1=3557andData=CountandSearchText=AlgomaandSearchType=BeginsandB1=AllandGeoLevel=PRandGeoCode=3557andSEX_ID=1andAGE_ID=1andRESGEO_ID=1#fnb1 (accessed February 13, 2021).

Szklarski, C. (2020). Canada's higher COVID-19 death rate tied to better chronic disease control. *The Canadian Press.*·Posted: Jul 16, 2020. Available online at: https://www.cbc.ca/news/health/covid-19-heart-stroke-1.5652003 (accessed July 30, 2020).

United Nations Press Briefing (1999). *Press Conference by Members of Guatemalan Historical Clarification Commission.* March 1, 2020. Available online at: https://www.un.org/press/en/1999/19990301.guate.brf.html (accessed September 16, 2020).

WHO, ICM, and FIGO (2004). *Making Pregnancy Safer: The Critical Role of the Skilled Attendant. A Joint Statement.* Geneva: WHO, ICM, and FIGO.

World Bank (2018). *Life Expectancy.* Available online at: https://data.worldbank.org/indicator/SP.DYN.LE00.IN?locations=GT (accessed September 11, 2020).

Wright, T. (2020). Violence against Indigenous women during COVID-19 sparks calls for MMIWG plan. *The Canadian Press.* May 10, 202. Available online at: https://www.ctvnews.ca/canada/violence-against-indigenous-women-during-covid-19-sparks-calls-for-mmiwg-plan-1.4932833 (accessed November 16, 2020).

16

Maternity Care Preferences for Future Pregnancies Among United States Childbearers: The Impacts of COVID-19

Theresa E. Gildner[1,2] and Zaneta M. Thayer[1,3]*

[1]Department of Anthropology, Dartmouth College, Hanover, NH, United States, [2]Department of Anthropology, Washington University in St. Louis, St. Louis, MO, United States, [3]Ecology, Evolution, Environment and Society Program, Dartmouth College, Hanover, NH, United States

***Correspondence:**
Theresa E. Gildner
gildner@wustl.edu

The COVID-19 pandemic has impacted maternity care decisions, including plans to change providers or delivery location due to pandemic-related restrictions and fears. A relatively unexplored question, however, is how the pandemic may shape future maternity care preferences post-pandemic. Here, we use data collected from an online convenience survey of 980 women living in the United States to evaluate how and why the pandemic has affected women's future care preferences. We hypothesize that while the majority of women will express a continued interest in hospital birth and OB/GYN care due to perceived safety of medicalized birth, a subset of women will express a new interest in out-of-hospital or "community" care in future pregnancies. However, factors such as local provider and facility availability, insurance coverage, and out-of-pocket cost could limit access to such future preferred care options. Among our predominately white, educated, and high-income sample, a total of 58 participants (5.9% of the sample) reported a novel preference for community care during future pregnancies. While the pandemic prompted the exploration of non-hospital options, the reasons women preferred community care were mostly consistent with factors described in pre-pandemic studies, (e.g. a preference for a natural birth model and a desire for more person-centered care). However, a relatively high percentage (34.5%) of participants with novel preference for community care indicated that they expected limitations in their ability to access these services. These findings highlight how the pandemic has potentially influenced maternity care preferences, with implications for how providers and policy makers should anticipate and respond to future care needs.

Keywords: out of hospital, homebirth, birth center, midwife, barriers to care

INTRODUCTION: FACTORS SHAPING MATERNITY CARE PREFERENCES AND BARRIERS TO PREFERRED CARE

Several factors are known to impact maternity care preferences among women living in the United States, particularly concerns about safety and risk during delivery (Klein et al., 2006; Miller and Shriver, 2012). There is a general cultural perception that technology-intensive birth in a hospital setting is the safest option, (i.e. compared to an out-of-hospital birth); a perception reinforced by the media, most prenatal educational material, and conversations with loved ones

(Klein et al., 2006; Miller and Shriver, 2012). In addition, anxiety about pain during delivery can contribute to an increased preference for cesarean birth, epidural anesthesia, and other types of pharmaceutical pain management not available outside of a hospital (Klein et al., 2006; Cheyney, 2008; Caughey and Cheyney, 2019). Unsurprisingly then, the vast majority of births in the United States (98.4%) occur in hospital settings (MacDorman and Declercq, 2019).

Yet growing evidence demonstrates the safety and benefits of "community" care and birth—defined as maternity care and birth experiences physically centered within a community and outside of a hospital (Davis-Floyd and Cheyney, 2019)—for low-risk pregnancies when attended by skilled midwives or (a very few) holistic obstetricians (Cheyney et al., 2014; Hutton et al., 2016; Rossi and Prefumo, 2018). Women seeking community care generally elect to give birth at home or in a freestanding birth center (as opposed to a hospital-based birth center, which is directly affiliated with, and usually inside, a hospital). The freestanding birth center offers a space designed to support women during labor and delivery, while keeping low-risk women out of the hospital (Caughey and Cheyney, 2019). Whether at home or in a birth center, women who choose community birth are attended by a midwife, barring serious complications that require hospital transfer, which occurs in around 11% of planned community births (Cheyney et al., 2014). The majority of midwives attending community deliveries in the United States are Certified Professional Midwives (CPMs), who are trained either by apprenticeship or in vocational midwifery schools, and are required to pass a national exam by demonstrating that they have the knowledge and skills required to attend out-of-hospital/community births (Davis-Floyd, 2018). There are approximately 3,000 practicing CPMs in the United States and its territories (Ida Darragh, NARM Board Chair, personal communication, September. 2020), and 13,024 CNMs—certified nurse-midwives—of whom only around 200 presently attend community births (American College of Nurse-Midwives(ACNM), 2020).

In the past few decades, recognition of the services offered by community midwives has slowly grown, resulting in a small but significant increase in women seeking community births across the United States (MacDorman et al., 2014; Caughey and Cheyney, 2019). Many women report choosing a community delivery because they wish to have more autonomy and control over their birth experience, avoid unnecessary medical interventions, experience provider care continuity, and give birth in what they perceive as a safe, familiar environment (Boucher et al., 2009; Zielinski et al., 2015). The CPMs who primarily attend such births have an approach to maternity care that is explicitly person-centered. "Person-centered care" has been defined in this context as services that account for the values, experiences, and circumstances unique to each individual, while also encouraging the participation of women (and their families) in care decisions (Kozhimannil et al., 2015). Midwifery care aligns well with these goals, usually leading to positive perinatal experiences, including increased comfort discussing care and greater client satisfaction with providers (Kozhimannil et al., 2015; Mattison et al., 2018). In addition, women of color are increasingly seeking community care in order to avoid the structural racism experienced in many hospital settings (Thompson, 2016; Davis, 2019).

Despite the benefits of community care for low-risk women, structural factors limit access to it. Specifically, local availability of care options and socioeconomic position have been shown to influence ability to use preferred providers and care facilities (Miller and Shriver, 2012). Individuals living in areas with few local care options may have to travel farther to access desired care, a pattern also linked with reduced prenatal care (Kitsantas et al., 2012; Meyer et al., 2016). Certain provider and facility types may also be completely inaccessible in some locations. As of 2017, 12 states had fewer than 20 freestanding birthing centers across the entire state, with some states having none (MacDorman and Declercq, 2019). Laws regulating midwifery practice within the United States also vary by state. For example, CPMs can practice legally in only 36 states, though they do practice outside the law in many other states, where they are striving for legalization (Davis-Floyd, 2018). Their questionable legal status in 14 states and low numbers in general potentially limit access to CPMs as primary care providers and curtail some women's ability to plan a community birth (Suarez and Bolton, 2018).

Geographic barriers to maternity care access are also compounded by socioeconomic factors. For instance, community care and delivery options are often not fully covered by insurance plans, further limiting women's choices (MacDorman and Declercq, 2019). Home births and birth center deliveries are typically much less expensive than hospital deliveries. The average cost for the full course of perinatal care and an uncomplicated home birth with a midwife is $2,870; for birth centers, the average cost is $7,240; for hospitals, the average cost for an uncomplicated vaginal birth is $12,156 (Anderson, Daviss, and Johnson, 2021). Many insurance plans will cover hospital-based care but not all community care options (MacDorman and Declercq, 2019). One recent study using United States national birth certificate data found that in the year 2017, approximately two-thirds of planned home births and one-third of birth center deliveries were self-paid by the mother, compared to only 3% of hospital deliveries (MacDorman and Declercq, 2019). Thus, a community birth is likely to be cost-prohibitive for many because it would have to be covered out-of-pocket, as is evident among individuals on Medicaid. In 2017, Medicaid covered just 8.6% of planned home births and 17.9% of birth center births, compared with 43.4% of hospital births (MacDorman and Declercq, 2019). Coverage also varies by state, with some states, (i.e. Alaska, Rhode Island, Vermont, and Washington) exhibiting much lower rates, (i.e. under 20%) of home births paid for out-of-pocket (MacDorman and Declercq, 2019). Both geographic and socioeconomic factors, along with provider accessibility, therefore appear to influence individual ability to access preferred care.

Women's ability to access preferred maternity care providers and facilities is important for improving maternal agency and satisfaction (Peters et al., 2019; Vedam et al., 2019). In addition, provider type can heavily influence birth experience. For instance, midwife use has been linked with reduced fear surrounding birth, increased information sharing by providers, and more individual autonomy (Hildingsson et al., 2019). Care satisfaction has also been shown to significantly impact birth outcomes, such that mothers who report being satisfied with their prenatal care are less likely to use pain relief in labor, deliver healthier babies, and are at lower risk of postpartum depression (Nicoloro-SantaBarbara et al., 2017). Conversely, women reporting dissatisfaction with their maternity care have reported increased pain during delivery. This is a concerning pattern, as poor birth experiences have been linked with elevated risk of postpartum depression (Bell and Andersson, 2016). Since prenatal care satisfaction is essential for optimizing labor and delivery outcomes and maternal mental health, it is important to understand and facilitate maternity care preferences, as well as factors that shape and constrain access to favored providers and facilities.

The complex factors influencing maternity care preferences and care access are currently in flux due to the ongoing COVID-19 pandemic, which has dramatically impacted all aspects of United States maternity care. Partners and support persons, including doulas, have not been allowed to attend prenatal appointments in hospitals and have even been barred from attending deliveries (Davis-Floyd, Gutschow, and Schwartz, 2020; Diamond et al., 2020; Gildner and Thayer, 2020). In many cases, newborns have been separated from mothers with confirmed COVID-19 as part of hospital policy (Davis-Floyd, Gutschow, and Schwartz, 2020; Diamond et al., 2020). Women also report increased fear of viral exposure when attending appointments or laboring in a hospital setting, and may alter their pain management strategy, (e.g. going without an epidural or nitrous oxide) to reduce perceived risk of exposure (Gildner and Thayer, 2020). Cumulatively, these factors have led many women in the United States to consider community care during the pandemic (Davis-Floyd, Gutschow, and Schwartz, 2020; Gildner and Thayer, 2020; Rocca-Ihenacho and Alonso, 2020).

Although preliminary, current evidence suggests that the increase in women preferring community care during the COVID-19 pandemic may be substantial. For example, our previous work using a sample of 1,400 pregnant women living in the United States found that participants displayed a substantially higher preference for community births than the national average before the COVID-19 pandemic (5.4% vs. 1.6%, respectively) (Gildner and Thayer, 2020). Interestingly, this percentage is also relatively high among those 667 participants who had previously given birth. Of those, 3.1% reported a community delivery for at least one of their previous births, but 5.1% of these same women now reported planning for a community delivery (Gildner and Thayer, 2020). These findings suggest that the documented increased preference for community birth is likely at least partly due to the COVID-19 pandemic, although it is unclear whether these altered maternity care preferences will persist beyond this lengthy period of public health crisis.

Additionally, altered care preferences may not be met due to the aforementioned geographic and socioeconomic barriers to preferred community care. Pre-existing care barriers may also be exacerbated during the pandemic. For instance, the current high rates of pandemic-related unemployment are linked with lost health insurance (Gangopadhyaya and Garrett, 2020), potentially inhibiting ability to afford needed maternity care. Reduced provider hours and clinic closures during the pandemic may also prevent women from accessing their preferred care services (Gildner and Thayer, 2020). Given this background, we consider how the COVID-19 pandemic may alter future maternity care preferences, and whether women anticipate barriers to accessing preferred care. Assessing how the pandemic has influenced women's care preferences will provide insight into the future needs of the United States healthcare system. Our study speaks to this nexus of scientific research and public health policy. Our driving questions are: Has the COVID-19 pandemic impacted future preferences for prenatal care? Specifically, do women express an increased interest in seeking community care during future pregnancies, after the pandemic subsides? Additionally, do women who used community care for the first time during their most recent pregnancy because of the pandemic indicate a preference for community care in future pregnancies, even once the pandemic is under control? What factors or experiences have contributed to altered preferences? And finally, what are the most commonly reported anticipated barriers to accessing preferred care in future pregnancies?

MATERIALS AND METHODS

To explore factors influencing altered care preferences and potential barriers to care access, we designed the "COVID-19 And Reproductive Effects" (CARE) study. We posted the CARE study on social media platforms (Facebook, Twitter) and distributed it via email to contacts working in maternity care and public health. Pregnant women over the age of 18 and living in the United States were eligible to participate. In order to increase sample diversity, we shared the study information with Indigenous, Black, and Latinx pregnancy groups, and reached out to contacts working in different geographic regions of the United States Participants who completed the prenatal survey and agreed to be re-contacted received a postnatal survey four weeks after their due date. The postnatal data presented here were collected between June 5–December 15, 2020. This study received ethical approval from Dartmouth College (STUDY00032045). We obtained informed consent from all participants. The survey was administered in REDCap, which automatically captures survey responses. The survey completion rate was 92.9% (1,092/1,175 participants). Survey questions regarding future care preferences were added following the start of data collection, after approximately 100 participants had already filled out the postnatal questionnaire, leading to the completion of 980 questionnaires with these responses.

Key Variables

Novel preference for community birth: A novel preference for community care was defined as women who used community care for the first time during the pandemic and indicated a continued preference for this care model during future pregnancies, as well as women who did not use community care in their most recent pregnancy but intended to during future pregnancies. Participants were asked whether they had changed to a community birth during their most recent pregnancy due to the COVID-19 pandemic. Participants were also asked to select which facility option they would prefer in a future pregnancy from the following list:

TABLE 1 | Codes generated based on common themes identified across participant qualitative descriptions of reasons for care preferences during future pregnancies.

Code name	Code description
Trust	Trust this care type based on previous experience, reputation, and/or level of provider training and expertize
Person-centered	Desire for more person-centered care (greater autonomy, provider communication, and more personalized care)
Holistic/natural	More holistic/natural care model used (fewer interventions and less medicalized)
Safety	Desire to feel safe, comfortable, taken care of, and/or less stressed
Pain	Want access to the pain management option(s) available with this type of care
Risk	High-risk pregnancy or previous cesarean section so feel must deliver using this option and/or want access to emergency care in case of complications
Disease exposure	Feel there is a low risk of disease exposure with this care type

- I would want to give birth in the same type of facility I used for this pregnancy;
- I would now want to give birth in a hospital;
- I would now want to give birth in a hospital-based birth center;
- I would now want to give birth in a freestanding birth center;
- I would now want to give birth at home.

For our analysis, individuals were coded as exhibiting a novel preference for community birth (in their most recent or a future pregnancy): 1) if they indicated that they had changed to a community birth during their most recent pregnancy due to the pandemic and also specified that they wanted a community birth in the future, (i.e. they do not plan to switch back to a hospital birth once the pandemic subsides), or 2) if they stated that in the future they wanted to give birth in a freestanding birth center or at home (but had not delivered in these facility types previously, including their most recent pregnancy).

Reasons for preferring this care option: Respondents were asked why they would select their listed preferred facility type for future pregnancies. For our qualitative content analysis, we used a conventional approach of open followed by focused coding, (e.g. Hsieh and Shannon. 2005; Saldaña, 2009). Specifically, first author Theresa Gildner read through all participant responses and took notes on keywords or phrases that were repeatedly used. She then generated preliminary codes she shared with co-author Zaneta Thayer, who then reviewed a subset of responses using these codes, adding new codes when no existing code matched the data (**Table 1**). Two Dartmouth undergraduate research assistants, Amanda Lu and Cecily Craighead, then independently coded the responses. Disagreements were discussed and reconciled between the two coders and Gildner to ensure consistency.

Expected barriers to preferred care during future pregnancies: Participants were asked if they anticipated any factors limiting access to their preferred facility type in a future pregnancy (Yes/No). If participants selected "Yes," they also indicated which of the following factors were expected to limit their access (selecting all that applied):

- My preferred care type is not available in my area;
- My preferred care type is not covered by my insurance;
- My preferred care type is too expensive;
- Other, describe.

Sample Characteristics

As described elsewhere (Thayer and Gildner, 2020), demographic data were collected on participant age, race/ethnicity, household income, education, zip code, and prior birth(s). Rural-Urban Continuum Codes (RUCC) were generated from zip code data to assess local population size (Gildner et al., 2020). Briefly, the RUCC is based on the county located at the zip code center point, with each participant receiving a code reflecting local population size and whether the area is classified as metropolitan or non-metropolitan (USDA, 2013). To assess insurance coverage, respondents were asked if they currently had any form of medical insurance (Yes/No), and whether their current insurance plan covered their preferred maternity care (Yes/No). Additionally, participants reported whether they were on Medicaid (Yes/No). For those participants who had given birth previously, prior birth location was also reported and coded as community (home or freestanding birth clinic) or in-hospital (hospital or hospital-based birth center). Finally, respondents reported where they had given birth during their most recent pregnancy (during the pandemic).

Analytic Approach

We conducted data analyses using Stata 14, generating sample descriptive statistics and assessing participant responses to address the primary study questions listed above.

Question 1: We calculated the frequency of women in the sample reporting a preference for community care during future pregnancies. Additionally, as described above, we coded the reasons given by women for these preferences to identify common themes and assessed the frequency of these coded responses within the sample (**Table 1**).

Question 2: We measured the percentage of participants who reported anticipated barriers to preferred future care, as well as the frequency with which each barrier type was selected from the provided list.

RESULTS

Sample Characteristics

Sample descriptive statistics are presented in **Table 2**. Participants lived in all 50 United States states and the District of Columbia.

TABLE 2 | Descriptive statistics of study sample. Sample means (with standard deviation and range) or frequency (percent) of model variables, for 980 participants.

Variable	Mean (SD; range)
Age (years)	31.9 (3.99; 18–47)
	Frequency (%)
Race/ethnicity	
White	868 (88.6%)
Hispanic, Latinx, or Spanish origin	48 (4.90%)
Black or African American	10 (1.02%)
Asian	28 (2.86%)
American Indian or Alaskan native	6 (0.61%)
Native Hawaiian or other Pacific Islander	3 (0.31%)
Other	17 (1.73%)
Location	
Metropolitan area, >1,000,000	583 (61.8%)
Metropolitan area, 250,000–1,000,000	209 (22.2%)
Metropolitan area, <250,000	70 (7.42%)
Non-metropolitan area	81 (8.59%)
Household income	
< $49,999	86 (8.86%)
$50,000–$99,999	298 (30.7%)
$100,000+	587 (60.5%)
Education level	
Less than a bachelor's degree	146 (14.9%)
Bachelor's degree	356 (36.4%)
Degree beyond a bachelor's degree	477 (48.7%)
Insurance coverage	
No	6 (0.61%)
Yes	974 (99.4%)
Insurance cover preferred maternity care	
No	48 (4.94%)
Yes	924 (95.1%)
Medicaid coverage	
No	908 (93.3%)
Yes	65 (6.68%)
Previous birth (before pandemic)	
No	496 (50.7%)
Yes	482 (49.3%)
Ever given birth at this location (before pandemic)	
Hospital or hospital-based birth center	464 (96.3%)
Home or freestanding birth clinic	18 (3.73%)
Birth location during the COVID-19 pandemic	
Hospital or hospital-based birth center	939 (95.8%)
Home or freestanding birth clinic	39 (3.98%)
In a car	2 (0.20%)
Novel future preference for community birth	
No	922 (94.1%)
Yes	58 (5.92%)
Anticipate barriers to future care	
No	930 (94.9%)
Yes	50 (5.10%)

Altered Care Preferences During Future Pregnancies

A total of 58 participants (5.92%) in the sample reported a novel preference for community birth following the onset of the COVID-19 pandemic, compared to 22 participants who had already preferred community care (even prior to the onset of the pandemic)–an over 200% increase in preference for community care. There was a clear overlap between preference for community delivery and midwifery care (51 participants preferred midwifery care, 87.9% of participants had a new preference for community care). Out of the participants exhibiting a novel preference for community care, 18 of the 20 women who reported changing from a hospital to a community birth during the pandemic also indicated they would prefer a community delivery during future pregnancies as well.

Of these 18 participants, 14 indicated they switched because they were concerned about hospital limits on support persons being able to attend delivery, and therefore having to labor alone. Thirteen of these women also reported being worried about being separated from their baby in a hospital setting, while 13 also indicated they were afraid of contracting COVID-19 at the hospital. Another 13 of these women indicated that they were concerned about restrictive hospital policies, (e.g. being forced to wear a mask during active labor). In addition to the 18 participants who chose a community birth for their most recent pregnancy and indicated they would also seek community care during future pregnancies, 40 women reported that they planned to opt for a community birth during future pregnancies (after the pandemic), resulting in a total of 58 participants exhibiting a novel preference for community care. When asked why they would select a community location for future deliveries, some common themes emerged. Of the subset of 53 participants with a novel preference for community care who described the reasons behind this partiality, 34.0% (18/53) stated that they perceived these care options to adhere to a more "natural" birth model, with less reliance on medical interventions or medications to speed up delivery, and more holistic and continuous care throughout pregnancy and the postpartum period. Similarly, 30.2% (16/53) of these participants reported that they felt these options would be more person-centered, (e.g. more effective provider communication, greater respect for the autonomy of the women and her birth plan, and more personalized care). In addition, 11.3% (6/53) of these respondents preferred a community delivery due to a lower perceived risk of pathogen exposure, while 37.7% (20/53) of participants described preferring community care because they felt safe and well cared for in these settings.

Participants who expressed a preference for in-hospital deliveries during future pregnancies were also asked to describe why they favored this option. A total of 900 participants indicated they preferred an in-hospital delivery, (i.e. hospital or hospital-based birth center). Of the 620 participants who described why they preferred an in-hospital birth, 46.5% (288/620) reported a desire to deliver in a hospital to ensure easy access to medical interventions, either due to personal risk factors, (e.g. previous cesarean birth) or in case of complications during delivery. Likewise, 32.6% (202/620) of these respondents stated that they felt most safe and well cared for in a hospital. Medicalized pain management also appeared to be a consideration for some women; 4.5% (28/620) of participants indicated that this was a primary motivation for seeking an in-hospital delivery in the future. Finally, 44.0% (273/620) of these respondents reported preferring an in-hospital delivery because they trusted the experience and training of medical staff, (e.g. due to personal experience in past deliveries or facility reputation).

Anticipated Barriers to Accessing Preferred Care During Future Pregnancies

Fifty participants (5.1% of the sample) reported that they expected barriers in accessing their preferred future care provider or facility type. Of those reporting a novel preference for community delivery, 34.5% (20/58) stated that they anticipated barriers that could prevent them from accessing their preferred care. We asked these respondents to indicate which factors may inhibit their care access. Seven participants reported that their preferred community care type was not available locally (was located too far away), eight stated that their preferred care type was not covered by their insurance, and eight said that it was too expensive. All other participants reported barriers that could be classified as reflecting high-risk pregnancies; specifically, six women reported they would likely be unable to access preferred care due to underlying medical conditions, age restrictions, or because they had previously delivered by cesarean.

DISCUSSION: NOVEL PREFERENCES FOR COMMUNITY CARE AND BARRIERS TO ACCESS

While the overwhelming majority of births in the United States occur within hospital settings, there has been an increase in community births in recent years. Our findings support the idea that the COVID-19 pandemic may have further accelerated this shift in maternity care preferences. These novel preferences were evident both among women who changed their birth plans during the pandemic and among those who were unable to alter their birth plans during this most recent pregnancy, but who stated that they intend to seek community care in future pregnancies. Notably, while the pandemic was the impetus for many women to explore out-of-hospital birthing options, the reasons why women stated that they preferred community births were largely consistent with reasons found in studies prior to the pandemic, including patient-centered care and preference for less medical intervention. Although the majority of these participants did not report any anticipated barriers to accessing their community care preferences, a relatively high proportion (over one-third) did indicate that they expected such limitations. This finding shows that there are perceived and real barriers to community care access in the United States Since our sample was whiter, wealthier, and more educated than the general population, it is likely that the prevalence of barriers would be even higher among a nationally representative sample of birthing mothers, particularly one that included more women of color.

Pandemic-Related Changes in Care Preferences

Of the 20 women who switched to community care during the pandemic, 18 reported that they would prefer a community birth during future pregnancies (while the other two indicated they would prefer an in-hospital birth in the future), even once the pandemic subsides. This suggests that their community-based perinatal experiences during this most recent pregnancy were positive, reinforcing their desire to use community care going forward (all respondents quoted below are white, reflecting the great majority of our sample). For example, one woman who switched to a community delivery during the pandemic stated:

Switching to the birthing center and midwife care was a blessing in disguise. They were totally aligned with our birthing goals and helped to facilitate the experience we wanted far better than a hospital and/or our previous provider could have (33-year-old, primigravid participant with a Bachelor's degree, living in a metro area of over one million people).

Likewise, a second participant described the benefits resulting from this unexpected birth plan change, affirming her desire to use community care during any future pregnancies:

Home birth was a wonderful and less stressful experience than my previous two hospital births—simply because I was at home which was a significantly less stimulating environment and I was surrounded exclusively by known people who I have established trusting relationships with (36-year-old, multigravid participant with a Master's degree, living in a metro area of over one million people).

Such participant experiences, which are representative of others, highlight how altered birth plans in response to the pandemic may lead to a continued preference for community deliveries in the future. Pandemic-related fears, (i.e. restrictive hospital policies, limited support during labor, separation from their infant, and disease exposure in a hospital setting) appear to have led women to assess the merits of community care options, altering their birth plans in some cases as they learned more about these previously unconsidered options and leading to lasting changes in care preference. While shifts towards community birth existed prior to the pandemic (MacDorman et al., 2014; Caughey and Cheyney, 2019), these results suggest that the pandemic may have served to further accelerate this shift. Several participants described how the pandemic had made them more aware of community care options:

Home birth was a great experience that I may not have tried without the pandemic (28-year-old, multigravid participant with a PhD, living in a metro area with a population of 250,000-—one million people).

Because of Covid and limitations in place, I have educated myself on other options and feel they meet my needs and the type of birth experience I want (32-year-old, multigravid participant with a Master's degree, living in a metro area of over one million people).

Some participants went further, describing how the pandemic led them to consider alternative birth models. As one respondent said:

While I was born at home myself, had not really considered home birth until the COVID-19 pandemic hit and it became possible that hospital facilities could be overwhelmed and my partner would not be permitted to attend me. In considering home birth for those reasons, I also became more concerned by the medicalization of the birth experience that can be associated with a hospital experience (36-year-old, primigravid participant with a Bachelor's degree, living in a non-metro area).

Concern about the medicalization of hospital birth was common throughout the subset of women reporting a new preference for community deliveries, as was a preference for a more holistic, natural birth model (34.0% of the subset). Women also asserted that they believed community births to be safer, both because community care prevented pathogen exposure (relative to a hospital setting) and/or because they felt most comfortable delivering in a less-medicalized environment (11.3% and 37.7% of the subset, respectively). Participants also reported a preference for community care due the belief that it is more person-centered (30.2% of the subset), thereby alleviating stress and enhancing their autonomy. As respondents noted:

I also love the idea of staying in the comfort of home and having a skilled birth [attendant] come to me instead of having to worry about when to leave for the hospital. And I find driving home with a newborn stressful, but birthing at home removes that factor (37-year-old, multigravid participant with a professional degree, living in a metro area of under 250,000 people).

Homebirths are AMAZING!!! I got to co-sleep and do what I wanted to do . . . (32-year-old, multigravid participant with a Bachelor's degree, living in a metro area of over one million people).

Nevertheless, as noted above, of the 900 participants who described why they would prefer an in-hospital birth during a future pregnancy, nearly half (46.5%) stated that this was because it afforded ready access to medical interventions in case of complications. Furthermore, in contrast to the women who reported feeling safest outside of a hospital, nearly one-third (32.6%) of the participants preferring in-hospital care described feeling more secure and cared for in a medical environment. These findings cumulatively suggest that most U. S. women still perceive community deliveries as inherently more dangerous than giving birth in a hospital—a concern that could outweigh competing desires to avoid hospital delivery during the pandemic. Yet it is interesting to note that although participants used similar terms ("safe," "secure," "less dangerous," etc.) to describe their preferences, individuals appeared to have very dissimilar perceptions of what these terms could mean in different circumstances and how these concepts applied to maternity care. A subset of women clearly defined "safe maternity care" as more medicalized, with easily available interventions and OB/GYNs. In contrast, other participants considered less-medicalized community care with fewer interventions to be the "safer" option.

These opposing views are likely due to a range of factors, including personal experience, stories from friends and family, exposure to various maternity care models in the media, and knowledge about the benefits and risks associated with each option (Klein et al., 2006; Sunil et al., 2010; Miller and Shriver, 2012; Smith et al., 2018). Many of these proximal factors may reflect the normative acceptance of the biomedicalization of childbirth in United States contexts (Jordan, 1993; Davis-Floyd, 2003, 2005; Wendland, 2007). However, as with so much else during the COVID-19 pandemic, this moment may represent an inflection point for some women, causing them to reassess their previous perceptions regarding the safety of hospital vs. community care. Indeed, the fact that 5.92% of the sample exhibited a novel preference for community deliveries is meaningful. Although birth center births more than doubled and home births increased by 77% between 2004 and 2017 in the United States, only one of every 62 births (1.61%) was classified as a community delivery in 2017 (MacDorman and Declercq, 2019). Thus, the 5.92% novel preference for community births during the pandemic in our sample could represent a substantial increase within the United States birthing population as a whole. These altered preferences may subsequently foster a greater demand for midwifery-led person-centered care models in community settings in the coming years, even after the pandemic ends, leading to better birth outcomes and large cost-savings (Anderson, Daviss, and Johnson 2021).

Barriers to Accessing Preferred Future Care

Only 50 respondents (5.1% of the sample) indicated that they anticipated barriers in accessing preferred future care types. Yet a relatively high percentage (34.5%) of participants expressing a novel preference for community deliveries reported that they expected barriers in accessing these new care preferences. Reported barriers, (e.g. lack of insurance coverage) may become more common in coming years, as evidenced by recent changes in maternity care costs. Out-of-pocket maternity care costs for all services have risen in the last decade, including for women with employer-based insurance and those in higher-income brackets (Moniz et al., 2020). Specifically, the Affordable Care Act requires employer-based insurance plans to cover maternity care, but plans are allowed to impose high deductibles and copayments for these services.

As a result, out-of-pocket service costs rose between 2008–2015, despite the cost of care remaining the same; a pattern largely attributed to rising deductibles (Moniz et al., 2020). These higher costs may lead women to delay or avoid needed care, which could subsequently lead to poor maternal and infant health outcomes. Thus, while the relatively affluent women in this sample may have been able to afford these higher out-of-pocket costs, evidence suggests a current trend of rising service costs for all women living in the United States--a pattern that is especially concerning given the growing unemployment rates, lost insurance coverage, and financial stress associated with the COVID-19 pandemic. If out-of-pocket maternity care costs continue to increase as the economic consequences of the pandemic persist, it seems likely that a larger portion of the pregnant women living in the United States will be unable to access preferred and needed services. This will be particularly evident for lower income women, who are more likely to be women of color.

Medical Care and Policy Implications

Even prior to the pandemic, United States maternity care outcomes were troubling. Recent estimates indicate that the United States spends roughly 17.8% of national gross domestic product (GDP) on health care, significantly higher than other high-income nations, which tend to range between 9.6 and 12.4% (Papanicolas et al., 2018; Martin et al., 2019a). Despite this high investment in health care, the United States consistently reports worse health outcomes relative to other high-income countries, with fewer people accessing health insurance, lower life expectancies, and higher maternal and infant mortality rates (especially among Black women) (Gunja et al., 2018; Papanicolas et al., 2018). These poor outcomes have led to active calls for healthcare reform in the United States. (e.g. an increased interest in "Medicare for all")--demands expected to be bolstered by the economic and medical fallout of the COVID-19 pandemic (King, 2020).

There are already signs of shifts in medical care services and insurance coverage. To take one example, Medicaid and other insurance types have recently expanded coverage to include telehealth appointments–including for maternity care–during the pandemic (Fryer et al., 2020). These changes are likely to also impact access to maternity care options, potentially enhancing the availability of community care services. For instance, in June 2020 the New York State COVID-19 Maternity Task Force announced that New York Governor Andrew Cuomo had directed the State Department of Health to allow freestanding birth centers run by midwives to operate independently for the first time in state history (New York State Government, 2020), providing pregnant women in New York State with more care options to meet their specific needs. Moreover, the task force moved to expedite the licensure process required to certify midwife-led freestanding birth centers (New York State Government, 2020).

Similar efforts to expand access to community births and midwifery care during the pandemic are also evident in other states, (e.g. Maine, New Jersey, Pennsylvania, Tennessee, and Texas) (Platt, 2020). These changes may have the added benefit of addressing the anticipated shortage of OB/GYN providers expected in coming years as a high proportion of doctors retire amidst a national shortage of younger doctors. This expected shortage has been attributed to a range of factors, including fewer ON/GYNs providing around-the-clock care and more maternity care doctors practicing subspecialties that do not involve routine deliveries (Ollove, 2016). More readily available midwifery community-based care may consequently address expected rising national demands for maternity care providers.

Study Limitations

Important study limitations exist. First, as previously mentioned, these data are not representative of the United States population as a whole. Women in our sample were older (31.9 years vs a national average of 29.0 in 2018), more likely to be white (88.6% in this sample vs 51.6% nationally), highly educated with at least Bachelor's degree (85.1% vs 33.0%), and were slightly more likely to live in a metropolitan area (91.4% vs 86.5%) (Centers for Disease Control and Prevention (CDC), 2020; Martin et al., 2019b). These demographic differences may contribute to variation in community care preferences and access. Evidence indicates that lower education levels are associated with limited knowledge of all care options (Sunil et al., 2010; Smith et al., 2018), resulting in higher rates of community births among well-educated women (Boucher et al., 2009), who are also more likely to be able to afford them. The high education levels evident in this sample may predispose participants to consider and seek out community care options.

In addition, rates of community birth are higher among white women than women of color (MacDorman and Declercq, 2019). This pattern has been attributed to a range of reasons, including financial barriers to preferred care and racial and ethnic disparities in high-risk pregnancy diagnoses, (e.g. preeclampsia and diabetes) that may increase the likelihood of delivery in a hospital setting for women of color (Howell, 2018; Onwuzurike et al., 2020). Still, the potential value of community births for women of color in particular is being increasingly recognized, as culturally centered community care can reduce exposure to structural racism and customize care to the needs of the individual (Hardeman et al., 2020; Tilden et al., 2020). Future care preference alterations should consequently be explored in more diverse study populations, which may experience greater barriers to learning about and accessing community care, especially during the pandemic.

For example, women of color appear more likely to experience pandemic-related maternity care disruptions for a variety of reasons linked with underlying structural inequities. These factors include less reliable access to phone and internet services needed for telehealth appointments, a greater reliance on public transportation to access care (which may be cut back due to the pandemic), and an increased likelihood of working in essential services (which may curtail their flexibility in scheduling healthcare appointments) (Onwuzurike et al., 2020). It is therefore necessary to consider how pandemic-related care disruptions and healthcare policy changes may exacerbate existing inequities, particularly among minority communities that have historically experienced inferior maternity care, less provider information sharing, and poorer birth outcomes (Niles et al., 2020; Onwuzurike et al., 2020), ultimately diminishing women's autonomy and their direct involvement in healthcare decisions (Altman et al., 2019). These disparities may consequently influence women's care preferences and the barriers they may face to accessing their preferred provider or facility.

Another study limitation is that we did not explicitly ask about home-to-hospital transfers; therefore, we do not have data on how many of our participants who planned community births ended up transferring to the hospital. This is an important issue, as other data show that while unforeseen complications are a primary driver of hospital transfers (Caughey and Cheyney. 2019), childbearers who are not fully ideologically committed to home birth do sometimes transfer to hospitals during labor, primarily for labor dystocia/failure to progress, because they feel safest in hospitals (Davis-Floyd, Gutschow, and Schwartz 2020).

CONCLUSION: ANTICIPATING FUTURE NEEDS

As women reassess their birth plans in response to pandemic-related concerns and limitations, it appears that some are learning more about community care options, with implications for current and future decisions. Our findings suggest that positive community delivery experiences during the pandemic, negative perceptions of in-hospital services, and a greater appreciation for the benefits of person-centered care may all contribute to shifting preferences among at least a subset of women living in the United States, and that these altered care preferences may persist beyond the COVID-19 pandemic. If true, this social shift will likely necessitate greater investment in CPM training, legalization, and licensing, as well as expanded insurance coverage to include community care services. Greater availability of community, person-centered care models for low-risk pregnancies may also represent a cost-effective strategy for reducing the current relatively high rates of maternal and infant mortality. Specifically, community care is linked with lower rates of poor birth outcomes, (i.e. preterm birth, low birth weight infants, and neonatal death) (Vedam et al., 2018). The maternity care experiences and preferences of women during the COVID-19 pandemic may therefore offer a view into how care decisions are changing in response to novel conditions, with implications for anticipating and responding to future needs.

ETHICS STATEMENT

The studies involving human participants were reviewed and approved by Dartmouth College (No. STUDY00032045). The patients/participants provided their written informed consent to participate in this study.

AUTHOR CONTRIBUTIONS

TG is a co-PI of the CARE project, conducted the analyses presented here, and drafted the manuscript. ZT is a co-PI of the CARE project, assisted in analysis design, and helped to edit the manuscript. Both authors read and approved the final manuscript.

ACKNOWLEDGMENTS

We would like to thank Sienna Craig, Chelsey Kivland, Robbie Davis-Floyd and Kim Gutschow for their invaluable feedback on this article. We are also grateful for Nadia Clement's assistance building the online survey and designing the recruitment flyers. We would also like to thank Margaret Sherin, Glorieuse Uwizeye, and Chlöe Sweetman for their useful feedback on the questionnaire during development. Further, we express our gratitude to Grace Alston, Cecily Craighead, Amanda Lu, and Rebecca Milner for their assistance in data coding and literature review.

REFERENCES

Altman, M. R., Oseguera, T., McLemore, M. R., Kantrowitz-Gordon, I., Franck, L. S., and Lyndon, A. (2019). Information and power: women of color's experiences interacting with health care providers in pregnancy and birth. *Soc. Sci. Med.* 238, 112491. doi:10.1016/j.socscimed.2019.112491

American College of Nurse-Midwives (ACNM) (2020). www.midwife.org.

Anderson, D. A., Daviss, B. A., and Johnson, K. C. (2021). "What if another 10% of deliveries in the United States occurred at home or in a birth center? Safety, economics, and politics," in *Birthing models on the human rights frontier: speaking truth to power.* Editors B. A. Daviss and R. Davis-Floyd (London, United Kingdom: Routledge).

Bell, A. F., and Andersson, E. (2016). The birth experience and women's postnatal depression: a systematic review. *Midwifery* 39, 112–123. doi:10.1016/j.midw.2016.04.014

Boucher, D., Bennett, C., McFarlin, B., and Freeze, R. (2009). Staying home to give birth: why women in the United States choose home birth. *J. Midwifery Wom. Health* 54 (2), 119–126. doi:10.1016/j.jmwh.2008.09.006

Caughey, A. B., and Cheyney, M. (2019). Home and birth center birth in the United States: time for greater collaboration across models of care. *Obstet. Gynecol.* 133 (5), 1033–1050. doi:10.1097/AOG.0000000000003215

Centers for Disease Control and Prevention (CDC) (2020). *Natality, 2016-2019 expanded results.* Available: https://wonder.cdc.gov/natality-expanded-current.html.

Cheyney, M., Bovbjerg, M., Everson, C., Gordon, W., Hannibal, D., and Vedam, S. (2014). Outcomes of care for 16,924 planned home births in the United States: the midwives alliance of north America statistics project, 2004 to 2009. *J. Midwifery Wom. Health* 59 (1), 17–27. doi:10.1111/jmwh.12172

Cheyney, M. J. (2008). Homebirth as systems-challenging praxis: knowledge, power, and intimacy in the birthplace. *Qual. Health Res.* 18 (2), 254–267. doi:10.1177/1049732307312393

Davis, D. A. (2019). Obstetric racism: the racial politics of pregnancy, labor, and birthing. *Med. Anthropol.* 38(7), 560–573. doi:10.1080/01459740.2018.1549389

Davis-Floyd, R., Gutschow, K., and Schwartz, D. A. (2020). Pregnancy, birth and the COVID-19 pandemic in the United States. *Med. Anthropol.* 39 (5), 413–427. doi:10.1080/01459740.2020.1761804

Davis-Floyd, R. (2018). American midwifery: a brief anthropological overview. *Ways of knowing about birth: mothers, midwives, medicine, and birth activism by Robbie davis-floyd.* Long Grove IL, United States: Waveland Press, 165–188.

Davis-Floyd, R. (2005). Anthropology and birth activism: what do we know? *Anthropol. News* 45 (5), 37–38. doi:10.1525/an.2005.46.5.37

Davis-Floyd, R. (2003). *Birth as an American rite of passage.* Berkeley CA, United States: University of California Press.

Davis-Floyd, R., and Cheyney, M. (2019). *Birth in eight cultures.* Long Grove IL, United States: Waveland Press.

Diamond, R. M., Brown, K. S., and Miranda, J. (2020). Impact of COVID-19 on the perinatal period through a biopsychosocial systemic framework. *Contemp. Fam. Ther.* 42 (3), 205–216. doi:10.1007/s10591-020-09544-8

Fryer, K., Delgado, A., Foti, T., Reid, C. N., and Marshall, J. (2020). Implementation of obstetric telehealth during COVID-19 and beyond. *Matern. Child Health J.* 24 (9), 1104–1110. doi:10.1007/s10995-020-02967-7

Gangopadhyaya, A., and Garrett, A. B. (2020). Unemployment, health insurance, and the COVID-19 recession. *SSRN Electronic Journal.*, 1–8. doi:10.2139/ssrn.3568489

Gildner, T. E., Laugier, E. J., and Thayer, Z. M. (2020). Exercise routine change is associated with prenatal depression scores during the COVID-19 pandemic among pregnant women across the United States. *PloS One* 15 (12), e0243188. doi:10.1371/journal.pone.0243188

Gildner, T. E., and Thayer, Z. M. (2020). Birth plan alterations among American women in response to COVID-19. *Health Expect.* 23(4), 969–971. doi:10.1111/hex.13077

Gunja, M. Z., Tikkanen, R., Seervai, S., and Collins, S. (2018). *What is the status of women's health and health care in the US compared to ten other countries.* New York, NY, United States: Commonwealth Fund.

Hardeman, R. R., Karbeah, J., Almanza, J., and Kozhimannil, K. B. (2020). Roots Community Birth Center: a culturally-centered care model for improving value and equity in childbirth. *Health*, 8(1), 100367. doi:10.1016/j.hjdsi.2019.100367

Hildingsson, I., Rubertsson, C., Karlström, A., and Haines, H. (2019). A known midwife can make a difference for women with fear of childbirth- birth outcome and women's experiences of intrapartum care. *Sexual and Reproductive Healthcare* 21, 33–38. doi:10.1016/j.srhc.2019.06.004

Howell, E. A. (2018). Reducing disparities in severe maternal morbidity and mortality. *Clin. Obstet. Gynecol.* 61 (2), 387. doi:10.1097/GRF.0000000000000349

Hsieh, H. F., and Shannon, S. E. (2005). Three approaches to qualitative content analysis. *Qual. Health Res.* 15 (9), 1277–1288. doi:10.1177/1049732305276687

Hutton, E. K., Cappelletti, A., Reitsma, A. H., Simioni, J., Horne, J., McGregor, C., et al. (2016). Outcomes associated with planned place of birth among women with low-risk pregnancies. *CMAJ (Can. Med. Assoc. J.)* 188 (5), E80–E90. doi:10.1503/cmaj.150564

Jordan, B. (1993). *Birth in four cultures: a crosscultural investigation of childbirth in yucatan, holland, Sweden, and the United States.* Long Grove, IL, United States: Waveland Press.

King, J. S. (2020). Covid-19 and the need for health care reform. *N. Engl. J. Med.* 382 (26), e104. doi:10.1056/NEJMp2000821

Kitsantas, P., Gaffney, K. F., and Cheema, J. (2012). Life stressors and barriers to timely prenatal care for women with high-risk pregnancies residing in rural and nonrural areas. *Wom. Health Issues* 22 (5), e455–60. doi:10.1016/j.whi.2012.06.003

Klein, M. C., Sakala, C., Simkin, P., Davis-Floyd, R., Rooks, J. P., and Pincus, J. (2006). Why do women go along with this stuff?. *Birth* 33 (3), 245–250. doi:10.1111/j.1523-536X.2006.00110.x

Kozhimannil, K. B., Attanasio, L. B., Yang, Y. T., Avery, M. D., and Declercq, E. (2015). Midwifery care and patient-provider communication in maternity decisions in the United States. *Matern. Child Health J.* 19 (7), 1608–1615. doi:10.1007/s10995-015-1671-8

MacDorman, M. F., and Declercq, E. (2019). Trends and state variations in out-of-hospital births in the United States, 2004-2017. *Birth* 46 (2), 279–288. doi:10.1111/birt.12411

MacDorman, M. F., Mathews, T. J., and Declercq, E. (2014). Trends in out-of-hospital births in the United States, 1990-2012. *NCHS Data Brief.* 144, 1–8. doi:10.1097/01.ogx.0000499836.04602.b3

Martin, A. B., Hartman, M., Washington, B., and Catlin, A. (2019a). National health care spending in 2017: growth slows to post-great recession rates; share of GDP stabilizes. *Health Aff.* 38 (1), 101377hlthaff201805085. doi:10.1377/hlthaff10.1377/hlthaff.2018.05085

Martin, J. A., Hamilton, B. E., Osterman, M. J., and Driscoll, A. K. (2019b). *Births: final data for 2018* Available: https://www.cdc.gov/nchs/data/nvsr/nvsr68/nvsr68_13-508.pdf.

Mattison, C. A., Dion, M. L., Lavis, J. N., Hutton, E. K., and Wilson, M. G. (2018). Midwifery and obstetrics: factors influencing mothers' satisfaction with the birth experience. *Birth* 45 (3), 322–327. doi:10.1111/birt.12352

Meyer, E., Hennink, M., Rochat, R., Julian, Z., Pinto, M., Zertuche, A. D., et al. (2016). Working towards safe motherhood: delays and barriers to prenatal care for women in rural and peri-urban areas of Georgia. *Matern. Child Health J.* 20 (7), 1358–1365. doi:10.1007/s10995-016-1997-x

Miller, A. C., and Shriver, T. E. (2012). Women's childbirth preferences and practices in the United States. *Soc. Sci. Med.* 75 (4), 709–716. doi:10.1016/j.socscimed.2012.03.051

Moniz, M. H., Fendrick, A. M., Kolenic, G. E., Tilea, A., Admon, L. K., and Dalton, V. K. (2020). Out-of-pocket spending for maternity care among women with employer-based insurance, 2008-15. *Health Aff.* 39 (1), 18–23. doi:10.1377/hlthaff.2019.00296

New York State Government (2020). *Governor Cuomo and COVID-19 maternity task force Chair melissa DeRosa announce increased access to midwife-led birth centers amid COVID-19 pandemic.* Governor Andrew M. Cuomo: https://www.governor.ny.gov/news/governor-cuomo-covid-19-maternity-task-force-chair-melissa-derosa-announce-increased-access.

Nicoloro-SantaBarbara, J., Rosenthal, L., Auerbach, M. V., Kocis, C., Busso, C., and Lobel, M. (2017). Patient-provider communication, maternal anxiety, and self-care in pregnancy. *Soc. Sci. Med.* 190, 133–140. doi:10.1016/j.socscimed.2017.08.011

Niles, P. M., Asiodu, I. V., Crear-Perry, J., Julian, Z., Lyndon, A., McLemore, M. R., et al. (2020). Reflecting on equity in perinatal care during a pandemic. *Health Equity* 4 (1), 330–333. doi:10.1089/heq.2020.0022

Ollove, M. (2016). *A shortage in the nation's maternal health care.* Washington, DC, United States: Pew Charitable Trusts. Online at: www.pewtrusts.org.

Onwuzurike, C., Meadows, A. R., and Nour, N. M. (2020). Examining inequities associated with changes in obstetric and gynecologic care delivery during the coronavirus disease 2019 (COVID-19) pandemic. *Obstet. Gynecol.* 136 (1), 37–41. doi:10.1097/AOG.0000000000003933

Papanicolas, I., Woskie, L. R., and Jha, A. K. (2018). Health care spending in the United States and other high-income countries. *Jama* 319 (10), 1024–1039. doi:10.1001/jama.2018.1150

Peters, I. A., Posthumus, A. G., Steegers, E. A. P., and Denktaş, S. (2019). Satisfaction with obstetric care in a population of low-educated native Dutch and non-western minority women. Focus group research. *PloS One* 14 (1), e0210506. doi:10.1371/journal.pone.0210506

Platt, T. (2020). *States implement strategies to safeguard pregnant women during the COVID-19 pandemic – the national academy for state health policy* https://www.nashp.org/states-implement-strategies-to-safeguard-pregnant-women-during-the-covid-19-pandemic/.

Rocca-Ihenacho, L., and Alonso, C. (2020). Where do women birth during a pandemic? Changing perspectives on Safe Motherhood during the COVID-19 pandemic. *Journal of Global Health Science* 2 (1), e4. doi:10.35500/jghs.2020.2.e4

Rossi, A. C., and Prefumo, F. (2018). Planned home versus planned hospital births in women at low-risk pregnancy: a systematic review with meta-analysis. *Eur. J. Obstet. Gynecol. Reprod. Biol.* 222, 102–108. doi:10.1016/j.ejogrb.2018.01.016

Saldaña, J. (2009). An introduction to codes and coding. *The coding manual for qualitative researchers* 3. 3rd Ed, Thousand Oaks, CA:SAGE publishers

Smith, J. N., Taylor, B., Shaw, K., Hewison, A., and Kenyon, S. (2018). "I didn't think you were allowed that, they didn't mention that." A qualitative study exploring women's perceptions of home birth. *BMC Pregnancy Childbirth* 18 (1), 1–11. doi:10.1186/s12884-018-1733-1

Suarez, A., and Bolton, M. (2018). Catching babies in prohibition states: midwives' accounts for an illegal profession. *Symbolic Interact.* 41 (2), 165–184. doi:10.1002/symb.339

Sunil, T. S., Spears, W. D., Hook, L., Castillo, J., and Torres, C. (2010). Initiation of and barriers to prenatal care use among low-income women in san antonio, Texas. *Matern. Child Health J.* 14 (1), 133–140. doi:10.1007/s10995-008-0419-0

Thayer, Z. M., and Gildner, T. E. (2020). COVID-19-related financial stress associated with higher likelihood of depression among pregnant women living in the United States. *Am. J. Hum. Biol.*, e23508. doi:10.1002/ajhb.23508

Thompson, D. (2016). Midwives and pregnant women of color: why We need to understand intersectional changes in midwifery to reclaim home birth. *Columbia Journal of Race and Law.* United States Department of Agriculture(USDA). Rural-Urban Continuum Codes. 2013. Available: https://www.ers.usda.gov/data-products/rural-urban-continuum-codes.aspx. 6, 27. doi:10.7916/D8V69JX0

Tilden, E. L., Phillippi, J. C., and Snowden, J. M. (2020). COVID-19 and perinatal care: facing challenges, seizing opportunities. *J. Midwifery Wom. Health.* doi:10.1111/jmwh.13193

United States Census Bureau (2019). *Fertility of women in the United States: 2018. Table 7: household income and income per household member among women with a birth in the past year by marital status: 2017.* Available: https://www.census.gov/data/tables/2018/demo/fertility/women-fertility.html#par_reference_1.

Vedam, S., Stoll, K., MacDorman, M., Declercq, E., Cramer, R., Cheyney, M., et al. (2018). Mapping integration of midwives across the United States: impact on access, equity, and outcomes. *PloS One* 13 (2), e0192523. doi:10.1371/journal.pone.0192523

Vedam, S., Stoll, K., McRae, D. N., Korchinski, M., Velasquez, R., Wang, J., et al. (2019). Patient-led decision making: measuring autonomy and respect in Canadian maternity care. *Patient Educ. Counsel.* 102 (3), 586–594. doi:10.1016/j.pec.2018.10.023

Wendland, C. L. (2007). The vanishing mother: cesarean section and "evidence-based obstetrics". *Med. Anthropol. Q.* 21 (2), 218–233. doi:10.1525/maq.2007.21.2.218

Zielinski, R., Ackerson, K., and Kane Low, L. (2015). Planned home birth: benefits, risks, and opportunities. *Int J Womens Health* 7, 361–377. doi:10.2147/IJWH.S55561

17

Birthing Between the "Traditional" and the "Modern": *Daī* Practices and Childbearing Women's Choices During COVID-19 in Pakistan

Inayat Ali[1]*, *Salma Sadique*[2], *Shahbaz Ali*[3] *and Robbie Davis-Floyd*[4]

[1]Department of Social and Cultural Anthropology, University of Vienna, Vienna, VIE, Austria, [2]Department of Community Health Sciences, Peoples University of Medical and Health Sciences for Women (PUMHSW), Sindh, Pakistan, [3]Independent Researcher, Islamabad, Pakistan, [4]Department of Anthropology, Rice University, Houston, TX, United States

Correspondence:
Inayat Ali
inayat_qau@yahoo.com

Pregnancy and birth are biological phenomena that carry heavy cultural overlays, and pregnant and birthing women need care and attention during both ordinary and extraordinary times. Most Pakistani pregnant women now go to doctors and hospitals for their perinatal care. Yet traditional community midwives, called *Dāī* in the singular and *Dāyūn* in the plural, still attend 24% of all Pakistani births, primarily in rural areas. In this article, *via* data collected from 16 interviews—5 with Dāyūn and 11 with mothers, we explore a maternity care system in tension between the past and the present, the Dāī and the doctor. We ask, what does the maternity care provided by the Dāyūn look like during times of normalcy, and how does it differ during COVID-19? We look at the roles the Dāī has traditionally performed and how these roles have been changing, both in ordinary and in Covidian circumstances. Presenting the words of the Dāyūn we interviewed, all from Pakistan's Sindh Province, we demonstrate their practices and show that these have not changed during this present pandemic, as these Dāyūn, like many others in Sindh Province, do not believe that COVID-19 is real—or are at least suspect that it is not. To contextualize the Dāyūn, we also briefly present local mother's perceptions of the Dāyūn in their regions, which vary between extremely positive and extremely negative. Employing the theoretical frameworks of "authoritative knowledge" and of critical medical anthropology, we highlight the dominance of "modern" biomedicine over "traditional" healthcare systems and its effects on the Dāyūn and their roles within their communities. Positioning this article within Pakistan's national profile, we propose formally training and institutionalizing the Dāyūn in order to alleviate the overwhelming burdens that pandemics—present and future—place on this country's fragile maternity care system, to give mothers more—and more viable—options at *all* times, and to counterbalance the rising tide of biomedical hegemony over pregnancy and birth.

Keywords: COVID-19, traditional midwives, Dāī, maternity care, Sindh Province, Pakistan

INTRODUCTION

Pregnancy is a biological phenomenon that is always, as Brigitte Jordan (1993) famously noted, "culturally marked and shaped." Thus many social scientists, and especially anthropologists, have paid significant attention to this cultural marking and shaping of birth (see for examples Davis-Floyd and Sargent, 1997; Ram and Jolly, 1998; De Vries et al., 2001; Lukere and Jolly, 2002; Davis-Floyd 2018; Cheyney and Davis-Floyd, 2019; Ali et al., 2020). How this biological phenomenon is affected during the challenges of COVID-19 (C-19) is currently being widely researched, as indicated in the articles in this Special Issue and many others. Yet little of that research to date has focused on the challenges C-19 poses to traditional midwives, and particularly in Pakistan, where they are known as *Dāyūn* in the plural and *Dāī* in the singular.

Empirically situated within Pakistan, mostly Sindh Province, this article aims to present: 1) the perceptions and practices of Dāyūn during ordinary times; 2) the Dāyūns' perceptions of and (non)practices around COVID-19; and 3) local mothers' perceptions of the Dāyūn working in these mothers' regions.

METHODS AND MATERIALS

Research Design

The article builds on various data resources, mainly ethnographic observations and fieldwork conducted during the COVID-19 pandemic, which was initially reported in Pakistan in February 2020. From March to October 2020, we adopted a qualitative research study design with an interview guide to gather data, study and comprehend the perspectives of Dāyūn and mothers dealing with the pandemic. Reproductive anthropologist Robbie Davis-Floyd added her considerable international expertise in midwifery and birth to generating the questions we asked the Dāyūn and worked with Inayat Ali to prepare the interview guide for the questions asked of the Dāyūn and the mothers.

Participants and Sampling

We used the purposive sampling method to select interlocutors. We conducted 16 virtual and in-person interviews: 5 with Dāyūn (from Sindh Province) and 11 with mothers who have used these midwives' services. All interlocutors were informed about the project and asked to give their consent. Since the first three authors conducted their previous ethnographic research in Sindh Province, they were aware of the Dāyūn but did not know them personally. We reached them via our pre-existing social contacts—family and acquaintances. The data generated from these five interviews proved sufficient for this article, as we reached saturation in terms of themes and information provided. These five Dāyūn are highly representative of the other Dāyūn practicing in Sindh Province because they all practice according to the same cultural traditions and share in the same belief system/worldview. It is impossible for us to guess their number, given that there is no official record available.

Data Collection

Using the interview guide, we focused our interviews with the Dāyūn on our central questions for them: How do they practice in ordinary times, and how have they dealt with the effects of the COVID-19 pandemic in Pakistan? Each specific question we asked is listed below above their responses to that question. Additionally, we carried out content and document analysis of news reports and various surveys, mainly government reports, to contextualize the pandemic in Pakistan as background for understanding our interview results. Using the Sindhi language, the first three authors conducted the interviews with the Dāyūn and the mothers in person at homes and as telephone conversations. We conducted the interviews with the mothers in the same ways. Our primary questions for them had to do with their perceptions of the Dāyūn and their practices. Later, we first three authors transcribed the data verbatim into English.

This article forms part of a larger project on COVID-19 in Pakistan, principally led by Inayat Ali and approved by the National Bioethics Committee of Pakistan (reference No. 4-87/NBC-471-COVID-19-09/20/). The names of interlocutors have been anonymized to maintain confidentiality. Moreover, the three authors also draw on their previous long-term ethnographic fieldwork in Pakistan, mainly in Sindh Province—Inayat Ali (2005-present), Salma Sadique (2013-present), and Shahbaz Ali (2012-present)—to supply qualitative data as background information.

Data Analysis

Data analysis was ongoing from the first interview. Data gathered from interviews and media were subjected to content analysis. Authors Inayat Ali, Salma Sadique and Shahbaz Ali continually read and re-read the obtained data to gain familiarity with it and allow for iteration. During these processes, salient themes were identified. The first three authors worked on the first draft. Then Inayat Ali and Davis-Floyd revised the article to refine the highlighted themes and played central roles in this article's crafting, most especially the discussion and analysis sections. The data obtained were eventually organized in terms of questions and interlocutors' verbatim responses, which we present below.

THEORETICAL FRAMEWORKS: AUTHORITATIVE KNOWLEDGE AND CRITICAL MEDICAL ANTHROPOLOGY

Health and ill-health are embedded in socio-cultural, political, economic and ideological structures and processes, as these factors influence specific health-seeking attitudes and behaviors. To understand a health-seeking action, it is essential to situate it within these contexts. Paying close attention to such health-seeking attitudes and behaviors shows subtle and complicated power dynamics at play not only in individuals but also in systems of knowledges and practices. Some knowledge systems come to dominate all others (Jordan, 1993). That is the case with the Western biomedical system, which has managed to achieve near-global hegemony and against which all other healthcare knowledge systems are evaluated. Thus such knowledge systems are often called "complementary," or "alternative"—meaning complementary or alternative to biomedicine, despite the fact that these systems may be primary sources of authoritative knowledge in their societies.

A bit of history is relevant here. When the British colonizers invaded old India (which then included what is now Pakistan), they affected every institution, including the extant medical systems, by enforcing their ideas, styles and methods of healthcare and what is now termed "biomedicine." Biomedicine (also referred to as "Western medicine," "conventional medicine," or "mainstream medicine") focuses on human biology and physiology in research and clinical practice, with treatment administered via formally trained doctors, nurses, and other such licensed practitioners (Banerji, 1974; Zaidi, 1988; Gaines and Davis-Floyd, 2004). As a result, the pre-existing local medical systems were governmentally neglected, rendered unable to retain their previous cultural authority, and re-considered as "alternative" (Ali, 2020b).

In lower resource countries, such alternative knowledge systems are usually called "traditional," and contrasted with "modern," meaning "biomedical," systems. Therefore, we employ Brigitte Jordan's (1993, 1997) helpful and widely used concept of *authoritative knowledge* as one of our analytical entry points. By "authoritative knowledge," Jordan specifically did not mean only the knowledge of "the authorities," though her concept is often used in this way. She meant any knowledge system considered authoritative by its users, on the basis of which people make decisions and take actions. Hence, authoritative knowledge can be held by individuals or entire communities; it can be the knowledge of the authorities or can be communally shared within cultures or groups.

Our ethnographic research for the prior projects described above shows that in Pakistan's Sindh Province, many rural people reject the notion that the knowledge held by governmental or by biomedical practitioners is always authoritative, especially during COVID-19. They prefer instead to rely on shared community ways of knowing, which in their case tend to insist that COVID-19 is not a real disease but rather a government plot to gain more foreign aid. For context, we note that this suspicion and/or outright rejection of governmental and "Western" authoritative knowledge have also specifically emerged in relation to vaccines and vaccination campaigns (Ali, 2020b; Ali, 2020c). People in Pakistan, including those of Sindh Province, have demonstrated extreme resentment and rejection of both—ever since the fake vaccination campaign carried out in 2011 by the US CIA to discover the whereabouts of Osama bin Ladin. These rural people also are suspicious of the ingredients of vaccines, given that some (malnourished and stunted) children have become extremely ill or have died from vaccine administration. Thus, since 2011, many vaccinators and their security guards have been attacked, and over 100 vaccinators have been killed (ibid).

We provide this information to illustrate some of the many reasons why the rural peoples of Sindh Province are so suspicious of governmental authoritative knowledge about COVID-19 and believe that it is a government "plot." The Dāyūn interviewed for this article share these same suspicions, which for them sometimes do and sometimes do not extend to the biomedical care of pregnant and birthing women. These midwives often prefer to trust their own authoritative knowledge about birth, including during COVID-19. Yet they are willing to transfer their clients to biomedical facilities when they face complications they cannot handle, considering the practitioners in these facilities to be the ultimate sources of authoritative knowledge (AK) about birth—though not for normal, uncomplicated births or for birth complications such as breech presentations, which they believe they are competent to handle themselves.

In Pakistan, there are significant differences between the multiple medical pluralisms that are considered meaningful sources of AK among the populace and the national healthcare system, which the government and biomedical practitioners have successfully made into the primary source of AK about injuries and diseases (Ali, 2020b). These other highly culturally regarded sources of medical (not including "biomedical") authoritative knowledge include Ayurveda, which some believe had its earliest origins in the region (3300–1300 BCE), while others place the origin of the first Ayurvedic text at around 550 CE), *Unami-Tib* (see below) and various folk medical knowledge systems, which are considered by the government not only as "alternative" but also as inferior (ibid). This national-level authority provided to Western-style biomedicine results in various structured forms of disparities, in which certain countries of the Global North and their cultures are globally dominant, and thus their "modern" standards of living and their systems of AK—most especially biomedical systems—are supposed to be striven for by low-resource, marginalized, and "pre-modern" countries.

This striving is expected by international development agencies such as the World Health Organization (WHO), the United Nations International Children's Emergency Fund (UNICEF), and the United States Agency for International Development (USAID), which tend to make the colonialist assumption that the more modern and biomedical they can help a low-resource country to become, the better off it will be. Thus the governments of low-income countries like Pakistan are urged to extensively support biomedicalization, and are given no support for their own "traditional" healthcare systems such as, again, Ayurveda and Unanī-Tib, which is an ancient system of medicine based on the teachings of Hippocrates and Galen, subsequently developed into a comprehensive and integrative healthcare system by Arabic and other practitioners. It is now, like the more well-known Ayurvedic system, also practiced extensively in Western nations and considered to be a form of holistic, "integrative" (a term used by holistic practitioners to contradict and critique the use of the terms "complementary" and "alternative") healing based on supporting and augmenting the body's own ability to heal itself. Although Unanī-Tib is now slightly institutionalized in Pakistan, and is taught in several university programs in India, it confronts significant issues in terms of resources to conduct research and operationalize it as a valued source of AK. For one example of such issues, most biomedical practitioners consider both Ayurveda and Unanī-Tib to be "quackery," as they also do for homeopathy and various other non-biomedical healing modalities (Davis-Floyd and St John 1998; Ali, 2020b). Another significant issue in Pakistan is who chooses to be a biomedical doctor (*Ddākdār*): usually, due to the high status, prestige, and financial benefits attached to the biomedical profession, many who wish to practice some form of medicine do not opt for Unanī-Tib or for Ayurveda, but for Western biomedicine and its system of authoritative knowledge.

The Dāyūn tend to follow the principles of Indigenous or "traditional" healthcare systems and mostly recommend medicines from Ayurveda, Unanī-Tib, or made by themselves at home. They used to be prestigious members of their communities, and some still are, as we discuss below. However, their status has significantly decreased in the country overall due to the high value now placed on biomedical maternity care. A few decades ago, the government of Pakistan, following guidelines from WHO, started a "lady health worker" (LHW) program to biomedically train local women to attend births. Because of this training, an LHW has more prestige and power than a Dāī, especially in those social circles that are economically well-off and have formal education.

As we shall show, a Dāī is still honorifically termed and perceived as a "mother" in villages, where biomedical healthcare facilities are still either unaffordable, inaccessible, or ineffective despite substantial attention from the government and global stakeholders. In such settings, a Dāī plays a pivotal role that can be seen against the backdrop of the structured socio-cultural, economic, and (geo-)political disparities prevailing in Pakistan. How such disparities shape health-seeking behaviors has been extensively studied and theorized by critical medical anthropologists (see Farmer, 1996; Briggs and Nichter, 2009; Biehl, 2016; Singer and Baer, 2018; Ali and Ali, 2020; Ali, 2020b) while other anthropologists have used authoritative knowledge as an effective analytical entry point and theoretical framework (for multiple examples, see Davis-Floyd and Sargent, 1997).

Herein we utilize both of these—critical medical anthropology (CMA) and the concept of authoritative knowledge (AK)—to form a cohesive theoretical framework for our data presentation and analysis and in order to illustrate the authoritative hegemony of Pakistani biomedicine, the institutionalized forms of disparities that affect the practices of the Dāyūn, and the conflicts and similarities between their systems of AK and that of Pakistani biomedicine. To accomplish the latter, below we examine the practices of the Dāyūn in biomedical terms and in terms of scientific evidence. (These two are discrepant; see Davis-Floyd, 2003a; Miller et al., 2016 for thorough analyses of the lack of a scientific evidence base for standard obstetric procedures for labor and birth).

PAKISTAN'S PROFILE: DEMOGRAPHIC, SOCIOCULTURAL AND HEALTH-SEEKING BEHAVIORS

The fifth most populated country in the world, with a total population of 22.23 million, Pakistan reports a total fertility rate of 3.6 births per woman (National Institute of Population Studies (NIPS) [Pakistan] and ICF, 2019)—higher than those of its neighboring countries. On average, mothers living in rural areas bear one child more than mothers in urban areas (3.9 vs. 2.9 births per woman) (ibid.) To provide maternal and child health care, Pakistan has Emergency Obstetric and Neonatal Care (EmONC) services in 275 hospitals and 550 health facilities, and family planning services in every health facility. Despite all that, the maternal mortality rate (MMR) is 170/100,000, still remarkably high compared to the other countries in the region (Government of Pakistan, 2019). Skilled practitioners (doctors, nurses, midwives, and female health visitors) provide antenatal care (ANC). Skilled attendant deliveries, the vast majority of which are assisted by doctors, have increased from 26% in 1990–91 to 69% in 2017–18, while the proportion of births attended by Dāyūn has concomitantly decreased from 41% in 1990–91 to 24% in 2017–18 (NIPS and ICF, 2019). According to one study published in 2008, around 70% of births took place at home at that time, usually assisted by a Dāī (Bhutta et al., 2008). Although there are no specific current statistics on the number of births attended by a Dāī in Sindh, studies report that it is substantial (Mcnojia et al., 2020).

The significant overall decrease in utilization of the Dāyūn's services can best be seen as a result of the Pakistani government's desire to phase out their traditional or Indigenous midwives—referred to in the international agency lexicon as "traditional birth attendants"—by providing more hospitals and smaller maternity homes/clinics, as is also being done in many other low-income countries. Anthropologists in general strongly prefer the term "traditional midwife" to acknowledge these practitioners' recognition in their communities as midwives (Davis-Floyd, 2018). In Pakistan, they practice almost exclusively in rural areas. Almost 4 decades ago, as in other countries, Dāī training programs were started in Pakistan, but were ultimately discontinued (Bhutta et al., 2008) because these trainings did not result in lowered maternal mortality rates. Yet these trainings were not offered in culturally appropriate ways, but rather in didactic, biomedical ways that failed to take into account and work with the culturally embedded authoritative knowledge of the Dāyūn. Additionally, these programs were not based on experiential learning—the primary learning mode of the Dāyūn, but rather on didactic, biomedical ways of teaching to which the Dāyūn could not relate (see Jordan, 1993; Cheyney et al., 2021 on the importance of experiential learning, which is the primary learning mode of all humans, including obstetricians and other medical personnel).

The Healthcare System in Pakistan

In Pakistan, medical pluralism prevails; as partially noted above, it includes biomedicine, Ayurveda, Unanī-Tib, homemade remedies and verbal healing *via* prayers and supplications (Ali, 2020b). Despite substantial efforts by the Pakistani government to shape people's perceptions and practices related to perinatal care, there is still a dearth of required facilities and skilled providers (Ali and Ali, 2020). Its biomedical system contains dispensaries, basic health units (BHUs), rural health centers (RHCs), and referral hospitals called District Headquarters (DHQs) and Tehsil

Headquarters (THQs). Pakistan has approximately 1,300 public sector hospitals, 5,530 BHUs, 700 RHCs, and 5,680 dispensaries, (which are the smallest primary biomedical healthcare units in Pakistan) (ibid.). There is one doctor per around 970 people, one dentist per around 9,450, and one hospital bed per 1,610 people (ibid)—resulting in extreme hospital and practitioner overwhelm when COVID-19 patients came flooding in, especially in urban areas. There is a significant difference in healthcare provision between rural and urban areas; urban areas have enough and more proper facilities than rural populations—a phenomenon labeled "urban bias" in healthcare policies (Zaidi, 1985; Ali, 2020b). Moreover, biomedical facilities in rural areas have inadequate and less qualified staff, and THQs and DHQs function poorly, partly due to syndemic corruption (Ali and Ali, 2020; Ali 2020b). And local-level healthcare facilities such as BHUs and dispensaries only function until 14:00 h during the week and are closed on Sundays.

For dealing with reproductive health, as previously noted, the Pakistani government introduced the LHW program in 1994 (Bhutta et al., 2008), into which local women with at least 8 years of formal education were recruited. After receiving 6 months of training to deliver care in the home, each LHW is responsible for about 1,000 people (approximately 200 families). There are over 100,000 LHWs in the country to provide maternal health care, family planning, and primary care in rural areas. Although they do not routinely attend deliveries at home as they have no such training, they maintain birth records, provide promotive and preventive educational services, manage milder illnesses (such as respiratory infections), refer people to healthcare facilities, provide oral polio vaccines, and promote routine immunization (Bhutta et al., 2008). Despite their significant workload, LHWs receive low salaries of approximately US $30 per month (ibid.; Ali 2020b) and often, they do not receive their salaries on time, as the Pakistani media has continually reported over the last decade.

The Pandemic in Pakistan: A Brief Overview

After reporting its first COVID-19 infection on February 26, 2020, statistics show that the coronavirus had infected over 535,000 Pakistanis and had caused over 11,300 deaths as of January 2021. In Sindh Province, there have been around 241,200 reported cases of COVID-19 and approximately 4,000 deaths. To deal with the outbreak, Pakistan implemented measures such as lockdowns, suspending international and national travel, opening quarantine centers, and deploying armed forces and police to implement these measures (Ali and Ali, 2020). Similar to measles and vaccinations in Pakistan (Ali, 2020a; Ali, 2020b; Ali, 2020c; Ali, 2020d), varying local perceptions of the existence or non-existence of COVID-19 and its causes and treatments resulted in the circulation of various rumors and conspiracy theories that often led to rural people being highly suspicious of, and not following, government-imposed restrictions on travel and gathering in groups, nor preventive measures like mask-wearing and frequent handwashing (Ali, 2020a; Ali, 2020e; Ali and Ali, 2020; Ali et al., 2020).

Socio-Economic Profiles of the Dāyūn

In this section, before we present the voices of the Dāyūn themselves, we offer their socio-economic profiles, explaining where they live, what type of communities they serve, their roles in those communities (which can be multiple, as they also often serve as healers), and who can become a Dāī. We also describe a few of their practices during pregnancy, as the following section focuses on their roles in birth.

All Dāyūn are female, married or widowed, and with no formal education. To become a Dāī, one must have already given birth to several children and received training from an elder, experienced Dāī—usually a family member, as is true for all of our Dāī interlocutors. In most cases, these learned skills are transferred from their mothers. Their socioeconomic status is low, and their ages usually range from 35 to 80 or even 90 years. Each Dāī has a defined area to practice in, demarcated either by her extended family, ethnic group or subgroup, or geographical access; most geographical areas are inherited. Within their areas, most of the Dāyūn are relatives.

In Sindh Province, the Dāyūn enjoy significant prestige, as indicated by the honorific term by which they are often called—*Dāī Aman* ("Aman" means "mother"). In this patriarchal society where most women cannot leave home alone, a Dāī can easily visit her field without any companion, and she never faces any gender-related harassment. Although this role has decreased over time, the Dāyūn also still often work as healers, especially for *Aurtānnī Bīmārī* (diseases of women). (Due to sociocultural, and primarily religious, reasons, people avoid saying the names of specific diseases pertaining to sexual health, irrespective of gender.)

During pregnancy, the Dāyūn use a specific herbal medicine prepared by the *Hakim* (herbalist), called *Batrīho,* which literally means "32" in the Sindhi language. Although it is available at a *Pansārī* (a grocery store that sells herbal medicines), *Batrīho* is also sold at biomedical pharmacies (locally called "medical stores"). With a mixture of 32 herbs, it is usually used in raw resin or syrup forms for multiple pregnancy issues, including inducing contractions at term, relieving false labor pains, or treating antepartum or postpartum hemorrhage. It is also used in a ground form applied to the vagina with cotton tied with a thread, as the belief is that if a baby is due (full-term), then labor pains will increase; otherwise, false pains will subside (Fatmi et al., 2005). The Dāyūn of Sindh Province attend a substantial number of the births in their allotted regions; the exact number is not known.

THE DāYūN OF SINDH: VIEWS, PRACTICES, THE GOVERNMENT, AND COVID-19

In what follows, after first introducing them (using anonymized names), we present the voices of the Dāyūn; we will provide discussion and analysis later on. Please note that sometimes, when we are quoting the Dāyūn, at a reviewer's request Inayat Ali provides the actual Sindhi words used, then offers literal translations and, when needed, their connotational meanings. Here we note that all Dāyūn have worked as a Dāī for many decades, are of low socioeconomic status, and have no formal education. The names we have given them are Sara, Mai Razul, Marvi, Gulan, and Zainab. All are Muslim—the predominant religion in Pakistan—with the exception of Sara, who is Hindu.

Sara is around 65 years of age. She has five children and 16 family members; her family income is around US$50 per month. Mai Razul does not remember her exact age, but guesses that she is around 70. She has nine children and lives in a joint family with 25 members. Their monthly income is around US$60; it increases if she attends some deliveries. For each birth she attends, she earns from US$20 to US$60, depending on the gender of the child, its place in the family order, and the socio-economic condition of the family. If it is a male baby, the first child, and the family is relatively well off, she may receive around US$60, which significantly helps her family with their daily life expenditures. Marvi is 90 years old. She has nine children and lives in a joint family with 18 family members. Her monthly income is around US$60. Gulan is 50 years old. She has three children and lives in a joint family with 15 family members. Her monthly income ranges from US$30 to US$50. Zainab is around 45 years old and lives in a joint family with her six children. She earns around US$40-50 monthly, depending greatly upon the number of deliveries she attends.

Questions Asked and Answered

Where did you receive your midwifery knowledge and training?

Sara received her midwifery education from her aunt, an experienced Daī in that community; Razul from her mother and her husband's first wife—the three currently work together; Marvi from her grandmother and from her own births: she said, "When I was young, my grandmother often asked me to dissect a hen to see its internal parts (especially the ovary) because this resembles a woman's internal part[1]. I have also delivered my own babies without the help of anyone." Gulan learned from her mother, who trained her "to examine the mother during pregnancy, conduct deliveries, and protect the baby." And Gulan's mother learned from her mother. Zainab said, "It is our family occupation that we have continued for many generations."

Is the government trying to push you out of practice? Does the government try to make you send women to facilities for birth? Does it help you in any way, such as by offering training?

None of these Dāyūn received any help from the *Hakūmat* (government) in any form, but all said that they wished the government would provide them with additional training. Razul did receive a 5-day training from the NGO Agha Khan, which she said helped her greatly. Zainab pointed out:

> Although I do not see any particular movement by the government to push us out directly, some efforts have affected our occupation significantly. In the surroundings, now there are maternity homes where [biomedically] trained women assist in deliveries and earn double the money that we do. Despite massive charges, many economically advantaged women prefer to go there.

And Razul noted, "Nowadays, there is hardly a role of a Dāī in delivery. Since hospitals have been established everywhere, most women prefer hospitals to a Dāī for delivery." Gulan agreed:

> Dāyūn used to play an essential role in the past, but now most of the community members prefer a hospital for delivery. There are a few families who call me to administer a delivery while believing that home is much better than a hospital because giving birth at a hospital is too economically expensive. Many people cannot afford these high hospital expenses because *Ddākdār ta gharīban khy kūhan thā* [Doctors are slaughtering the poor].

How many births do you think you have attended in your lifetime? Have any mothers and babies died under your care?

> *Sara:* I don't remember the exact number of births I have attended but there have been many. As I remember, around 15 women and 20 newborns have died at the time of birth. When I observe it is beyond my expertise, I inform the woman's mother-in-law and husband to take the woman to a hospital for delivery. Sometimes the family does not take her to a hospital because they follow *Pothī* and do not go against it [Pothī is a Hindu religious ritual used to decide whether the delivery should be at a hospital or at home].
>
> *Razul*: I have attended over 2,000 births, and never lost a woman or child during birth.
>
> *Marvi*: I am working as a Dāī for an exceedingly long time. Although I don't remember the number, I have attended more than a thousand *Wayam* (births). During my 25 years of work, *Char Māyon Āllah Sāin Khy Piyārun Thī Wayun* [literally meaning: "four women were loved by Allah." The connotational meaning is that "four women have died"] at the time of birth, and 10 babies were stillborn (*Katcā bbār'rra*), and five more died after the first week of birth.
>
> *Gulan*: I have attended so many *Wayam* (deliveries), that I don't remember the exact number. Two mothers died on the second day of delivery and five died after seven days. More than 10 newborns died during birth.

[1]These questions are from an etic perspective, whereas to explore roles, perceptions and practices during ordinary and extraordinary Covidian times, we used a Sindhi version—the emic version—of the interview guide, which asked these questions in locally comprehensible terms.

Zainab: I have helped in a few thousand deliveries. Around five women have died and some infants.

Do you provide prenatal, birth, and postpartum care? What is your care like, what does it consist of? (e.g., massage, palpating the baby to determine size and position, etc?)

Sara: Yes, I provide care during *Umaidwarī* [the prenatal period], *Wayam* [birth], and *Ādh-sut* [postpartum care]. I confirm the pregnancy of women. I do prenatal massage and give some herbs for standard vaginal delivery. I primarily provide services during delivery and the first week of a baby's life.

Razul: Some women call us for *Ādh-sut* [postpartum care], for their baby's body massage, clothes washing, and sometimes for their home chores if they live in a nuclear family. However, if I am called to monitor an *Umaidwārī* [pregnancy], then I give some *Dawā* [medicine] to women such as crystallized sugar and cardamon mixed in milk and black tea, which increase the strength of the labor pains. In the postpartum period, I put *Thāl* [a big steel plate] and three to four bricks on the women's belly for 1 hour, which helps to bring the *Bbachydānī* [uterus] to its regular place and reduce belly fat.

Marvi: I don't provide such services anymore due to being too old. When I was young, I did *Ādh-sut* [massage] of a woman and child. Presently, I only deliver a baby. Mostly, women come to my home, or I go in the case of an emergency.

Gulan: Yes, I provide prenatal, birth, and postpartum care to women. In prenatal care, I provide abdominal massage until delivery. In our community, women in their *Pakan Mahīnan* [third trimester] require oil massage of the entire body. I also provide postpartum care until the *Chathī* [a ritual arranged to name the baby on the sixth day, in which a specific food is cooked, especially sweet rice; relatives participate and give some money[2]]. After delivery I massage the mother's whole body and wash her *Gandā Kāprā* [literally "dirty clothes" but it signifies clothes with blood that are considered highly impure]. I also massage the newborn during this time. In some cases, I offer this care during *Chālīiho* [40 days] as in our *Sindhī* culture, baby massage is important because it makes the baby's features beautiful and the baby can sleep easily. On the second day after the birth, I keep an old traditional *Āttā Chākki* [a typical grinder made of coarse stone used to grind wheat flour] on the abdomen of the woman for half an hour, because *Chākki* is heavier and due to this heaviness *Bāchēdāni pēhji jāi tē bēhāndi* [the uterus returns to its usual position], and abdominal fat will not increase. I do this in the morning and ask women not to take breakfast.

Zainab: There are a few villages in the surrounding where people call me for assisting in *Wayam.* I pay a visit to these villages often to know about any woman conceiving so that I can guide her right from the beginning. That means I offer prenatal, birth, and postpartum care. I provide massage to the pregnant woman as well as palpating the baby to determine size and position. Many women also go for an ultrasound to determine the gender of the baby.

How much do you charge for your care? Can you make a living from your midwifery work?

Sara: With no demand for much money, I happily accept whatever is paid. People may pay around [US$5-10] in addition to clothes and sometimes grains or vegetables. It highly depends on how much they have. Sometimes, a mother pays in certain installments. *Bus Hin Kam Sān Asān Jo Guzar Safar Thi Wanjjy Tho.* [This work, although it is not sufficiently paid, helps to make our living].

Razul: We do not demand money from them. They give us money of their own will. Some give us [US$10-20] and some pay [US$40]. Yet others may give money, rations as well as clothes to us. The economically well-off women also give us around [US$1-2] daily that helps us in our daily life expenditures. Such an amount is not enough for everything we need, but it helps us lead a satisfying life.

Marvi: I am not doing *Dāīpo* [midwifery] for any economic incentives; thus, I don't ask for money. I just take *Mithāī* [this can be interpreted as sweets or sometimes as money that is paid without demand] on the birth of a baby. I cannot make it as living.

Gulan: In my case, it is up to the family how much it pays. Some families just give us new clothes and *Mubārkī* [the amount of money received by relatives at the naming ceremony of an infant] of Chathī and a few women give around [US$20] per delivery, including clothes and rations such as sugar, flour, milk, and rice. We are provided with these goods, are provided with a *Busrī* [a locally prepared sweet bread], and people say: Dāī *Mūnh Mithō Krē* [the Dāī should make her mouth sweet].

Zainab: We make this work as our main profession to make our livelihood. Our men do other labor, while we adult women after producing some children work as a Dāī. You know, unmarried girls cannot do this due to our culture. [This can be seen in the entire culture of the country, in which reproduction is a highly private matter, rarely

[2]Concerning the details of Chathī, please see Ali, 2020b.

discussed even among one's close family.] Our older generations train us when we are married and have given birth to a few children.

Are you trusted and respected in your community? Or are you regarded as outdated?

Sara: Since I am much closer to the community, they have been trusting and respecting me as a *Hakim* [herbalist, local healer] of their community. This is because I have been taking care of them during challenging times without charging them much money. In contrast, [biomedical] *Dākdār* [doctors] charge them significant amounts.

Marvi: I am still being trusted and respected in our community. People do love, respect, and take care of me.

Gulan: Those who call me, they see me as a trustworthy person and treat me as a mother.

Zainab: Yes, we are highly trusted and respected by people. People of all ages and genders call us *Dāī Aman* and they give us prestige equal to their biological mothers. Even those who visit maternity homes to deliver their babies give respect to us, because these older generations were assisted in birth by our older generations.

Razul: Being a Dāī, we are still being trusted and respected in our community. They call us *Dāī Aman* [Mother Dāī]. There was a time when Dāī attended all deliveries. Nevertheless, that time is no more, as some families perceive us as *Jāhil* [illiterate people who know nothing].

Where do the women you attend give birth? In their own homes with you in attendance or someplace you use for birth? What do you do about cleanliness?

Sara: Pregnant mothers come to my hut for delivery, but sometimes I have to go to their home in case of an emergency. When a woman is in labor pain, she sends anyone from the family (especially an older woman, husband, brother, or children) and calls *Jāpo walī* [a term used for the Daī in the Bāggrrī community']. I immediately visit that house for delivery. Houses are not clean like a hospital, but I try to keep that place clean. I wash my hands before and after delivery.

Razul: Usually, women give birth in their own homes. They call us before delivery, and then we examine whether we should do the delivery or refer her to a hospital. Before delivery, we make sure that everything should be *Sāf suthrī* [clean]. We also wash our hands before and after delivery.

Marvi: Pregnant women visit my home for delivery. In case of an emergency, I go to a woman's home. I keep the delivery place clean, and I wash my hands with soap twice or thrice before and after delivery.

Gulan: When a woman feels some *Sūr* [labor pain], she sends her husband. If the husband is not present during that time, then she sends an elder woman or child to inform me while saying: *Māi or amā khē bār jā sūr Āhin* [the wife or mother is in labor pain]. I immediately visit that house, even overnight or if it is raining. Most deliveries occur in a woman's house in a separate room, yet sometimes in my hut. Since in our village houses are mostly *Kachā* [made of mud and bricks], it is rather challenging to keep that place clean, but we do our best. I wash my hands twice prior to and post-delivery.

Zainab: I regularly visit villages in my surroundings. I know about the *Mahīnā* [months that can be called trimesters] of women and remain attentive about those who are in their *Pakā Mahīnā* [mature or final months]. I am called by the family to their house to administer the delivery.

Can you handle birth complications like stuck shoulders and breech birth (baby coming bottom- or feet-first)?

Sara: Yes, I can handle the birth complications, such as *Ūbto Bbār* [breech position of the baby][3]. In our *Bāggārrī* community, it is obligatory to ask for a goddess through a specific ritual called *Pothī* performed by a *Bhopā* [a religious leader] or an older person at home. Since we practice Hinduism *via* this ritual, we seek supernatural help and permission for delivery: either it will be a standard vaginal delivery or not. If not, then please allow us to visit a doctor. If it is a normal delivery, then we present *Parsād* [a devotional offering made to a god or a goddess that mostly contains food and is shared among people] in the name of our goddess, which may include animals, money, and sweets. Moreover, if the baby comes bottom-first, then I put oil with fingers on the uterus [oil lubrication] and do massage of the abdomen that helps the fetus to change its position immediately.

Razul: Before delivery, we examine the pregnant woman to know if there is any *Khatro* [danger or complication] or not. If yes, we recommend our women go to a hospital for delivery. Yet, if during delivery, we have to face such complications, we handle such cases very carefully and deliver the baby.

Marvi: If there is *Ūbto Bbār* [breech position], I usually recommend the family bring the mother to a hospital for delivery. Nonetheless, if such cases emerge during delivery, then I deal with these complications carefully.

Zainab: Since we are highly trained, based on our experiences and family orientation, I can handle any complications. Nonetheless, if it is truly out of my control, then I accompany the woman to a maternity home to assist the delivery.

[3] These Dāyon as well as mothers use a term called *Bbār* that in English translates as "baby" not "fetus."

Gulan: Yes, I know the *Sūbto ya Sidho Bbār* [head-first] and *Ūbto ya Ansidhu Bbār* [breech position of the fetus]. I can handle the birth complication. When there is *Ūbto Bbār* [baby coming bottom-first], I with my crossed fingers, after dipping them in oil, do the abdominal massage of the woman and apply oil lubrication to her uterus. Owing to this, the baby gradually changes its position and standard vaginal delivery happens within half an hour. During such hard situations, I also inform the mothers' family that the delivery is difficult, and the baby may die in the abdomen. Therefore, there is a need to use my *Dawā* [her prepared medicines] such as white and black glycerin mixed with mustard oil to dip cotton pouches in and to keep them in the woman's uterus. This helps control the adverse effects, especially *Zahar* [poison], caused by a *Mual Bbār* [dead baby] in the *Bbachydānī* of a woman during the delivery.

I also give milk or black tea mixed with castor oil to pregnant women to drink, which increases the labor pain [contraction strength] and helps deliver the baby easily. I know stillbirth *via* abdominal checking. *Pait mē bāar ggōrhō thē wēēndō āhā* [the fetus becomes in a ball or round shape in the uterus]. In that case, I ask the mother about the baby's movement. Moreover, if the delivery complications become worse, then I inform to the mother's family that I cannot manage it. Despite making many efforts, if I fail to conduct the delivery, then I refer the pregnant woman to a nearby hospital.

In response to Gulan's comments, we must note that actual hospitals with the required technology, medicine and a trained obstetrician are usually not located in the rural areas of Pakistan, including Sindh Province. The available biomedical facilities are *Wayam Ghar* (maternity homes) run by skilled midwives, whom laypeople call *Dākdār* or *Mandam* (a local version of "madam" used for female birth practitioners) as they cannot differentiate between an obstetrician and a skilled midwife. In some cases, a laboring woman experiencing complications can be brought to a dispensary or a private clinic run by a physician or maybe by a dispenser (a biomedical technician working at a dispensary).

What do you do if a baby is born and does not breathe?

All Dāyūn shared the following in common to deal with a baby who does not breathe: to blow *Phuk* (breath) in the baby's mouth, keep the newborn upside down to let any fluids drain from the mouth, or slap the baby's back (also to release fluids) until the baby cries. However, a few Dāyūn also described other strategies. Sara added, "I give ash to mix with cow urine in the child's mouth." Gulan stated, "We massage the baby with warm mustard oil. If the baby still does not breathe, then we put the *Nārro* [the umbilical cord] after cutting on the *Tawā* [a steel plate used for making chapatti] to heat until it becomes black. Yet, if the measures do not work, then I refer the baby to a nearby hospital to put them on a *Sāh Wārī Machine* [a machine that gives breath, denoting a ventilator]." All these measures help the baby to breathe.

How long do you wait to cut the cord? Until it stops pulsing, or right away? What instrument do you use to cut the cord, and do you sterilize it first?

Sara: I prefer to cut *Nārro* [the cord] as soon as the baby and placenta are delivered. Most often, I cut the cord with a broken piece of mirror that I think needs not to be sterilized.

Razul: We cut *Nārro* between 30 and 60 seconds after birth for improved maternal and infant health and nutrition outcomes. Since I use a new blade or scissor to cut the cord, there is no need to sterilize it.

Marvi: Usually, I cut *Nārro* after 1 min while considering that it is better for maternal and infant health. I use a new blade and sometimes an old blade to cut the cord. If I use the old blade, then I put it in boiling water for 5–10 min.

Gulan: I immediately cut the cord since a delay in cutting is not good for the mother's health. I use shaving blades to cut it. I prefer to use a new blade to cut the cord so I don't need to sterilize it.

Zainab: If it is a healthy baby, then I cut the cord right after the birth; otherwise, I can wait for a few minutes to do so [the baby can get more oxygenated blood through the cord]. I always use a new blade.

Will you attend the birth of a woman with a previous cesarean?

Sara: I have delivered a few women with a previous *operation* [the laypeople in Sindh, including the Dāyūn, use the English word "operation" to mean "cesarean")[4].

Razul: If a woman with a previous operation faces no complications, we attend the delivery ... Once, there was a woman [with a previous cesarean] who was waiting for a vehicle to go to the hospital for delivery but owing to unavailability of transport on time she could not go. At that time, she called me immediately to administer the delivery and by the grace of Almighty Allah, I successfully delivered the baby without any complications.

Marvi: I have assisted cases of a woman with a previous operation many times. Yet, I am vigilant to make sure that woman faces no complications; otherwise, I refuse.

Gulan: It depends on the baby's position. I have delivered many women successfully who were previously delivered by operation.

[4]Moreover, the word "operation" is also used for any small or large surgical biomedical intervention. Laypeople also use this term for women who get a tubal ligation to prevent them from conceiving in the interests of family planning.

Zainab: If a woman has an operation history, then I avoid assisting her. Yet I offer my postnatal services, such as massage, washing clothes, and arranging *Chatthī*.

Can you deal successfully with postpartum hemorrhage (excessive bleeding after birth)? If yes, how do you handle that? What do you do?

Sara: Yes, many times I have dealt with postpartum hemorrhage. I put a cotton pouch in the woman's uterus to control the bleeding, but if it is excessive and does not stop, then I refer the woman to the hospital for blood transfusion.

Razul: To control postpartum hemorrhage, I advise women to walk and to be given *Kuttī* [a local sweet made from dry fruit, honey, butter, crystallized sugar, cardamom, and wheat bread]. If due to physical weakness, the bleeding does not stop, *Kuttī* helps to reduce the excessive blood.

Marvi: To control the excessive bleeding, I give the mother cold things such as water or any cold drink. This coldness helps to stop bleeding. If bleeding does not stop, then I refer her to the hospital for treatment.

Gulan: If excessive bleeding happens, I massage the upper and lower abdomen of women. After the massage, I put an old but clean rug or cloth in the woman's uterus to reduce the bleeding.

Zainab: I make my best efforts to control the excessive bleeding. But I soon realize if I cannot handle otherwise, I promptly bring the lady to a hospital.

Has the number of women coming to you increased since COVID-19? If so, by how much? How many births do you usually attend per month? How many per month since COVID-19?

Sara: There is no significant impact of coronavirus to increase the number of women to come for delivery.[5] It is usual to conduct seven to eight deliveries per month as it was prior to the pandemic.

Razul: Most women go to doctors as before. As I am old, I can't go outside the village for the conduct of delivery. During regular times, I attend four to five deliveries per month. In contrast, during coronavirus, that number has increased to six or seven deliveries since women fear becoming ill due to this virus.

Marvi: There is some impact of coronavirus on the number of women to visit me. I usually conduct two to three deliveries per month whilst nowadays it has increased to around six deliveries.

Gulan: Due to the coronavirus, many women have preferred home delivery. They share that if they visit a hospital for Wayum [birth], the government may put their name on the list of corona patients and they may die there[6]. Consequently, I have attended over 30 births since the coronavirus started, which is a higher number than usual. Women also think that, if they go to a hospital for delivery, their delivery will only happen by operation instead of a normal delivery.

Zainab: It is hard to say. Although the coronavirus has not made a significant difference, I attended to a few more women. In contrast, a few women assisted by me in their previous deliveries and during their pregnancy visited a maternity home to deliver their babies. Those who were my clients and economically poor called me to deliver their babies at their home.

Do you feel that COVID-19 is a dangerous disease? Do you ask women to get tested for COVID before birth? What precautions, if any, do you take to keep you and your clients from getting infected? Do you have any access to personal protective equipment (PPE)? Does the government help you with that at all, or support you in any way?

Sara: I heard for many months that coronavirus is a dangerous disease, and those infected can die. Honestly, no one has been infected with this virus in our community. Therefore, it is not a disease, but these are only *Afwāhūn* (rumors) by the government to get funds from other countries. I don't follow the government recommended measures. Nevertheless, I wash my hands prior to and after delivery. There is neither availability of *Hifāzatī Sāmān*[7] nor provision by the government. We even don't receive any funds during normal times under Ihsās and the Benazir Income Support Program [BISP[8]] by the government. The government only gives funds to Muslim communities [and we are Hindu].

Razul: Coronavirus is just an *Afwāh* [rumor]. That is why we do not wear a mask during the delivery, but yes, we wash our hands, which we also do during normal times. We do not have any kind of PPE. The available rags and equipment at home are used during the delivery.

Marvi: I am skeptical of whether coronavirus exists or not. Without following the specific measures recommended by the government, I thoroughly wash

[5]They don't call it "COVID-19" or a "pandemic." Instead, they use the terms "corona," "coronavirus," or *Wabā* (an infectious disease). Concerning the language of the pandemic in Pakistan, please see Ali and Davis-Floyd, 2020.

[6]In studying such rumors, Inayat Ali (2021b) has found that many people in Pakistan believe that "whoever goes to a hospital during coronavirus never returns alive." Such rumors spread quickly in the country (see also Ali, 2020c; Ali, 2020e; Ali, 2021a).

[7]Our interlocutors were unaware of the acronym "PPE." Instead, they called it Hifāzatī Sāmān, which literally translates as "preventive stuff."

[8]These are government funded programs to support the economically poor.

my hands. Also, the government has not provided me with any Hifāzatī Sāmān [PPE].

Gulan: Although I have heard that coronavirus is a dangerous disease, I have not seen any infected person in my village. I believe that it is propaganda by non-Muslim people. I don't wear any mask. Actually, no one in our village wears a mask or keeps a physical distance. Everyone in our village has participated in all gatherings such as religious processions, marriage, and funerals. We don't have any fear of corona. We live our lives as usual. Yet, I am delighted that due to fear of coronavirus, many women have visited me for delivery. To attend them, I have adopted the usual measures—cleaning the place and washing my hands. It would make no sense to ask a woman to wear a mask when she is going through enormous pain and she needs to be able to breathe. I have not received any support from the government, such as Hifāzatī Sāmān [PPE kits]. To practice safe delivery at home, I buy blades, scissors and threads myself from the bazaar.

Zainab: There are many stories circulating about this *Wabā* [infectious disease] of coronavirus. Some say it is true and some refute it. I maintain the same preventive measures that I have been used to—washing my hands, cleaning the space where the woman will deliver the baby, giving a warm bath to the baby. Normally, when a woman is in labor pain, she stays in a room along with a few women—mostly her mother or mother-in-law, or grandmother—and her news of delivery is kept secret. We believe that making it public makes the birth complicated. Often, when I was assisting a delivery, we were a few women there and we kept our hands washed. No, I neither received any Hifāzatī Sāmān (PPE) nor I could afford to buy it.

Has the government at all recognized the value of home births during the coronavirus, or do they still want all women to go to clinics or hospitals for birth?

Razul: The government has no role in deciding or implementing a decision to deliver at home or hospital. The pregnant woman or her family usually decides whether she should go to a hospital or call a Dāī for the delivery. No woman who delivered a baby during COVID-19 informed me that they had been recommended by the government to visit a Dāī.

Marvi: The woman or her family makes these decisions. There is no role of the government. Moreover, no one was recommended by the government to visit me.

Gulan: The government is not in favor of home delivery. If women give birth at home, the number of coronavirus patients will decrease [and the hospital will make less money]; therefore, the government is interested in hospitals rather than home.

Zainab: I think the government encourages women to deliver their babies at a hospital. Yet, in my villages, I did not hear anything from women that they have been directed to visit a hospital. And there were some women who were conscious not to visit a hospital due to the risk of being infected.

Are you training apprentices to follow in your footsteps, or will your knowledge die with you?

Razul and Marvi are not training anyone; they say that no younger women want to be midwives, preferring more professional jobs. Sara is training her daughter-in-law, and Gulan is training her daughter "because I want our family to provide the services of Dāī till *Qayāmat* [the Day of Judgment]. When I die, hopefully, my daughter transfers this *Ddaihī* [Indigenous] knowledge to the coming generation." Zainab wishes to train others, but states that "there are significant impacts of several maternity homes run by nurses in our area." Yet she is sure that "no one can take away our right to lead a *Chathī* [again, a ritual arranged to name the baby on the sixth day], or to provide our postnatal services.

Discussion and Analysis of Dāyūn's Practices and Perceptions

In sum, the Dāyūn we interviewed are all older women with children, most of whom need the financial help that working as a Dāī provides them. They were all trained by older female relatives and some, like Gulan and Zainab, are determined to carry forward this multi-generational knowledge and skillset within their families. In contrast, others, like Marvi and Razul, understand that their knowledge will die with them because, as they noted, younger girls today are not interested in midwifery. Receiving no institutional support, these Dāyūn carry on as best they can. They charge little for their services and often receive even less; nevertheless, whatever they receive from families helps a great deal with their family income. And it also helps those families, as biomedical practitioners charge high prices for their services, including those who run the maternity homes—charges that can be avoided if the mother goes to a Dāī. All report that they are still highly respected in their communities, yet Razul noted that some now perceive Dāyūn as "illiterate people who know nothing."

In general, their practices consist of prenatal massage, delivery attendance (which had been diminishing for some until COVID-19 sent more women to some of them), and postpartum care consisting of baby massage, washing bloody clothes considered highly polluting, helping with home chores, and leading the baby-naming ceremony—which, as Zainab points out, culturally cannot be taken away from them even if births are. Their delivery skills include the ability to turn the baby *in utero* into a better position for birth—something few, if any, hospital practitioners know how to do; they simply perform cesareans instead (Daviss and Bisits 2021). And it should be noted that most obstetricians today have lost the skills for attending vaginal breech birth (ibid.), while these Dāyūn are preserving them. In addition, "modern" homebirth midwives in high-resource countries, where homebirth rates hover between 1 and 2% and the usual number of births homebirth midwives attend per month is around 4 (personal correspondence with US midwives Vicki Penwell and Marimikel Potter, December 2020) would consider it extremely challenging to take on as many deliveries per month (often as many as 8) as these Dāyūn are accustomed to doing—although, during the coronavirus pandemic, many US homebirth midwives are doing exactly that (ibid).

Concerning COVID-19, like many in Sindh Province (Ali, 2020e; Ali and Ali, 2020), these Dāyūn perceive this disease as propaganda generated by the government to meet its vested interests, such as controlling the population and receiving additional foreign aid. Their belief or strong suspicion that COVID-19 is not real led them to take no extra precautions in addition to the ones they already used. These Dāyūn made it clear that whether the birth takes place in their homes or in the birthing women's homes, they strive for cleanliness and wash their hands pre- and post-birth. Yet they are happy about this "non-real" COVID-19, as some of them have seen an uptick in clients (who do believe that is real) fleeing hospital contagion. Although they insist that they can handle birth complications, at the same time they seem fine with referring women to local maternity homes or clinics when the Dāī feels that the situation has gone beyond her ability to handle it.

It is beyond the scope of this article to investigate each and every practice these midwives describe. However, after a quick internet search, we can say that some of their remedies, which may seem ridiculous on the surface, do turn out to have scientifically demonstrated efficacy. For example, placing cotton pouches dipped in glycerin and mustard oil inside the uterus to prevent infection from a dead fetus may actually be effective, as mustard oil possesses powerful antimicrobial properties and may help block the growth of certain types of harmful bacteria. And cardamom is also an anti-bacterial and immune system booster, while castor oil, which has strong anti-inflammatory effects, has long been used by US homebirth midwives to help induce labor—a practice initiated as far back as ancient Egypt. A randomized controlled trial found that "Castor oil is effective for labor induction, in post-date multiparous women in outpatient settings" (Gilad et al., 2018:1).

Cow urine, which Sara mentioned that she uses for neonatal resuscitation, has long been used in Ayurveda, as the cow is considered sacred in India, but we could find no evidence of its efficacy. We thought that perhaps this practice was to make the baby gag and therefore breathe, but according to experienced midwife Vicki Penwell (personal communication January 26, 2021):

> Anything more solid than a liquid that is put far enough back to elicit a gag reflex would be a potential hazard to block the airway; it is contraindicated to put anything in the mouth of an unconscious person, unless you are actually inserting an airway or intubating... I can see no benefit and lots of potential harm in this practice.

In contrast, patting the baby's back and delivering mouth-to-mouth resuscitation are generally effective for babies who do not immediately breathe. Waiting to cut the cord for 1–2 min, as almost all of these Dāyūn do, is consistent with international guidelines on delayed cord clamping, which allows more oxygenated blood to flow from the placenta to the newborn. Yet placing an old, though "clean," cloth or piece of rug into the uterus to stop post-partum hemorrhage (PPH) is a dangerous practice that can produce infection. Abdominal massage for stopping PPH is indeed helpful, yet having the mother drink cold water or walk to stop PPH are unproven and likely ineffective techniques—walking especially is likely to increase the bleeding—unless the bleeding is due to a retained placenta and walking helps it to come out. (We did not specifically ask what the Dāyūn do for retained placentas.) Yet all our Dāyūn interlocutors do try to bring hemorrhaging women to a biomedical facility if they themselves cannot stop the bleeding, although sometimes, as Sara described, the Hindu family does not allow it if the Pothī ritual says "no," demonstrating the strong influence that religious beliefs can have on birth.

Certainly, baby massage is likely to help the infant sleep. As for the rest of their practices, such as placing something heavy on the mother's abdomen to "bring the uterus to its regular place and reduce belly fat," and invoking Allah or a certain goddess and performing certain rituals, these are culturally embedded and meaningful to both the Dāyūn and their clients. Thus, the care they provide is socioculturally, if not always medically, safe. For example, ritually invoking the help of a goddess in whom all present believe can help to replace fear with a sense of safety and control, as rituals are so good at doing (Davis-Floyd and Laughlin, 2016).

Yet clearly, the practices of these Dāyūn are a mixed bag regarding medical efficacy. We recommend further research on the efficacy of traditional midwives' practices everywhere before they are gone, as around the world, they are being phased out of practice or dying without passing on their knowledge and skills to future generations. For as we have shown, some of their practices are indeed efficacious and could be useful to contemporary practitioners. For a bit of cross-cultural comparison, traditional midwives in Mexico have for centuries rubbed the mother's own birth blood onto her belly to stop a post-partum hemorrhage (Davis-Floyd, 2018), and professional Japanese independent midwives use a turkey baster to inject that blood into her rectum for quicker absorption (ibid.)—both of which may seem as ridiculous at first glance as some of the practices of the Sindh Dāyūn—until one realizes that this blood contains high levels of oxytocin, which helps the uterus clamp down and stop the bleeding. Thus, it is clear that such practices should be investigated for possible efficacy, rather than simply being dismissed as vestiges of an outdated past.

MOTHERS' PERCEPTIONS OF THE DāYūN

The excerpts and information we present herein from our 11 interviews with mothers (whose names are anonymized) are designed to provide sociocultural context for the practices and cultural positionings of the Dāyūn of Sindh; thus they are focused on these mothers' beliefs about and usages or non-usages of Dāyūn. Some of these mothers emphatically preferred delivery with a Dāī. Two of them, both of whom lived in a small village with some formal education (which their husbands also had) and limited resources, were each planning to deliver their fifth child in their homes assisted by a family Dāī, as they had previously done. They stated, "Our Dāī Aman is caring and knowledgeable. She has not only assisted us but has also assisted our mothers and grandmothers in delivering all their children." One of these women noted that her mother-in-law had birthed 10 babies with the assistance of a Dāī Aman. And one woman with a Master's degree stated that she visits a hospital for antenatal care (ANC) but prefers to be assisted by a Dāī for labor and birth during COVID-19 because she fears hospital infection. Another woman, 30 year-old Sumbal, who received no formal education, had recently lost her baby during ANC. She shared her painful story, "I was interested in giving birth at a hospital but due to careless doctors, I lost my baby [prenatally]. It would have been better to stay at home. Now in the future, I will never go to a hospital for any prenatal care [or for birth, but will use my local Dāī Aman]."

In contrast, Sania, who has a grade 12 education and a husband who is a government employee, stated that she did not believe in the Dāyūn "because they are not fully trained." Likewise, Sumaira, who is in her 30 s with a Master's degree and has a private job and a self-employed husband, delivered her first two babies at home with a Dāī, but found that these births were "very painful," so she chose a maternity home run by "an intelligent and caring" nurse, whom she called a *Dākdāryānnī* (a term used for a female doctor) for her next three deliveries. The last one was during the pandemic, and the nurse "took extra care. She was wearing a mask and cleaning her hands repeatedly," but she did not require Sumaira to wear a mask "because it was difficult for me to breathe." Yet after the delivery, Sumaira "called our family Dāī Aman to massage my baby and me as well as washing my clothes and arranging the ritual of *Chathī*. We paid her around US$30, including some food and the money people paid during *Chathī*. I still think to pay her more." Yet Sumaira did not trust this Dāī to deliver a baby, saying:

> Recently, one woman lost her son due to this Dāī's inappropriate handling. When it was not possible anymore to assist the delivery, she brought the woman to the nearby maternity home where I deliver my babies. The nurse was shocked because it was not possible to save the baby, and there were risks involved that the mother might die, too. The nurse [did her best and] luckily, the mother survived.
>
> Similarly, she mishandled another mother and brought her to the same nurse when the mother's situation was already too complicated. The nurse saved the mother and the baby. However, the mother died after almost three weeks. The underlying reasons in both cases were that she [the Dāī] uses some medicine that she puts in the *Bbachydānī* [this term is used interchangeably for vagina and uterus]....My mother and grandmothers delivered their babies assisted by the grand generations of these Dāī, but they were more intelligent and skillful [than those of today].

What Sumaira says about the greater skills of the "grand generations" of these Dāyūn may well be true, as these former generations had no medical backup at all and so had to rely entirely on their own authoritative knowledge and skills in handling birth complications. In contrast, today's Dāyūn know that they can refer clients with complications to the nearby medical facilities and that their knowledge and skills are denigrated by medical authorities and some members of their own communities, and thus their knowledge no longer counts as authoritative in the eyes of many.

In these mothers' words and in the words of some of the Dāyūn whom we quote, we can detect the gradual demise of the Dāī in Pakistan. As maternity homes and hospitals become more readily available, a growing number of pregnant women are choosing this much more modern mode of care, and indeed, as Dāī Razul stated, many are now indeed viewing the Dāyūn as illiterate and premodern vestiges of the past.

STUDY LIMITATIONS

This study has a specific limitation: due to word length requirements, we were not able to include the full results of all of our 11 interviews with the mothers. Nevertheless, these case studies provide unique insights into two largely unresearched arenas: the practices of the Dāyūn of Sindh, and the roles of the Dāī during the COVID-19 pandemic—which, in our study, turned out to have only to do with the ways in which they already practiced. And we trust that the limitation of our small number of interlocutors is counterbalanced by the first three local authors' lengthy and detailed ethnographic research in the Province, especially on health, illness, vaccination, and, most recently, maternity care—all of which have informed the background and context we provide in this article.

CONCLUSION: RECOMMENDING TRAINING AND FULL INTEGRATION FOR THE DāYūN

In this article, we have presented the voices and choices of both Dāyūn and childbearing women regarding childbirth practices, facility birth, and the now globally syndemic COVID-19, placing primary focus on the voices of the Dāyūn and more limited focus on mothers' perspectives on their practices. After briefly situating this article within Pakistan's socio-cultural, economic, and political landscape, we have shown that the government has made substantial efforts to shape people's perceptions and practices related to perinatal care and to COVID-19 by foregrounding the authoritative knowledge and the authority of biomedicine as practiced in Pakistan. And we have illustrated Pakistan's medical pluralism, its lack of governmental support, and how the Dāyūn incorporate aspects of integrative modalities like Ayurveda and Unami-Tib, along with their own remedies as passed down to them through generations.

Although Dāyūn have historically attended the vast majority of births in the country, today pregnant women are increasingly choosing medical facilities for antenatal care and delivery as part of the modernizing process that is sweeping over low- and middle-income countries and that leads to the perception of traditional midwives as premodern vestiges of the past (Davis-Floyd, 2018). Yet as we have shown, a significant percentage of rural women in Pakistan still choose Dāyūn for delivery, and the Dāyūn maintain their status as providers of the valuable pre- and postnatal services described above, which include abdominal massage; turning the baby *in utero* (called "external version")—a skill many obstetricians do not have; the administration of certain medicinal remedies with varying degrees of efficacy; the washing of clothes considered too impure for others to touch; baby massage; and leading the *Chathī*—the baby-naming ceremony.

As we have shown, Dāyūn learn their knowledge and skills from other Dāyūn, usually older family members, but seem very open to receiving formal training, although no such government training has been offered to our interlocutors (an NGO did offer one training, which one of them benefited from, thereby demonstrating the need for more). They assist delivery either at their home or at the mother's. Out of the five Dāyūn we interviewed, two are teaching these skills to the younger generation, while the others recognize that their knowledge will die with them. These Dāyūn claim that they can handle all pregnancy- and birth-related complications, including vaginal breech deliveries, but clearly, given their statements that they do refer women to medical facilities, sometimes they need biomedical help—in addition to the supernatural help they seek via ritual performance. Some of their practices seem scientifically questionable, while others have clear benefits, as described above.

Unfortunately, it is not possible to know their statistical outcomes, as the government does not keep these; thus we have no way of quantitively assessing the results of their practices. Should such records begin to be kept, they might or might not show efficacy. Our five Dāyūn interlocutors shared that around 31 women have died over the decades of their care. Perhaps some or all of these deaths could have been prevented had the Dāyūn been given formal training. Yet statistics show that thousands of pregnant women die during their hospital deliveries. As noted earlier, the overall MMR in Pakistan is high, at 170/100,000, and cannot be blamed entirely on the Dāyūn, as they account for only 24% of the births in that country.

Regarding baby deaths, these Dāyūn report more than 40 among them, while some did not remember, so let's guess high, around 80 in total. If we guess that on average, each Dāī has attended around 1,500 births (though some attended less and some more), that would be 7,500 lifetime births for our five Dāyūn with a perinatal mortality rate of 80 perinatal deaths per 7,500 births, or 10/1,000. That rate is far lower than the overall Pakistani perinatal mortality rate, which is 57/1,000 (NIPS and ICF, 2019).

Like many others in Sindh Province, these Dāyūn consider COVID-19 to be government propaganda, perhaps an attempt by the Pakistani government to secure more foreign funding. Since they do not take COVID seriously, they have not adapted their practices to using preventive measures nor PPE, beyond their normal practices of cleanliness. Nevertheless and somewhat ironically, they have seen an increase in the numbers of women seeking their services both for ANC and for birth in order to avoid hospital contagion. For that reason, these Dāyūn have welcomed the advent of this "fake" disease.

Given that in normal times, around 24% of Pakistani women, especially those living in rural areas, still prefer the Dāyūn for their perinatal care, and that during a pandemic, more pregnant women than usual seek their care, we stress that these Dāyūn should be given additional, formal training to better prepare them for successful birth attendance at all times. For example, although it is not possible to project an MMR from 31 maternal deaths out of 7,500 births, as the numbers are too low (MMRs are determined by X amount of deaths per 100,000), nevertheless 31 is a very high number for 7,500 births (Yet it is important to remember that many of the women these Dāyūn attend are malnourished and thus are often stunted and have weakened immune systems). It remains clear that these Dāyūn truly need advanced training to prevent maternal deaths—for example, in the administration of misoprostol/Cytotec to stop PPH after the baby is born and the placenta is out, as has been successfully done in Afghanistan by Canadian midwife Betty-Anne Daviss and her team (see Daviss, 2021) and in Ethiopia *via* the Home-Based Lifesaving Skills program (described in Buffington et al., 2021).

We must consider the numerous and critical roles of these Dāyūn, the ongoing preferences of many women for their care, and the acceptance of their knowledge as authoritative by many in their communities. We foreground these considerations within the contexts of the challenges posed by COVID-19 and the structural disparities of the country, which result in better biomedical care and better-equipped and staffed biomedical facilities for the urban yet not for the rural poor. (As we have shown, some of the biomedical clinics available in Sindh Province are staffed by only one person.) Thus we strongly suggest that the government, in addition to supplying these Dāyūn with the requisite skills and tools to better deal with birth complications, should also formally link them to a particular medical facility for client transfer when needed. And we suggest that this facility should welcome such transfers of care from Dāyūn and should encourage them to stay throughout labor and birth to provide culturally safe continuity of care (see Barclay, 2009 for a description of such a successful program in Samoa). This would provide what Davis-Floyd (2003b) has called "seamless articulation" during transport, as contrasted with the "fractured articulations" that occur when the transporting midwives are disregarded or actively shamed by biomedical personnel for not using a biomedical facility in the first place.

Instead of suffering from syndemic structural disparities in a health care system aligned against them and that fails to adequately serve the rural and Indigenous poor, thereby perpetuating the legacies of colonization (Foucault, 1973; Banerji, 1974; Banerji, 1981; Zaidi, 1988; Farmer, 1996; Singer and Baer, 2018; Ali, 2020a; Ali, 2020b; Ali, 2020c; Ali and Ali, 2020; Ali and Davis-Floyd, 2020; Ali et al., 2020), Dāyūn should become officially recognized and integrated frontline caregivers in their areas. This will help to lessen the overwhelming impacts on the insufficient healthcare system of the country during this present pandemic and future emergencies to come; will assist the economically poor to receive appropriate and affordable treatment; and will help these Dāyūn themselves to make a viable living. We strongly propose institutionalizing these practitioners at the grassroots level to improve their skills (thereby potentially saving lives) and to mitigate both the unnecessary over-medicalization and commodification of pregnancy and birth and the rising hegemony of the biomedical healthcare system and its system of authoritative knowledge. Integrating the Dāyūn, with their knowledge of "alternative" healthcare systems, would also help to facilitate the growth of medical pluralism in Pakistan and to reduce its population's increasing dependency on biomedicine. Given that Ayurvedic medicine and Unami-Tib are efficacious enough to have gained popularity in many countries of the Global North (though they—and especially Ayurveda—are regarded by biomedical doctors and researchers as ineffective and even dangerous), it seems only reasonable that they should also be fostered in their countries of origin in the Global South, and that the home remedies of the Dāyūn that are efficacious should also be researched, recorded, and transmitted.

As previously noted, biomedicine is only one among many healing modalities, and it only makes sense that the authoritative knowledge systems of other, integrative modalities should be preserved, as the Pakistani Dāyūn are doing. Especially given that these "alternative" and "complementary" knowledge systems are far cheaper and much lower-tech and less carbon-intensive than Western-style biomedicine, we argue that they should be further integrated and augmented. In this Anthropocene Era, the onrushing Climate Crisis is poised to cause multiple disasters and future pandemics that may well overwhelm biomedical facilities and prove the necessity of flexible, community-based, "low-tech, skilled touch" (Davis-Floyd et al., 2021) models of care such as those provided by many community midwives around the world (ibid). The Dāyūn of Pakistan, if given the additional training they need and fully integrated into the healthcare system, can become just such providers, who will be greatly needed in the uncertain future to come.

ETHICS STATEMENT

The studies involving human participants were reviewed and approved by the National Bioethics Committee of Pakistan. Written informed consent for participation was not required for this study in accordance with the national legislation and the institutional requirements.

AUTHOR CONTRIBUTIONS

IA and RD-F: conception, research design, methodology, theoretical framework, analysis, discussion, and editing. IA, SS, and SA: Data collection and translation. IA, SS, SA, and RD-F: drafting article and proof reading. All authors contributed to the article and approve the submitted version.

ACKNOWLEDGMENTS

We are highly thankful to our interlocutors who gave their precious time and shared important data.

REFERENCES

Ali, I. (2020a). Anthropology in emergencies: the roles of anthropologists during the COVID-19 pandemic. *Pract. Anthropol.* 42, 16–22. doi:10.17730/0888-4552.42.4.20

Ali, I. (2020b). Constructing and negotiating measles: the case of Sindh Province of Pakistan. PhD thesis. Vienna (Austria): University of Vienna.

Ali, I. (2020c). The COVID-19 pandemic: making sense of rumor and fear. *Med. Anthropol.* 39, 376–379. doi:10.1080/01459740.2020.1745481

Ali, I. (2020d). Impact of COVID-19 on vaccination programs: adverse or positive? *Hum. Vaccines Immunother.* 16 (11), 2594–2600. doi:10.1080/21645515.2020.1787065

Ali, I. (2020e). Impacts of rumors and conspiracy theories surrounding COVID-19 on preparedness programs. *Disaster Med. Public Health Prep.* 1–6. doi:10.1017/dmp.2020.325

Ali, I., and Ali, S. (2020). Why may COVID-19 overwhelm low-income countries like Pakistan? *Disaster Med. Public Health Prep.* 1–5. doi:10.1017/dmp.2020.329

Ali, I., and Davis-Floyd, R. (2020). The interplay of words and politics during COVID-19: contextualizing the universal pandemic vocabulary. *Pract. Anthropol.* 42 (4), 20–24. doi:10.17730/0888-4552.42.4.20

Ali, I., Sadique, S., and Ali, S. (2020). COVID-19 significantly affects maternal health: a rapid-response investigation from Pakistan. *Front. Glob. Women's Health* 1, 1–8. doi:10.3389/fgwh.2020.591809

Ali, I. (2021a). "COVID-19 amid rumours and conspiracy theories: the interplay between local and global worlds," in *Coronavirus disease (COVID-19). Advances in experimental Medicine and biology (AEMB).* Editor N. Rezaei. (New York, NY: Springer).

Ali, I. (2021b). Rituals of containment: many pandemics, body politics, and social dramas during COVID-19 in Pakistan. *Front. Sociol.* doi:10.3389/fsoc.2021.648149

Banerji, D. (1974). Social and cultural foundations of health services systems. *Econ. Polit. Wkly.* 9, 1333–1346. Available at: https://www.jstor.org/stable/4363912.

Banerji, D. (1981). The place of indigenous and western systems of medicine in the health services of India. *Soc. Sci. Med.* 15 (2), 109–114. doi:10.1016/0271-7123(81)90030-4

Barclay, L. U. (2009). "Samoan midwives' stories: joining social and professional midwives in new models of birth," in *Birth models that work*. Editors R. Davis-Floyd, L. Barclay, B. A. Daviss, and J. Tritten (Berkeley CA: University of California Press), 119–139.

Bhutta, Z. A., Memon, Z. A., Soofi, S., Salat, M. S., Cousens, S., and Martines, J. (2008). Implementing community-based perinatal care: results from a pilot study in rural Pakistan. *Bull. World Health Organ.* 86, 452–459. doi:10.2471/blt.07.045849

Biehl, J. (2016). Theorizing global health. *Med. Anthropol. Theor.* 3, 127–142. doi:10.17157/mat.3.2.434

Briggs, C. L., and Nichter, M. (2009). Biocommunicability and the biopolitics of pandemic threats. *Med. Anthropol.* 28, 189–198. doi:10.1080/01459740903070410

Buffington, S., Sibley, L., Armbruster, D., Beck, D., Lori, J., Dynes, M., et al. (2021). "Home-based lifesaving skills: working with local leaders and families to prevent maternal and perinatal mortality," in *Birthing models on the human rights frontier: speaking truth to power*. Editors B. A. Daviss and R. Davis-Floyd (London, United Kingdom: Routledge).

Cheyney, M., and Davis-Floyd, R. (2019). "Birth as culturally marked and shaped," in *Birth in eight cultures*. Editors R. Davis-Floyd and M. Cheyney (Long Grove IL: Waveland Press), 1–16.

Cheyney, M., Davis-Floyd, R., and Jordan, B. (2021). Authoritative knowledge: ways of doing, teaching, and learning about birth. A tribute to Brigitte Jordan. *Pract. Anthropol.* 43 (1), 41–48. doi:10.17730/0888-4552.43.1.41

Davis-Floyd, R. (2003a). *Birth as an American rite of passage*. Berkeley, CA: University of California Press.

Davis-Floyd, R. (2003b). "Homebirth emergencies in the US and Mexico: the trouble with transport," in *Reproduction gone awry, a special issue of social science and medicine*, Editors G. Jenkins and M. Inhorn. 56, 1913–1931. doi:10.1016/s0277-9536(02)00213-7

Davis-Floyd, R. (2018). *Ways of knowing about birth: mothers, midwives, medicine, and birth activism*. Long Grove IL: Waveland Press.

Davis-Floyd, R., and Laughlin, C. D. (2016). *The power of ritual*. Brisbane, Australia: Daīly Grail Press.

Davis-Floyd, R., Lim, R., Penwell, V., and Ivry, T. (2021). "Effective maternity disaster care: low-tech, skilled touch," in *Sustainable birth in disruptive times*. Editors K. Gutschow, R. Davis-Floyd, and B. A. Daviss (New York, NY: Springer Nature).

Davis-Floyd, R., and Sargent, C. (Editors) (1997). *Childbirth and authoritative knowledge: cross-cultural perspectives*. Berkeley CA: University of California Press.

Davis-Floyd, R., and St John, G. (1998). *From doctor to healer: the transformative journey*. New Brunswick, NJ: Rutgers University Press.

Daviss, B. A. (2021). "Are top down or grassroots' solutions better in conflict areas? Two approaches to foreign aid in Afghanistan," in *Birthing models on the human rights frontier: speaking truth to power*. Editors B. A. Daviss and R. Davis-Floyd (London, United Kingdom: Routledge).

Daviss, B. A., and Bisits, A. (2021). "Bringing back breech: dismantling hierarchies and re-skilling practitioners," in *Birthing models on the human rights frontier: speaking truth to power*, Editors B. A. Daviss and R. Davis-Floyd (London, United Kingdom: Routledge).

De Vries, R., Wrede, S., Van Teijlingen, E., and Benoit, C. (2001). *Birth by design: pregnancy, maternity care and midwifery in North America and Europe*. London, United Kingdom: Routledge.

Farmer, P. (1996). Social inequalities and emerging infectious diseases. *Emerg. Infect. Dis.* 2, 259. doi:10.3201/eid0204.960402

Fatmi, Z., Gulzar, A. Z., and Kazi, A. (2005). Maternal and newborn care: practices and beliefs of traditional birth attendants in Sindh, Pakistan. *East. Mediterr. Health J.* 11, 226–234.

Gaines, A. D., and Davis-Floyd, R. (2004). "Biomedicine," in *Encyclopedia of medical anthropology*. Editors R. C. R. Ember and M. Ember (Berlin, Germany: Springer Science and Business Media), 95–109.

Gilad, R., Hochner, H., Savitsky, B., Porat, S., and Hochner-Celnikier, D. (2018). Castor oil for induction of labor in post-date pregnancies: a randomized controlled trial. *Women Birth* 31 (1), e26–e31. doi:10.1016/j.wombi.2017.06.010

Government of Pakistan (2019). *Pakistan economic survey 2018-19*. Islamabad, Pakistan: Ministry of Finance.

Jordan, B. (1993). *Birth in four cultures: a crosscultural investigation of childbirth in Yucatan, Holland, Sweden, and the United States*. Long Grove IL: Waveland Press.

Jordan, B. (1997). "Authoritative knowledge and its construction," in *Childbirth and authoritative knowledge: cross-cultural perspectives*. Editors R, Davis-Floyd and C. Sargent (Berkeley, CA: University of California Press), 55–79.

Leslie, C. M. (1989). Indigenous pharmaceuticals, the capitalist world system, and civilization. *Kroeber Anthropol. Soc.* 69, 23–31.

V. Lukere and M. Jolly (Editors) (2002). *Birthing in the pacific: beyond tradition and modernity?* Honolulu, HI: University of Hawai'i Press.

Mcnojia, S. Z., Saleem, S., Feroz, A., Khan, K. S., Naqvi, F., Tikmani, S. S., et al. (2020). Exploring women and traditional birth attendants' perceptions and experiences of stillbirths in district Thatta, Sindh, Pakistan: a qualitative study. *Reprod. Health* 17 (1), 3–11. doi:10.1186/s12978-020-0852-0

Miller, S., Abalos, E., Chamillard, M., Ciapponi, A., Colaci, D., Comandé, D., et al. (2016). Beyond too little, too late and too much, too soon: a pathway towards evidence-based, respectful maternity care worldwide. *Lancet* 388 (10056), 2176–2192. doi:10.1016/S0140-6736(16)31472-6

National Institute of Population Studies (NIPS) [Pakistan] and ICF (2019). *Pakistan demographic and health survey 2017-18*. Islamabad, Pakistan, and Rockville, Maryland, United States: NIPS and ICF.

K. Ram and M. Jolly (Editors) (1998). *Maternities and modernities: colonial and postcolonial experiences in Asia and the Pacific*. Cambridge, United Kingdom: Cambridge University Press.

Singer, M., and Baer, H. (2018). *Critical medical anthropology*. Boca Raton, FL: CRC Press.

Zaidi, S. A. (1985). The urban bias in health facilities in Pakistan. *Soc. Sci. Med.* 20 (5), 473–482. doi:10.1016/0277-9536(85)90362-4

Zaidi, S. A. (1988). *The political economy of health care in Pakistan*. Lahore, Pakistan: Vanguard.

18

Perinatal Depression of Exposed Maternal Women in the COVID-19 Pandemic in Wuhan, China

Guoqiang Sun [1†], Qi Wang [2†], Ying Lin [1], Ruyan Li [1], Lijun Yang [1], Xian Liu [1], Min Peng [1], Hongyan Wang [1], Xuewen Yang [1], Wei Ren [1], Hui Yang [1] and Yao Cheng [1]*

[1] *Obstetrics Department, Maternal and Child Health Hospital of Hubei Province, Huazhong University of Science and Technology, Wuhan, China,* [2] *Department of Epidemiology and Biostatistics, School of Public Health, Tongji Medical College, Huazhong University of Science and Technology, Wuhan, China*

***Correspondence:**
Yao Cheng
chengyao2014@sina.com*

[†] These authors have contributed equally to this work.

Objective: This study aims to investigate perinatal depression in women who gave birth during the COVID-19 pandemic in Wuhan, and to evaluate the effect of the pandemic on perinatal depression prevalence.

Methods: A cross-sectional investigation was conducted into women hospitalized for delivery in Hubei Maternity and Child Healthcare Hospital from December 31, 2019 to March 22, 2020, a period which encompasses the entire time frame of the COVID-19 pandemic in Wuhan. The Edinburgh Postnatal Depression Scale (EPDS) was adopted to evaluate perinatal depression status. A Chi-square test and logistic regression model were utilized for data analysis.

Results: A total of 2,883 participants were included, 33.71% of whom were found to suffer from depressive symptoms. In detail, 27.02%, 5.24%, and 1.46% were designated as having mild, moderate, and severe depressive symptoms, respectively. The perinatal depression prevalence increased as the COVID-19 pandemic worsened. Compared to the period from December 31, 2019 to January 12, 2020, perinatal depression risk significantly decreased within the 3 weeks of March 2–22, 2020 (1st week: OR = 0.39, 95% CI: 0.20, 0.78; 2nd week: OR = 0.35, 95% CI: 0.17, 0.73; and 3rd week: OR = 0.48, 95% CI: 0.25, 0.94); and the postnatal depression risk significantly rose within the four weeks of January 27-February 23, 2020 (1st week: OR = 1.78, 95% CI: 1.18, 2.68; 2nd week: OR = 2.03, 95% CI: 1.35, 3.04; 3rd week: OR = 1.48, 95% CI: 1.02, 2.14; and 4th week: OR = 1.73, 95% CI: 1.20, 2.48).

Conclusion: The dynamic change of perinatal depression was associated with the progression of the COVID-19 pandemic among new mothers who were exposed to the pandemic. An elevated risk of postnatal depression was also observed during the COVID-19 pandemic.

Keywords: COVID-19, EPDS, prenatal, postnatal, depression

INTRODUCTION

In December 2019, a novel virus, officially named SARS-CoV-2, caused an outbreak of pneumonia in Wuhan. The disease was named coronavirus disease 2019 (COVID-19) by the WHO. The newly identified SARS-CoV-2 virus was one of high transmissibility (1). The COVID-19 pandemic has since spread across China and around the world. On January 30, 2020, the WHO declared the virus a public health emergency of international concern, and then a worldwide pandemic on March 12, 2020 (2). The ongoing pandemic has posed a great threat to the physical and mental health of affected individuals.

Chinese governments have taken extensive and efficient actions to control the pandemic. Many provinces and regions in China implemented highest-level public health measures in response to the emergency. The *Guidance Manual on the Prevention and Control of Novel Coronavirus-Infection Pneumonia in the Community* issued by the national government on January 28, 2020, suggested traffic restrictions, home quarantine, and other social distancing measures (3). Besides, to avoid cross-infection opportunities in hospitals, designated hospitals and medical centers were established to exclusively treat the SARS-CoV-2 infection.

Global public health emergencies may promote psychological disorders in affected individuals. The severe acute respiratory syndrome (SARS), which caused a worldwide epidemic in 2003, equipped China with valuable lessons on how to control and prevent COVID-19, and has evidenced the importance of public psychological crisis management in the control of major public health events (4). The SARS epidemic was demonstrated to have negative psychological effects on infected patients (5), health professionals (6), students (7), and the general public (8). Scholars have called for attention to be drawn to the psychological disorders related to COVID-19 pandemic exposure (9). To tackle the potential psychological problems of affected individuals, the Chinese Center for Disease Control and Prevention issued the *Guiding Principles for Intervention in Emergency Psychological Crises during the Novel Coronavirus-Infection Pneumonia Epidemic*, and announced that an intervention of psychological crises should be involved in the whole deployment of COVID-19 pandemic prevention and control (10). Moreover, some hospitals and psychologists provided free online courses on psychological crisis treatment for COVID-19 affected individuals (11).

However, there are limited mental health services available for maternal women, as well as evidence for efficient management against the psychological effect of the pandemic. As a vulnerable group affected by high levels of estrogen and progesterone, the upper respiratory tract mucosa of pregnant women thickens causing edema and mild congestion, which are prone to respiratory infection. And SARS-CoV-2 infected pregnant patients were presented to have poor prognoses. Therefore, perinatal mothers deserve priority in psychological health guarantees (12). Maternal depression is one of the most common complications among perinatal women, which may result in devastating life events to mothers, infants, and families (13). Perinatal depression may have negative effects on offspring well-being throughout their whole life (14–16). The mortality rate attributed to perinatal depression-resulted suicide even exceeds that caused by postpartum hemorrhage and pregnancy induced hypertension (17). New mothers need delivery-related medical services in hospitals where they may be confronted with nosocomial SARS-CoV-2 infection, which possibly increases their psychological crisis during the perinatal period. With all this in mind, the perinatal depression status of maternal women is worthy of assessment during the entire COVID-19 pandemic period.

This study aims to investigate the prevalence of perinatal depression in hospitalized maternal women and to evaluate the depression risk in relation to COVID-19 pandemic exposure. The findings of our study will provide helpful experiences for the handling of subsequent large-scale psychological crises among perinatal women.

METHODS

Data Sources and Study Population

The participants were general healthy pregnant women receiving delivery services at Hubei Maternity and Child Healthcare Hospital in Wuhan, one of the largest cities in central China. The hospital is the largest Class III Grade A maternity center in Hubei Province. In 2018, one out of five newborns in Wuhan were expected to be delivered in this hospital. Their delivery help services mainly provided for women not infected with COVID-19 during the pandemic.

The study conducted included hospitalized individuals with a gestation of 28 weeks and above or $\leq$7 days after delivery (as of the perinatal period). Our study was approved by the Ethics Committee of the hospital. The cross-sectional study was implemented from December 31, 2019 to March 22, 2020, a period that spanned the whole COVID-19 pandemic in Wuhan. All participants provided oral informed consent before the investigation, in line with the Declaration of Helsinki regarding human participation. The questionnaire survey was mainly completed online using the WeChat-based survey program Questionnaire Star (questionnaire link: https://www.wjx.cn/jq/55187836.aspx), which was wildly used during the COVID-19 pandemic. A total of 5% of the participants completed a paper questionnaire with the exact same items due to the temporary unavailability of their mobile phone in hospital.

Variable Definitions

Exposure Variable

The COVID-19 pandemic was regarded as an exposure variable. The daily reported number of confirmed COVID-19 patients was key to the psychological responses of the exposed new mothers, manifesting perinatal depression during the entire epidemic period. Sequential events occurred with the updated measures against the pandemic, including: 1) the first reported patients with unknown pneumonia on December 31, 2019; 2) newly reported patients with an onset of January 16, 2020 on January 18, 2020; 3) the official announcement of the human-to-human transmission on January 20, 2020; 4) the beginning of inner-city traffic restrictions and home quarantine on January

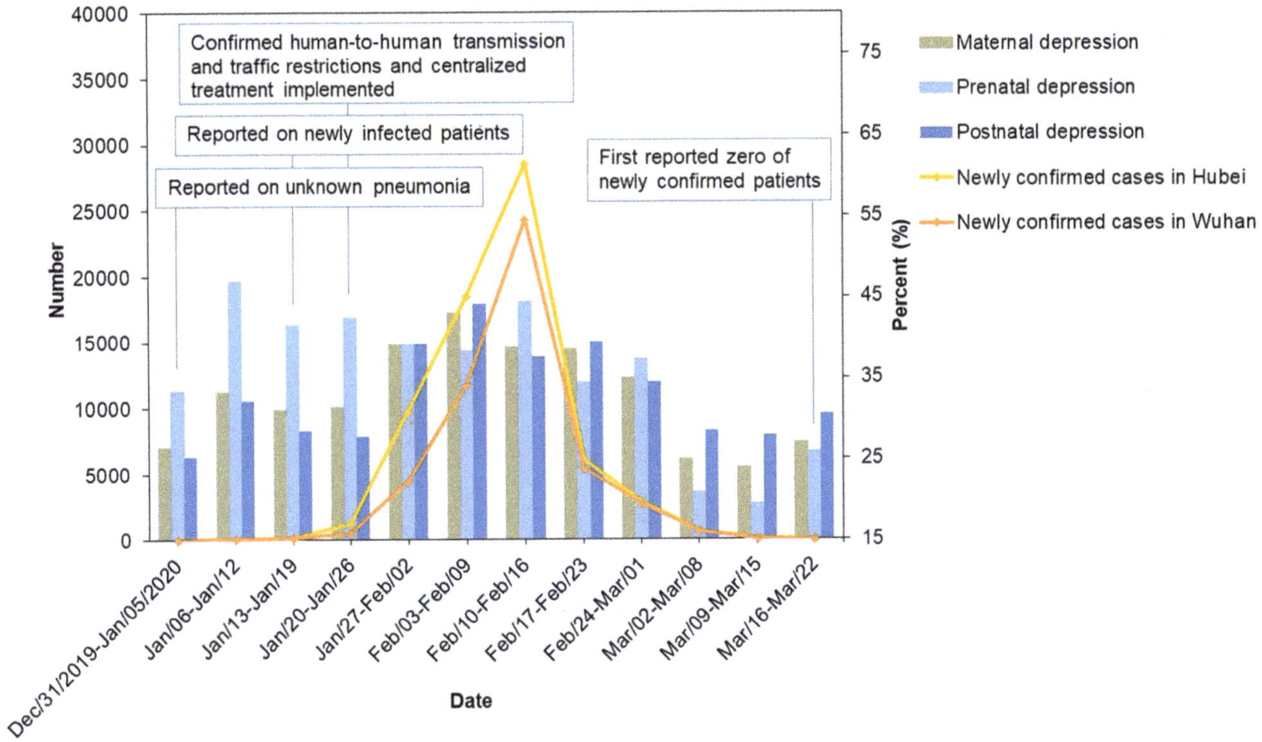

FIGURE 1 | The newly confirmed cases of COVID-19 and the prevalence of perinatal depression in Wuhan from December 31, 2019 to March 22, 2020. Surveillance data of COVID-19 were obtained from the official website of the Health Commission of Hubei Province (http://wjw.hubei.gov.cn/fbjd/dtyw/).

23, 2020; 5) centralized treatment and quarantine strategies to the confirmed patients, suspected patients, patients with a fever symptom, and close contacts; and 6) the first reported zero number of new COVID-19 patients up to March 18, 2020 on March 19, 2020 (18, 19). In response to the concurrent COVID-19 pandemic, maternal women may suffer a different degree of perinatal depression throughout several time intervals.

Covariates

Covariates included sociodemographic variables such as age (< 25, 25–29, 30–34, and > 34), ethnicity (Han and other), education (junior high or below, senior high, and college or above), Hukou (urban and rural), annual family income (<50,000 ¥, 50,000–100,000 ¥, more than 100,000 ¥, and unknown), delivery status (prenatal and postnatal), gravidity (1, 2–3, and ≥4), parity (0–1 and ≥2), gestational age (<37 and ≥37), health-related behaviors like prior history of traumatic delivery experiences (yes and no), sleep quality (good, fair, and poor), smoking (no, yes, and passive smoking), alcohol drinking (no and yes), and exercise (no and yes) during pregnancy.

Otherwise, most mothers lived with their family and family members played an important role in their social interaction. An Adaptation, Partnership, Growth, Affection, and Resolution Scale (APGAR) was used to evaluate the family function of each respondent. The scale was developed by Smilkstein and has been widely used (20, 21). It consists of five dimensions (adaptation, partnership, growth, affection, and resolution) (22). Each item was rated on a scale from 0 (*hardly ever*) to 2 (*almost always*). The APGAR scale was translated into Chinese in this study and was confirmed to be of good internal consistency (Cronbach's $\alpha = 0.80$). A final summarized score of 0–3, 4–6, and 7–10 indicated poor, fair, and good family functions (23).

Dependent Variables

The Edinburgh Postnatal Depression Scale (EPDS) was used for perinatal depression assessment. The EPDS was compiled by Cox et al. (24) and has been proven to have good reliability and validity, and be suitable for depression assessment during pregnancy and postpartum periods. The scale comprises 10 items, each of which is scored on a four-point scale ranging from 0 to 3 by severity. Finally, the summarized score is classified into four grades, with 0–9, 10–16, 17–21, and 22–30 points indicating none, mild, moderate, and severe depression levels, respectively (25). The internal consistency of this scale was good in our study (Cronbach's $\alpha = 0.92$).

Statistical Analysis

The statistical analyses were performed using SAS 9.4 for Windows. A Chi-square test was used to analyze differences in categorical variables, including sociodemographic variables, health behavior factors, and the exposure variable. Multiple logistic regression models adjusted for the mentioned covariates were used to evaluate the dependency of perinatal depression risks on the exposures. Results of the multiple logistic regression

TABLE 1 | Descriptive statistics for the sociodemographic variables of participants.

Variables	No depression N (%)	Depression N (%)	Total N (%)	χ^2	P
Age				7.9910	0.0462
<25	86 (4.50)	40 (4.12)	126 (4.37)		
25-29	789 (41.29)	405 (41.67)	1,194 (41.42)		
30-34	791 (41.39)	368 (37.86)	1,159 (40.20)		
>34	245 (12.82)	159 (16.36)	404 (14.01)		
Total	1,911 (66.29)	972 (33.71)	2,883 (100.00)		
Ethnicity				0.1006	0.7511
Han	1,857 (97.23)	947 (97.43)	2,804 (97.29)		
Other	53 (2.77)	25 (2.57)	78 (2.71)		
Education					
Junior high or below	136 (7.12)	69 (7.10)	205 (7.11)	0.4932	0.7814
Senior high	259 (13.55)	141 (14.51)	400 (13.87)		
College or more	1,516 (79.33)	762 (78.40)	2,278 (79.01)		
Hukou				0.0008	0.9775
Rural	676 (35.37)	344 (35.43)	1,020 (35.39)		
Urban	1,235 (64.63)	627 (64.57)	1,862 (64.61)		
Family income (¥)				3.2618	0.3530
<50,000	233 (12.19)	127 (13.07)	360 (12.49)		
50,000-100,000	419 (21.93)	232 (23.87)	651 (22.58)		
≥100,000	1,017 (53.22)	483 (49.69)	1,500 (52.03)		
Unclear	242 (12.66)	130 (13.37)	372 (12.90)		
Delivery status				1.4369	0.2306
Prenatal	504 (26.78)	234 (24.68)	738 (26.08)		
Postnatal	1,378 (73.22)	714 (75.32)	2,092 (73.92)		
Gravidity				0.3191	0.5721
1	852 (46.18)	449 (47.26)	1,301 (46.55)		
2-3	799 (43.31)	405 (42.63)	1204 (43.08)		
≥4	194 (10.51)	96 (10.11)	290 (10.38)		
Parity				0.1639	0.6856
0-1	1,225 (66.40)	638 (67.16)	1,863 (66.65)		
≥2	620 (33.60)	312 (32.84)	932 (33.35)		
Gestational age (weeks)				7.5788	0.0059
<37	168 (9.11)	118 (12.45)	286 (10.24)		
≥37	1,676 (90.89)	830 (87.55)	2,506 (89.76)		

No depression: EPDS score 0-9; depression: EPDS score 10-30.

model were reported as adjusted odds ratios (OR) and corresponding 95% confidence intervals (CI). All analyses were two-sided and a p-value of <0.05 was considered statistically significant.

RESULTS

A total of 4,895 inpatients in the hospital were eligible during the study period, and 2,937 of them agreed to participate in the survey. After removing those with incomplete data ($n = 18$) and with prior depression ($n = 36$), 2,883 participants were included in the statistical analysis. **Figure 1** shows the number of daily confirmed COVID-19 cases and the perinatal depression prevalence per week during the study period. From the end of 2019 when the first COVID-19 cases emerged in Wuhan, the perinatal depression prevalence continued to increase along with the increasing number of daily reported COVID-19 cases. During the time intervals of January 13–19 and February 3–9, the daily reported number of new cases increased rapidly in Wuhan. Meanwhile, the depression prevalence rose from 30.99% within the week of January 13–19 to 42.98% within the week of February 3–9. The highest prenatal depression value was 46.97% within the week of January 6–12. And the highest postnatal value was 44.15% within the week of February 3–9. As the emergence of SARS-CoV-2 infections slowed down, the perinatal depression prevalence showed a downward trend from 42.98% during February 3–9 to 23.85% during March 9–15.

Table 1 and **Supplementary Table 1** show the sociodemographic characteristics of participants stratified by depression levels. In total, 33.71% of all participants were

TABLE 2 | Descriptive statistics for the health behavior factors of participants during pregnancy.

Variables	No depression N (%)	Depression N (%)	Total N (%)	χ^2	P
Traumatic delivery experience				16.8512	<0.0001
Yes	115 (6.08)	100 (10.36)	215 (7.53)		
No	1,777 (93.92)	865 (89.64)	2,642 (92.47)		
Sleep quality				193.2296	<0.0001
Good	1,156 (60.94)	345 (35.60)	1,501 (52.37)		
Fair	661 (34.84)	495 (51.08)	1,156 (40.33)		
Poor	80 (4.22)	129 (13.31)	209 (7.29)		
Smoking				10.3242	0.0013
No	1,840 (97.05)	916 (94.63)	2,756 (96.23)		
Yes	56 (2.95)	52 (5.37)	108 (3.77)		
Drinking				0.7171	0.3971
No	1,851 (97.63)	937 (97.10)	2,788 (97.45)		
Yes	45 (2.37)	28 (2.90)	73 (2.55)		
Exercise				15.2252	<0.0001
No	706 (37.26)	432 (44.81)	1,138 (39.80)		
Yes	1,189 (62.74)	532 (55.19)	1,721 (60.20)		
Family function				77.5428	<0.0001
Poor	29 (1.52)	24 (2.47)	53 (1.84)		
Fair	73 (3.82)	143 (14.71)	216 (7.49)		
Good	1,809 (94.66)	805 (82.82)	2,614 (90.67)		

No depression: EPDS score 0-9; depression: EPDS score 10-30.

TABLE 3 | Descriptive statistics for independent variables of participants during the COVID-19 epidemic.

Variables	No depression N (%)	Depression N (%)	Total N (%)	χ^2	P
Period of COVID-19 epidemic				45.4120	<0.0001
December 31, 2019–January 5, 2020	78 (4.08)	28 (2.88)	106 (3.68)		
January 6–January 12	177 (9.26)	88 (9.05)	265 (9.19)		
January 13–January 19	167 (8.74)	75 (7.72)	242 (8.39)		
January 20–January 26	103 (5.39)	47 (4.84)	150 (5.20)		
January 27–February 2	143 (7.48)	92 (9.47)	235 (8.15)		
February 3–February 9	134 (7.01)	101 (10.39)	235 (8.15)		
February 10–February 16	213 (11.15)	135 (13.89)	348 (12.07)		
February 17–February 23	223 (11.67)	140 (14.40)	363 (12.59)		
February 24–March 1	203 (10.62)	109 (11.21)	312 (10.82)		
March 2–March 8	193 (10.10)	64 (6.58)	257 (8.91)		
March 9–March 15	166 (8.69)	52 (5.35)	218 (7.56)		
March 16–March 22	111 (5.81)	41 (4.22)	152 (5.27)		

No depression: EPDS score 0-9; depression: EPDS score 10-30.

found to have depressive symptoms, 27.02, 5.24, and 1.46% of which were indicative of mild, moderate, and severe depression, respectively (**Supplementary Table 1**). The majority of participants were aged 25–29 (41.42%), of Han race (97.29%), highly educated (79.01%), urban (64.61%), and had a family income of ≥ 100,000 ¥ (52.03%). The depression prevalence was higher (of marginal significance) in the participants over 34 years of age than those of ≤ 34 years (16.36 vs. 12.82%, $p = 0.0462$).

Table 2 and **Supplementary Table 2** show the health behavior factors stratified by depression levels. Most of the participants (92.47%) reported no previous traumatic delivery experience; and those who experienced a traumatic delivery had a higher depression prevalence (10.36 vs. 6.08%, $p < 0.0001$). Only 52.37% of participants reported a good sleep quality during pregnancy. Participants with a poor or fair sleep quality had significantly higher depression prevalence than those with a good sleep quality. Moreover, most participants did not smoke or drink alcohol during gestation. Compared to those without smoking habits, the participants who smoked either actively or passively had higher depression prevalence (5.37 vs. 2.95%, $p = 0.0013$). Participants who did not exercise during pregnancy had more prevalent depression than those who exercised regularly (44.81

TABLE 4 | Logistic regression analysis for the effects of independent variables on prenatal depression and postnatal depression.

Variables	Prenatal depression			Postnatal depression		
	Crude OR (95% CI)	Adjusted OR (95% CI)[a]	Adjusted OR (95% CI)[b]	Crude OR (95% CI)	Adjusted OR (95% CI)[a]	Adjusted OR (95% CI)[b]
Period of COVID-19 epidemic (in reference to December 31, 2019–January 5, 2020)						
January 13–January 19	0.84 (0.42, 1.66)	0.89 (0.43, 1.84)	0.75 (0.36, 1.56)	0.93 (0.62, 1.40)	0.92 (0.61, 1.39)	0.98 (0.64, 1.50)
January 20–January 26	0.84 (0.36, 1.95)	1.19 (0.46, 3.08)	0.85 (0.35, 2.08)	0.92 (0.57, 1.48)	0.89 (0.55, 1.43)	0.90 (0.55, 1.48)
January 27–February 2	0.92 (0.43, 1.95)	1.01 (0.46, 2.19)	1.06 (0.48, 2.37)	1.67 (1.13, 2.48)*	1.67 (1.12, 2.47)*	1.78 (1.18, 2.68)**
February 3–February 9	0.86 (0.41, 1.82)	0.94 (0.43, 2.07)	1.02 (0.45, 2.31)	2.05 (1.39, 3.03)***	2.03 (1.37, 3.00)***	2.03 (1.35, 3.04)***
February 10–February 16	1.07 (0.54, 2.11)	1.38 (0.68, 2.82)	1.37 (0.65, 2.89)	1.54 (1.08, 2.19)*	1.53 (1.07, 2.19)*	1.48 (1.02, 2.14)*
February 17–February 23	0.71 (0.35, 1.44)	0.77 (0.36, 1.62)	0.77 (0.36, 1.65)	1.71 (1.21, 2.42)**	1.71 (1.20, 2.42)**	1.73 (1.20, 2.48)**
February 24–March 1	0.80 (0.40, 1.63)	0.86 (0.41, 1.79)	0.85 (0.39, 1.83)	1.40 (0.97, 2.02)	1.41 (0.97, 2.04)	1.42 (0.96, 2.09)
March 2–March 8	0.35 (0.18, 0.66)**	0.36 (0.18, 0.71)**	0.39 (0.20, 0.78)**	1.08 (0.68, 1.70)	1.08 (0.69, 1.71)	1.08 (0.67, 1.73)
March 9–March 15	0.34 (0.17, 0.67)**	0.38 (0.19, 0.79)**	0.35 (0.17, 0.73)**	0.95 (0.58, 1.54)	0.93 (0.57, 1.52)	0.90 (0.54, 1.50)
March 16–March 22	0.44 (0.24, 0.83)*	0.49 (0.25, 0.95)*	0.48 (0.25, 0.94)*	1.24 (0.58, 2.64)	1.18 (0.55, 2.53)	1.27 (0.58, 2.79)

[a]*Adjusted for sociodemographic variables including age, ethnicity, education, Hukou, family income, delivery status, gravidity, parity, and gestational age;*
[b]*Adjusted for sociodemographic and health behavior factors including age, ethnicity, education, Hukou, family income, delivery status, gravidity, parity, gestational age, traumatic delivery experience, sleep quality, smoking, drinking, exercise, and family function.*
***$p < 0.001$, **$p < 0.01$, *$p < 0.05$.

vs. 37.26%, $p < 0.0001$). The majority of participants (90.67%) reported good family functions, and those reporting poor or fair family functions had significantly higher depression prevalence.

Table 3 and **Supplementary Table 3** show the dynamic changes of exposures and depression levels of participants. The depression prevalence in the participants was significantly different during several time intervals throughout the COVID-19 pandemic.

Table 4 shows the results of the logistic regression model for the effects of the COVID-19 pandemic on perinatal depression. Compared to the 1st week (December 31, 2019–January 12, 2020) of the pandemic, the prenatal depression risk was significantly decreased during the 3 week period starting from March 2, 2020 (1st week: OR = 0.39, 95% CI: 0.20, 0.78; 2nd week: OR = 0.35, 95% CI: 0.17, 0.73; and 3rd week: OR = 0.48, 95% CI: 0.25, 0.94), whereas the postnatal depression risk significantly rose during the 4 weeks between January 27 and February 23, 2020 (1st week: OR = 1.78, 95% CI: 1.18, 2.68; 2nd week: OR = 2.03, 95% CI: 1.35, 3.04; 3rd week: OR = 1.48, 95% CI: 1.02, 2.14; and 4th week: OR = 1.73, 95% CI: 1.20, 2.48).

DISCUSSION

In this study, the prevalence rate of perinatal depression was reported among the hospitalized pregnant women exposed to the COVID-19 pandemic in Wuhan. The prevalence of perinatal depression per week ranged from 23.85 to 42.98%. The overall prevalence of perinatal depression was higher in low- and middle-income countries (19–25%), than that in developed countries (7–15%) (26, 27). It should be noticed that a population-based participant enrolment method was adopted in other studies, whereas a hospital-based method was used in our study. Participants enrolled using the different methods possibly differ in general characteristics, and hence differ in perinatal depression risk. Moreover, the participants had just experienced or were about to experience a delivery, which might cause an increased risk of perinatal depression for them.

The prevalence of prenatal depression was at a high level during the COVID-19 pandemic in Wuhan. Okagbue et al. performed a review study of 26 articles, observing that the prevalence of EPDS-evaluated prenatal depression was 23.8% in pregnant women in their third trimester (28). Huang et al. conducted a cross-sectional survey of 320 pregnant women in their second and third trimesters in Wuhan, reporting a depression prevalence of 29.06% (29). Another study reported that prenatal depression prevalence ranged from 22.10 to 31.94% in Shiyan City, Hubei Province (30, 31). The prenatal depression prevalence in this study was higher than Western China (14.2%) and lower than Eastern China (34.9–36.8%) (32–35).

These results are a warning that the COVID-19 pandemic may possibly bring negative mental impacts to pregnant women all over the world. Controlling for sociodemographic and health behavior variables, the risk of prenatal depression decreased during the period of March 2–22, 2020 compared with the counterpart value at the beginning of the pandemic (December 31, 2019–12 January 12, 2020). The obscure and confusing public information about the pandemic during January 6–12, 2020 may have contributed to the high prenatal depression prevalence in this period. The first report of COVID-19 was published on December 31, 2019; however, the official announcement of the human-to-human transmission of COVID-19 did not occur until January 20, 2020. With implementations of public health measures against the pandemic, including isolation, quarantine, social distancing, and community containment, etc., the daily reported number of new onsets continued to decline, which was smaller than 200 per day after March 1, 2020 (18). This achievement in the prevention and control of the pandemic may be a reason for the decreased prenatal depression prevalence during that period. Flowers et al. studied the biopsychosocial effect of influenza pandemics, showing that pregnant women were vulnerable to a sense of pressure concerning influenza pandemics and death from influenza (36). As a negative and stressful life event, the COVID-19 pandemic probably increased mental depression. It was found that negative life events during pregnancy were associated with increased depression in the third trimester (37–39). The previous SARS outbreak which caused an international public health crisis, has been proven to have had adverse effects on people's mental health, especially in the severely affected areas (40, 41). Otherwise, the Wuhan city quarantine measure started on January 23, 2020 may also have increased postnatal psychological pressure.

This study is the first to reveal the prevalence of perinatal depression in individuals exposed to the COVID-19 pandemic. Some limitations of the study should be noted. First, as a cross-sectional study, it was not able to confirm a causal relationship between the COVID-19 pandemic and depression risks. Second, we enrolled generally healthy prenatal and postnatal women without SARS-CoV-2 infection in this study. And all participants were from a single maternity institution located in the seriously affected area (with respect to the number of COVID-19 cases). Prudence is needed to extend the research conclusions to those SARS-CoV-2 infected individuals and other areas. Third, the study was hospital-based, which possibly resulted in the limited representability of participants and hence limited the extensionality of our conclusions. Forth, this study included only the inpatient participants recruited in perinatal periods. The mental health effects of exposures in the first and second trimesters still need to be studied in the COVID-19 pandemic.

During the COVID-19 pandemic, intervention measures against perinatal depression are crucial for the well-being of new mothers and babies. The dynamic change of perinatal depression was associated with COVID-19 pandemic progression among the maternal women studied. An elevated risk of postnatal depression was also observed during the COVID-19 pandemic.

ETHICS STATEMENT

The studies involving human participants were reviewed and approved by the Ethics Committee of Hubei Maternal and Child Health Care Hospital. Written informed consent for participation was not required for this study in accordance with the national legislation and the institutional requirements.

AUTHOR CONTRIBUTIONS

GS: design, data collection, and manuscript editing. QW: data collection, data interpretation, and literature search. YC: manuscript draft, design, data collection, and data analysis. YL, RL, LY, and XL: data collection, data interpretation, and manuscript review. MP, HW, and XY: data collection, manuscript review, and visualization. WR and HY: data collection, data validation, and manuscript revision. All of the authors gave final approval of the version to be submitted, and agree to be accountable for all aspects of the work.

ACKNOWLEDGMENTS

We would like to express our gratitude to all the medical staff of the Department of Obstetrics for their responsible work during the COVID-19 pandemic to ensure the safety of maternal inpatients. We are also grateful to all the inpatients who participated in this study.

REFERENCES

Lai CC, Shih TP, Ko. WC, Tang HJ, Hsueh PR. Severe acute respiratory syndrome coronavirus 2 (SARS-CoV-2) and coronavirus disease-2019 (COVID-19): the epidemic and the challenges. *Int J Antimicrob Agents.* (2020) 55:105924. doi: 10.1016/j.ijantimicag.2020.105924

World Health Organization. *Coronavirus Disease (COVID-2019) Situation Reports.* World Health Organization (2020). Available online at: https://www.who.int/emergencies/diseases/novel-coronavirus-2019/situation-reports/ (accessed March 30, 2020).

Health Commission of Hubei Province. *Community Novel Coronavirus Infection Prevention and Control Guidance Manual (trial version).* Health Commission of Hubei Province (2020). Available online at: http://wjw.hubei. gov.cn/bmdt/ztzl/fkxxgzbdgrfyyq/xxfb/202001/t20200128_2015727.shtml (accessed March 30, 2020).

Yip PS, Cheung YT, Chau PH, Law YW. The impact of epidemic outbreak: the case of severe acute respiratory syndrome (SARS) and suicide among older adults in Hong Kong. *Crisis.* (2010) 31:86–92. doi: 10.1027/0227-5910/a0 00015

Montemurro N. The emotional impact of COVID-19: from medical staff to common people. *Brain Behav Immun.* (2020) 87:23–4. doi: 10.1016/j.bbi.2020.03.032

Lung FW, Lu YC, Chang YY, Shu BC. Mental symptoms in different health professionals during the sars attack: a follow-up study. *Psychiatr Q.* (2009) 80:107–16. doi: 10.1007/s11126-009-9095-5

Main A, Zhou Q, Ma Y, Luecken LJ, Liu X. Relations of SARS-related stressors and coping to Chinese college students' psychological adjustment during the 2003 beijing SARS epidemic. *J Couns Psychol.* (2011) 58:410– 23. doi: 10.1037/a0023632

Peng EY, Lee MB, Tsai ST, Yang CC, Morisky DE, Tsai LT, et al. Population-based post-crisis psychological distress: an example from the SARS outbreak in Taiwan. *J Formos Med Assoc.* (2010) 109:524– 32. doi: 10.1016/S0929-6646(10)60087-3

Bao Y, Sun Y, Meng S, Shi J, Lu L. 2019-nCoV epidemic: address mental health care to empower society. *Lancet.* (2020) 395:e37–8. doi: 10.1016/S0140-6736(20)30309-3

National Health Commission of the People's Republic of China. *Notice on Issuing novel Coronavirus Infection Pneumonia Emergency Psychological Crisis Intervention Guidelines.* National Health Commission of the People's Republic of China (2020). Available online at: http://wwwnhcgovcn/jkj/s3577/202001/6adc08b966594253b2b791be5c3b9467shtml (accessed March 30, 2020).

Liu S, Yang L, Zhang C, Xiang YT, Liu Z, Hu S, et al. Online mental health services in China during the COVID-19 outbreak. *Lancet Psychiatry.* (2020) 7:e17–8. doi: 10.1016/S2215-0366(20)30077-8

Rasmussen SA, Smulian JC, Lednicky JA, Wen TS, Jamieson DJ. Coronavirus disease 2019 (COVID-19) and pregnancy: what obstetricians need to know. *Am Obstetr Gynecol.* (2020) 222:415–26. doi: 10.1097/01.aoa.0000719440.84472.52

Rafferty J, Mattson G, Earls MF, Yogman MW. Incorporating recognition and management of perinatal depression into pediatric practice. *Pediatrics.* (2019) 143:e20183260. doi: 10.1542/peds.2018-3260

Buthmann J, Finik J, Ventura G, Zhang W, Shereen AD, Nomura Y. The children of superstorm sandy: maternal prenatal depression blunts offspring electrodermal activity. *Biol Psychol.* (2019) 146:107716. doi: 10.1016/j.biopsycho.2019.107716

Hannigan LJ, Eilertsen EM, Gjerde LC, Reichborn-Kjennerud T, Eley TC, Rijsdijk FV, et al. Maternal prenatal depressive symptoms and risk for early-life psychopathology in offspring: genetic analyses in the Norwegian mother and child birth cohort study. *Lancet Psychiatry.* (2018) 5:808– 15. doi: 10.1016/S2215-0366(18)30225-6

Schuez-Havupalo L, Lahti E, Junttila N, Toivonen L, Aromaa M, Pautava P, et al. Parents' depression and loneliness during pregnancy and respiratory infections in the offspring: a prospective birth cohort study. *PLoS ONE.* (2018) 13:e0203650. doi: 10.1371/journal.pone.0203650

Khalifeh H, Hunt IM, Appleby L, Howard LM. Suicide in perinatal and non-perinatal women in contact with psychiatric services: 15 year findings from a UK national inquiry. *Lancet Psychiatry.* (2019) 3:233– 42. doi: 10.1016/S2215-0366(16)00003-1

National Health Commission of China. *Up to March 23, 2020 Novel Coronavirus Pneumonia Epidemic.* National Health Commission of China (2020). Available online at: http://www.nhc.gov.cn/xcs/yqtb/202003/5819f3e13ff6413ba05fdb45b55b66ba.shtml (accessed March 1, 2020).

Pan A, Liu L, Wang C, Guo H, Hao X, Wang Q, et al. Association of public health interventions with the epidemiology of the covid-19 outbreak in Wuhan, China. *JAMA.* (2020) 323:1915–23. doi: 10.1001/jama.2020.6130

Smilkstein G. The family APGAR: a proposal for a family function test and its use by physicians. *J Fam Pract.* (1978) 6:1231–9.

Cheng Y, Zhang L, Wang F, Zhang P, Ye B, Liang Y. The effects of family structure and function on mental health during China's transition: a cross-sectional analysis. *BMC Fam Pract.* (2017) 18:59. doi: 10.1186/s12875-017-0630-4

Pérez PA, García OL, Rodríguez SE, Losada BA, Porras SN, Gómez MMA. Family function and the mental health of the caregiver of dependent relatives. *Aten Primaria.* (2009) 41:621–8. doi: 10.1016/j.aprim.2009.03.005

Lu C, Yuan L, Lin W, Zhou Y, Pan S. Depression and resilience mediates the effect of family function on quality of life of the elderly. *Arch Gerontol Geriatr.* (2017) 71:34–42. doi: 10.1016/j.archger.2017.02.011

Cox JL, Holden JM, Sagovsky R. Detection of postnatal depression. Development of the 10-item Edinburgh postnatal depression scale. *Br J Psychiatry.* (1987) 150:782–6. doi: 10.1192/bjp.150.6.782

Shrestha SD, Pradhan R, Tran TD, Gualano RC, Fisher JRW. Reliability and validity of the Edinburgh Postnatal Depression Scale (EPDS) for detecting perinatal common mental disorders (PCMDs) among women in low- and lower-middle-income countries: a systematic review. *BMC Pregnancy Childbirth.* (2016) 16:72. doi: 10.1186/s12884-016- 0859-2

Gelaye B, Rondon MB, Araya R, Williams MA. Epidemiology of maternal depression, risk factors, and child outcomes in low-income and middle-income countries. *Lancet Psychiatry.* (2016) 3:973–82. doi: 10.1016/S2215-0366(16)30284-X

Woody CA, Ferrari AJ, Siskind DJ, Whiteford HA, Harris MG. A systematic review and meta-regression of the prevalence and incidence of perinatal depression. *J Affect Disord.* (2017) 219:86–92. doi: 10.1016/j.jad.2017.05.003

Okagbue HI, Adamu PI, Bishop SA, Oguntunde PE, Opanuga AA, Akhmetshin EM. Systematic review of prevalence of antepartum depressi on during the trimesters of pregnancy. *Open Access Maced J Med Sci.* (2019) 7:1555–60. doi: 10.3889/oamjms.2019.270

Huang Z, Yin L, Zhang M, Xu Y. Analysis of the status and influencing factors of perinatal depression of pregnant and lying in women in Wuhan. *Mater Child Health Care China.* (2015) 30:5347–50. doi: 10.7620/zgfybj.j.issn.1001-4411.2015.31.17

Wu D. Depressive symptoms of pregnant women in Shiyan area and risk factors. *China J Health Psychol.* (2018) 26:349–51. doi: 10.13342/j.cnki.cjhp.2018.03.009

Mei R, Wang Y. Analysis of psychological depression and anxiety of pregnant women and related factors. *Chin Med Factory Mine.* (2015) 28:752–4. doi: 10.13429/j.cnki.cjcr.2015.06.021

Wu J, Zhang Y, Jiang W, Hu M, Huang M, Yu Y, et al. Association between prenatal depression and gestational body weight gain. *Dis Surveill.* (2016) 31:781–5. doi: 10.3784/j.issn.1003-9961.2016.09.016

Dong Q, Li Y, Miao H, Ma Y, Zhao Q. Depression symptoms during different period of pregnancy and influencing factors. *Chin J Reprod Health.* (2017) 28:106–9. doi: 10.3969/j.issn.1671-878X.2017.02.002

Cheng W, Xue H, Wang X. The study on depression and anxiety factors among pregnant women in Shenyang. *Mater Child Health Care China.* (2019) 34:4058–61. doi: 10.7620/zgfybj.j.issn.1001-4411.2019.17.57

Xie Y, Pan X, Zhao Z, Yang X, Zhao F, Wen Y, et al. Prevalence of antenatal and predictors of antenatal depression in Chengdu. *Chin J Family Plann Gynecotokol.* (2019) 11:36–40. doi: 10.3969/j.issn.1674-4020.2019.12.12

Flowers P, Davis M, Lohm D, Waller E, Stephenson N. Understanding pandemic influenza behaviour: an exploratory biopsychosocial study. *J Health Psychol.* (2016) 21:759–69. doi: 10.1177/1359105314537542

Xiao M, Liu D, Yang D, Yan C, Lei J. Effect of family function and pregnancy life events on second child pregnant women in their third trimesters. *Chin J Nursing.* (2019) 54:1354–8. doi: 10.3761/j.issn.0254-1769.2019.09.014

Li X, Wang A, Du S, Wang M, Zhou C. Effect of life events on the emotion of pregnant women. *Mater Child Health Care China.* (2011) 26:1303–5.

Mitchell SJ, Ronzio CR. Violence and other stressful life events as triggers of depression and anxiety: what psychosocial resources protect African American mothers? *Matern Child Health J.* (2011) 15:1272– 81. doi: 10.1007/s10995-010-0668-6

Hawryluck L, Gold WL, Robinson S, Pogorski S, Galea S, Styra R. SARS control and psychological effects of quarantine, Toronto, Canada. *Emerg Infect Dis.* (2004) 10:1206–12. doi: 10.3201/eid1007.030703

Lee TM, Chi I, Chung LW, Chou KL. Ageing and psychological response during the post-SARS period. *Aging Ment Health.* (2006) 10:303– 11. doi: 10.1080/13607860600638545

19

Opinion Review of Socioeconomic Impact of COVID-2019 on Women's Health

Victory U. Salami[1], *Stanley I. R. Okoduwa*[2,3*], *Aimee O. Chris*[2], *Susannah I. Ayilara*[1] *and Ugochi J. Okoduwa*[4]

[1] *Scientific and Industrial Research Department, National Research Institute for Chemical Technology, Zaria, Nigeria,* [2] *Department of Biochemistry, Babcock University, Ilishan-Remo, Nigeria,* [3] *Directorate of Research and Development, Nigerian Institute of Leather and Science Technology, Zaria, Nigeria,* [4] *Industrial and Environmental Pollution Department, National Research Institute for Chemical Technology, Zaria, Nigeria*

***Correspondence:**
Stanley I. R. Okoduwa
siroplc@gmail.com;
okoduwas@babcock.edu.ng

The global battle to survive the onslaughts of the Coronavirus Disease 2019 (COVID-19) started in December 2019 and continues today. Women and girls have borne the brunt of the hardship resulting from the health crises. This paper examined the effects of COVID-19 on women. Socioeconomic factors resulting from the pandemic, especially in relation to women's health, were discussed after studying published articles. They include gender specificity and COVID-19, the economic toll of COVID-19 on women, pregnancy and COVID-19, gender-based violence due to COVID-19, and health-care impacts of COVID-19. Making up the majority in the healthcare workforce, women were at higher risk of infection with COVID-19 due to their exposure as caregivers to infected patients. The pandemic took its toll on them as part of the greater population in the informal sector of the economy due to the lockdown directive, as many experienced severe monetary shortages and job losses. Pregnant women infected with COVID-19 were prone to severe diseases, maternal complications, and death due to their weakened immunity and exposure during clinical procedures. Gender-based violence was observed to have increased across the globe for women. The results of this review strongly indicate that women are disproportionately affected by the ongoing COVID-19 health crisis. This review will help health-care professionals and policymakers arrive at properly-thought-through decisions to better manage health crises. Governments and all key players should address the challenge by devising effective policies with a gendered view.

Keywords: SARS-CoV2, COVID-19, women's health, socio-economic status, coronavirus

INTRODUCTION

Severe Acute Respiratory Syndrome Coronavirus-2 (SARS-CoV2), also called COVID-19, is a new coronavirus infection identified in December 2019 originating from Wuhan, China (1). Since its outbreak, it has spread to more than 220 countries in the world with rising cases of fatality. Some regions have overcome the third wave of the crisis and are facing the start of a fourth (2). As of February 1, 2021, 13:00 GMT, the weekly update of the World Health Organization reports that there have been over 100 million confirmed cases with more than two million confirmed deaths globally (3). This disease has initiated a fast-growing global crisis that has taken researchers and policymakers without notice, thus leaving them scrambling to collect and analyze data so that its true impact on affected countries can be grasped (4).

As the world begins vaccination to manage the COVID-19 pandemic, preventive measures have been advocated, including physical distancing. The current pandemic and the imposed physical/social distancing policy are emphasizing health inequalities based on gender, socioeconomic status, and race (5–9), thereby highlighting the discrimination of other marginalized groups, such as internally displaced people, those in extreme poverty, people with disabilities, migrants, and the refugees whose majority are women and children (10). The gendered effect of COVID-19 on women presents a huge challenge that cannot be ignored. Deliberations about the health effects of COVID-19 should include unique conditions that make women more at risk (11).

In this review, research findings from publications retrieved online were used to highlight some health and socioeconomic challenges due to the COVID-19 pandemic that are particular to women. The discussion was based on COVID-19 in relation to five key factors: (1) gender specificity (is COVID-19 neutral to men and women?), (2) economic toll (has COVID-19 affected the economic life of women?), (3) pregnancy (does COVID-19 affect pregnant women more than non-pregnant women?), (4) gender-based violence (has COVID-19 affected the rate of gender-based violence?), and (5) health care (how have women fared in accessing sexual and reproductive health care during the COVID-19 pandemic?). If the items discussed in this paper are properly taken into consideration, the likelihood of future health crises would be better managed.

METHODS

The study employed a literature search of majorly published journal articles written in English from electronic databases such as ScienceDirect, PubMed, and Google Scholar. Information from the World Health Organization and the United Nations Women databases was also accessed. The literature search was performed by all authors listed on the paper between July 15, 2020, and February 3, 2021. Articles were searched using the following keywords: women; COVID-19; impacts of COVID-19 or effects of COVID-19; economic impacts of COVID-19; social effects of COVID-19; health impacts of COVID-19; COVID-19 pandemic; SARS Cov-2; and Coronavirus.

Population

Females in this article refer to women and girls. The ages of the females who participated in the studies included in this review ranged from 13 years old and above.

Selection Criteria

Reports and full-text articles related to the health, social, and economic impacts of COVID-19 on women were selected. The study excluded reports and articles that excluded the impacts/effects of COVID-19 on women, articles not written in English, as well as information derived from blogs and other unverifiable sources.

RESULT AND DISCUSSION

A total of 1,518 records were identified based on selection criteria of key search words: 1,006 from the databases searched and 512 from other sources. After screening to remove articles that did not capture the context of interest, duplicates, and articles not written in the English Language, a total of 291 articles were selected. Of the 291 selected articles, 266 were not suitable because they were misleading in context and were thus excluded. The remaining 25 selected articles were then included for analysis.

Gender Specificity and COVID-19

Gender is a path upon which the COVID-19 pandemic is widening health inequalities (11). Years before this pandemic, women typically reported more physically unhealthy days than men even though they used more preventive care services (12). Women have poorer results for widespread diseases such as myocardial infarction (13), asthma (12), and diabetes (14). This health discrimination is aggravated for women of low socioeconomic status, older age, physical disability, lower education, residence in rural geographic locations, and those who are not white (11). In a recent web-based survey of 780,961 participants from 183 countries, a major risk association for infection with COVID-19 was observed for people who were of the female gender, aged above 60 years, and those who had preexisting disease conditions, such as heart disease, kidney disease, diabetes, and liver disease (15). Women are at greater risk of mental health challenges and exhibit more psychological distress than men (16). Based on the available literature, COVID-19 health crises will likely distress women mentally to a higher degree (16). In a study on mood, empathy, and sleep quality during the isolation period due to COVID-19 in Canada, the authors discovered that women suffered more due to trauma symptoms, depression, and increased anxiety (17). Many health-care staff members could develop posttraumatic stress disorder due to burnout, depression, and anxiety during and after the pandemic, and this is another factor supporting the weightier impact of the pandemic on women (18).

COVID-19 does not discriminate against gender (male or female), health status (healthy or immuno-compromised), or age (although infection in children is less common, most affected adults are between 25 and 89 years old) (19, 20). Initial reports indicated that men were at greater risk of severe disease and death from COVID-19 infection compared with women (7, 21, 22). Researchers warned that those early investigations were to be treated with caution because they are incomplete and inconsistent across countries (23, 24). Current statistics of sex-disintegrated data (which is presently incomplete) show that more women test positive for COVID-19 compared to men (25). Recognizing the direct and indirect effects of the disease on women will assist in providing effective responses for similar health crises in the future (26).

Across the globe, about 70% of health-care workers (doctors, nurses, midwives, community health workers, cleaners, caterers, and launderers) are women, of which 80% are nurses in most countries. These women are particularly at risk of infection through contact with sick patients (23). Factors associated with fatalities of patients with COVID-19 include older age, obesity, diabetes mellitus, hypertension, and cardiovascular diseases (27).

The Economic Toll of COVID-19 on Women

Although physical distancing slows down the transmission of COVID-19, the advantage of this measure needs to be balanced with its effects on the informal sector of the economy (8). The implementation of the lockdown measure in developing countries (particularly in Africa where poverty, weak health-care systems, and overcrowding exists) has taken its toll on all (especially women) (8). Many women in the non-formal sector have limited access to social security, and, as such, widespread job losses will have a long-term impact on their economic independence and security (4).

An estimated 740 million women are employed in the informal sector of the economy, which includes tourism, hospitality, and retail. In developing countries, this workforce constitutes more than two-thirds of women. To make a living, they rely on open public space, which is at present being limited to curb the spread of the virus. Therefore, severe monetary shortfalls are very much felt by these women who earn less, save less, and hold more insecure jobs compared to their male counterparts (7, 28).

COVID-19 and the restrictions put in place to curtail its spread have interrupted markets and businesses and many have lost their means of living (29). In April 2020, The International Labour Organization (ILO) projected that lockdown will distress about 3 billion employees (81% of the global labor force) and that the COVID-19 pandemic could cost between 5 million and 25 million jobs (7). Recently, the ILO posits that estimations of revenue losses from labor show a global decline of 10.7% during the first three quarters of 2020 compared with the corresponding period in 2019, which amounts to 3.5 trillion United States dollars (5.5% global gross domestic product) (30). The International Monetary Fund projected a major shrinkage of global output in 2020 (31).

According to Clare Wenham, assistant professor of Global Health Policy, London School of Economics and Political Science, the economic toll the COVID-19 pandemic has on women is an indirect consequence, coming not from being infected but from being affected (28). Despite a major limitation from the fact that not all countries provide sex-disaggregated data, a clear trend of the pandemic's indirect effect on women has appeared (28). Women have less access to social protection, and most single-parent households are women. The capability of women to absorb economic shocks is less than that of men (28). The Institute for Fiscal Studies found that women in the United Kingdom were 1.5 times more likely than men to have either quit their job or lost it during the lockdown (28). As countries experienced lockdown, jobs were lost with disastrous consequences on the holders.

The care burden on women has increased due to the imposed lockdown—care for the sick and elderly, care for children forced to stay at home because their schools have been ordered to stop, and care for other family members who are all locked down at home. Consequently, during the pandemic, women are the leading participators in an unnoticed economy as unpaid caregivers in the family. This unnoticed economy has actual consequences on the economy and lives of women. It is strongly recommended that governments offer inclusive social security for all caregivers to lessen the burden on unpaid care workers (7, 32).

Pregnancy and COVID-19

Several studies have been conducted, and they unanimously agree that pregnant women could be more prone to contracting COVID-19 due to their weakened immune systems (33–35). Pregnant women who are infected with the COVID-19 virus are at more risk of serious diseases and greater risk of being hospitalized, subjected to mechanical ventilation, and being admitted to the intensive care unit compared with non-pregnant women with COVID-19 (36). This observed susceptibility in pregnant women is probably partly due to exposure risk from clinical settings and practices as well as the physiological changes that occur in pregnancy (11). In infected pregnant women, there is no proof of vertical transmission of the virus to the unborn child; however, there are higher incidences of preterm deliveries (37, 38). Furthermore, several authors reported severe maternal complications related to pregnant women with COVID-19 (39–41) and even deaths (42, 43). After systematically reviewing 19 studies of pregnant women with severe acute respiratory syndrome (SARS), middle east respiratory syndrome (MERS), or COVID-19, Di-Mascio and his fellow researchers revealed that infected pregnant women had more cases of Cesarean delivery, preeclampsia, preterm birth, and maternal death (34, 35, 44, 45).

Data on COVID-19 infections in pregnancy have been mainly from North America and Europe. Early confirmation from low and middle-income countries such as Nepal and Uganda shows that though the rate of infection is not high among the population, imposed restrictions due to the pandemic are distressing maternal-child outcomes, showing a severe drop in maternal facility births (up to 50% in Nepal) and amplified neonatal and maternal morbidity (46, 47).

Gender-Based Violence Due to COVID-19

Crises (natural disasters, war, or epidemics) accentuate incidences of gender-based violence against women (48, 49). This was the trend during the Ebola (2014) and Zika (2016) outbreaks (50). The existing challenge of physical abuse against women will expectedly worsen with COVID-19. Developing data indicate that since the pandemic broke out, domestic and sexual violence have risen in many regions and will likely escalate (51–53). As health, security, and financial challenges cause tension and strain in families, confinement because of the lockdown directive intensifies this pressure and makes people (particularly men, angered and frustrated by their lack of money) more prone to domestic violence toward their female partners (54–56). Some of the risk factors underlying gender-based violence include the narrowness of accommodation due to overcrowding, social isolation, fear of dying, low income, reduced access to services, decreased peer support, increased consumption of addictive substances, and male aggression (7, 51, 57–60). Since the implementation of the lockdown by governments around the world, many countries have observed an upsurge in cases of gender-based violence. Government authorities, civil society groups, and women's rights activists have indicated rising cases of gender-based violence across the globe (51, 52). The Refuge website has equally reported that calls about gender-based violence have increased by 150% (61). Intimate partner violence was reported to have increased by 30% in France and Cyprus, 33% in Singapore, and 25% in Argentina (53). Different states in the US also reported an intimate partner violence increase of 21–35% (62). Increased gender-based violence and demand for emergency shelter were also reported in Spain, Canada, Germany, and UK (53). In Nigeria, with the initial lockdown of three major states—Lagos, Ogun, and the Federal Capital Territory—throughout April 2020, gender-based violence significantly increased by 56% (49). During the first 2 weeks of lockdown, gender-based violence cases rose from 346 to 794 (40).

Health-care services are currently inundated with COVID-19 cases. In places where basic vital services are sustained, a breakdown in harmonized response from important sectors such as health, justice, police, and social services coupled with the physical/social distancing measure implies that sectors will be limited to provide satisfactory care to women who are suffering violence (7). That is to say, though shelters are available for women experiencing violence to take refuge, the lockdown order has compelled bodies such as judicial courts (in which the legal advocacy work for these victims are to be conducted) to close (11). Health-care services and police that are first-line responders are hardly available as they are overwhelmed too (48).

Due to the existing gender digital divide (62, 63), women in several nations, particularly those facing many forms of inequity, might be unable to access help services by cell phone or internet (owing to the lack of it). Even if these women have access to these means, they might be unable to use them because they are being closely watched by their perpetrators of violence. A Delhi-based NGO in India witnessed a 50% drop in calls on its helplines despite increased incidences of gender-based violence. This may have been due to the fear of getting discovered by their offenders (63, 64). As the use of online platforms has increased, women's rights experts and other bodies have reported an increase in varied forms of online violence against women, including bullying, stalking, sex-trolling, and sexual harassment (51, 53, 65).

The Ebola crisis with its resultant school closures showed that several forms of violence had worsened during the national health emergency, such as sexual exploitation and abuse of girls of reproductive age, child marriage, and trafficking (66, 67), and COVID-19 is following a comparable trend (68). The global cost of violence against women is bound to increase as gender-based violence increases during the pandemic and will sadly keep rising in the aftermath (7, 51).

Health-Care Impacts of COVID-19

Epidemics limit access to the healthcare system particularly preventive and reproductive health care (11). Evidence from previous health crises reveals that obstetric care is particularly compromised (11). During a widespread health crisis, such as COVID-19, the unique health needs of women are more unlikely to be met as access to satisfactory health services, reproductive and maternal health care, essential medicines, and vaccines are undermined. The availability of maternal health care with sexual and reproductive health services and gender-based violence-linked services is crucial to the health, welfare, and rights of women. When resources are diverted from these provisions/services, increased maternal mortality and morbidity are the result (7).

The upsurge in cases of COVID-19 is seriously hurting both the wealthiest and most sophisticated health systems. With the ongoing pandemic, honest fears arise about the survival capability of less-developed countries (with frail health systems) (7). From previous national health crises, the diversion of funds from important but less urgent health services, such as maternal care and gender-based violence response, to focus on the health emergency at hand is the advantageous approach, yet important services need not be completely abandoned even at such critical times (8, 11). Conceding the reproductive and sexual health of girls and women during the ongoing pandemic implies many will likely experience pregnancy. According to Guttmacher Institute modeling estimates, a reduction by 10% in short- and long-term use of contraceptives could result in more than 15 million unintended pregnancies across 132 low- and middle-income countries (69).

Limitations of the Study

The study was primarily based on published literature obtained from only three major databases. However, the non-systematic nature of the review represents a limitation in terms of the validity of the findings. Reports from unverifiable sources such as blog sites that were not documented in a verifiable source were not analyzed. The limited evidence for undeveloped/developing regions, or the general unawareness and even blackout regarding gender disparities and inequalities in COVID-19 crises were limitation factors in this study. Nevertheless, the strength of the study lies on the review of parameters that relate to women in the current COVID-19 health crisis. These included gender specificity, economic toll, pregnancy, gender-based violence, and the health-care impacts of COVID-19 on the health status of women around the globe.

CONCLUSION

This article has reviewed some parameters as it relates to women in the current COVID-19 health crisis. Women are at a higher risk of infection with the COVID-19 virus due to their exposure as caregivers. COVID-19-infected pregnant women are at greater risk of other severe diseases including hospitalizations. This is most likely due to the physiological changes and exposure risks during antenatal care and childbirth. More women than men work in the informal sector of the economy, which was the worst hit by the lockdown directive that followed the outbreak of the pandemic. Many women became pregnant during the lockdown as a result of not being able to go to their places of work. Couples spent more time together, and this led to pregnancies for even some who did not plan on getting pregnant (9). The unpaid care burden for the sick, elderly, children, and adults locked down at home fell disproportionately on women. The gender-based violence increased across the globe as physical distancing measures were taken to limit the spread of COVID-19. The unique healthcare needs of women, which include sexual and reproductive health care, maternal health care (antenatal and postnatal care), essential medicines, immunization, and gender-based violence-linked services should not be downplayed during health emergencies. The approach by key players to tackle the impacts of the COVID-19 pandemic will be inefficient if it does not have a gendered stance considering the peculiar needs of women. Governments should therefore provide social security to ease their burden.

Recommendations

Further research in the future is recommended to provide insight on how cultural and racial differences as well as other determinants of health (such as community, education, and the neighborhood) are impacting women during the COVID-19 pandemic. As useful data emerges with time, more investigations to understand the impact of COVID-19 pandemic on women's health across a broader geographic area (especially comparing more developed countries with those of the less developed countries) is imperative. Additional systematic studies to comprehend the overall effect of the COVID-19 pandemic on women's health is important to improve the wealth of scientific knowledge.

AUTHOR CONTRIBUTIONS

SO carried out the concept, design, and main interpretation of the study. VS, AC, SA, and UO conducted the electronic searches. VS drafted the manuscript and participated in the literature search and paper analysis. SO and VS critically reviewed and revised the manuscript for important intellectual content. UO participated in the proof editing. All authors made substantial, direct, and intellectual contributions to the work. The final version of the manuscript was read by all authors before giving their consent for its publication.

ACKNOWLEDGMENTS

The authors are grateful to the management of the Training and Consultancy Department, SIRONigeria Global Limited, Abuja, Nigeria for their kind assistance in the proofreading and English language editing services of the revised version of this paper.

REFERENCES

World Health Organization. *Protocol for Assessment of Potential Risk Factors for Coronavirus Disease 2019 (COVID-19) Among Health Workers in a Health Care Setting, 23 March, 2020.* World Health Organization (2020).

Fisayo T, Tsukagoshi S. Three waves of the COVID-19 pandemic. *Postgrad Med J.* (2020). doi: 10.1136/postgradmedj-2020-138564. [Epub ahead of print].

Guo YR, Cao QD, Hong ZS, Tan YY, Chen SD, Jin HJ, et al. The origin, transmission and clinical therapies on coronavirus disease 2019 (COVID-19) outbreak–an update on the status. *Military Med Res.* (2020) 7:11. doi: 10.1186/s40779-020-00240-0

Jin JM, Bai P, He W, Wu F, Liu XF, Han DM, et al. Gender differences in patients with COVID-19: focus on severity and mortality. *Front Public Health.* (2020) 8:152. doi: 10.3389/fpubh.2020.00152

Yaya S, Yeboah H, Charles CH, Otu A, Labonte R. Ethnic and racial disparities in COVID-19-related deaths: counting the trees, hiding the forest. *BMJ Global Health.* (2020) 5:e002913. doi: 10.1136/bmjgh-2020-002913

Ravi K. Ethnic disparities in COVID-19 mortality: are comorbidities to blame? *Lancet.* (2020) 396:22. doi: 10.1016/S0140-6736(20)31423-9

World Health Organization. *Gender and COVID-19: Advocacy Brief, 14 May, 2020 (No. WHO/2019-nCoV/Advocacy_brief/Gender/2020.1).* World Health Organization (2020).

Bamidele JO, Daniel OJ. Epidemiology of Coronavirus Disease (COVID-19) in Nigeria. *Ann Health Res.* (2020) 6:125–32. doi: 10.30442/ahr.0602-01-74

Ozili P. COVID-19 in Africa: socio-economic impact, policy response and opportunities. *Int J Soc Soc Policy.* (2020). doi: 10.1108/IJSSP-05-2020-0171. [Epub ahead of print].

World Bank. *Informing the Refugee Policy Response in Uganda: Results From the Uganda Refugee and Host Communities 2018 Household Survey. Informing the Refugee Policy Response in Uganda.* Washington, DC (2019). Available online at: www.worldbank.org

Connor J, Madhavan S, Mokashi M, Amanuel H, Johnson NR, Pace LE, et al. Health risks and outcomes that disproportionately affect women during the COVID-19 pandemic. A review. *Soc Sci Med.* (2020) 266:113364. doi: 10.1016/j.socscimed.2020.113364

CDC, Centers for Disease Control and Prevention 2013. CDC health disparities and inequalities report — United States, 2013. *Morb Mortal Wkly Rep.* (2013) 62:85–154. Available online at: https://www.cdc.gov/mmwr/pdf/ other/su6203.pdf (Accessed July 31, 2020).

Mehta L, Beckie T, DeVon H, Grines C, Krumholz H, Johnson M, et al. Acute myocardial infarction in women. *Circulation.* (2016) 133:916– 47. doi: 10.1161/CIR.0000000000000351

Roche MM, Wang PP. Sex differences in all-cause and cardiovascular mortality, hospitalization for individuals with and without diabetes, and patients with diabetes diagnosed early and late. *Diabetes Care.* (2013) 36:2582– 90. doi: 10.2337/dc12-1272

Alam MR, Kabir MR, Reza S. Comorbidities might be a risk factor for the incidence of COVID-19: evidence from a web-based survey. *Prev Med Rep.* (2021) 21:101319. doi: 10.1016/j.pmedr.2021.101319

Sáenz-Herrero M, López-Atanes M, Recio-Barbero M. Female corporality, gender roles, and their influence on women's mental health in times of COVID-19. *Front Glob Women's Health.* (2020) 1:563209. doi: 10.3389/fgwh.2020.563209

Guadagni V, Umilta A, Iaria G. Sleep quality, empathy, and mood during the isolation period of the COVID-19 pandemic in the Canadian population: females and women suffered the most. *Front Glob Women's Health.* (2020) 1:563209. doi: 10.3389/fgwh.2020.585938

Boniol M, McIsaac M, Xu L, Wuliji T, Diallo K, Campbell J. Gender equity in the health workforce: analysis of 104 countries. *Working Paper 1.* Geneva: World Health Organization (2019).

Elena BM, Samuel MC, Salvador PM. *Economic Gender Gap in the Global South: How Institutional Quality Matters.* United Nations University- Maastricht Economic and Social Research Institute on Innovation and Technology (MERIT) (2020).

Liu Z, Bing X, Zhi XZ. Novel coronavirus pneumonia emergency response epidemiology team. The epidemiological characteristics of an outbreak of 2019 coronavirus diseases (COVID-19) in China. *Zhonghua Liu Xing Bing Xue Za Zhi.* (2020) 41:145–51. doi: 10.46234/ccdcw2020.032

Purdie A, Hawkes S, Buse K, Onarheim K, Aftab W, Low N, et al. *Sex, Gender and COVID-19: Disaggregated Data and Health Disparities*. BMJ Global Health Blog (2020). Available online at: https://blogs.bmj.com/bmjgh/2020/03/24/sex-gender-and-covid-19-disaggregated-data-and-health-disparities/ (accessed July 27, 2020).

Richardson S, Hirsch JS, Narasimhan M, Crawford JM, McGinn T, Davidson KW, et al. Presenting characteristics, comorbidities, and outcomes among 5700 patients hospitalized with COVID-19 in the New York city area. *J Am Med Assoc.* (2020) 323:2052–9. doi: 10.1001/jama.2020.6775

WHO Gender Equity in the Health Workforce: Analysis of 104 Countries. (2019). Available online at: https://apps.who.int/iris/bitstream/handle/10665/ 31134/ WHO-HIS-HWF-Gender-WPI-2019.1-eng.pdf?Ua=1 (accessed February 3, 2021).

Wenham C, Smith J, Morgan R. COVID-19: the gendered impacts of the outbreak. *Lancet.* (2020) 395:846–8. doi: 10.1016/S0140-6736(20)30526-2

Global Health. *COVID-19 Sex-Disaggregated Data Tracker: Sex, Gender and COVID19 USA.* (2020). Available online at: https://globalhealth5050.org/covid19/sex-disaggregated-data-tracker/ (accessed July 30, 2020).

Simba N, Ngcobo S. Are pandemics gender neutral? Women's health and COVID-19. *Front. Glob. Womens Health.* (2020) 1:570666. doi: 10.3389/fgwh.2020.570666

Zhou F, Yu T, Du R, Fan G, Liu Z. Clinical course and risk factors for mortality of adult inpatients with COVID-19 in Wuhan, China: a retrospective cohort study. *Lancet.* (2020) 395:1054–62. doi: 10.1016/S0140-6736(20)30566-3

Burki T. The indirect impact of COVID-19 on women.. (2020) 20:904– 5. doi: 10.1016/S1473-3099(20)30568-5

UNITED NATIONS (UN). *Shared Responsibility, Global Solidarity: Responding to the Socio-economic Impacts of Covid-19.* UN (2020). Available online at: https://www.Un2.Un.Org/Files/Sg_Report_Socio-Economic_ Impact_Of_Covid19.Pdf

International Labour Organisation Monitor: COVID-19 and the World of Work, 6th ed. Updated Estimates and Analysis (2020). Available online at: http://oit.org/wcmsp5/groups/public/---dgreports/---dcomm/documents/ briefingnote/wcms_743146.pdf

Bluedorn J, Gopinath G, Sandri D. *An Early View of the Economic Impact of the Pandemic in 5 Charts.* IMFBlog: Website (2020). Available online at: https://blogs.imf.org/2020/04/06/an-early-view-of-the-economic- impact-of-the-pandemic-in-5-charts (accessed February 8, 2021).

Nanthini S, Nair T. *United Nations. COVID-19: SG Op-ed on COVID-19's Impact on Women.* (2020). Available online at: https://www.jstor.org/stable/ pdf/resrep26875.pdf (accessed May 28, 2020).

Phoswa WN, Khaliq OP. Is pregnancy a risk factor of COVID-19? *Eur J Obstetr Gynecol.* (2020) 252:605–9. doi: 10.1016/j.ejogrb.2020.06.058

Di-Mascio D, Khalil A, Saccone G, Rizzo G, Buca D, Liberati M, et al. Outcome of Coronavirus spectrum infections (SARS, MERS, COVID-19) during pregnancy: a systematic review and meta-analysis. *Am J Obstetr Gynecol.* (2020) 2:100107. doi: 10.1016/j.ajogmf.2020.100107

Chen H, Guo J, Wang C. Clinical characteristics and intrauterine vertical transmission potential of COVID-19 infection in 9 pregnant women: a retrospective review of medical records. *Lancet.* (2020) 395:809– 15. doi: 10.1016/S0140-6736(20)30360-3

Ellington S, Strid P, Tong VT, Woodworth K, Galang RR, Zambrano LD et al. Characteristics of women of reproductive age with laboratory- confirmed SARS-CoV-2 infection by pregnancy status—United States, January 22–June 7, 2020. *Morb Mortal Wkly Rep.* (2020) 69:769– 75. doi: 10.15585/mmwr.mm6925a1

Liu H, Wang L, Zhao S, Kwak-kim J, Mor G, Liao A. Why are pregnant women susceptible to COVID-19? An immunological viewpoint. *J Reprod Immunol.* (2020) 139:103122. doi: 10.1016/j.jri.2020.103122

Sentilhes L, De-Marcillac F, Jouffrieau C, Kuhn P, Thuet V, Hansmann Y, et al. COVID-19 in Pregnancy was associated with maternal morbidity and preterm birth. *Am J Obstetr Gynecol.* (2020) 223:914–e1. doi: 10.1016/j.ajog.2020.06.22

Liu Y, Chen H, Tang K, Guo Y. Clinical manifestations and outcome of SARS-COV-2 infection during pregnancy. *J Infect.* (2020). doi: 10.1016/j.jinf.2020.02.028

Breslin N, Baptiste C, Miller R, Fuchs K, Goffman D, Gyamfi-Bannerman C, et al. COVID-19 in pregnancy: early lessons. *Am J Obstetr Gynecol.* (2020) 2:100111. doi: 10.1016/j.ajogmf.2020.100111

Noelle B, Caitlin B, Cynthia GB, Russell M, Rebecca M, Kyra B, et al. COVID-19 infection among asymptomatic and symptomatic pregnant women. Two weeks of confirmed presentations to an affiliated pair of New York City hospitals. *Am J Obstetr Gynecol.* (2020) 2:100118. doi: 10.1016/j.ajogmf.2020.100118

Hantoushzadeh S, Shamshirsaz AA, Aleyasin A, Seferovic MD, Aski SK, Arian SE, et al. Maternal death due to COVID-19. *Am J Obstetr Gynecol.* (2020) 223:109-e1. doi: 10.1016/j.ajog.2020. 04.030

Ramos Amorim MM., Soligo Takemoto ML., Fonseca E.B. Maternal deaths with COVID-19: a different outcome from mid to low resource countries. *Am J Obstetr Gynecol.* (2020) 223:298–9. doi: 10.1016/j.ajog.2020. 04.023

Assiri A, Abedi GR, Al Masri M, Bin Saeed A, Gerber SI, Watson JT. Middle East Respiratory Syndrome coronavirus infection during pregnancy: a report of 5 cases from Saudi Arabia. *Clin Infect Dis.* (2016) 63:951– 3. doi: 10.1093/cid/ciw412

Stockman LJ, Lowther SA, Coy K, Saw J, Parashar UD. SARS during pregnancy United States. *Emerg Infect Dis.* (2004) 10:1689–90 doi: 10.3201/eid1009.040244

McDonald CR, Weckman AM, Wright JK, Conroy AL, Kain KC. Pregnant women in low and middle-income countries require a special focus during the COVID-19 pandemic. *Front Glob Women's Health.* (2020) 1:564560. doi: 10.3389/fgwh.2020.564560

Ashisk KC, Gurung R, Kinney MV, Sunny AK, Moinuddin M, Basnet O, et al. Effect of the COVID-19 pandemic response on intrapartum care, stillbirth, and neonatal mortality outcomes in Nepal: a prospective observational study. *Lancet Glob Health.* (2020) 8:e1273–81. doi: 10.1016/S2214-109X(20)3 0345-4

Thibaut F, van Wijngaarden-Cremers PJM. Women's mental health in the time of Covid-19 pandemic. *Front Glob Women's Health.* (2020) 1:17. doi: 10.3389/fgwh.2020.588372

Fawole OI, Okedare OO, Reed E. Home was not a safe haven: women's experiences of intimate partner violence during the COVID-19 lockdown in Nigeria. *BMC Women's Health.* (2021) 21:32. doi: 10.1186/s12905-021-01177-9

Davies SE, Bennett BA. Gendered human rights analysis of Ebola and Zika: locating gender in global health emergencies. *Int Affairs.* (2016) 92:1041– 60. doi: 10.1111/1468-2346.12704

Amadasun S. COVID-19 palaver: ending rights violations of vulnerable groups in Africa. *World Dev.* (2020) 134:105054. doi: 10.1016/j.worlddev.2020.105054

Sánchez OR, Vale DB, Rodrigues L, Surita FG. Violence against women during the COVID-19 pandemic: an integrative review. *Int J Gynecol Obstetr.* (2020) 151:180–7. doi: 10.1002/ijgo.13365

United Nations. *Global Humanitarian Response Plan Covid-19. United Nations Coordinated Appeal. April–December 2020.* New York, NY (2020). Available online at: https://www.humanitarianresponse.info/sites/www.humanitarianresponse.info/files/documents/files/global_humanitarian_response_plan_covid-19_1.pdf

Fore HH. A wake-up call: COVID-19 and its impact on children's health and wellbeing. *Lancet Glob Health.* (2020) 8:e861-2. doi: 10.1016/S2214-109X(20)30238-2

United Nations. *Covid-19 and Women's Human Rights: Guidance-What Is the Impact of Covid-19 on Gender-Based Violence?* New York, NY: (2020). Available online at: www.ohchr.org

Parkinson D, Zara C. The hidden disaster: domestic violence in the aftermath of natural disaster. *Aust J Emerg Manage.* (2013) 28:28– 35. Available online at: http://www.scopus.com/inward/record.url?scp= 84884969994&partnerID=8YFLogxK

Schneider D, Harknett K McLanahan S. Intimate partner violence in the great recession. *Demography.* (2016) 53:471–505. doi: 10.1007/s13524-016-0462-1

Roesch E, Amin A, Gupta J, García-Moreno C. Violence against women during covid-19 pandemic restrictions. *BMJ.* (2020) 369:m1712. doi: 10.1136/bmj.m1712

Phillips B, Jenkins P, Enarson E. Violence and disaster vulnerabilty. In: Phillips B, Thomas D, Fothergill A, Blinn-Pike L, editors. *Social Vulnerability to Disasters.* Boca Raton, FL: CRC Press (2019) p. 279–303.

Kelly J, Morgan T. Coronavirus: domestic abuse calls up 25% since lockdown, charity says. *BBC NEWS.* (2020). Available online at: https://www.bbc.com/news/uk-52157620

Wagers S. Domestic violence growing in wake of coronavirus outbreak. *The Conversation.* (2020). Available online at: https://theconversation. com/ domestic-violence-growing-in-wake-of-coronavirus-outbreak-135598 (accessed August 10, 2020).

Cadena MV. Gender job gaps and challenges in the digital economy: findings from global governance entities. *Cuadernos Administr.* (2020) 36:158–71. Available online at: https://cuadernosdeadministracion.univalle.edu.co/index. php/ cuadernos_de_administracion/article/view/8767

Chris AO, James G, Okoduwa S.I.R. Attitude towards access and utilization of maternal health services by women at Sabon-Gari local government area, Kaduna, Nigeria. *Int J Women's Health Care.* (2019) 4:1– 5. doi: 10.33140/ IJWHC.04.01.01

Chandra J. COVID 19 lockdown rise in domestic violence, Police Apathy: NCW. *The Hindu.* (2020, April 2). Retrieved from: www.thehindu.com/ news/ national/COVID-19-lockdown-spike-in-domestic-violence-says~ ncw/ article31238659.ece

Davies S. *Risk of Online Sex Trolling Rises as Coronavirus Prompts Home Working.* (2020). Available online at: https://www.reuters.com/article/us- women-rights-cyberflashing.trfn-idUSKBN2153HG (accessed February 3, 2021).

UNGA A/70/723. *Protecting Humanity from Future Health Crises: Report of the High Level Panel on the Global Response to Health Crises.* UNICEF Helpdesk, 'GBV in Emergencies: Emergency Responses to Public Health Outbreaks' (2018). p. 2.

UNESCO. *COVID-19 School Closures Around the World Will Hit Girls Hardest.* (2020). Available online at: https://en.unesco.org/news/covid-19- school-closures-around-world-will-hit-girls-hardest (accessed August 11, 2020).

IASC. *Guidelines for Integrating Gender-Based Violence Interventions in Humanitarian Action: Food Security and Agriculture, UNGA A/70/723. Protecting Humanity From Future Health Crises: Report of the High Level Panel on the Global Response to Health Crises* (2015).

Riley T, Sully E, Ahmed Z, Biddlecom A. Estimates of the potential impact of the COVID-19 pandemic on sexual and reproductive health in low- and middle-income countries. *Int Perspect Sex Reprod Health.* (2020) 46:73– 6. doi: 10.1363/46e9020

20

COVID-19 Effect on Access to Maternal Health Services in Kenya

Jackline Oluoch-Aridi[1,2*], *Tecla Chelagat*[2], *Mary M. Nyikuri*[2], *Joseph Onyango*[2], *Danice Guzman*[1], *Cindy Makanga*[1], *Laura Miller-Graff*[1,3] *and Robert Dowd*[1]

[1] *The Ford Family Program in Human Development Studies and Solidarity, Kellogg Institute for International Studies, University of Notre Dame, Notre Dame, IN, United States,* [2] *Strathmore Business School, Institute of Healthcare Management, Strathmore University, Nairobi, Kenya,* [3] *Department of Psychology, The Kroc Institute of Peace Studies, University of Notre Dame, Notre Dame, IN, United States*

***Correspondence:**
Jackline Oluoch-Aridi
joluocha@nd.edu

Introduction: Maternal mortality continues to be one of the biggest challenges of the health system in Kenya. Informal settlements in Kenya have been known to have higher rates of maternal mortality and also receive maternity services of varied quality. Data assessing progress on key maternal health indicators within informal settlements are also often scarce. The COVID-19 pandemic hit Kenya in March this year and so far, the impact of the pandemic on access to maternal health has not been established. This study aims to add to the body of knowledge by investigating the effects of the COVID-19 pandemic and mitigation strategies on access to health care services in informal settlements.

Methods: Qualitative methods using in-depth interviews were used to assess women's experiences of maternity care during the COVID-19 era and the impact of proposed mitigation strategies such as the lockdown and the curfew. Other aspects of the maternity experience such as women's knowledge of COVID-19, their perceived risk of infection, access to health facilities, perceived quality of care were assessed. Challenges that women facing as a result of the lockdown and curfew with respect to maternal health access and quality were also assessed.

Results: Our findings illustrate that there was a high awareness of the symptoms and preventative measures for COVID-19 amongst women in informal settlements. Our findings also show that women's perception of risk to themselves was high, whereas risk to family and friends, and in their neighborhood was perceived as low. Less than half of women reported reduced access due to fear of contracting Coronavirus, Deprioritization of health services, economic constraints, and psychosocial effects were reported due to the imposed lockdown and curfew. Most respondents perceived improvements in quality of care due to short-waiting times, hygiene measures, and responsive health personnel. However, this was only reported for the outpatient services and not in-patient services.

Conclusion: The most important recommendation was for the Government to provide food followed by financial support and other basic amenities. This has implications for the Government's mitigation measures that are focused on public health measures and lack social safety-net approaches for the most vulnerable communities.

Keywords: COVID-19, informal settlements, Kenya, women, maternity services, access

INTRODUCTION

The Novel Coronavirus disease, commonly referred as COVID-19, was declared a public health emergency of international concern on 30th January 2020 and declared a global pandemic on the 11th March 2020 (1). Previous research has indicated that pandemics, such as Ebola in West Africa, can devastate the provision of maternal health services in low-resilience health systems (2–4). A study modeling the coverage of essential maternal and child health interventions estimated a 8.3–38.6% increase in maternal deaths per month across 118 low- and middle-income countries (LMICs) during the COVID-19 pandemic (5). The COVID-19 pandemic reached Kenya on March 15, 2020. Currently (as per 25th August 2020) the number of cases in Kenya is estimated at 32,577 infections, with 18,895 recoveries and 554 deaths (6). Nairobi City in Kenya is estimated to have the highest the number of COVID infections in the country with at 342 as per July 2020 with ~30% of new infections in peri-urban settings (7). It is estimated that about 70% of Nairobi's more than 4 million residents reside in urban slums (8–10).

As a preventive response, Kenya imposed strict curfews and lockdown rules to prevent the spread of COVID-19. The Kenyan Government banned international flights, closed schools, and banned large social gatherings; mass prayer gatherings, large weddings and funerals, in order to prevent the accelerated transmission of the virus (11). In addition to this, the Government issued a 30-day lock down as a mitigation measure to COVID-19 transmission. This was accompanied by a curfew that was initially restricted movement between 7.00 p.m. and 4.00 a.m. but was subsequently extended to 9.00 p.m. to 5.00 a.m. These government directives pose a huge dilemma, as they have disrupted access to health services by mothers (12). Despite the fact that expectant mothers have been allowed to leave their houses and go to health facilities to access delivery care during emergencies. They have however had challenges with transportation to health facilities during the curfew. These restrictions may disproportionately affect those living in informal settlements within large cities. Recent evidence has shown that women face access challenges that are both structural, such as transportation to health facilities, and social, such as fear of health care workers (13). These settings also have already existing challenges with regard to the quality of maternal health care services and women report receiving maternal health services of varied quality (13).

Studies that have focused in informal settlements have assessed residents' perceptions of government directives to contain the pandemic and concluded that the Government measures to mitigate COVID-19 need to have communication channels that are targeted at reaching less-educated households (14). Other studies have shown that although COVID-19 mitigation strategies are needed, they are known to have an indirect negative impact on women's well-being, for example many hospitals have put restrictions on visits by partners and relatives during admission at the hospitals for delivery (15). This is despite the fact that women are normally denied companionship during delivery in most hospitals due to privacy concerns (16). The COVID period presents new challenges for women with the lockdowns and curfews instilling fear and necessitating the need for birth companionship. Lockdowns have also result in varied economic consequences such as job loss, food and housing insecurity further aggravating health outcomes (17, 18). It is possible that within informal settlements the impact of the job losses might indirectly affect women's ability to access health care due to economic hardship, subsequently reducing access to health facilities.

A review of the existing literature demonstrates an information gap on the impact of pandemic on maternal well-being especially in a resource-scarce setting where marginalized women often receive poor quality of care (19, 20). A population survey in 60 LMICs suggest a declining trend on utilization of maternal and child health (MCH) services such as delivery, antenatal care (ANC) attendance and child immunization (21). Studies have established that health workers in other sub-Saharan African settings are not well-prepared to provide treatment for COVID patients and insufficiently prepared to meet the demands of the women (22). These limitations may have serious implications for women's health. For example, a recent study modeling the coverage of essential maternal and child health interventions estimated a 8.3–38.6% increase in maternal deaths per month across 118 low- and middle-income countries (LMICs) during the COVID-19 pandemic (5).

This study aimed to assess the extent of the impact of the imposed lockdowns and curfew on access to maternal health services for women living in informal settlements. We also assessed women's knowledge of the signs and symptoms of COVID-19, women's perceived risk of infection to further understand how the virus affects women and their health during the pandemic. These findings provide a critical information for frontline health workers and policy makers who are seeking to quickly develop pandemic responsive programs and strategies that are relevant, person-centered and context friendly. By incorporating women's voices, Ministries of Health and other non-state health care providers can be better able conduct targeted care and minimize the negative consequences of COVID-19.

METHODS

Study Setting

This qualitative study focused on women's experiences with person-centered maternity care amongst women living in the informal settlements in the Embakasi area in Nairobi City, Kenya. The study area has an estimated population of almost one million people, in mostly low-income housing and informal settlements. Residents in Embakasi experience widespread poverty and high unemployment and belong to the lowest wealth quintile in Kenya. The health system consists of both primary public health centers and several private health facilities and mission health facilities. The main referral health facility is a secondary maternity hospital.

Data Collection

Study Design, Recruitment, and Participants

Participants were drawn from an ongoing longitudinal study focused on assesses quality of maternal care services in the Embakasi region of Nairobi, capital of Kenya. For the current study, a subsample of women was selected to completed telephonic interviews (71), which were conducted by four researchers in the months May-June 2020 with women who had received services for childbirth in the past 6 weeks from public, private and missionary hospitals in this region.

The first author is a trained public health specialist and the research assistants were trained on qualitative research methods. The facilities were purposively selected to represent both health centers and secondary maternities. They also represented three types of health facilities present in Kenya: public, private, and mission health facilities. The health facilities in the study were chosen in collaboration with the first author.

Women were recruited during child welfare clinics. The inclusion criteria were women who were aged between 18 and 49 and had delivered their babies within the identified facilities in the past 6 weeks. Verbal informed consent was obtained from all the women after providing information about the study and the potential benefits and risks of their involvement in the study via a phone call. The interviews were conducted by phone to mitigate the risk to participants due to COVID-19. During the phone interviews women were asked whether they had been to the health facility during the COVID-19 pandemic and to share their experiences during this time. A semi-structured interview guide was used (See **Appendix 1**). Interviews were conducted in Kiswahili, a language commonly spoken by women in this setting. The discussions were recorded and transcribed verbatim in Kiswahili. The transcripts were then, translated into English by the sixth author (CM) who is a native speaker of Kiswahili. The transcripts were back translated from Kiswahili to English by the first author also a native speaker of Kiswahili to ensure that the meaning was maintained. A total of 82 women who met the criteria were approached via phone calls. Nine of them were in an area with very poor mobile phone connectivity. Two women were unavailable. Therefore only 71 interviews were conducted. Ethical review approval from Strathmore University IRB, University of Notre Dame IRB and permission to conduct the research from The National Commission on Science Technology and Innovation (NACOSTI).

TABLE 1 | Sociodemographic characteristics of the participants.

Participant characteristics	Percentage $N = 71$
Age (Mean)	28 (5.3)
Parity	
Primiparous	16 (23%)
Multiparous	55 (77%)
Marital Status	
Married	61 (86%)
Single	10 (14%)
Education	
Primary	18 (25%)
Secondary	43 (61%)
College	10 (14%)
Occupation	
Employed	10 (14%)
Unemployed	61 (86%)
Type of health facility	
Mission health facility	29 (41%)
Public health facility	25 (53%)
Private health facility	17 (24%)
Delivery history	
All deliveries in a health facility	61 (86%)
At least one delivery outside health facility	10 (14%)

Data Analysis

We read all the transcripts to gain familiarization with the data. We iteratively coded line-by-line across the entire data set. We then analyzed the data applying emerging codes. We then compared these codes to those in the coding framework that we established a priori from the interview guide. We followed Braun and Clark's (23) thematic analysis to analyze the data. We grouped codes into categories, reviewed the themes for patterns, defined the themes. Four coders compared the themes and discussed the themes. We reviewed transcripts and analyzed the data until we reached data saturation and we could not identify any new themes. An Additional **Appendix 2** to show how open codes were used to generate categories and themes.

RESULTS

The characteristics of the women respondents are contained in **Table 1** below.

The mean age of the women was 28 years. Seventy seven percentage of the women were multiparous with a majority (88%) of the women were married. A vast majority of the women were unemployed (86%). The rest of the characteristics are contained in **Table 1**. We identified four main themes in the data: (1) Awareness and risk perception on COVID-19. In this theme we discuss women's ability to identify at least three symptoms of COVID-19, key prevention measures as well as their perceived risk of infection (2) perceived quality of health services. This theme describes our findings regarding women's perceived changes in the quality of maternal health services during the COVID-19 pandemic. (3) Economic challenges. This theme identifies women's several accounts of economic struggles where they describe their experiences with loss of income generation and this resulting in their in ability to afford transportation to the health facility and (4) mitigation strategies. This theme identifies strategies that women used to try and mitigate the impacts of the COVID-19 pandemic that would allow them to increase access to health facilities.

Awareness and Risk Perception on COVID-19

Most of the respondents with about 60% had a high awareness of the key symptoms and preventative measures employed to reduce the spread of the COVID-19. They were able to mention key symptoms such as high body temperature, persistent cough, and fever. Most women were aware of preventative measures including frequent washing of hands, sanitizing, wearing face masks and maintaining social distance.

> *"...The symptoms include: fever, severe coughing and also an increase in the body temperature. I know it is a dangerous disease whose preventive measures include: frequent washing of hands, sanitizing, wearing face masks and maintaining social distance of one meter away when interacting with other people..." (Respondent #44)*

Perceived Risk of Contracting COVID-19

Respondents were asked about their risk of contracting COVID-19 to self, family and friends and their neighborhood. A majority of the women—~56% of those women interviewed—perceived a high risk of the virus to their health. They viewed it as serious and anticipated getting infected if they left their residence. They undertook the necessary precautions to prevent infection such as using sanitizer and washing their hands regularly and wearing face masks. They also reported practicing social distancing.

> *"...From my perception I think this Corona issue is serious and that's why I have sanitizer in my house, washing my hands and I ensure I wear a mask whenever I leave the house..." (Respondent #38)*

> *"...According to me it is serious. I don't leave the house to go anywhere, because if I go out, I might meet anyone and contract the disease and infect my baby. So, I just sit in the house and take care of the baby, maybe I send someone to get me something..." (Respondent #40)*

In extreme cases women, were aware that the COVID-19 carried a risk of mortality if precautions were not taken and one was in a crowded setting.

> *"...Coronavirus can cause death if you do not take care of yourself. If you do not take preventative measures when you leave home or are in a crowded place, you can easily get coronavirus..." (Respondent #16)*

On the other hand, a majority of women perceived a low threat of infection to friends and family with 68% mentioned that they perceived their friends and family at a low risk of getting infected by COVID-19. They attributed this to their friends and family being careful and following Government measures to contain the virus.

> *"...If you look at my friends, they are really careful. They are trying their best to follow all the rules put in place so that they do not get sick. Then if you look at my family, they are also careful. I do not think anyone will get it unless...for this person who is always going out. But so far I feel they are all being careful and following the rules..." (Respondent#36)*

They described them as taking precautions such as handwashing, sanitizing and wearing of masks when out in the public. These measures led them to believe that most of their friends and family were at a low risk of infection

> *"...I don't think they might get infected because I have seen the way they take steps and precautions to prevent that. They wash their hands and sanitize regularly and they also take their clothes off whenever they come from out. So, I cannot say they can get the disease because all of them have masks ..." (Respondent #40)*

Almost half of the women perceived a low threat of infection with the virus within their residences. They attribute this low perceived threat to not knowing anyone who had contracted the virus in their neighborhood

> *"... I have heard that this disease is killing a lot of people, but I have not heard about anybody contracting this disease in my area." (Respondent #16)*
> *I don't think it is that serious because so far, I haven't heard of any coronavirus confirmed cases here at our place and the residents are observing all the preventive measures put in place by the government through the Ministry of health. (Respondent #43)*

Perceived Quality of Health Services

The respondents reported varying levels of perceived change in access and quality of services provided as a result of measures put in place due to COVID-19. About half of the women (51%) indicated that they were accessing health services normally and would continue to go to the health facility despite the risk of exposure to the virus.

> *"...I haven't changed the way I access the health care services. I'm just going the way I used to, and also as instructed by the nurse in charge of my baby, although I am fearful and worried of who I might meet at the health facility..." (Respondent# 23)*

Respondents perceived quality of care to have improved due to hygiene, caution, attentiveness, privacy, low patient-load, restricted movements, increased numbers of nurses, and shorter turn-around time for patient attendance.

> *"...I will say that the quality of service delivered has changed for the better because the Health workers are more vigilant when attending to the patients unlike before when they weren't that*

much cautious such as observing good hygiene all the time..." (Respondent #41) "*...I will also say that the social distancing rule put in place whereby each patient is attended to one by one has made the patients to be more free to the doctors and tell them what they are really undergoing through because in the past, patients could be congested in one room and make the other patient fear to speak up what he or she is going through...*" (Respondent #44)

The change in the health facility culture was perceived to be contributing to improved quality of care. There was an observed change in how COVID-19 preventative measures were enforced by the security at the entrance of the health facility as well as by health workers such as doctors and nurses.

> "*...I will say that the quality of service has changed for the better because even the watch man and every health worker is observing all the hygienic measures put in place thus the patients feel safer... they wear masks, protective clothes which they were not using before*" (Respondent #45)
> "*...Yes there has been a change in the quality of service e delivered because the health workers are more cautious when handling patients and also the patients are attended to one by one unlike before where three patients could congest in one room....and the way they handle patients is totally different because they handle shifts to prevent overcrowding*" (Respondent #46)

Although most facilities were strict in enforcing the COVID-19 mitigation measures, some respondents reported that experiences at the health facilities they attended as not taking seriously the mitigation measures against COVID-19

> "*...they just kept telling us to have our masks on, but it was not that serious. They were not taking this Corona thing seriously. But in facility X you always had to have your mask on. For me I did not see anything different in the facility Y....*" (Respondent #36)

Perceptions of time taken at the facility were mixed. Women described health services that were delivered efficiently at times, and slower health services at other times. Less time was attributed to fewer patients as well as hastened health services.

> "*...when I left my home for the hospital, the services were quicker than before because during this COVID-19 period there were fewer patients at the health facility.... the duration taken in the facility was very little and the nurses were fast in their services...*" (Respondent #19)

Although most respondents seemed pleased with the change in the quality of services, some mentioned changes to routine prenatal services. One woman who had taken her baby for immunization witnessed other women who had taken their babies for growth monitoring been turned away by the health care workers. She overheard them been informed that it was unnecessary during the COVID-19 times.

> "*... I visited the hospital when I took my baby for immunization; at the hospital I observed mothers whose babies were to be weighed were turned back by the nurses who said it is not necessary at this time of COVID-19 they were avoiding crowds...*" (Respondent #15)

Other women also described been turned back because of the large number of people being served

> "*...It is because sometimes you can't come there at the hospital because you will not even be served. You see people are many so you go and you are told to go and come back some other day...*" (Respondent #41)

On the other hand, COVID-19 transmission mitigation strategies such as mandatory temperature checks and sanitization at every station were perceived to increase time spent at the facility. The respondents attributed the long waiting time due to health personnel constantly changing their protective gears.

> "*.... Before we just used to enter, they write something for you, you go somewhere else but now you see you must be tested first then you go sanitize before you now go inside the hospital...*" (Respondent #24)

Although COVID-19 mitigation strategies had led to perceived improvements in quality at the outpatient department, the inpatient services seemed to have remained the same. There were also incidences of slower services and overcrowding public maternity hospital wards.

> "*...That one was tough, because there were many people. When I went to the ward, if any one of us in there would have been having corona, all of us would have contracted it. One bed three people, there's no space to turn, that was a challenge, because those giving birth were many, those undergoing CS were many. There was nowhere to rest, you are just told to go to room three. where you ask for some space on a bed to put your baby, then you can sit on the bench after undergoing the CS. It was quite a challenge....*" (Respondent #40)

Fear of Infection With COVID-19

While nearly half reported that they were able to access the health facilities, slightly less than half (40%) were hesitant to visit health facilities due to fear, they indicated that their main reason for not going into a health facility was fear. They described uncertainty regarding meeting people with COVID-19 at the health facility and risking exposure to the virus.

> "*...I'm going less times compared to non-COVID-19 times. First of all it is because of fear, I'm worried that maybe if I go to the Hospital more often I may get exposed to the people who are infected with coronavirus and unluckily I get infected with the disease too..I am also afraid of exposing my child to the Corona virus when I frequently visit the hospital...*" (Respondent #43)

They further expressed fear of contracting COVID- 19 from health care workers who were regularly being exposed and risked infecting them.

> "*... I will be afraid because I don't know if the nurse or the doctor, I find at the facility has the disease. So, I will be afraid...*" (Respondent #2)

This fear of the health facility resulted into some women foregoing scheduled visits to the health facility

> *"...It has reduced. I go a few times now. I cannot say it is because of money for me. It is just because I fear to get this disease. It is not easy for me to go to hospital because I fear. I would just stay in the house and wait to feel better. I would just take medicine until I feel better... " (Respondent #36)*

Some respondents also feared to be deemed to be COVID positive if captured by the temperature screening processes that could find their temperature to be high.

> *"...You know right now, you do not even want to go to hospital, even when the baby is sick you become scared. You see how they say when you have corona your temperature is high; they might say that you have corona ... " (Respondent #36)*

Some of the mitigation measures put in place for COVID-19 were reported to instill fear among community members and the employers of casual laborers which could easily resort to stigma. This stigma resulted into unemployment for some people.

> *"...Keeping distance has also made people fear each other......employers are afraid that you might infect them with COVID-19." (Respondent #33)*

Economic and Food Security Challenges

Some women identified economic reasons for not accessing health services. They said that they were unemployed and loss their sources of income and lacked money for transportation to health facilities. They therefore prioritized essential provisions such as purchasing food over going to the health facility.

> *".... As a result of COVID 19. I don't have a job, so the little that we get we prioritize for food then health will come after." (Respondent #43)*

For those who had some money to purchase food items, they found them to be very expensive because the supply was low.

> *".... you will go to the shop especially to the groceries and they tell you this curfew and lockdown has affected the supply chain and food stuffs are overpriced... " (Respondent #6)*

Reports of food insecurity were also reported as a result of loss of income.

> *"...So, there is low income.... sometimes we don't consume the way we used to, we have to minimize the expenditure on the house, food, getting food and something to eat is a challenge ... " (Respondent #6)*

The lockdown together with the curfew that was initially put at 7.00 p.m. affected businesses with most of them closing as early as 5.00 p.m. This resulted in a significant loss of gainful income.

> *"...Things have become difficult... because going for stuff to come and sell is an issue. I have been staying in the house, I have spent all the money, it is over. If it is time to close work, I have told you I just sell vegetables so these hours of leaving have become stressful. You must close early before 7.00 p.m. Things have become difficult now... " (Respondent #22)*

These difficult economic situations resulted in challenges with psychosocial well-being.

> *"...Stress, stress is there because of these lockdowns because business is not there and there is no money and you see I now have 4 children... " (Respondent #5)*
> *"...Am stressed with the children, I am the one is blamed by my husband if anything goes wrong in the house, I am also stressed when my baby doesn't get enough milk to breastfeed, all this is happening because of the lockdown and curfew..."*

Children being at home was mentioned as a challenge.

> *"... the challenge that I face is that all my children are back at home and none of them is in school... " (Respondent #62)*

The Government initiated curfews to reinforce social distancing not only constrained access to health care services but also led women to attend health facilities unaccompanied. Reports of support companions being denied entry at the health facilities when women sought delivery services.

> *"...when my labor started, I went to the hospital x with my cousin and neighbor but could not be allowed in. Unfortunately, this was way past curfew hours (7 pm). However, they couldn't go back to the home and had to stay at the hospital. I had to pretend that I couldn't walk so that the watchman could allow them to help me walk back to the hospital building. After I went inside the maternity they were not allowed inside." (Respondent #40)*

Coping With the Challenges Brought About COVID-19

Following the challenges described above, several coping strategies were reported by the respondents. Most of the strategies came from non-governmental organizations and the local administration to cope with loss of livelihood. Non-governmental organizations commenced food distribution to the affected families. In one of the settlements, respondents reported receiving food rations twice a week.

> *"...There were people getting aid at the centre A. They were receiving assorted food items. So, for someone like me with a child and I have a very big demand, I queue and then get some food stuff. They come twice a week... " (Respondent #66)*

Other non-governmental organizations distributed items such as soap and money

> *"...one day we were given a bar of soap with an organization called H"... "I have received a little support in terms of funds and am so thankful for that." (Respondent # 035)*

Some respondents however mentioned favoritism in food distribution, citing a lack of transparency and clear criteria.

> *"...Have not seen anything or maybe it's given and am not aware because I hear from people food is distributed at night to those who are known to the people concerned... " (Respondent # 62)*

However, the support received from the local administration fell below community members' expectations. They expected economic support, but the support they received was often advisory and related to COVID-19 containment measures. The area administration and landlords were reported to have teamed up to enforce curfew measures.

> *"...The Member of County Assembly (MCA), and the Chief, even the landlords have also helped when it came to warning and enforcing the restrictions. He used to call and warn people about letting strangers in and encouraging people to report anyone who does it... they should give food to people like us who can't go to work because I wash clothes for people but now, they can't allow us in the house. Food is very expensive at the moment people are taking advantage by adding the prices of items. Because you know food is the reason you will go get infected with these diseases because you are going look for food." (Respondent #24)*

Recommendations by Women to the Government

Our respondents were mostly concerned about food, basic supplies, rent. and financial assistance. They made no recommendations regarding their access to health services. The most important recommendation was for the Government to provide food with one third of the women recommending this. They suggested that the Government should support families economically by providing food items so that people don't have to go look for work and thus endanger their families.

> *"... providing essential needs such as food...talking to the landlords at least yeah the rent issue is also a problem for so many of us... If they can get someone to help us with pads because there are no pads." (Respondent # 6)*

In addition, some saw the role of the Government as going beyond food items to encompass provision of hand sanitizers and masks; as well as ensuring that families were not evicted from their houses due to lack of rent.

> *"...The government should buy for people mask and sanitizer, there is no money paying for house rent is a problem the government should talk to the owners of the house to make them understand what people are going through, those people who work their time is limited because of curfew..." (Respondent # 65)*

DISCUSSION

Our study sought to explore the maternity experiences women residing in informal settlements during the COVID-19 pandemic. Specifically, we assessed women's knowledge of COVID-19, their perceived risk of infection, access to health facilities, perceived quality of care and challenges experienced as a result of the COVID-19 pandemic mitigation measures. Overall, the findings revealed important effects of the pandemic on maternity care and access, suggesting some improvements in quality of care as well as some continued challenges with access and quality that were further exacerbated by the pandemic. In addition to their reflections on maternity care, specifically, women also commonly reported more general concerns and economic stressors about the effects of the pandemic that have important implications for how multisystemic supports might be put into place to support perinatal women.

The findings revealed that women continued to access health facilities and would continue to do so despite the perceived risks of infection by COVID-19. Less than half of women reported reduced access due to fear of contracting the coronavirus, deprioritization of health services, economic constraints, psychosocial effects due to the imposed lockdown and curfews. Some of the reduced access was due to new hospital policies that restricted women's entry to the health facility. These changes resulted in hospital policies that dictated for certain routine services such as growth monitoring were unimportant during this time due to the risk of contracting COVID-19. Other restrictions included prohibition of friends and family accompanying women to the health facility at a time when they were needed most by the women. Jolivet et al. (24) emphasizes that respectful care and human rights need to be upheld even at times of a pandemic such as the COVID-19. They call for the use of ethical guidelines in access to proven practices during maternity care.

Most of the respondents perceived improvements in quality of care due to short-waiting times, hygiene measures and responsive health personnel. However, this was only reported for the outpatient services as some in-patient services remained overcrowded. While the Government measures to contain COVID-19 were lauded and appreciated by all, there were several effects; some were unintended. This includes fear of exposure to the virus, economic constraints and effects on psychosocial well-being. While nearly half reported that they were able to access the health facilities, slightly less than half (40%) were hesitant to visit health facilities due to fear, stigma, and reported lack of proper COVID-19 preventive measures at the facilities. This is in line with findings of a study in West Africa conducted during the Ebola outbreak that illustrated that the outbreak disrupted services and fear of seeking treatment (2). There were reports of overcrowding especially in the inpatient department and most mothers were scared due to lack of physical distancing which is one of the measures for preventing COVID-19 infections

Women's positive response to the increased attention and privacy their received during care highlight that the COVID pandemic mitigation measures at health facilities might have led to better experiences of patient centered maternity care and dignified care particularly during outpatient care. Studies focused on women experiences during facility-based delivery highlight High quality patient centered maternity care as represented by dignified care including privacy (25).

Our findings also illustrate that awareness of the symptoms and preventative measures for COVID-19 was high. These findings are consistent with a study by the Population Council to assess COVID-19 knowledge attitude and practices in informal settlement in Nairobi showed that knowledge on COVID-19 symptoms was high and respondents could name several preventative methods (14). Our findings however differ from other studies conducted by White Ribbon Alliance (WRA) in selected counties in Kenya between April and May 2020 to determine the impact of COVID-19 on reproductive, maternal, and newborn health services. Whereas our study reported high levels of knowledge on COVID-19, this study found out that many citizens who live in slums in other parts of Kenya, did not know about the curfew. This was attributed to women lacking phones or radios, and the fact that information takes time to disseminate particularly in rural areas. This might also possibly be due to the changing demographics that indicate that women in informal settings are increasingly younger and possess secondary education (26). Our study was also conducted 2 months later which could possibly explain the learning curve. Findings show that women's perception of risk to themselves was high, but that perception of risk to family and friends, and in their neighborhood was low.

A majority of the participants had lost their jobs and their source of livelihoods and were struggling with access to income. Consequently, there were reports of lack of food, lack of rent and stress. To cope with these challenges, some women reported receiving support from the non-governmental organizations as well as government local administration. However, they reported that government support was focused on enforcing COVID-19 preventative measures while women's priority was food and rent. Our findings conform with other studies that have been conducted during the COVID-pandemic that indicate that effects of the lockdown have been primarily economic (14). In the case of women's access to maternity services, the primary access difficulty may therefore be women's in ability to pay for costs associated with accessing health care, despite its ongoing availability and women's overall willingness to use it. Evidence from the Ebola virus outbreak in 2013–2016 in Western Africa shows the negative indirect effects that such crises can have on sexual and reproductive health (2).

A major cross cutting issue from our study was stress related to the loss of livelihoods and severe economic constraints. Women reported being stressed due to unemployment, food security, rent, and sudden school closures. This economic hardship led to some women reducing their access to health care by prioritizing their finances to basic provisions as opposed to using it for transportation costs to the health facility thus reducing access to health services overall. We recommend that state and non-state actors should focus efforts on the impacts of income loss and food security, with special attention to women. This can be achieved by ensuring that those most at need of assistance are the ones receiving it by considering that assistance is getting into the hands of women given their increased experience of social and economic impacts.

A major limitation of the study was that the first lock-down which had restrictions on movement after 7 p.m. and before 4.00 a.m. greatly limited travel. The only plausible means to communicate effectively with the women was via mobile phones. The penetration of mobile phones is reasonably high within the urban slums of Nairobi. However, this might have limited the population we interviewed to women who are slightly economically stronger because of the ability to afford and use a mobile phone.

CONCLUSION

It is likely that despite the best efforts of health professionals, that an upward surge in the numbers of COVID-19 related deaths in women of reproductive age, including pregnant and post-natal women, will take place. It is crucial, however, to continue every effort as a vital contribution to safe childbirth and high-quality maternal care, and to continue to work toward the achievement of sustainable development goals. Although the Kenyan Ministry of Health (MOH) launched a COVID-19 Taskforce to steer the country's prevention, containment and mitigation measures, there is need to include additional measures to prevent the devastating health, social and economic impact of a COVID-19 outbreak particularly among women living in informal settlements.

ETHICS STATEMENT

The studies involving human participants were reviewed and approved by Strathmore University IRB Ethics Committe. The patients/participants provided their written informed consent to participate in this study.

AUTHOR CONTRIBUTIONS

JO-A, LM-G, and RD conceptualized the study. JO-A, TC, CM, and MN analysed the data. JO-A, TC, and MN wrote the manuscript. JO, DG, and LM-G provided critical feedback to the manuscript. All authors read and approved the manuscript prior to publication.

REFERENCES

World Health Organization. *WHO Director-General's Statement on IHR Emergency Committee on Novel Ciribavurys (2019-nCoV).* Geneva: WHO (2020).

Camara BS, Delamou A, Diro E, Béavogui AH, El AM. Effect of the 2014 / 2015 Ebola outbreak on reproductive health services in a rural district of Guinea : an ecological study. *Trans R Soc Trop.* (2017) 111:22–9. doi: 10.1093/trstmh/trx009

Delamou A, Ayadi AM, El Sidibe S, Delvaux T, Camara BS, Sandouno SD, et al. Articles Effect of Ebola virus disease on maternal and child health services in Guinea : a retrospective observational cohort study. *Lancet Glob Health.* (2017) 5:e448–57. doi: 10.1016/S2214-109X(17)30078-5

Sochas L, Channon AA, Nam S. Counting indirect crisis-related deaths in the context of a low-resilience health system : the case of maternal and neonatal health during the Ebola epidemic in Sierra Leone. *Health Policy Plan.* (2017) 32:32–9. doi: 10.1093/heapol/czx108

Roberton T, Carter ED, Chou VB, Stegmuller AR, Jackson BD, Tam Y, et al. Articles early estimates of the indirect effects of the COVID-19 pandemic on maternal and child mortality in low-income and middle- income countries : a modelling study. *Lancet Glob Health.* (2020) 8:e901–8. doi: 10.1016/S2214-109X(20)30229-1

Corona Tracker (2020). Available online at: https://www.coronatracker.com/country/kenya/ (accessed November 9, 2020).

Ministry of Health Kenya. Press Releases. *Ministry of Health Kenya* (2020). Available online at: https://www.health.go.ke/press-releases/ (accessed July 22, 2020).

Nyadera IN, Onditi F. COVID-19 experience among slum dwellers in Nairobi: a double tragedy or useful lesson for public health reforms? *Int Soc Work.* (2020) 63:838–41. doi: 10.1177/0020872820944997

Kenya National Bureau of Standards. *Kenya Integrated Household Budget Survey 2015-2016* (2018). Available online at: http://54.213.151.253/nada/ index.php/catalog/88

UN Habitat. *Kenya Habitat Country Programme Document 2018-2021 (No. 978-92-1-132772-4)* (2018). Available online at: https://unhabitat.org/sites/ default/files/2019/09/hcpd_kenya_2018_-_2021_0.pdf

Tanui C. *Church services, mosque gatherings banned as govt moves to contain COVID-19.* Capital News. (2020). Available online at: https://www.capitalfm.co.ke/news/2020/03/22

Onditi F, Obimbo MM, Kinyanjui SM, Nyadera IN. Rejection of containment policy in the management of COVID-19 in Kenyan Slums : is social geometry an option? *Res Square [Preprint].* (2020). doi: 10.21203/rs.3.rs-40952/v1

Naanyu V, Mujumdar V, Ahearn C, McConnell M, Cohen J, et al. Why do women deliver where they had not planned to go? A qualitative study from peri-urban Nairobi Kenya. *BMC Pregnancy Childbirth.* (2020) 20:30. doi: 10.1186/s12884-019-2695-7

Austrian K, Pinchoff J, Tidwell JB, White C, Abuya T, Kangwana B, et al. COVID-19 related knowledge, attitudes, practices and needs of households in informal settlements in Nairobi, Kenya. *Bull World Health Organ [Preprint].* (2020). doi: 10.2471/BLT.20.260281

Pallangyo E, Nakate MG, Maina R, Fleming V. The impact of covid-19 on midwives' practice in Kenya, Uganda and Tanzania: A reflective account. *Midwifery.* (2020). 89:102775. doi: 10.1016/j.midw.2020.102775

Afulani P, Kusi C, Kirumbi L, Walker D. Companionship during facility- based childbirth: Results from a mixed-methods study with recently delivered women and providers in Kenya. *BMC Pregnancy Childbirth.* (2018) 18:1–28. doi: 10.1186/s12884-018-1806-1

Shupler M, Mwitari J, Gohole A, Anderson de Cuevas R, Puzzolo E, Cukic I, et al. COVID-19 lockdown in a Kenyan informal settlement: impacts on household energy and food security. *medRxiv [Preprint].* (2020). doi: 10.1101/2020.05.27.20115113

Zar HJ, Dawa J, Bueno G, Castro-rodriguez JA. Challenges of COVID-19 in children in low- and middle-income countries. *Paediatr Respir Rev.* (2020) 35:70–4. doi: 10.1016/j.prrv.2020.06.016

Miller S, Abalos E, Chamillard M, Ciapponi A, Colaci D, Comandé D, et al. Beyond too little, too late and too much, too soon: a pathway towards evidence-based, respectful maternity care worldwide. *Lancet.* (2016) 388:2176–92. doi: 10.1016/S0140-6736(16)3 1472-6

Mwamuye MK, Nyamu HM. Devolution of health care system in Kenya: a strategic approach and its implementation in Mombasa County, Kenya. *Int J Adv Res.* 2:263–68. (2014).

Semaan A, Audet C, Huysmans E, Afolabi B, Blencowe H, Assarag B, et al. Voices from the frontline : findings from a thematic analysis of a rapid online global survey of maternal and newborn health professionals facing the COVID-19 pandemic. *BMJ Glob Health.* (2020) 5:e002967. doi: 10.1136/bmjgh-2020-002967

Afulani PA, Gyamerah AO, Aborigo R, Nutor J, Malechi H, Laar A, et al. Perceived preparedness to respond to the COVID-19 pandemic: a study with healthcare workers in Ghana. *medRxiv [Preprint].* (2020) doi:10.1101/2020.07.10.20151142

Braune V, Clark V. Using thematic analysis in psychology. *Qual Res Psychol.* (2006) 3:77–101.

Jolivet RR, Warren CE, Sripad P, Ateva E, Gausman J, Mitchell K, et al. Upholding Rights Under COVID-19: the respectful maternity care charter. *Health Hum Rights.* (2020) 22:391–4.

Afulani PA, Kirumbi L, Lyndon A. What makes or mars the facility- based childbirth experience : thematic analysis of women's childbirth experiences in western Kenya. (2017) 14:180. doi: 10.1186/s12978-017- 0446-7

African Population and Health Research Center (APHRC). *Population and Health Dynamics in Nairobi's Informal Settlements: Report of the Nairobi Cross-Sectional Slums Survey (NCSS) 2012.* Nairobi: APHRC (2014), 1–185.

Austrian K, Pinchoff J, Tidwell JB, White C, Abuya T, Kangwana B, et al. COVID-19 related knowledge, attitudes, practices and needs of households in informal settlements in Nairobi, Kenya. *SSRN Electron J.* (2020). doi: 10.2139/ssrn.3576785

21

COVID-19 Lockdown Increased the Risk of Preterm Birth

Ting-ting Lin[1†], Chen Zhang[1,2†], Lei Chen[1], Li Jin[2], Xian-hua Lin[2], Jie-xue Pan[2], Cindy-Lee Dennis[3], Ben W. Mol[4,5], He-feng Huang[1,2] and Yan-ting Wu[2*]*

[1] Shanghai Key Laboratory of Embryo Original Diseases, The International Peace Maternity and Child Health Hospital, School of Medicine, Shanghai Jiao Tong University, Shanghai, China, [2] Research Department, Institute of Reproduction and Development, Obstetrics and Gynecology Hospital, Fudan University, Shanghai, China, [3] Lawrence S. Bloomberg Faculty of Nursing, University of Toronto, Toronto, ON, Canada, [4] Monash University Monash Medical Centre, Clayton, VIC, Australia, [5] Aberdeen Centre for Women's Health Research, University of Aberdeen, Aberdeen, United Kingdom

***Correspondence:**
He-feng Huang
huanghefg@sjtu.edu.cn
Yan-ting Wu
yanting_wu@163.com

† These authors have contributed equally to this work and share first authorship

Purpose: To estimate whether the city-specific lockdown in Shanghai induced by the COVID-19 pandemic affected preterm birth rates among uninfected pregnant women in different trimesters.

Methods: The population-based retrospective cohort study was conducted in the International Peace Maternity and Child Health Hospital (IPMCH) in Shanghai, China. Pregnant women without COVID-19 received perinatal healthcare during lockdown (from January 24, 2020 to March 24, 2020) and non-lockdown (from January 24, 2019 to March 24, 2019) period and giving birth to a live infant at IPMCH were enrolled. 1:1 propensity score matching and Inverse probability of treatment weighting were used to evaluate preterm birth (<37 weeks), very preterm birth (<34 weeks), preterm birth with premature rupture of membranes (PROM-PTB), spontaneous preterm birth with intact membranes (S-PTB), and medically induced preterm birth (MI-PTB) between two groups.

Results: 8,270 pregnant women were in the lockdown group, and 9,815 were in the non-lockdown group. Pregnant women in second trimester during lockdown had a higher risk of PTB than those during the non-lockdown period [OR: 1.43 (CI 1.01–2.02), ARD: 1.7% (CI 0.04–3.4%), $p = 0.045$]. Furthermore, pregnant women in third trimester during lockdown had a higher risk of PROM-PTB than those during the non-lockdown period [OR: 1.64 (CI 1.09–2.47), ARD: 0.9% (CI 0.2–1.6%), $p = 0.02$]; no group differences were found related to rates of VPTB, S-PTB or MI-PTB.

Conclusion: In this cohort study in China, we found that there was an increased risk in preterm birth for non-infected women in COVID-19 lockdown who were in their second trimester.

Keywords: COVID-19, lockdown, preterm birth, very preterm birth, premature rupture of membranes

INTRODUCTION

Coronavirus disease 2019 (COVID-19) is a highly infectious disease with a significant mortality rate that has limited effective treatment options (1). In late 2019, hospitals in Wuhan City in Hubei Province admitted multiple patients with unexplained pneumonia with a history of exposure to the South China Seafood Market, and these cases of pneumonia have since been confirmed as

COVID-19. COVID-19 was officially identified as a type B infectious disease with human-to-human transmission by the National Health Council on January 20, 2020 (2). Due to the high contagiousness of COVID-19 and the population's general susceptibility, a city-wide lockdown was declared in Shanghai on January 24, 2020 and ended on March 24 (3), 2020. During the lockdown, (1) childcare facilities, schools and universities were closed; (2) all non-emergency workers were required to work from home; (3) gatherings of more than 10 people were banned; and (4) industrial production was almost at a standstill (3). Rates of anxiety and depression increased rapidly among the general population (4, 5).

Preterm birth (PTB) is a significant cause of infant mortality and morbidity (6). Infants born preterm are at higher risk for various health problems and developmental delays, often resulting in emotional and financial difficulties for families and an increased use of health and social services (7). Previous research suggests that societal lockdown procedures implemented by governments to mitigate the impact of the COVID-19 pandemic on population health may result in reduced rates of preterm birth, particularly among those occurring at very low gestational ages (8–10). In a US study examining hospital birth data, there was a significant decrease in the incidence of PTB in 2020 during the COVID-19 pandemic compared with the rates during the 2019 pre–COVID-19 period (9.9 vs. 12.6%; OR, 0.76; 95% CI, 0.58–0.99). There was also a significant decrease in PTB at <34 weeks gestation (2.5 vs. 4.7%; aOR, 0.51; 95% CI, 0.31–0.82) and PTB at <28 weeks gestation (0.6 vs. 1.5%; aOR, 0.37; 95% CI, 0.15–0.93) in 2020 compared with the rates in 2019 (9). In an Irish study where regional data covering most of the 2020 lockdown period were compared with historical regional and national data, an unprecedented reduction in births of very low birthweight (VLBW) and extremely low birthweight (ELBW) infants was observed coinciding with the COVID-19 lockdown (10). In a national quasi-experimental study conducted in the Netherlands, the initial implementation of COVID-19 mitigation measures in early March 2020 was associated with a substantial reduction in the incidence of preterm births in the following months (8). Although these studies have reached similar conclusions, they only compared the outcomes among pregnant women in their third trimester during the lockdown period. It remains unknown whether the pregnancy outcomes of women in their first or second trimester are affected by the COVID-19 lockdown.

The purpose of this study was to follow uninfected pregnant women in all three trimesters of pregnancy during the COVID-19 lockdown in Shanghai to determine whether the lockdown independently affected PTB rates.

MATERIALS AND METHODS

Patient Enrollment

This retrospective cohort study was conducted at the International Peace Maternity and Child Health Hospital (IPMCH), which is a university-affiliated hospital in which ~20% of all births in Shanghai, China. Eligible pregnant women were those who had negative nasopharyngeal swab nucleic acid test when they attended routine obstetrics clinic during pregnancy and at time of delivery (11); and who received perinatal healthcare during the lockdown period. Furthermore, they had to have given birth to an infant with a gestational age >20 weeks at IPMCH. Women were excluded if they underwent *in vitro* fertilization, had a twin or multiple birth and were not of the Han race. The start of the lockdown in Shanghai was officially declared on January 24, 2020 (3), and the city-specific lockdown ended on March 24, 2020, when the Shanghai government adjusted the public health emergency response from level one to level two (12).

Data Collection

For all eligible pregnant women, the following data were collected by hospital staff and recorded in the electronic medical file: maternal age, marital status, pre-pregnancy body weight and height, smoking status, current alcohol consumption, maternal education level, parity, preterm birth history, pregnancy complications, date of last menstrual period (LMP), paternal age, paternal education level, neonatal birth weight, Apgar score, and electronic fetal heart rate monitoring records. Maternal and paternal educational levels were defined as the years of education after graduation from primary school and were categorized as <6 years (low), 6 to 10 years (middle) and >10 years (high). Height and pre-pregnancy weight were used to obtain BMI scores which calculated by dividing the weight obtained above by the square of the height and categorized as low weight (<18.5), normal weight (18.5–23.9), overweight or obese (≥24.0). Marital status, smoking status and current consumption of alcohol were self-reported and categorized as yes or no. Parity was defined as the number of previous pregnancies resulting in at least one live birth, and was categorized as nulliparous (None) and multiparous (≥1). Preterm birth history was defined as a history of one or more live births at <37 weeks of gestation. The gestational age of all eligible women was estimated according to the date of the last menstrual period and was adjusted according to routinely performed ultrasonography in the first trimester. The gestational phase during the lockdown period induced by the COVID-19 pandemic was defined as (1) first trimester (pregnant women who were in their first trimester during the lockdown period); (2) first to second trimester (pregnant women who were in their first trimester when the lockdown started and were in second trimester when the lockdown ended); (3) second trimester (pregnant women who were in their second trimester during the lockdown period); (4) second to third trimester (pregnant women who were in their second trimester when the lockdown started and were in their third trimester when the lockdown ended); and (5) third trimester (pregnant women who were in their third trimester during the lockdown period) (**Figure 2**).

Diagnostic Criteria

In this study, preterm birth (PTB) was defined as a birth before 37 weeks of gestation. Very early preterm birth (VPTB) was defined as a birth before 34 weeks of gestation. PTB was classified into spontaneous PTB and medically induced preterm birth (MI-PTB) according to clinical presentation, and spontaneous PTBs were further categorized as preterm birth with premature rupture of membranes (PROM-PTB) or spontaneous preterm birth with intact membranes (S-PTB). The classification criteria were as follows: (1) PROM-PTB was defined as PTB with spontaneous rupture of the membranes at <37 weeks of gestation and before the onset of contractions; (2) S-PTB was defined as spontaneous PTB with intact membranes; and (3) MI-PTB was defined as PTB after labor induction or cesarean delivery for maternal or fetal indications (13). Pregnancy complications included gestational diabetes and pregnancy-induced hypertension. Gestational diabetes mellitus (GDM) was defined as diabetes diagnosed in the second or third trimester of pregnancy that was not clearly identified as overt diabetes prior to gestation (14). Pregnancy-induced hypertension (PIH) was defined as systolic blood pressure (SBP) >140 mmHg and diastolic blood pressure (DBP) >90 mmHg during pregnancy and was classified into three conditions: (1) gestational hypertension and preeclampsia (PE); (2) pre-existing hypertension plus superimposed gestational hypertension with proteinuria; and (3) unclassifiable hypertension during pregnancy (15). Stillbirth was defined as a baby born with no signs of life at a gestational age of 24 weeks or more. Abnormal Apgar score was defined as a 5-min Apgar score of 7 or less. Fetal distress, also named as "non-reassuring fetal status" by the recommendation of ACOG Committee on Obstetrics Practice, was defined as a pathophysiological condition in which fetus was suffering from insufficient oxygen supply, which was diagnosed through electronic fetal heart rate (FHR) monitoring (16). Low birth

TABLE 1 | Baseline characteristics total sample, unweighted sample, propensity score-matched sample, and inverse probability of treatment-weighted sample.

	Unweighted Sample			Propensity 1:1 Matching			Inverse probability of treatment weighting		
	Lockdown (*N* = 8,270)	**Non-lockdown (*N* = 9,815)**	***P*-value**	**Lockdown (*N* = 8,268)**	**Non-lockdown (*N* = 8,268)**	***P*-value**	**Lockdown (*N* = 18,088)**	**Non-lockdown (*N* = 18,084)**	***P*-value**
Maternal Demographics									
Age, median (Q1-Q3), y	31 (29–34)	31 (29–34)	<0.001	31 (29–34)	31 (29–34)	0.06	31 (29–34)	31 (29–34)	<0.001
Marital Status									
Married	8,220 (99.4)	9,709 (98.9)	0.001	8,218 (99.4)	8,218 (99.4)	1.00	17,920 (99.1)	17,927 (99.1)	0.54
Single or divorced	50 (0.6)	106 (1.1)		50 (0.6)	50 (0.6)		168 (0.9)	157 (0.9)	
Body mass index, median (Q1–Q3),kg/m^2	20.8 (19.3–22.8)	20.7 (19.2–22.6)	0.009	20.8 (19.3–22.8)	20.8 (19.3–22.8)	0.08	20.8 (19.3–22.7)	20.8 (19.3–22.7)	<0.001
Body mass index									
Low	1,106 (13.4)	1,381 (14.1)	0.02	1,106 (13.4)	1,188 (14.4)	0.07	2,530 (14.0)	2,458 (13.6)	0.25
Normal	5,863 (70.9)	7,026 (71.6)		5,863 (70.9)	5,857 (70.8)		12,808 (70.8)	12,947 (71.6)	
Overweight or Obesity	1,301 (15.7)	1,408 (14.3)		1,299 (15.7)	1,223 (14.8)		2,751 (15.2)	2,678 (14.8)	
Current smoker (yes)	31 (0.4)	51 (0.6)	0.04	33 (0.4)	42 (0.5)	0.30	106 (0.6)	96 (0.5)	0.48
Current alcohol consumption (yes)	63 (0.8)	254 (2.6)	<0.001	63 (0.8)	69 (0.8)	0.60	319 (1.8)	317 (1.8)	0.94
Education level									
Low	610 (7.4)	743 (7.6)	<0.001	610 (7.4)	579 (7.0)	0.27	1,447 (8.0)	1,288 (7.1)	<0.001
Middle	5,655 (68.4)	6,972 (71.0)		5,655 (68.4)	5,749 (69.5)		12,442 (68.8)	12,762 (70.6)	
High	2,005 (24.2)	2,100 (21.4)		2,003 (24.2)	1,940 (23.5)		4,200 (23.2)	4,034 (22.3)	
Parity									
Nulliparous	5,763 (69.7)	6,789 (69.1)	0.43	5,761 (69.7)	5,730 (69.3)	0.60	12,548 (69.4)	12,547 (69.4)	0.99
Multiparous	2,507 (30.3)	3,029 (30.9)		2,507 (30.3)	2,538 (30.7)		5,541 (30.6)	5,537 (30.6)	
Preterm birth history (yes)	13 (0.2)	55 (0.6)	<0.001	13 (0.2)	6 (0.1)	0.11	28 (0.2)	39 (0.2)	0.18
Gestational phase during COVID-19 lockdown									
First trimester	280 (3.4)	325 (3.3)	0.001	280 (3.4)	268 (3.2)	0.73	620 (3.4)	592 (3.3)	<0.001
First to second trimester	2,088 (25.2)	2,403 (24.5)		2,088 (25.3)	2,060 (24.9)		4,630 (25.6)	4,389 (24.3)	
Second trimester	1,313 (15.9)	1,735 (17.7)0		1,313 (15.9)	1,367 (16.5)		2,888 (16.0)	3,181 (17.6)	
Second to third trimester	1,942 (23.5)	2,414 (24.6)		1,941 (23.5)	1,968 (23.8)		4,234 (23.4)	4,454 (24.6)	
Third trimester	2,647 (32.0)	2,938 (29.9)		2,646 (32.0)	2,605 (31.5)		5,716 (31.6)	5,467 (30.2)	
Paternal demographics									
Age, median (Q1–Q3), y	32 (30–35)	32 (29–35)	<0.001	32 (30–35)	32 (29–35)	0.06	32 (29–35)	32 (29–35)	<0.001
Education level									
Low	609 (7.4)	718 (7.3)	0.002	609 (7.4)	597 (7.2)	0.07	1,411 (7.8)	1,263 (7.0)	0.001
Middle	5,482 (66.3)	6,734 (68.6)		5,482 (66.3)	5,617 (67.9)		12,050 (66.6)	12,349 (68.3)	
High	2,179 (26.3)	2,363 (24.1)		2,177 (26.3)	2,054 (24.8)		4,627 (25.6)	4,473 (24.7)	

weight (LBW) was defined as newborn whose birth weight was <2,500 g. Very low birth weight (VLBW) was defined as newborn whose birth weight was <1,500 g. Macrosomia was defined as newborn whose birth weight was more than 4,000 g.

Statistical Analyses

Considering the differences in baseline characteristics between the two groups of participants (**Table 1**), we used propensity score matching to generate a cohort with similar baseline characteristics. The propensity score is the conditional probability of having a specific exposure level (lockdown vs. non-lockdown) under a given set of baseline covariates (17, 18). A multivariate logistic regression model was used to estimate propensity scores, and all baseline characteristics listed in **Table 1** were included as covariates (1) using a 1:1 matching protocol with no replacement for matching with a caliper width equal to 0.005 and (2) evaluating the *P*-values of all baseline covariates before and after matching to assess whether they were balanced. Standard differences of <5% indicated a relatively small imbalance. There were no missing data for the variables in the matched cohort.

Inverse probability of treatment weighting (IPTW) was used to investigate the COVID-19 exposure among the entire population of pregnant women when this population hypothetically moved from no COVID-19 exposure (non-lockdown) to exposure (lockdown) in different pregnancy phases. Participants were weighted by the inverse of the probability of exposure to the COVID-19 lockdown. The association between COVID-19 lockdown and PTB was estimated using the Odds Ratio (OR) obtained from log binomial regression and the Absolute Risk Difference (ARD) obtained from identity link binomial regression. In both groups, the IPTW weights were used with a quasibinomial model to obtain robust variance estimates. To avoid convergence issues, the R package glm2 was used. Group differences were assessed by calculating IPTW proportions, weighted medians, and standardized mean differences.

The differences in the distribution of maternal characteristics between lockdown and non-lockdown groups were evaluated by the chi-square test for categorical variables and the Mann–Whitney *U*-test for continuous variables. Time to delivery was evaluated through Kaplan-Meier estimates, and differences between the groups were tested with a log rank test. Logistic regression was performed to calculate crude and adjusted odds ratios (aORs) and 95% confidence intervals (CIs). Potential confounders included maternal age, parity, preterm birth history, GDM, PIH, and paternal age. The selection of potential confounders was based on biological plausibility, identification of a variable as a confounder in previous studies, changes in the effect estimate of interest, or reduction in the residual variability of the outcome. Sensitivity analysis was used to evaluate the difference in PTB in each subgroup between the matched lockdown and non-lockdown groups to identify potential bias. A two-sided *P*-value of <0.05 was considered statistically significant. All statistical tests were conducted using SPSS version 24.0 and R version 3.6.

RESULTS

Baseline Characteristics

A total of 9,213 pregnant women were consecutively enrolled from January 24th, 2020, to March 24th, 2020 (lockdown), and

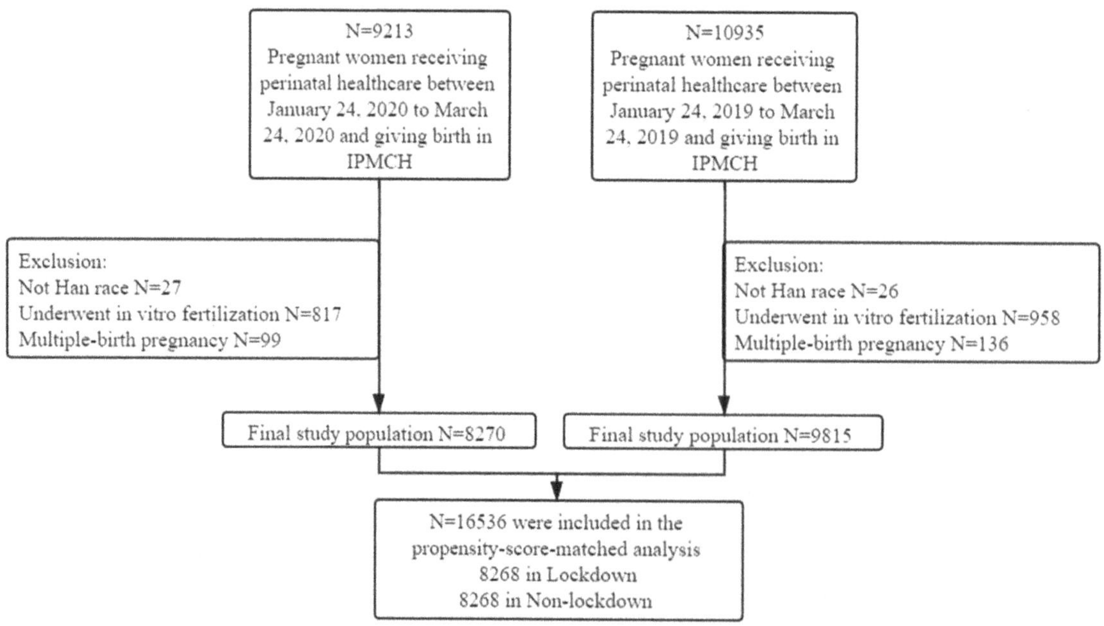

FIGURE 1 | Flow chart of the study population.

10935 were enrolled from January 24th, 2019, to March 24th, 2019 (non-lockdown). After the implementation of the exclusion criteria, 8,270 pregnant women in the lockdown group and 9,815 pregnant women in the non-lockdown group remained in the final study population (**Figure 1**).

Table 1 shows the baseline characteristics between the two groups in the unweighted sample analysis, propensity score-matched analysis, and inverse probability treatment weighting analysis. Compared with the non-lockdown group, women in the lockdown group were more likely to be married (99.4 vs. 98.9%, $P = 0.001$), have a higher BMI (20.8 vs. 20.7 kg/m^2, $P = 0.009$), have a higher education level (24.2 vs. 21.4%, $P < 0.001$). They were also less likely to be current smokers (0.4 vs. 0.6%, $P = 0.04$), have current alcohol consumption (0.8 vs. 2.6%, $P < 0.001$) and have a preterm birth history (0.2 vs. 0.6%, $P < 0.001$). Through the use of propensity score matching, 8,268 women in the lockdown group were matched with 8,268 women in the non-lockdown group. After matching, the *P*-values of all variables were >0.05, indicating that no significant differences existed between the two groups. Through the use of IPTW, marital status, maternal BMI distribution, smoking and alcohol consumption, and preterm birth history were balanced between the two groups (**Table 1**).

Risk of PTB and VPTB in Different Pregnancy Phases

Although there was no group difference in the prevalence of PTB (5.7 vs. 5.3%, $P = 0.71$) or VPTB (1.3 vs. 1.2%, $P = 0.78$) in the total sample (**Supplementary Table 1**). Women in lockdown during their second trimester had a higher rate of PTB (unweighted sample: 5.9 vs. 4.6%, $P = 0.08$; matched: 5.9 vs. 4.2%, $P = 0.045$; IPTW: 6.0 vs. 4.6%, $P = 0.02$) (**Table 2**; **Figure 2**) and a non-significantly higher rate of VPTB (unweighted sample: 1.9 vs. 1.4%, $P = 0.32$; matched: 1.9 vs. 1.2%, $P = 0.12$; IPTW: 2.0 vs. 1.4%, $P = 0.11$) (**Table 2**) than those in the non-lockdown period. After adjusting for maternal age, parity, GDM, and paternal age, women in their second trimester during lockdown had a higher risk of PTB [unweighted sample: OR: 1.34 (CI 0.97–1.86), ARD: 1.3 (CI 0.3–2.9), $p = 0.08$; matched: OR: 1.43 (CI 1.01–2.02), ARD: 1.7 (CI 0.04–3.4), $p = 0.045$; IPTW: OR: 1.32 (CI 1.05–1.65), ARD: 1.4 (CI 0.3–2.5), $p = 0.02$] (**Table 2**) and a non-significantly higher risk of VPTB [unweighted sample: OR: 1.33 (CI 0.76–2.32), ARD: 0.5 (CI −0.4 to 1.4), $p = 0.32$; matched: OR: 1.63 (CI 0.85–3.12), ARD: 0.7 (CI −0.2 to 1.6), $P = 0.14$; IPTW: OR: 1.37 (CI 0.93–2.03), ARD: 0.6 (CI −0.05 to 1.3), $p = 0.11$] than those in non-lockdown cohort (**Table 2**). There were no significant differences between the two groups in PTB or VPTB rates during the other pregnancy phases (first, first to second, second to third and third trimesters) (**Supplementary Table 2**).

The Association Between COVID-19 Lockdown and Subtypes of PTB in Different Pregnancy Phases

We further explored the risk of different clinical subtypes of PTB (PROM-PTB, S-PTB, and MI-PTB) associated with COVID-19 lockdown in different pregnancy phases. The prevalence

TABLE 2 | Analysis of PTB and Subtypes of PTB in Women Exposed in Their Second or Third Trimester.

	Unweighted Sample					Propensity 1:1 Matching					Inverse probability of treatment weighting				
	No. (AR, %)		ARD, % (96% CI)	OR (95%CI)	*P*-value	No. (AR, %)		ARD, % (96% CI)	OR (95% CI)	*P*-value	No. (AR, %)		ARD, % (96% CI)	OR (95% CI)	*P*-value
	Lock down	Non-lock down				Lock down	Non-lock down				Lock down	Non-lock down			
Second trimester															
PTB	78 (5.9)	79 (4.6)	1.3 (−0.3 to 2.9)	1.34 (0.97–1.86)	0.08	78 (5.9)	58 (4.2)	1.7 (0.04–3.4)	1.43 (1.01–2.02)	0.04	172 (6.0)	146 (4.6)	1.4 (0.3–2.5)	1.32 (1.05–1.65)	0.02
VPTB	25 (1.9)	25 (1.4)	0.5 (−0.4 to 1.4)	1.33 (0.76–2.32)	0.32	25 (1.9)	16 (1.2)	0.7 (−0.2 to 1.6)	1.63 (0.85–3.12)	0.14	57 (2.0)	46 (1.4)	0.6 (−0.05 to 1.3)	1.37 (0.93–2.03)	0.11
PROM-PTB	33 (2.5)	30 (1.7)	0.8 (−0.2 to 1.8)	1.47 (0.89–2.42)	0.13	33 (2.5)	25 (1.8)	0.7 (−0.4 to 1.8)	1.25 (0.73–2.15)	0.42	72 (2.5)	55 (1.7)	0.8 (0.07–1.5)	1.42 (0.99–2.03)	0.06
S-PTB	21 (1.6)	21 (1.2)	0.4 (−0.5 to 1.3)	1.33 (0.72–2.44)	0.36	21 (1.6)	12 (0.9)	0.7 (−0.1 to 1.5)	1.81 (0.87–3.76)	0.11	49 (1.7)	38 (1.2)	0.5 (−0.1 to 1.1)	1.43 (0.93–2.19)	0.10
MI-PTB	24 (1.8)	28 (1.6)	0.2 (−0.7 to 1.1)	1.14 (0.66–1.97)	0.65	24 (1.8)	21 (1.5)	0.3 (−0.7 to 1.3)	1.15 (0.63–2.12)	0.65	89 (3.1)	86 (2.7)	0.4 (−0.4 to 1.2)	1.14 (0.85–1.55)	0.38
Third trimester															
PTB	110 (4.2)	104 (3.5)	0.7 (−0.3 to 1.7)	1.18 (0.90–1.56)	0.23	110 (4.2)	90 (3.5)	0.7 (−0.3 to 1.7)	1.18 (0.89–1.58)	0.25	237 (4.1)	192 (3.5)	0.6 (−0.1 to 1.3)	1.19 (0.98–1.44)	0.08
VPTB	12 (0.5)	11 (0.4)	0.1 (−0.3 to 0.5)	1.21 (0.53–2.75)	0.65	12 (0.5)	10 (0.4)	0.1 (−0.3 to 0.5)	0.98 (0.41–2.32)	0.96	25 (0.4)	21 (0.4)	0 (−0.2 to 0.2)	1.14 (0.64–2.04)	0.66
PROM-PTB	61 (2.3)	45 (1.5)	0.8 (0.08–1.5)	1.52 (1.03–2.24)	0.04	61 (2.3)	37 (1.4)	0.9 (0.2–1.6)	1.64 (1.09–2.47)	0.02	130 (2.3)	83 (1.5)	0.8 (0.3–1.3)	1.51 (1.14–1.99)	0.003
S-PTB	18 (0.7)	25 (0.9)	−0.2 (−0.7 to 0.3)	0.80 (0.43–1.47)	0.47	18 (0.7)	21 (0.8)	−0.1 (−0.6 to 0.4)	0.84 (0.44–1.59)	0.59	38 (0.7)	45 (0.8)	−0.1 (−0.4 to 0.2)	0.81 (0.52–1.24)	0.33
MI-PTB	31 (1.2)	34 (1.2)	0 (−0.6 to 0.6)	1.01 (0.62–1.65)	0.96	31 (2.0)	32 (1.8)	0.2 (−0.5 to 0.9)	0.32 (0.56–1.54)	0.78	121 (2.1)	106 (1.9)	0.2 (−0.3 to 0.7)	1.09 (0.84–1.42)	0.51

AR, Absolute Risk; ARD, Absolute Risk Difference; OR, Odds Ratio; PTB, Preterm Birth; VPTB, Very Preterm Birth; PROM-PTB, preterm birth with premature rupture of membranes; S-PTB, spontaneous preterm birth with intact membranes; MI-PTB, medically induced preterm birth.

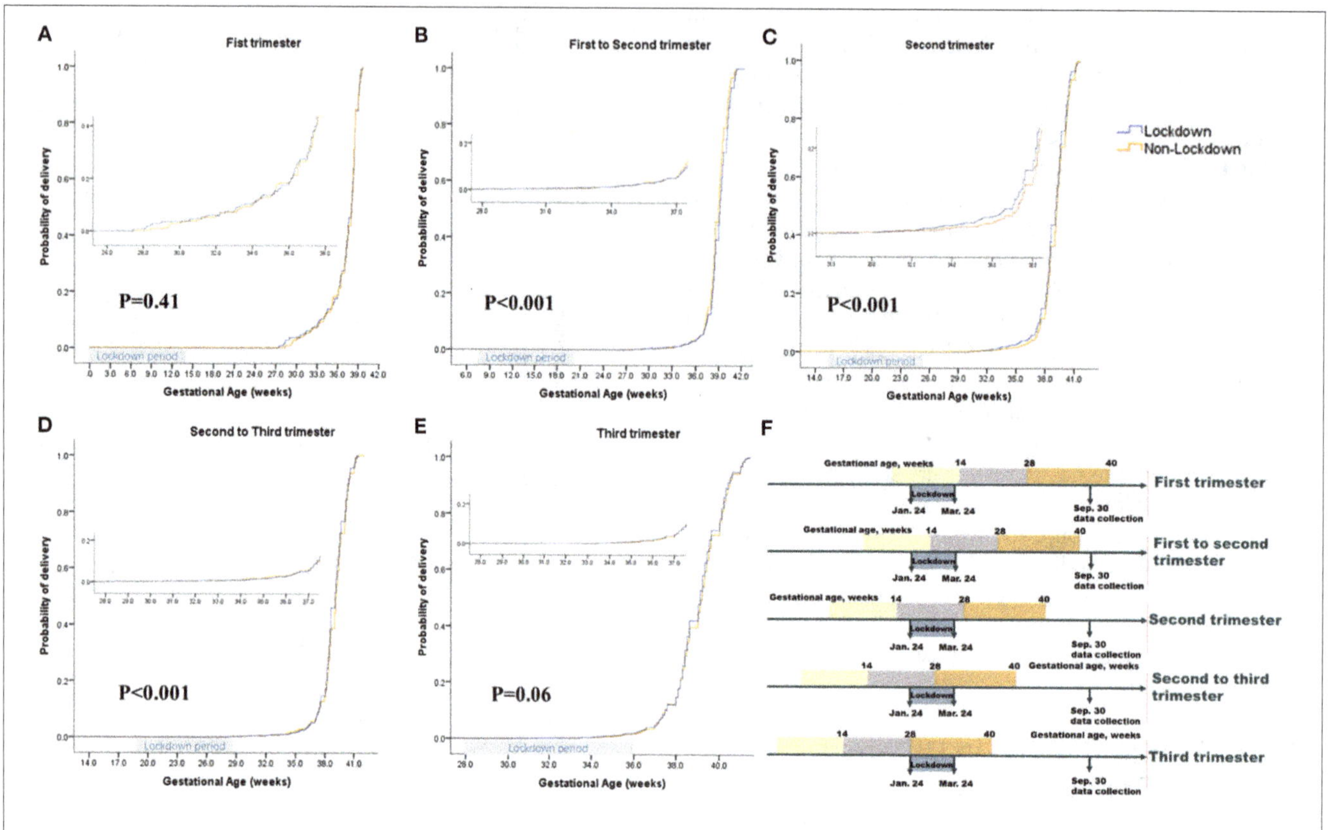

FIGURE 2 | Kaplan-Meier Curve for Lockdown and Non-Lockdown Groups in Propensity-Score-Matched Cohort and the Definition of Different Pregnancy Phases. This figure shows the probability of delivery among pregnant women who were in different pregnancy phases during Lockdown period in two groups. *P*-values were calculated through log rank test. The small picture in each picture is a partial enlarged picture of 28–37 weeks of gestation. **(A)**, Pregnant women who were in First trimester during Lockdown period. **(B)**, Pregnant women who were in First to Second trimester during Lockdown period. **(C)**. Pregnant women who were in Second trimester during Lockdown period. **(D)**. Pregnant women who were in Second to Third trimester during Lockdown period. **(E)**. Pregnant women who were in Third trimester during Lockdown period. **(F)** The definition of different pregnancy phases.

of PROM-PTB in the third trimester among women in lockdown was higher than that among those in non-lockdown (unweighted sample: 2.3 vs. 1.5%, $P = 0.04$; matched: 2.3 vs. 1.4%, $P = 0.02$; IPTW: 2.3 vs. 1.5%, $P = 0.003$) (**Table 2**; **Supplementary Figure 1**). After adjusting for maternal and paternal age and parity, among pregnant women in their third trimester, those in lockdown had an increased risk of PROM-PTB compared to those in non-lockdown [unweighted sample: OR: 1.52 (CI 1.03–2.24), ARD: 0.8 (CI 0.08–1.5), $P = 0.04$; matched: OR: 1.64 (CI 1.09–2.47), ARD: 0.9 (CI 0.2–1.6), $p = 0.02$; IPTW: OR: 1.51 (CI 1.14–1.99), ARD: 0.8 (CI 0.3–1.3), $P = 0.003$] (**Table 2**). The pregnant women in lockdown during their third trimester did not have an increased risk of S-PTB or MI-PTB in the three types of analysis (**Table 2**). There were no significant differences between the two groups in PROM-PTB, S-PTB, or MI-PTB rates in the other pregnancy phases (first, first to second, second and second to third trimesters) (**Supplementary Figure 1**; **Supplementary Table 3**).

Sensitivity Analyses

In sensitivity analyses, we divided pregnant women during their second trimester into a propensity score-matched cohort based on whether they had GDM, which resulted in 1,195 pregnant women without GDM and 172 with GDM in the non-lockdown group and 1,102 women without GDM and 211 with GDM in the lockdown group. The association between lockdown and PTB did not change substantially (**Supplementary Table 4**; **Supplementary Figure 2**). After adjusting for maternal and paternal age, and parity, pregnant women without or with GDM in lockdown had a higher risk of PTB [without GDM: OR: 1.27 (CI 0.86–1.88), $p = 0.24$; with GDM: OR: 1.73 (CI 0.68–4.40), $p = 0.25$] and VPTB [without GDM: OR: 1.55 (CI 0.77–3.11), $p = 0.22$; with GDM: OR: 3.27 (CI 0.46–23.28), $p = 0.24$] than those in non-lockdown, although the results did not reach statistical significance (**Supplementary Table 4**). Similar results were also found in the unweighted sample and through the use of IPTW (**Supplementary Table 4**). We also performed sensitivity analyses for the association between COVID-19 lockdown and PROM-PTB rates among pregnant women with or without GDM during their third trimester in the propensity score-matched cohort. Pregnant women in lockdown during their third trimester, with or without GDM, had a higher risk of PROM-PTB [without GDM: OR: 1.70 (CI 1.08–2.69), $p = 0.02$; with GDM: OR: 1.05 (CI 0.37–2.97), $p = 0.94$] than those in non-lockdown in the propensity score-matched analysis. Similar results were found in the unweighted sample and through the use of IPTW (**Supplementary Table 5; Supplementary Figure 3**).

DISCUSSION

This is the first study to examine the relationship between the COVID-19 lockdown and preterm birth among women who were affected by the lockdown in different trimesters. We found that exposure to the COVID-19 lockdown did not reduce, but increased the risk of PTB among pregnant women in their second trimester and increased the risk of PROM-PTB among those in their third trimester.

Previous evidence suggests that the COVID-19 pandemic and the lockdown measures taken by governments to mitigate its impact on population health were associated with reductions in PTBs (8–10, 19). However, these studies focused on the outcomes of pregnant women who were in their third trimester during the COVID-19 lockdown. In our study, we found that the PTB rate was stable among women in their third trimester, which is consistent with a retrospective study conducted in the United Kingdom (20). The difference with previous studies may be attributed to race and the national attitude toward the COVID-19 pandemic and need for lockdown measures. We further explored the impact of the COVID-19 lockdown on women during early or middle pregnancy and found that exposure to the lockdown led to a 1.42-fold risk of PTB among women in the second trimester and a 1.64-fold risk of PROM-PTB among women in the third trimester. Lockdown measures have a significant societal impact, as they lead to an increased risk for unemployment, low-income status, and family conflicts (21). These factors increase a pregnant woman's risk for anxiety and depression (21). Anxiety has been shown to enhance hypothalamus-pituitary-adrenal cortex (HPA) axis activity (22, 23). Studies have demonstrated that the levels of corticotropin-releasing hormone (CRH), which is released when anxiety stimulates the HPA axis, are significantly higher in women who have delivered a preterm infant than in those who gave birth at term (24). Alternatively, the increase in PTB rates among women exposed to the lockdown may have resulted from indirect effects such as reluctance to go to the hospital when needed (e.g., reduced fetal movements or mild vaginal infection) due to a fear of developing a COVID-19 infection or not wanting to increase the burden on the health care system (20). Changes in obstetrical care may also have played a role in the higher rates of PTB due to staff shortages and reduced number of antenatal visits, ultrasound scans, and screening procedures (25). It was consistent with the finding of a systematic review, in which the incidence of preterm birth occurred was similar among pregnant women who tested positive compared with negative for SARS-CoV-2 (26). The preterm birth rates in this review were thought influenced by transient changes in obstetric management (26). Other possible explanations for our findings include (1) changes in referral methods where more high-risk women were sent to the participating hospital or (2) more high-risk women choosing to deliver at the larger more specialized hospital (20). It is important to provide quality obstetric services that also included the effective management of anxiety and depression to try and mitigate the risk for preterm birth.

Our study has numerous strengths. This study provides the first evidence that the effects of the COVID-19 lockdown on the preterm birth rate have a trimester difference. Second, we used several statistical methods (unweighted sample, propensity score matching, and IPTW) to examine the association between exposure to the COVID-19 lockdown and risk for a PTB to ensure the accuracy of the study results. Some limitations also exist. First, we did not confirm the mental health status of participants during the COVID-19 lockdown. However, another study by our team evaluated the mental health of pregnant women in 25 hospitals in China before and during the pandemic and found significantly higher rates of depression and anxiety among those who were pregnant during the COVID-19 lockdown (23). Second, some pregnant women in their early pregnancy during the COVID-19 pandemic had not yet given birth when we completed the data analysis. As such, the sample size for those in their first trimester was slightly smaller. Furthermore, the number of gestational weeks for women examined in their first trimester was lower than that of those examined in other trimesters. Thus, those examined in their first trimester who had given birth and were included in our analyses were naturally more likely to have delivered a preterm infant. This explains why the PTB rate among women examined in their first trimester was higher than that among those examined later in their pregnancy. Last, although we controlled for as many PTB confounding factors as possible, there may be other unmeasured confounders that could have caused bias in our propensity score-matched cohort.

This is the first study to explore the relationship between COVID-19 lockdown and PTB among non-infected women in different trimesters. Different from previous research conclusions, our study suggests that women in their second trimester during the COVID-19 lockdown were at an increased risk for PTB and that those in their third trimester were at an increased risk for PROM-PTB. Sufficient prenatal care and education program should be emphasized for pregnant women during any society lockdown and warrant additional research.

ETHICS STATEMENT

The studies involving human participants were reviewed and approved by International Peace Maternity and Child Health Hospital review board (No. GKLW2019-51). The patients/participants provided their written informed consent participate in this study.

AUTHOR CONTRIBUTIONS

H-fH and Y-tW devised the study concept and design. T-tL and CZ drafted the manuscript and conducted the statistical analysis. LC, LJ, X-hL, and J-xP were responsible for the data collection and quality control. Y-tW, H-fH, C-LD, and BM critically revised the manuscript for important intellectual content. All authors provided administrative, technical, and material support and agreed with the final version of the article.

ACKNOWLEDGMENTS

We are extremely grateful to the pregnant women, doctors and nurses who participated in this study.

REFERENCES

Weiss P, Murdoch DR. Clinical course and mortality risk of severe COVID-19. *Lancet.* (2020) 395:1014–5. doi: 10.1016/S0140-6736(20)30633-4

China, t.N.H.C.o.t.P.s.R.o. *Announcement on Incorporating the COVID-19 into the Administration of Statutory Infectious Diseases.* (2020). Available online at: http://www.gov.cn/zhengce/zhengceku/2020-01/21/content_ 5471164.htm the National Health Commission of the People's Republic of China (accessed January 20, 2020).

government S. *Shanghai Launches Primary Response Mechanism for Major Public Health Emergencies.* (2020). Available online at: http://service.shanghai. gov.cn/SHVideo/newvideoshow.aspx?id=55A4E7A6E3D3A8C3 (accessed September 6, 2021).

Ettman CK, Abdalla SM, Cohen GH, Sampson L, Vivier PM, Galea S. Prevalence of depression symptoms in US adults before and during the COVID-19 pandemic. *JAMA Netw Open.* (2020) 3:e2019686. doi: 10.1001/jamanetworkopen.2020.19686

Liu S, Yang L, Zhang C, Xiang YT, Liu Z, Hu S, et al. Online mental health services in China during the COVID-19 outbreak. *Lancet Psychiatry.* (2020) 7:e17–8. doi: 10.1016/S2215-0366(20)30077-8

Glover AV, Manuck TA. Screening for spontaneous preterm birth and resultant therapies to reduce neonatal morbidity and mortality: a review. *Semin Fetal Neonatal Med.* (2018) 23:126–32. doi: 10.1016/j.siny.2017. 11.007

Chawanpaiboon S, Vogel JP, Moller AB, Lumbiganon P, Petzold M, Hogan D, et al. Global, regional, and national estimates of levels of preterm birth in 2014: a systematic review and modelling analysis. *Lancet Glob Health.* (2019) 7:e37–46. doi: 10.1016/S2214-109X(18)30451-0

Been JV, Burgos Ochoa L, Bertens LCM, Schoenmakers S, Steegers EAP, Reiss IKM. Impact of COVID-19 mitigation measures on the incidence of preterm birth: a national quasi-experimental study. *Lancet Public Health.* (2020) 5:e604–11. doi: 10.1016/S2468-2667(20)30223-1

Berghella V, Boelig R, Roman A, Burd J, Anderson K. Decreased incidence of preterm birth during coronavirus disease 2019 pandemic. *Am J Obstet Gynecol MFM.* (2020) 2:100258. doi: 10.1016/j.ajogmf.2020.100258

Philip RK, Purtill H, Reidy E, Daly M, Imcha M, McGrath D, et al. Unprecedented reduction in births of very low birthweight (VLBW) and extremely low birthweight (ELBW) infants during the COVID-19 lockdown in Ireland: a 'natural experiment' allowing analysis of data from the prior two decades. *BMJ Glob Health.* (2020) 5. doi: 10.1136/bmjgh-2020-0 03075

Chen H, Guo J, Wang C, Luo F, Yu X, Zhang W, et al. Clinical characteristics and intrauterine vertical transmission potential of COVID-19 infection in nine pregnant women: a retrospective review of medical records. *Lancet.* (2020) 395:809–15. doi: 10.1016/S0140-6736(20)30360-3

goverment S. *Shanghai Decided to Adjust the Primary Response to Major Public Health Emergencies to Secondary Response.* (2020). Available online at: http://www.shanghai.gov.cn/nw48635/20200826/0001-48635_64496.html (accessed March 24, 2020).

Goldenberg RL, Culhane JF, Iams JD, Romero R. Epidemiology and causes of preterm birth. *Lancet.* (2008) 371:75–84. doi: 10.1016/S0140-6736(08)60074-4

American Diabetes Association. 2. Classification and diagnosis of diabetes: standards of medical care in diabetes-2020. *Diabetes Care.* (2020) 43(Suppl. 1):S14–31. doi: 10.2337/dc20-S002

Kintiraki E, Papakatsika S, Kotronis G, Goulis DG, Kotsis V. Pregnancy-Induced hypertension. *Hormones.* (2015) 14:211– 23. doi: 10.14310/horm.2002.1582

ACOG Committee Opinion. Number 326, December 2005. Inappropriate use of the terms fetal distress and birth asphyxia. *Obstet Gynecol.* (2005) 106:1469–70. doi: 10.1097/00006250-200512000-00056

Rosenbaum PR, Rubin DB. The central role of the propensity score in observational studies for causal effects. *Biometrika.* (1983) 70:41– 55. doi: 10.1093/biomet/70.1.41

Rubin DB. Using propensity scores to help design observational studies: application to the tobacco litigation. *Health Serv Outcomes Res Methodol.* (2001) 2:169–88. doi: 10.1023/A:1020363010465

Hedermann G, Hedley PL, Bækvad-Hansen M, Hjalgrim H, Rostgaard K, Poorisrisak P, et al. Danish premature birth rates during the COVID-19 lockdown. *Arch Dis Child Fetal Neonatal Ed.* (2021) 106:93–5. doi: 10.1136/archdischild-2020-319990

Khalil A, von Dadelszen P, Draycott T, Ugwumadu A, O'Brien P, Magee L. Change in the incidence of stillbirth and preterm delivery during the COVID- 19 pandemic. *JAMA.* (2020) 324:705–6. doi: 10.1001/jama.2020.12746

Hamadani JD, Hasan MI, Baldi AJ, Hossain SJ, Shiraji S, Bhuiyan MSA, et al. Immediate impact of stay-at-home orders to control COVID-19 transmission on socioeconomic conditions, food insecurity, mental health, and intimate partner violence in bangladeshi women and their families: an interrupted time series. *Lancet Glob Health.* (2020) 8:e1380– 9. doi: 10.1016/S2214-109X(20)30366-1

Obel C, Hedegaard M, Henriksen TB, Secher NJ, Olsen J, Levine S. Stress and salivary cortisol during pregnancy. *Psychoneuroendocrinology.* (2005) 30:647–56. doi: 10.1016/j.psyneuen.2004.11.006

Wu Y, Zhang C, Liu H, Duan C, Li C, Fan J, et al. Perinatal depressive and anxiety symptoms of pregnant women during the coronavirus disease 2019 outbreak in China. *Am J Obstetr Gynecol.* (2020) 223:240.e241– 0.e249. doi: 10.1016/j.ajog.2020.05.009

Mancuso RA, Schetter CD, Rini CM, Roesch SC, Hobel CJ. Maternal prenatal anxiety and corticotropin-releasing hormone associated with timing of delivery. *Psychosom Med.* (2004) 66:762–9. doi: 10.1097/01.psy.0000138284.70670.d5

Kc A, Gurung R, Kinney MV, Sunny AK, Moinuddin M, Basnet O, et al. Effect of the COVID-19 pandemic response on intrapartum care, stillbirth, and neonatal mortality outcomes in nepal: a prospective observational study. *Lancet Glob Health.* (2020) 8:e1273–81. doi: 10.1016/S2214-109X(20)30345-4

Huntley BJF, Mulder IA, Di Mascio D, Vintzileos WS, Vintzileos AM, Berghella V, et al. Adverse pregnancy outcomes among individuals with and without severe acute respiratory syndrome coronavirus 2 (SARS-CoV- 2): a systematic review and meta-analysis. *Obstet Gynecol.* (2021) 137:585– 96. doi: 10.1097/AOG.0000000000004320

Permissions

All chapters in this book were first published by Frontiers; hereby published with permission under the Creative Commons Attribution License or equivalent. Every chapter published in this book has been scrutinized by our experts. Their significance has been extensively debated. The topics covered herein carry significant findings which will fuel the growth of the discipline. They may even be implemented as practical applications or may be referred to as a beginning point for another development.

The contributors of this book come from diverse backgrounds, making this book a truly international effort. This book will bring forth new frontiers with its revolutionizing research information and detailed analysis of the nascent developments around the world.

We would like to thank all the contributing authors for lending their expertise to make the book truly unique. They have played a crucial role in the development of this book. Without their invaluable contributions this book wouldn't have been possible. They have made vital efforts to compile up to date information on the varied aspects of this subject to make this book a valuable addition to the collection of many professionals and students.

This book was conceptualized with the vision of imparting up-to-date information and advanced data in this field. To ensure the same, a matchless editorial board was set up. Every individual on the board went through rigorous rounds of assessment to prove their worth. After which they invested a large part of their time researching and compiling the most relevant data for our readers.

The editorial board has been involved in producing this book since its inception. They have spent rigorous hours researching and exploring the diverse topics which have resulted in the successful publishing of this book. They have passed on their knowledge of decades through this book. To expedite this challenging task, the publisher supported the team at every step. A small team of assistant editors was also appointed to further simplify the editing procedure and attain best results for the readers.

Apart from the editorial board, the designing team has also invested a significant amount of their time in understanding the subject and creating the most relevant covers. They scrutinized every image to scout for the most suitable representation of the subject and create an appropriate cover for the book.

The publishing team has been an ardent support to the editorial, designing and production team. Their endless efforts to recruit the best for this project, has resulted in the accomplishment of this book. They are a veteran in the field of academics and their pool of knowledge is as vast as their experience in printing. Their expertise and guidance has proved useful at every step. Their uncompromising quality standards have made this book an exceptional effort. Their encouragement from time to time has been an inspiration for everyone.

The publisher and the editorial board hope that this book will prove to be a valuable piece of knowledge for researchers, students, practitioners and scholars across the globe.

List of Contributors

Sarah Rudrum
Department of Sociology, Acadia University, Wolfville, Canada

Inayat Ali
Department of Social and Cultural Anthropology, University of Vienna, Vienna, VIE, Austria

Salma Sadique
Department of Community Health Sciences, Peoples University of Medical and Health Sciences for Women (PUMHSW), Sindh, Pakistan

Shahbaz Ali
Independent Researcher, Islamabad, Pakistan

Julia Chinyere Oparah
Provost and dean of the faculty, Race, Gender and Sexuality Studies Department, Mills College, Oakland, CA, United States

Jennifer E. James
Institute for Health and Aging, University of California, San Francisco, CA, United States

Destany Barnett
School of Nursing, University of California, San Diego, CA, United States

Linda Marie Jones, Sayida Peprah and Jessica A. Walker
Black Women Birthing Justice Collective, Oakland, CA, United States

Daphina Melbourne
California Preterm Birth Initiative, University of California, San Francisco, CA, United States

Mariel Rivera
Department of Anthropology, Syracuse University, Syracuse, NY, United States

Emaline Reyes
Department of Anthropology, Temple University, Philadelphia, PA, United States

David A. Anderson
Centre College, Danville, KY, United States

Kenneth C. Johnson
School of Epidemiology and Public Health, Faculty of Medicine, University of Ottawa, Ottawa, ON, Canada

Sarah E. DeYoung
Disaster Research Center and Sociology and Criminal Justice, University of Delaware, Newark, DE, United States

Michaela Mangum
Disaster Research Center, Joseph R. Biden, Jr. School of Public Policy and Administration, University of Delaware, Newark, DE, United States

Theresa E. Gildner
Department of Anthropology, Dartmouth College, Hanover, NH, United States
Department of Anthropology, Washington University in St. Louis, St. Louis, MO, United States

Zaneta M. Thayer
Department of Anthropology, Dartmouth College, Hanover, NH, United States
Ecology, Evolution, Environment and Society Program, Dartmouth College, Hanover, NH, United States

Kim Gutschow
Departments of Anthropology and Religion, Williams College, Willliamstown, MA, United States

Robbie Davis-Floyd
Department of Anthropology, Rice University, Houston, TX, United States

Stephen Okumu Ombere
Department of Sociology and Anthropology, Maseno University, Maseno-Kisumu, Kenya

Betty-Anne Daviss
The Pauline Jewett Institute of Women's and Gender Studies, Faculty of Arts and Social Sciences, Carleton University, Ottawa, ON, Canada
l'Hôpital Montfort and The Ottawa Hospital, Midwifery Divisions, Ottawa, ON, Canada

Tammy Roberts
Independent Researcher, Elliot Lake, ON, Canada

Candace Leblanc and Angela Ashawasegai
Independent Researcher, Ottawa, ON, Canada

Iris Champet
Asociación para la Promoción, Investigación y Educación en salud en el Occidente de Guatemala (PIES), Quetzaltenango, Guatemala

Bernadette Betchi
Algonquin College, Ottawa, ON, Canada

Laura Gamez
Independent Researcher, Hamilton, ON, Canada

Cristina Alonso, Akane Sugimoto Storey, Ilse Fajardo and Hannah S. Borboleta
Luna Maya, San Cristobal de las Casas, Mexico

Camila López, Víctor Flores, Cristian Sierra and Susan Díaz
Maternity Dra. Eloísa Díaz - La Florida Hospital, Santiago, Chile

Christian Figueroa
Maternity Dra. Eloísa Díaz - La Florida Hospital, Santiago, Chile
Faculty of Medicine, Pontificia Universidad Católica de Chile, Santiago, Chile

Gonzalo Leiva
Maternity Dra. Eloísa Díaz - La Florida Hospital, Santiago, Chile
Faculty of Medicine, Pontificia Universidad Católica de Chile, Santiago, Chile
Chilean Observatory of Obstetric Violence, Santiago, Chile

Michelle Sadler
Chilean Observatory of Obstetric Violence, Santiago, Chile
Faculty of Liberal Arts, Universidad Adolfo Ibáñez, Santiago, Chile

Susana Quezada
International Consultant, Early Childhood Development and Maternal and Child Health, Washington, DC, United States

Brenda Benaglia
University of Bologna, Bologna, Italy

Daniela Canzini
Voci di Nascita Birth Community, Bologna, Italy

Anna Ozhiganova
Center of Medical Anthropology, Institute of Anthropology and Ethnology (RAS), Moscow, Russia

Susan Crowther, Andrea Gilkison and Judith McAra-Couper
Centre for Midwifery and Women's Health Research, Faculty of Health and Environmental Studies, AUT University, Auckland, New Zealand

Robyn Maude, Billie Bradford and Diana Austin
School of Nursing, Midwifery, and Health Practice, Te Herenga Waka Victoria University of Wellington, Wellington, New Zealand

Jayne Krisjanous
Wellington School of Business and Government, Te Herenga Waka Victoria University of Wellington, Wellington, New Zealand

Julie Johnson Searcy
Department of History and Anthropology, Butler University, Indianapolis, IN, United States

Angela N. Castañeda
Department of Sociology and Anthropology, DePauw University, Greencastle, IN, United States

Guoqiang Sun, Ying Lin, Ruyan Li, Lijun Yang, Xian Liu, Min Peng, Hongyan Wang, Xuewen Yang, Wei Ren, Hui Yang and Yao Cheng
Obstetrics Department, Maternal and Child Health Hospital of Hubei Province, Huazhong University of Science and Technology, Wuhan, China

Qi Wang
Department of Epidemiology and Biostatistics, School of Public Health, Tongji Medical College, Huazhong University of Science and Technology, Wuhan, China

Victory U. Salami and Susannah I. Ayilara
Scientific and Industrial Research Department, National Research Institute for Chemical Technology, Zaria, Nigeria

Aimee O. Chris
Department of Biochemistry, Babcock University, Ilishan-Remo, Nigeria

Stanley I. R. Okoduwa
Department of Biochemistry, Babcock University, Ilishan-Remo, Nigeria
Directorate of Research and Development, Nigerian Institute of Leather and Science Technology, Zaria, Nigeria

Ugochi J. Okoduwa
Industrial and Environmental Pollution Department, National Research Institute for Chemical Technology, Zaria, Nigeria

Danice Guzman, Cindy Makanga and Robert Dowd
The Ford Family Program in Human Development Studies and Solidarity, Kellogg Institute for International Studies, University of Notre Dame, Notre Dame, IN, United States

Jackline Oluoch-Aridi
The Ford Family Program in Human Development Studies and Solidarity, Kellogg Institute for International Studies, University of Notre Dame, Notre Dame, IN, United States
Strathmore Business School, Institute of Healthcare Management, Strathmore University, Nairobi, Kenya

Tecla Chelagat, Mary M. Nyikuri and Joseph Onyango
Strathmore Business School, Institute of Healthcare Management, Strathmore University, Nairobi, Kenya

Laura Miller-Graff
The Ford Family Program in Human Development Studies and Solidarity, Kellogg Institute for International Studies, University of Notre Dame, Notre Dame, IN, United States
Department of Psychology, The Kroc Institute of Peace Studies, University of Notre Dame, Notre Dame, IN, United States

Ting-ting Lin and Lei Chen
Shanghai Key Laboratory of Embryo Original Diseases, The International Peace Maternity and Child Health Hospital, School of Medicine, Shanghai Jiao Tong University, Shanghai, China

Chen Zhang and He-feng Huang
Shanghai Key Laboratory of Embryo Original Diseases, The International Peace Maternity and Child Health Hospital, School of Medicine, Shanghai Jiao Tong University, Shanghai, China
Research Department, Institute of Reproduction and Development, Obstetrics and Gynecology Hospital, Fudan University, Shanghai, China

Li Jin, Xian-hua Lin, Jie-xue Pan and Yan-ting Wu
Research Department, Institute of Reproduction and Development, Obstetrics and Gynecology Hospital, Fudan University, Shanghai, China

Cindy-Lee Dennis
Lawrence S. Bloomberg Faculty of Nursing, University of Toronto, Toronto, ON, Canada

Ben W. Mol
Monash University Monash Medical Centre, Clayton, VIC, Australia
Aberdeen Centre for Women's Health Research, University of Aberdeen, Aberdeen, United Kingdom

Index

Printed in the USA
CPSIA information can be obtained
at www.ICGtesting.com
LVHW080735221023
761596LV00011B/2135